MW01268270

ISCHEMIA-REPERFUSION IN CARDIAC SURGERY

Developments in Cardiovascular Medicine

VOLUME 142

The titles published in this series are listed at the end of this volume.

Ischemia-reperfusion in cardiac surgery

edited by

HANS MICHAEL PIPER
Institute of Physiology,
Heinrich-Heine-University, Düsseldorf, Germany

and

CLAUS J. PREUSSE
Department of Thoracic and Cardiovascular Surgery,
Heinrich-Heine-University, Düsseldorf, Germany

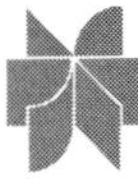

KLUWER ACADEMIC PUBLISHERS
DORDRECHT / BOSTON / LONDON

Library of Congress Cataloging-in-Publication Data

Ischemic-reperfusion in cardiac surgery / edited by Hans Michael Piper
and Claus J. Preusse.
p. cm. -- (Developments in cardiovascular medicine ; v. 142)
Includes index.
ISBN 0-7923-2241-X (hb. : alk. paper)
1. Cardiac arrest, Induced. 2. Heart--Preservation.
3. Myocardial reperfusion. 4. Reperfusion injury. I. Piper, Hans
Michael. II. Preusse, C. J. III. Series.
[DNLM: 1. Myocardial Ischemia--prevention & control.
2. Myocardial Ischemia--physiopathology. 3. Myocardial Reperfusion
Injury--prevention & control. 4. Myocardial Reperfusion. 5. Heart
Arrest, Induced. W1 DE997VME v. 142 1993 / WG 280 I77 1993]
RD598.35.I53I8 1993
617.4'12059--dc20
DNLM/DLC
for Library of Congress 93-16723
CIP

ISBN 0-7923-2241-X

Published by Kluwer Academic Publishers,
P.O. Box 17, 3300 AA Dordrecht, The Netherlands.

Kluwer Academic Publishers incorporates
the publishing programmes of
D. Reidel, Martinus Nijhoff, Dr W. Junk and MTP Press.

Sold and distributed in the U.S.A. and Canada
by Kluwer Academic Publishers,
101 Philip Drive, Norwell, MA 02061, U.S.A.

In all other countries, sold and distributed
by Kluwer Academic Publishers Group,
P.O. Box 322, 3300 AH Dordrecht, The Netherlands.

Printed on acid-free paper

Table of Contents

PART FOUR: Evaluation of cardioplegic methodology

List of contributors

CARY W. AKINS
Department of Surgery – White 503, Massachusetts General Hospital, Harvard Medical School, 23 Fruit Street, Boston, MA 02114, USA

ROBERTO BOLLI
Section of Cardiology, Baylor College of Medicine, The Methodist Hospital, 6535 Fannin, MS F-905, Houston, TX 77030, USA
Co-authors: Marcel E. Zughaib, Paul B. McCay, Mohamed 0. Jeroudi, Craig Hartley, Jian-Zhong Sun, Selim Sekili and Xiao-Ying Li

MARCEL BORGERS
Department of Morphology, Janssen Research Foundation, Turnhoutseweg 30, B-2340 Beerse, Belgium
Co-author: Willem Flameng

GERALD D. BUCKBERG
Department of Surgery, UCLA School of Medicine, B2-375 CHS, 10833 Le Conte Avenue, Los Angeles, CA 90024-1741, USA
Co-authors: Bradley S. Allen and Friedhelm Beyersdorf

DAVID J. CHAMBERS
Cardiac Surgical Research, The Rayne Institute, St. Thomas' Hospital, London SE1 7EH, UK
Co-author: Mark V. Baimbridge

SALLY DARRACOTT-CANKOVIC
The Transplant Unit, Papworth Hospital, Papworth Everard, Cambridge CB3 8RE, UK

JAN WILLEM DE JONG
Thorax Center, Ee2371, Erasmus University Rotterdam, The Netherlands
Co-authors: Tom Huizer, Maarten Janssen, Rob Krams, Monique Tavenier and Pieter D. Verdouw

SHARON L. HALE
The Heart Institute, Hospital of the Good Samaritan, 616 South Witmer Avenue, Los Angeles, CA 90017, USA
Co-author: Robert A. Kloner

GERD HEUSCH
Department of Pathophysiology, Center of Internal Medicine, University of Essen, Hufelandstraße 55, D-45147 Essen, Germany
Co-authors: Dietrich Baumgart, Rainer Schulz and Thomas Ehring

SHUKRI F. KHURI
Department of Surgery, Veterans Administration Medical Center, 1400 VFW Parkway, West Roxbury, MA 02132, USA
Co-author: Michael B. Tantillo

ERNST-GEORG KRAUSE
Department of Molecular Cardiology, MDC Max-Delbrück-Center, Berlin-Buch, Robert-Rössle-Strasse 10, D-13122 Berlin-Buch, Germany
Co-authors: Dorothea Pfeiffer, Ulla Wollenberger and Hans-Georg Wollert

SIDNEY LEVITSKY
Division of Cardiothoracic Surgery, New England Deaconess Hospital, Harvard Medical School, 110 Francis Street, Suite 2C, Boston, MA 02215, USA
Co-authors: Irvin B. Krukenkamp, Christopher A. Caldarone and paul Burns

FLAVIAN M. LUPINETTI
Section of Thoracic Surgery, University of Michigan, Taubman Health Care Center – Box 0344, Ann Arbor, MI 48109, USA

JOHN E. MAYER, Jr.
Department of Cardiac Surgery, Children's Hospital Boston, Rm 1319, 300 Longwood Avenue, Boston, MA 02115, USA

PHILIPPE MENASCHE
Department of Cardiovascular Surgery, Hôpital Lariboisière, 2 Rue Ambroise Paré, F-75475 Paris Cedex 10, France

HANS MICHAEL PIPER
Department of Cardiovascular Physiology, Physiological Institute, Heinrich-Heine-University, Postfach 101007, D-40001 Düsseldorf, Germany
Co-authors: Berthold Siegmund and Klaus-Dieter Schlüter

CLAUS J. PREUSSE
Department of Thoracic and Cardiovascular Surgery, Surgical Clinic, Heinrich-Heine-University, Postfach 101007, D-40001 Düsseldorf, Germany

HAGEN D. SCHULTE
Department of Thoracic and Cardiovascular Surgery, Surgical Clinic, Heinrich-Heine-University, Postfach 101007, D-40001 Düsseldorf, Germany

HIROYUKI SUGA
Department of Physiology II, Okayama University Medical School, 2 Shikatacho, Okayama, 700 Japan
Co-authors: Taketoshi Namba, Junichi Araki, Kazunari Ishioka, Haruo Ito, Takuji Akashi, Ling Yun Zhao, Dan Dan Zhao, Miao Liu, Wakako Fujii and Miyako Takaki

Preface

From the beginning of modern heart surgery, surgeons have routinely dealt with problems of myocardial ischemia and reperfusion. For cardiac surgeons, therefore, the phenomena of delayed post-ischemic recovery and irreversible ischemic myocardial injury (e.g., in the form of the "stone heart") have been familiar for a long time and, consequently, attempts to protect myocardium intraoperatively against ischemic injury have a long history. In many instances, however, the protocols for surgical interventions which require temporary ischemic conditions were initially designed without a secure knowledge of the underlying pathophysiological mechanisms. For a long time surgical practice had not been sufficiently supported by basic clinical or experimental research, and it is thus not surprising that many operative protocols had to be altered or even abandoned as this research developed. Even today, after three decades of open heart surgery and great progress in basic research, the methodological repertoire for myocardial protection in heart surgery is not optimal.

Myocardial protection in cardiac surgery is a problem of great complexity; this has many reasons. First, the heart is heterogeneous with respect to tissue type (e.g., ventricular myocardium vs. myocardium of the conduction system), tissue topology (e.g., subendocardial vs. subepicardial myocardium), and cell types which these tissues are composed of (e.g., endothelial cells, cardiomyocytes). Second, the cardiac surgeon is faced with individuals of different ages (from neonates to very old adults). Third, these individuals need heart surgery because of various kinds of congenital or acquired heart disease, in emergency or elective operations. It is unlikely that for all these different conditions a single procedure of intraoperative myocardial protection is equally optimal. Instead, there may be different requirements for optimal protection. But how different would these have to be, and what would they have in common? To answer these questions more clinical and experimental research is needed.

Experimental research has been very valuable for investigating basic principles of myocardial protection. It has the clear advantage over most clinical investigations in that circumstantial conditions can be better controlled and more powerful analytical procedures can be applied, thereby providing a more detailed causal analysis. The strength of experimental studies is the use of selected, but well-defined experimental models of reduced complexity.

Experimental work on whole hearts, isolated myocardial cells, and subcellular myocardial structures from large and small animals has greatly augmented the understanding of myocardial injury in ischemia and reperfusion. It has identified a number of key steps in the causal process that all models of the energy-depleted and -repleted myocardial cell seem to have in common. This basic knowledge has been and will be stimulating for the improvement of intraoperative techniques for myocardial protection.

From the early days of cardiac surgery up to the present, surgeons have concentrated on protecting the myocardium intraoperatively against damage caused by *ischemia*. The oldest method is hypothermia, a simple but effective way to provide protection against ischemia. Hypothermia has been combined with perfusion of the myocardium with various cristalloid, colloidal or blood containing solutions. The primary aim of all these approaches has been to achieve a reduction in myocardial energy demand during cardiac ischemia, since a slow-down in the depletion of myocardial stores of energy was found to delay the development of ischemic injury. During recent years cardiac surgeons have become aware that modifications of the conditions of ischemia itself are not the only possibilities in providing myocardial protection, modifications of the *pre- and post-ischemic conditions* may also be helpful. Thus, it may be beneficial to use a "preconditioning" protocol, i.e. submit the myocardium to a brief period of ischemia-reperfusion before starting the extended period of ischemia. In animal studies, "preconditioning" has been shown to increase the myocardial tolerance to prolonged ischemia. Experimental studies have also demonstrated that reperfusion of ischemic myocardium can add something to tissue injury as developed during the ischemic period ("reperfusion injury"). It seems now promising to investigate how myocardial preservation in heart surgery can be further improved by modifying the conditions of reperfusion so that "reperfusion injury" is reduced or even prevented.

"Protection" is a comparative term. Its use is dependent on suitable parameters. The problems in comparing different procedures for myocardial protection in today's heart surgery can also be understood as uncertainty about the quality and use of such parameters. The most widely used parameter for myocardial protection against ischemic injury is certainly post-ischemic myocardial performance. By many clinicians and basic scientists this parameter is regarded as the "gold standard" for evaluating protection, as protection against ischemic injury should, of course, lead to an improvement of the result of reperfusion. But what, exactly, is "the result of reperfusion"? The result may vary with time and the protocol for reperfusion. The cardiac performance found during the early phase of reperfusion is not a reliable predictor of the ultimate functional recovery and, thus, of efficiency of the method of protection applied to the ischemic-reperfused heart. The post-ischemic myocardium may be in a state of "stunning", i.e. transient post-ischemic malfunction, which will eventually disappear without any further treatment. Conversely, myocardial function may also deteriorate after an acceptable initial performance due to secondary causes of cell injury during ongoing reperfusion (e.g., myocardial attack by leukocytes). This argument illustrates that the selection of suitable parameters and the mode how they should be applied (e.g. in time) presupposes a detailed knowledge about the causal key events in ischemia-reperfusion. To a large extent this knowledge originates from experimental research.

We, the editors of this book, believe that progress in myocardial protection in heart surgery depends on close communication between clincians and experimental scientists. This book was planned to bring together the current views of basic scientists and cardiac surgeons on myocardial injury in ischemia-reperfusion with the aim to stimulate the further development of methods for myocardial protection.

H.M. Piper & C.J. Preusse
Düsseldorf, Germany

PART ONE

Pathophysiology of ischemia and reperfusion

1. Moderate ischemic injury and myocardial stunning

MARCEL E. ZUGHAIB, PAUL B. McCAY, MOHAMED O. JEROUDI, CRAIG HARTLEY, JIAN-ZHONG SUN, SELIM SEKILI, XIAO-YING LI, and ROBERTO BOLLI

Introduction

Reperfusion of acutely ischemic myocardium is associated with a constellation of characteristic structural and functional derangements, which range widely in severity [1]. At one end of the spectrum are transient, completely reversible abnormalities such as reperfusion arrhythmias and postischemic myocardial dysfunction or "myocardial stunning" [2–14]. At the other end are severe, irreversible abnormalities such as cell death (infarction). Thus, myocardial stunning should be considered as a mild, sublethal sequela of ischemia/reperfusion injury.

When myocardial stunning was first described by Vatner's group in 1975 [13], this phenomenon received relatively little attention because at that time coronary reperfusion was thought to be a rare occurrence. Myocardial stunning was regarded mostly as a laboratory curiosity. During the 1980s, however, postischemic dysfunction has become the focus of increasing interest both among experimentalists and clinicians because of two major reasons. First, coronary reperfusion by means of thrombolytic therapy, percutaneous transluminal coronary angioplasty, or bypass surgery has become a standard approach to the management of acute ischemic syndromes in patients with coronary artery disease. Second, several studies have demonstrated that many patients experience spontaneous reperfusion as a result of lysis of coronary thrombi or release of coronary spasm. Accordingly, it has become increasingly evident that postischemic myocardial stunning is a part of the natural history of coronary artery disease and may contribute significantly to the morbidity associated with this disorder.

Our knowledge regarding myocardial stunning has increased dramatically in the past decade. Rarely has so much work been done in such a little time. It is astonishing to compare what we knew about postischemic myocardial stunning ten years ago with what we know now. As we enter the 1990s, the intensity of interest in this phenomenon continues to grow, as does the amount of research invested into its basic and clinical facets. Cardiologists are becoming progressively more aware of the existence of stunning in patients and of its potential pathophysiological and therapeutic implications.

The purpose of this chapter is to summarize our current knowledge of the phenomenon of myocardial stunning. Specifically, we will attempt to (i)

H.M. Piper and C.J. Preusse (eds): Ischemia-reperfusion in cardiac surgery, 3–40.

define this phenomenon, (ii) classify its different pathophysiological settings, (iii) review critically the various mechanisms proposed for it, (iv) discuss its clinical implications, and (v) identify the major unresolved issues in areas for future research. Many of the concepts discussed in this chapter have been covered in a recent review [15].

What exactly is myocardial stunning?

It is not unusual to see the term "myocardial stunning" inappropriately applied to situations in which the persistence of contractile abnormalities could be explained by the occurrence of myocellular death. Incredible as it may seem, sometimes the distinction between myocardial stunning and myocardial infarction is still not clearly made, particularly by persons who do not specifically work in this area. This confusion (which obviously has deleterious effects) can be eliminated by using a simple, clear definition of myocardial stunning. Postischemic dysfunction, or myocardial stunning, is the mechanical dysfunction that persists after reperfusion *despite the absence of irreversible damage*. The essential point of this definition is that post-ischemic dysfunction, no matter how severe or prolonged, is a *fully reversible* abnormality. It follows that the diagnosis of myocardial stunning should not be made unless one can demonstrate that the tissue in question is entirely viable.

Accordingly, myocardial stunning is a relatively mild, sublethal injury that must be kept quite distinct from myocardial infarction. Whether these two conditions share a common mechanism is presently unknown. This chapter will discuss only results obtained in experimental preparations in which mechanical dysfunction is likely to be due to stunning rather than to cell death.

In which experimental setting does myocardial stunning occur?

Myocardial stunning, as defined above, is a 'syndrome' that has been observed in a wide variety of experimental settings with major pathophysiological differences. The common denominator to these heterogeneous settings is that in all of them the myocardium is exposed to a transient ischemic episode, not long enough to cause irreversible injury. Since the heterogeneity of the experimental models of stunning has been one of the major impediments to the full elucidation of the pathogenesis and pathophysiology of this abnormality, it is important to point out the differences among various settings.

The available observations can be classified into the following categories.

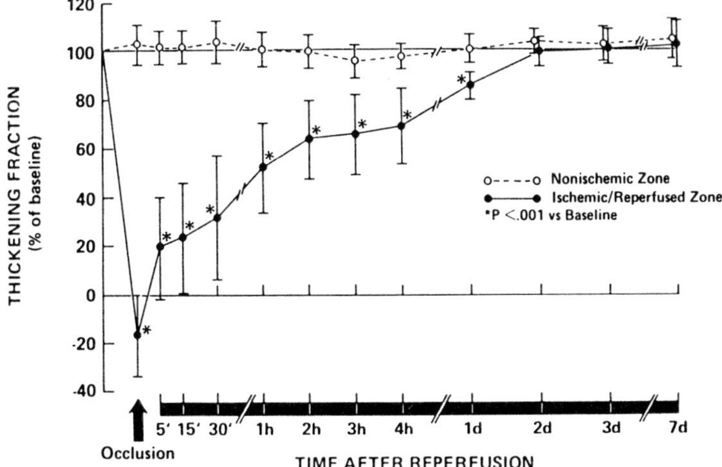

Figure 1.1. Changes in systolic wall thickening in conscious dogs undergoing a 15-min LAD occlusion and seven days of reperfusion. Regional myocardial function was measured as systolic thickening fraction, which is expressed as percent of baseline values. Data are mean % SD (n = 21). Contractile function in the reperfused myocardium recovered slowly; on the average, wall thickening was still significantly depressed at one day and returned to baseline at two days after reperfusion. Thus, a single 15-min coronary occlusion is sufficient to impair myocardial contractility for 24 h. Reproduced with permission from the American Journal of Physiology 1988; 254: H102–H114.

Myocardial stunning after a single, completely reversible ischemic episode

In the dog, a coronary occlusion lasting <20 min does not result in any myocardial necrosis [5,16], but upon reperfusion, the recovery of contractile performance in the previously ischemic myocardium is delayed for several hours [2,4,5,10–12,14]. This is the 'classic' model of myocardial stunning, the one where the phenomenon was originally described [14], and the one most commonly used in experimental investigations. The exact duration of postischemic contractile abnormalities in this model has varied in different experimental preparations [5,14]. Using a Doppler ultrasound probe that can assess function in different layers of the ventricular wall, we have shown that in conscious dogs, the average transmural systolic wall thickening (an integrated measure of function across the ventricular wall) remains depressed up to 24 h after a single 15-min coronary occlusion (Figure 1.1) [10]. Nevertheless, the rate of recovery is nonuniform and is faster in the subepicardium than in the subendocardium, so that thickening in the innermost layers may be impaired at a time when thickening in the outermost layers has returned to normal [12]. In addition, it appears that myocardial stunning is a global mechanical derangement that involves both systolic and diastolic functions [11].

Myocardial stunning after multiple, completely reversible ischemic episodes

Repeated brief (5 or 10 min) coronary occlusions have a cumulative effect on systolic function and result in prolonged contractile impairment despite absence of irreversible damage [17–22]. The largest impairment of contractility occurs after the first occlusion, with subsequent occlusions causing progressively smaller decrements in mechanical performance [23]. This model of myocardial stunning differs from the single 10- or 15-min occlusion model in that the mechanical dysfunction develops gradually and is associated with a considerably greater total ischemic burden (50–60 min vs. 10–15 min). Repetitive ischemia also has a cumulative effect on the time to complete recovery, but such effect has not been thoroughly studied.

Myocardial stunning after a single, partly irreversible ischemic episode (subendocardial infarction)

In the dog, when reperfusion is instituted after a period of coronary occlusion >20 min but <3 h, the subendocardial portion of the region at risk is generally found to be infarcted, whereas variable quantities of subepicardial tissue remain viable [16]. This subepicardial tissue salvaged by reperfusion may require days or weeks to recover its contractile function [3,5–9]. Thus, early reperfusion during acute myocardial infarction results in an admixture of infarcted subendocardium and stunned subepicardium (i.e., irreversible and reversible dysfunction, respectively).

Myocardial stunning after global ischemia in isolated hearts

Cellular viability in these preparations depends on many factors, including species, temperature, duration of ischemia, and perfusate composition. Although in these models the reversibility of the contractile abnormalities cannot be verified, under selected conditions isolated hearts reperfused after transient ischemia exhibit complete normalization of phosphocreatine content and intracellular pH [24–32], suggesting that viability is generally preserved. Accordingly, despite the numerous obvious differences from ischemia *in vivo*, myocardial stunning can be mimicked in selected isolated heart preparations. Nevertheless, the data must be taken with caution and verified in intact animal preparations before concluding that they are relevant to stunning. The relevance to stunning becomes obviously questionable in cases where these preparations are associated with significant cell death [33–42]. The indiscriminate use of isolated hearts as models of stunning has generated some confusion and should be avoided. It must be stressed that the isolated heart is inherently limited because one cannot usually demonstrate full recovery of function after reperfusion and because assessment of cellular viability is difficult. Isolated hearts can be quite useful, but the data should not be automatically extrapolated to the intact animal and should be confirmed in this latter model.

Myocardial stunning after global ischemia during cardioplegic arrest in vivo

Despite the use of hypothermic cardioplegia, global ischemia in intact animals is usually followed by prolonged contractile abnormalities [43–46]. The reversibility of these derangements has not been documented, but under carefully controlled conditions they are likely to be due mostly to stunning.

Myocardial stunning after exercise-induced ischemia

Increased myocardial oxygen demands (e.g., by exercise) is the face of limited supply (flow-limiting stenosis), may provoke myocardial ischemia and dysfunction in animals. These contractile abnormalities persist beyond cessation of exercise even if the stenosis is reversed [47]. Thus, myocardial stunning can also occur after high flow ischemia in which the primary problem is an increase in oxygen demands rather than a decrease in supply.

Because of the many significant pathophysiological differences among these situations, one cannot assume that observations made in one setting necessarily apply to the others. An important, unresolved issue is whether or not all forms of stunning share a common pathogenesis.

What determines the severity of myocardial stunning?

In conscious dogs undergoing a 15-min coronary occlusion there is a close coupling between the degree of myocardial dysfunction after reperfusion and collateral blood flow during the preceding period of ischemia, whereby even small differences in ischemic perfusion are associated with large differences in postischemic recovery [10]. Furthermore, as discussed above, the severity of stunning is greater in the inner layers of the left ventricular wall, which are the most severely ischemic, than in the outer layers [12,48]. Equally important is the duration of flow deprivation: the longer the ischemic period, the greater the ensuing mechanical abnormalities [14,49].

Thus, the severity of postischemic dysfunction is determined primarily by the severity and duration of the antecedent ischemia. This concept has two important implications. First, whatever the precise mechanism responsible for stunning may be, such mechanism must be initiated and modulated by perturbations associated with ischemia. Although stunning appears to be, in part, a form of 'reperfusion injury' (see below), it is ischemia that 'primes' the myocardium for the development of such injury. Second, any intervention that improves perfusion during ischemia would be expected to attenuate stunning after reflow. Reducing the severity of ischemia is probably the most effective way to reduce the severity of postischemic dysfunction.

What is the mechanism of myocardial stunning?

In very general terms, therefore, postischemic dysfunction is modulated by abnormalities occurring during ischemia. But what is the specific sequence of events whereby transient ischemia leads to prolonged depression of contractility?

Several different hypotheses, not necessarily exclusive, have been proposed.

Impaired energy production by mitochondria

ATP stores in the stunned myocardium are depressed and recover slowly [5,8,50–52], with a time course paralleling that of contractile function [5,8]. Thus, in the early 1980s the hypothesis was advanced [13,51,52] that postischemic dysfunction may result from an inability of the myocardium to resynthesize enough high energy phosphates to sustain contractile function, possibly because of washout of adenine nucleotide precursors. Numerous subsequent observations, however, have refuted this theory. First, recovery of contractility in several models of postischemic dysfunction was independent of myocardial ATP levels [24,25,53–56]. Second, the content of phosphocreatine in the stunned myocardium is normal or supranormal upon reperfusion ('phosphocreatine overshoot') [5,24,25,28,50,52,54,57], implying that the phosphorylation ability of the mitochondria remains intact. Third, the stunned myocardium is exquisitely responsive to inotropic stimuli with a marked and sustained increase in contractility [19,28,58–63]. This striking inotropic response occurs without a decrease in ATP or phosphocreatine stores [28,60], indicating that energy production is not inherently impaired and can keep pace with high metabolic demands. Fourth, manipulations that increase ATP levels in the stunned myocardium fail to improve mechanical performance [30,64].

In summary, the available evidence suggests that a defect ATP regeneration by the mitochondria is not the primary cause of myocardial stunning.

Impaired energy use by myofibrils

A decrease in myofibrillar creatine kinase activity [65] and a reduction of its substrate (free ADP) to produce ATP at the contraction site occur in stunned myocardium [28,65]. These abnormalities might disrupt normal energy use and thus have been postulated to contribute to postischemic dysfunction [65]. This hypothesis, however, does not explain the considerable contractile and metabolic reserve of the stunned myocardium [19,28,58–63] and is therefore considered implausible. Indeed, the reversal of postischemic dysfunction by inotropic stimuli implies that the residual activity of myofibrillar creatine kinase is still sufficient to run the myofibrillar ATPase reaction at normal or even supranormal rates.

Impairment of sympathetic neural responsiveness

There is conflicting evidence that postischemic dysfunction is associated with functional sympathetic denervation [66,67]. That this abnormality plays a major role in myocardial stunning seems unlikely at the present time.

Impairment of myocardial perfusion

Following a 15-min coronary occlusion, post-reperfusion subepicardial blood flow is normal whereas subendocardial flow is slightly decreased (~20%) [4,10–12,68–70]. The mechanism and significance of this phenomenon are unclear [69,70]. Arguably, the reduced subendocardial perfusion may contribute to the impaired mechanical performance [4]. However three considerations suggest that this is not the case: (1) there is no correlation between subendocardial blood flow and wall thickening in the postischemic myocardium [69,70]; (2) the loss of systolic function (dyskinesis or akinesis) is out of proportion to the slight (~20%) decrease in subendocardial perfusion [69,70]; and (3) the contractile reserve of the postischemic myocardium is normal or near-normal [19,62,63].

Damage of the extracellular collagen matrix

A structural defect, namely, the disruption of the mechanical coupling function provided by the extracellular collagen network, was postulated by Eng's group to explain myocardial stunning [71,72]. A recent study [73] however, has demonstrated that collagen is disrupted by twelve 5-min coronary occlusions but not by a single 15-min occlusion followed by reperfusion. Thus, collagen damage may contribute to myocardial stunning after multiple ischemic episodes, but is unlikely to be a causative factor after a single, completely reversible ischemic episode (Table 1.1).

Decreased sensitivity of myofilaments to calcium

In isolated ferret hearts subjected to 15 min of normothermic global ischemia, Kusuoka *et al.* [25] observed that the stunned myocardium exhibited decreased responsiveness to calcium, as manifested by a decrease in the maximal calcium-activated force and a decrease in the myocardial sensitivity to extracellular calcium. The authors speculated that the reduced sensitivity to extracellular calcium, in turn, could be due to either a decrease in the intracellular free Ca^{2+} concentration ($[Ca]_i$) transient or a decrease in the sensitivity of myofilaments to calcium [25]. Two recent studies refute the former theory [32,74] by demonstrating that the calcium transient is (paradoxically) increased in the stunned myocardium after 15 min [32] or 20 min [74] of global ischemia at 37°C in isolated ferret hearts. It was therefore proposed [32,74] that the fundamental mechanism for postischemic dysfunc-

Table 1.1. Classification of myocardial stunning and evidence for the various mechanisms proposed in experimental animals.

Experimental setting	Evidence for a pathogenetic role of				
	Oxygen radicals	Sarcoplasmic reticulum dysfunction	Calcium overload	Reduced calcium sensitivity	Damage of collagen matrix
Stunning due to decreased blood flow					
a) *Regional ischemia*					
1) Single, completely reversible ischemic episode	++	?	?	–	–
2) Multiple, completely reversible ischemic episodes	+	+	?	–	+
3) Single, partly irreversible	±	?	?	?	?
b) *Global ischemia*					
4) Isolated heart *in vitro*	+	?	+	+	?
5) Cardioplegic arrest *in vivo*	+	?	?	?	?
Stunning due to increased O_2 demands					
6) Exercise-induced ischemia	–	?	?	?	?

\+ Published studies support this mechanism.
++ Published studies from multiple laboratories consistently support this mechanism; evidence is also available in conscious animal preparations.
– Published studies do not support this mechanism.
? No data are available.

tion is reduced sensitivity of the contractile apparatus to calcium rather than insufficient availability of free cytosolic calcium during systole. One problem with this hypothesis derived from *in vitro* studies is that it does not explain two observations made *in vivo*: (1) the stunned myocardium exhibits a normal or near-normal contractile reserve when challenged with inotropic stimuli, [19,62,63], and (2) the apparent sensitivity of the stunned myocardium to intracoronary calcium is not decreased [62]. If the primary problem was a reduced sensitivity of myofilaments to calcium, then the contractile response to exogenous calcium or to other inotropic agents (which act by raising $[Ca]_i$) should be reduced.

In summary, although *in vitro* studies suggest that myocardial stunning is a result of reduced calcium sensitivity rather than of reduced calcium availability, *in vivo* studies are not readily reconcilable with this interpretation (Table 1.1).

Calcium overload

The concept that calcium overload is an important pathogenetic contributor to myocardial stunning is based on the following lines of evidence. First, postischemic contractile abnormalities are significantly attenuated in isolated ferret hearts subjected to 15 min of global normothermic ischemia and reperfused with solutions containing low concentrations of calcium [25]. The fact that no intervention was applied during ischemia indicates that calcium entry upon reperfusion may be an important mechanism of myocardial stunning. A decrease in the severity of stunning is also observed in hearts pretreated with ryanodine, an inhibitor of cellular calcium overload [27]. Second, mechanical and metabolic abnormalities similar to myocardial stunning are produced by exposure of isolated ferret hearts to a transient calcium overload in the absence of ischemia [75]. Third, transient intracellular acidosis during early reperfusion can prevent myocardial stunning in isolated ferret hearts [29] and in open-chest dogs [76] subjected to 15 min of ischemia. Since acidosis antagonizes not only the influx of calcium into cells (by inhibiting the Na^+-Ca^{2+} exchange and the slow calcium channels) but also the intracellular binding of calcium [29], these results provide indirect evidence that a transient calcium overload contributes to postischemic dysfunction. Fourth, recent studies [26,77,78] have shown that $[Ca]_i$ increases between 10 and 20 min of global ischemia in isolated hearts. This is the same duration of ischemia that results in myocardial stunning. In these models, $[Ca]_i$ appears to remain transiently elevated during very early reflow [74,79], but returns to normal values within few minutes after reperfusion [26,74,77]. It should be noted, however, that the measurements performed thus far have failed to show a post-reperfusion rise of $[Ca]_i$ to levels higher than those attained during ischemia. Thus, no direct evidence exists at present to support the reperfusion-induced $[Ca]_i$ overshoot postulated by the calcium overload theory.

How does $[Ca]_i$ rise during ischemia? One possibility is through decreased calcium uptake by the sarcoplasmic reticulum [80]. Na^+-Ca^{2+} exchange could also play a role with a rise in intracellular Na^+ during ischemia due both to metabolic inhibition of the Na^+-K^{2+}-ATPase, and to acidosis and consequent Na^+-H^+ exchange [81–83]. Since the Na^+-Ca^{2+} exchange is inhibited by acidosis and since intracellular pH in the stunned myocardium normalizes quickly after reflow [25,28–30,57], entry of calcium via the Na^+-Ca^{2+} exchange may be greatly increased upon reperfusion [81,83–85]. However, the above mechanisms remains speculative and further research will be necessary to elucidate the pathogenesis of calcium overload. In addition, the mechanism(s) by which a transient calcium overload induces prolonged contractile dysfunction is (are) also unclear, although it is known that elevation of cytosolic calcium could trigger production of oxygen radicals via xanthine oxidase [86] (see below), and that increased cytosolic calcium can activate phospholipases and other degradative enzymes [31,87].

At first sight, the calcium overload theory may appear paradoxical in view of the fact that exogenous calcium ameliorates function in the stunned myocardium [25,62]. However, this discrepancy is only apparent. The increase in $[Ca]_i$ is postulated to be a brief phenomenon occurring immediately after reflow, following which there may be either a normalization of $[Ca]_i$ transients or even a relative calcium deficiency (see below). The early excessive $[Ca]_i$ levels could damage intracellular organelles concerned with contraction and thereby produce prolonged mechanical dysfunction, which would persist as an after-effect at a time when $[Ca]_i$ is no longer elevated. Thus, there could be an 'early phase' of elevated $[Ca]_i$ followed by a 'late phase' of decreased $[Ca]_i$.

Calcium channel blockers have been used in an attempt to gain insights into the role of altered calcium homeostasis *in vivo*, but unfortunately the results are difficult to interpret. Verapamil [56], diltiazem [88], nifedipine [89], nitrendipine [90], and amlodipine [91] have been shown to improve recovery of function in regionally stunned myocardium in intact animals. However, it is unclear whether these beneficial effects reflected a direct protective action of the drugs or were mediated by favorable modifications of afterload, preload, heart rate, and regional myocardial blood flow, all of which could modulate the contractile performance of the stunned myocardium [18,56]. A recent study [92] demonstrated a direct protective action of nifedipine on functional recovery of the stunned myocardium independently of any effect on systemic hemodynamics or regional myocardial blood flow. However, interpretation of these results is problematic because the beneficial effects of nifedipine were noted even when treatment was started 30 min after reperfusion [92], whereas myocardial stunning has been suggested to result from disturbances occurring immediately after reflow [25]. It is unlikely that nifedipine acted in a specific way to decrease $[Ca]_i$ because administration of calcium or inotropic agents (which raise $[Ca]_i$) improves contractile function in the stunned myocardium [19,28,58–63]. The mechanism of action of nifedipine in this intriguing study [92] remains to be elucidated. A recent report by Heusch and coworkers indicates that nisoldipine attenuates myocardial stunning only when given before ischemia, not when given at reperfusion [93]. The reasons for the discrepancy between this study [93] and the nifedipine study mentioned above [92] are unknown.

In summary, considerable evidence suggests that a transient calcium overload during early reperfusion contributes to the pathogenesis of myocardial stunning after global ischemia *in vitro*. Further investigations are needed to establish the significance of this concept *in vivo*.

Excitation-contraction uncoupling due to sarcoplasmic reticulum dysfunction

This mechanism was investigated by Krause *et al.* [94] in a canine model of postischemic dysfunction produced by eight to twelve 5-min occlusions separated by 10–min reflow periods. Sarcoplasmic reticulum isolated from the stunned myocardium demonstrated a decrease in the ability to transport calcium, concomitant with a reduction in the activity of the Na^+, Mg^{2+}-ATPase [94]. Accordingly, a decrease in the amount of calcium stored in the sarcoplasmic reticulum as a result of a reduction in the calcium pump activity could conceivably diminish contractile protein activation via attenuated calcium release during systole [94].

Sarcoplasmic reticulum dysfunction with its attendant inadequate delivery of calcium to the contractile proteins is an attractive hypothesis that would be consistent with the observation that exogenous administration of calcium can reverse the postulated calcium deficiency and return contractile function of stunned myocardium to preischemic levels [62]. It would also be consistent with the notion that inotropic agents (which increase $[Ca]_i$) can reverse myocardial stunning [19,28,58–63]. However, since this hypothesis implies that the amplitude of the $[Ca]_i$ transient is decreased, it is not easily reconcilable with *in vitro* data [32,74] (see above). Considerable more work will be needed to determine whether similar dysfunction of the sarcoplasmic reticulum occurs in other models of myocardial stunning (Table 1.1) and whether it is associated with decreased $[Ca]_i$ transients *in vivo*. In addition, the factor(s) that cause injury to the sarcoplasmic reticulum remain to be elucidated.

Generation of oxygen-derived free radicals

Effect of antioxidants on myocardial stunning after a brief coronary occlusion

In the early 80s, a number of investigators, including ourselves, postulated that reactive oxygen metabolites (e.g., superoxide anion ($\cdot O_2^-$, hydrogen peroxide (H_2O), and hydroxyl radical ($\cdot OH$)) contribute to myocardial stunning. To test this hypothesis, we employed an open-chest dog preparation in which the left anterior descending coronary artery is occluded for 15 min (which is well established not to result in myocardial cell necrosis [16]) and then reperfused [95]. Hence, the mechanical derangements observed after reperfusion can be entirely ascribed to stunning. Such 15-min coronary occlusions result, in our experience, in reproducible severe myocardial stunning, such that the reperfused region remains dyskinetic or markedly hypokinetic for at least 4 h after reflow [15].

In an early study [96], we found that administration of superoxide dismutase (SOD) (which catalyzes the dismutation of $\cdot O_2^-$ to O_2 and H_2O_2) and catalase (which reduces H_2O_2 to O_2 and H_2O) significantly enhanced recovery of function after reperfusion. Similar findings with SOD and catalase were also observed by other investigators [54,97–99]. In a subsequent study [100], we found that neither enzyme alone significantly improved recovery of function in the stunned myocardium; however, when they were combined, contractile recovery was significantly greater than that observed in controls or in dogs receiving either agent alone. These results suggest that the combined administration of SOD and catalase is more likely to be effective against stunning than separate administration making the contribution of both $\cdot O_2^-$ and H_2O_2 to the cellular damage responsible for myocardial stunning equally important. Similar results were recently reported in rabbits [99]. The inability of SOD alone to mitigate postischemic dysfunction has also been observed in a pig model [101].

However, it remains uncertain whether $\cdot O_2^-$ and H_2O_2 contribute to stunning by direct cytotoxicity or via formation of other species like the highly reactive ·OH radical which is generated by their interaction through the metal-catalyzed Haber-Weiss reactions [102]. Consequently, the accumulation of $\cdot O_2^-$ and H_2O_2 could, at least in part, produce postischemic dysfunction indirectly through generation of ·OH. We used dimethylthiourea, (an ·OH scavenger that is more effective than traditional ·OH scavengers [103] and that does not react with $\cdot O_2$ or H_2O_2 *in vitro* [104]) to evaluate that possibility. We observed that dimethylthiourea produced a significant and sustained improvement in the function of the stunned myocardium [104]. These results were further corroborated by studies using N-2–mercaptopropionyl glycine (MPG). MPG is a powerful scavenger of ·OH with no effect on $\cdot O_2^-$ or H_2O_2 *in vitro* [105], readily enters the intracellular space, is active orally, and effectively attenuates myocardial stunning *in vivo* [105,106]. The protective effects of MPG against stunning have been recently confirmed in rabbits [99]. In addition, the iron chelator, desferrioxamine, was found to attenuate postischemic dysfunction [107,108], presumably through prevention of the iron-catalyzed formation of ·OH (through the Haber-Weiss or Fenton mechanisms) and of the propagation of ·OH-initiated lipid peroxidation [102]. Taken together, these results suggest that the ·OH radical (or one of its reactive products) is a mediator of postischemic dysfunction and that the beneficial effects of SOD and catalase previously demonstrated [54,96–98,100] are due in part to prevention of ·OH generation.

Other antioxidant therapies, such as probucol, have been recently shown to attenuate myocardial stunning in the rabbit [109].

The effectiveness of antioxidants that scavenge ·OH or prevent its generation should not be interpreted as evidence that all of the damage initiated by oxygen radicals is mediated via ·OH. It is generally agreed that H_2O_2 is a relatively inert species and that its toxicity may be largely due to its reduction to ·OH [102]. However, there is evidence that $\cdot O_2^-$ in itself can directly cause cellular toxicity *in vitro* [110; reviewed in ref. 111]. Furthermore, since catalase alone prevents formation of ·OH by removing H_2O_2, the fact that SOD has to be added to catalase to produce significant attenuation of stunning *in vivo* [100] implies the existence of a component of damage specifically due to $\cdot O_2^-$. It appears, therefore, that all three species ($\cdot O_2^-$, H_2O_2, and ·OH) are important in postischemic dysfunction ($\cdot O_2^-$ and ·OH as mediators of injury and H_2O_2 as a precursor of ·OH) [100].

The studies discussed above [54,96–100,104–109] consistently support the oxyradical hypothesis, but their significance is limited by the fact that they were all performed in open-chest animals. Thus, artifacts due to the combined effects of anesthesia, hypothermia, surgical trauma, volume and ionic imbalances, unphysiologic conditions and attending neuro-humoral perturbations, as well as other potentially confounding variables, cannot be excluded. Indeed, we [112] have recently demonstrated that the severity of myocardial stunning induced by a 15–min coronary occlusion is greatly exaggerated in open-chest as compared with conscious dogs, even when differences in collateral flow are taken into account and fundamental physiological variables in the open-chest preparation are carefully kept within normal limits. The striking differences between the two models indicate the presence of artifacts in the open-chest dog and raise the possibility that results obtained in this model may not be applicable to more physiological conditions. It was therefore essential that the oxyradical hypothesis be tested in conscious animal preparations. Recently, we [112] observed that the combined administration of SOD and catalase in conscious, unsedated dogs subjected to a 15-min coronary occlusion produced a significant enhancement of the recovery of function that was sustained for at least 6 h after reflow. No subsequent deterioration occurred, indicating that postischemic depression of contractility is not a useful 'protective' response to injury. Similar findings were obtained with desferrioxamine and MPG [113]. These results [112,113] indicate that the oxyradical hypothesis developed in open-chest models is applicable to conscious models.

In summary, numerous investigations from several independent laboratories [54,96–100,104–109,112] uniformly suggest that oxygen metabolites play a significant role in the genesis of myocardial stunning after a 15-min period of ischemia, both in open-chest and in conscious animals. It seems clear that a portion of the damage is mediated by ·OH. However, the available evidence suggests that myocardial stunning cannot be simplistically ascribed to a single oxygen species, and that all of the three initial metabolites of oxygen ($\cdot O_2^-$, H_2O_2 and ·OH) contribute to the cellular injury responsible for postischemic dysfunction. Iron also appears to play a role in stunning, presumably by catalyzing the formation of ·OH. The relative contributions of the various oxygen metabolites remain to be definitively established.

Direct evidence for the oxyradical hypothesis

The studies reviewed heretofore [54,96–100,104–109,112] are limited by the fact that the evidence for a causative role of oxygen metabolites in postischemic dysfunction was indirect and, therefore, inconclusive. None of these studies [54,96–100,104–109,112] demonstrated that oxygen radicals are indeed produced in stunned myocardium and that the antioxidants that attenuate stunning do so by inhibiting free radical reactions (rather than by some nonspecific mechanism). Therefore, in order to definitively validate the oxyradical hypothesis of stunning, it was necessary to directly demonstrate and quantitate free radical generation in the presence and absence of antioxidant interventions.

Free radical production had been directly demonstrated in isolated rabbit or rat hearts undergoing global ischemia and reperfusion [40,41,114–116], but because of the numerous important differences in experimental conditions, results obtained *in vitro* cannot necessarily be extrapolated to the intact animal. We used the spin trap, α-phenyl N-tert-butyl nitrone (PBN), and electron paramagnetic resonance (EPR) spectroscopy to detect and measure production of free radicals in our *in vivo* model of postischemic dysfunction (15-min coronary occlusion in open-chest dogs) [117]. Following infusion of PBN, EPR signals characteristic of PBN radical adducts were detected in the venous blood draining from the ischemic-reperfused vascular bed [118] (Figure 1.2). The EPR signals were consistent with a mixture of different secondary lipid radicals, such as alkyl and alkoxyl radicals. The myocardial production of radicals began during coronary occlusion but increased dramatically after reperfusion, peaking at 2 to 4 min (Figure 1.3). After this initial burst, production of radicals abated but did not cease, persisting up to 3 h after reflow [118] (Figure 1.3). Figure 1.4 demonstrates that there was a linear, positive relation between the magnitude of adduct production and the magnitude of ischemic flow reduction, indicating that the intensity of free radical generation after reflow is proportional to the severity of the antecedent ischemia [118]: the greater the degree of hypoperfusion, the greater the subsequent production of free radicals and, by inference, the severity of reperfusion injury. These findings imply that interventions aimed at improving perfusion during ischemia are likely to attenuate free radical reactions after reflow.

In a subsequent study [119], we found that SOD plus catalase suppressed the production of free radicals in the stunned myocardium (Figure 1.5), indicating that these radicals result from univalent reduction of oxygen. Importantly, the inhibition of free radical production was associated with improvement of myocardial stunning [119]. More recently, we observed that MPG [105] or desferrioxamine [120], administered just before reperfusion,

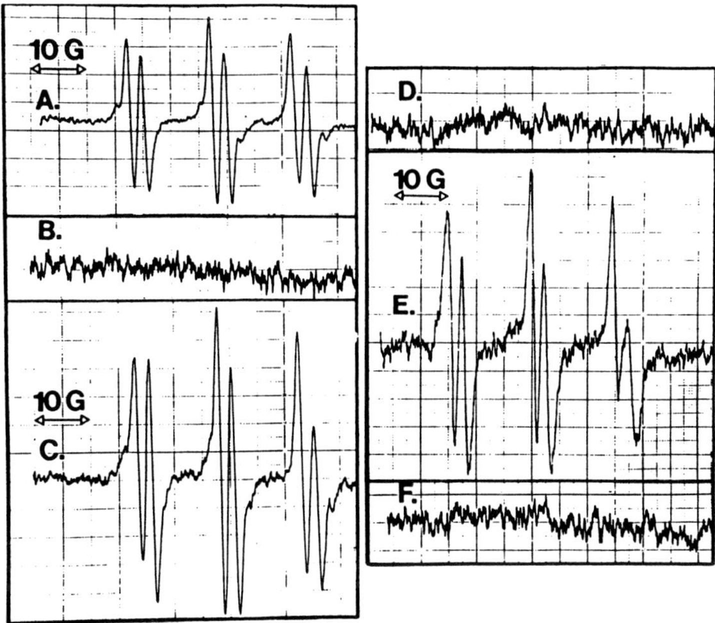

Figure 1.2. Representative electron paramagnetic resonance (EPR) spectra of PBN radical adducts detected in the coronary venous effluent blood in open-chest dogs. Dogs underwent a 15-min coronary occlusion followed by reperfusion. The spin trap, α-phenyl N-tert-butyl nitrone (PBN), was infused intracoronarily beginning 5 min before occlusion and continuing until 10 min after reperfusion (group I), beginning 20 s before reperfusion and continuing until 10 min after reperfusion (group II), or beginning 30-min after reperfusion and continuing until 40 min after reperfusion (group III). The average rate of infusion was 4.4 mg/min. Blood samples were obtained from a vein draining the ischemic/reperfused region and the plasma lipids were extracted by the Folch procedure and analyzed by EPR spectroscopy. Shown in this figure are signals from plasma samples obtained: (A) 3 min after reperfusion in a dog from group I (PBN infusion started 5 min before ischemia) ($a_N = 14.75$, $a_B^H = 2.69$ G; gain, 5×10^5); (B) at corresponding time after start of PBN infusion in a control dog (gain, 1×10^6); (C) 5 min after reperfusion in a dog in group II (PBN infusion started 20 s before reperfusion) ($a_N = 14.77$, $a_B^H = 2.69$ G; gain, 5×10^5); (D) at corresponding time after start of PBN in a second control dog (gain, 1×10^6); (E) 35 min after reperfusion in a dog in group III (PBN infusion started 30 min after reperfusion) ($a_N = 15.00$, $a_B^H = 2.78$ G; gain, 2×10^6); (F) at corresponding time after start of PBN in a third control dog (gain, 1×10^6). The signals observed are characteristic of radical adducts of PBN. These results demonstrate that free radicals are generated in the stunned myocardium in the intact dog. The spectrometer settings were as follows: microwave power, 19.7 mW; modulation amplitude, 1 G; time constant, 1.25 s; scan range, 100 G; and scan time, 8 min. All spectra were recorded at room temperature (25°C). Reproduced with permission from the Journal of Clinical Investigation 1988; 82: 476–85.

markedly attenuated myocardial stunning and the associated production of PBN adducts; however, the same agents given 1 min after reperfusion did not attenuate myocardial stunning or initial PBN adduct production (Figures 1.6 and 1.7). Thus, three different antioxidant interventions (SOD plus

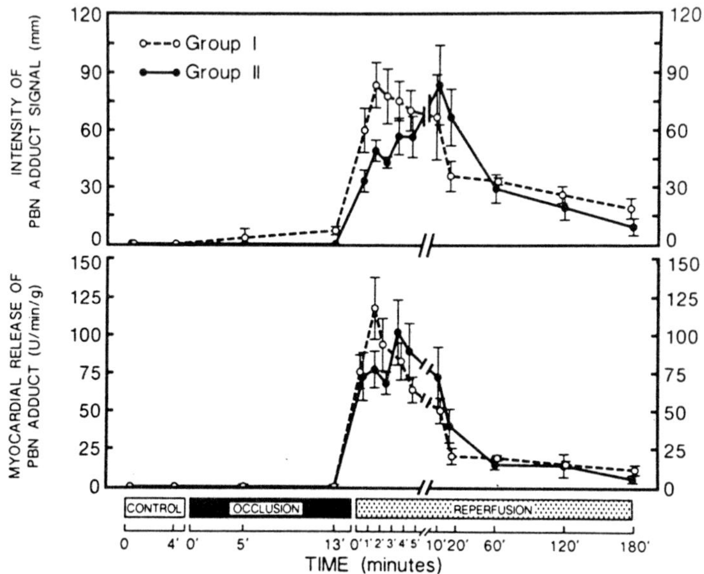

Figure 1.3. (Upper panel) Intensity of the electron paramagnetic resonance spectroscopy signals detected in the coronary venous effluent blood in groups I and II. (Lower panel) Time course of myocardial release of PBN adducts in groups I and II. Data are mean ± SEM. Open-chest dogs underwent a 15-min coronary occlusion followed by reperfusion. Group I received intracoronary PBN starting 5 min before occlusion and continuing until 10 min after reperfusion (n = 5); group II received intracoronary PBN starting at reperfusion and ending 10 min thereafter (n = 5). Reperfusion after 15 min of ischemia was associated with a burst of free radical generation, which abated by 10 min but continued up to 3 h after reflow. PBN, α-phenyl N-tert-butyl nitrone. Reproduced with permission from The Journal of Clinical Investigation 1988; 82: 476–85.

catalase, MPG, and desferrioxamine) reduced postischemic dysfunction at the same doses and under the same experimental conditions in which they reduced formation of PBN adducts. These circumstances strongly suggest that there is a cause-and-effect relationship between the production of free radicals in the stunned myocardium and the depression of contractility.

More recently, we have demonstrated, using PBN, that free radicals are also produced in the stunned myocardium in the conscious dog after a 15-min occlusion [121], with a time-course similar to that observed in the open-chest dog. These results [121] provide important evidence that the generation of free radicals observed in open-chest animals [105,117–120,122] is not an artifact due to the unphysiologic conditions associated with this preparation. In another recently reported study [123], we have used aromatic hydroxylation of phenylalanine to investigate whether the hydroxyl radical is generated in the stunned myocardium. We have found that hydroxylated derivatives of phenylalanine (ortho-, meta-, and para-tyrosine) are released

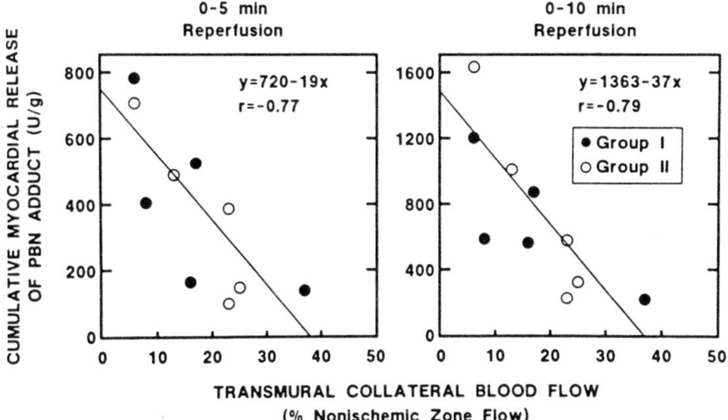

Figure 1.4. Relationship between mean transmural collateral blood flow to the ischemic region during coronary occlusion (horizontal axis) and total cumulative myocardial release of PBN adducts during the first 5-min (left) and 10-min (right) of reperfusion. Collateral flow is expressed as percentage of simultaneous nonischemic zone flow; adduct release is expressed in arbitrary units per gram of myocardium. Solid circles represent dogs in group I (PBN given before ischemia); open circles represent dogs in group II (PBN given at reperfusion). In both groups, the myocardial production of PBN adducts after coronary reperfusion was linearly and inversely related to collateral flow during the antecedent occlusion. These data suggest that the severity of the ischemic injury is the major determinant of the severity of the subsequent reperfusion injury. PBN, α-phenyl N-tert-butyl nitrone. Reproduced with permission from The Journal of Clinical Investigation 1988; 82: 476–85.

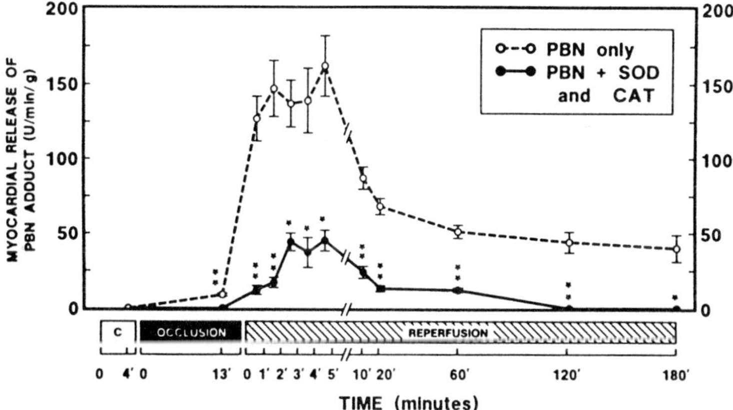

Figure 1.5. Time course of myocardial release of PBN adducts in group I (PBN only, n = 6) and group II (PBN plus superoxide dismutase and catalase, n = 6). Data are mean ± SEM. Administration of superoxide dismutase and catalase markedly inhibited production of free radicals in the stunned myocardium after 15 min of regional ischemia. $*P < 0.05$; $**P < 0.01$ vs. group I. PBN, α-phenyl N-tert-butyl nitrone. Reproduced from Proceedings of the National Academy of Sciences of the USA 1989; 86: 4695–9.

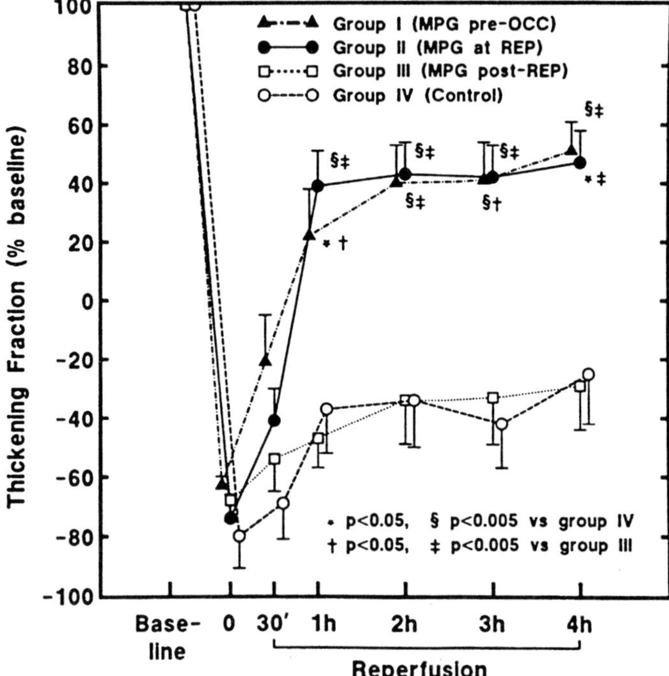

Figure 1.6. Systolic thickening fraction in the ischemic/reperfused region 5 min after coronary occlusion (O) and at selected times after reperfusion in the following groups: Group I (MPG infusion started 15 min before ischemia, n = 8), group II (MPG started 1 min before reperfusion, n = 9), group III (MPG infusion started 1 min after reperfusion, n = 10), and group IV (controls, n = 10). Thickening fraction is expressed as percent of baseline values. Data are mean ± SEM. MPG attenuated postischemic dysfunction to a similar extent irrespective of whether the infusion was started before ischemia or just before reperfusion; however, infusion started 1 min after reperfusion was ineffective, suggesting that the critical radical-mediated injury occurs in the first few moments after reperfusion. MPG, N-2-mercaptopropionyl glycine. Reproduced with permission of The American Heart Association from Circulation Research 1989; 65: 607–22.

in the local coronary venous blood during the first few minutes of reperfusion after a 15-min occlusion, both in open-chest and in conscious dogs [123], indicating that ·OH is produced in the stunned myocardium upon reperfusion. The similarity of the results obtained in our canine model of stunning with two completely different techniques (spin trapping [105,117–122] and aromatic hydroxylation [123]) further corroborates the concept that reactive oxygen species play a significant role in the pathogenesis of postischemic ventricular dysfunction.

In summary, measurements of free radicals in experimental models of stunned myocardium [105,117–123] provide direct evidence supporting a pathogenetic role of oxygen metabolites. Specifically, these studies indicate that (1) free radicals are produced in the stunned myocardium in both open-

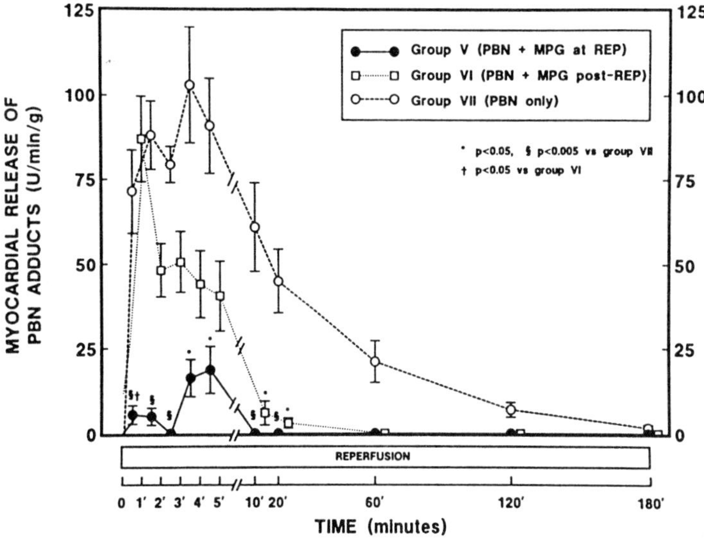

Figure 1.7. Time course of myocardial release of PBN adducts in group V (MPG infusion started 1 min after reperfusion, (n = 5), group VI (MPG infusion started 1 min after reperfusion, (n = 5), and group VII (controls, n = 6). Data are mean ± SEM. All groups received PBN by the intracoronary route. Infusion of MPG started 1 min before reperfusion markedly suppressed production of free radicals in the stunned myocardium. Infusion of MPG started 1 min after reperfusion did not affect the initial production of free radicals and produced a delayed suppression which became evident by 10 min of reflow. Since only MPG given as in group V attenuated postischemic dysfunction (whereas MPG given as in group VI did not) (see Figure 1.1), these data suggest that the free radicals important in myocardial stunning are those generated immediately after reperfusion. MPG, N-2-mercaptopropionyl glycine; PBN, α-phenyl N-tert-butyl nitrone. Reproduced with permission of The American Heart Association from Circulation Research 1989; 65: 607–22.

chest and conscious dogs after reversible regional ischemia; (2) the univalent pathway of reduction of oxygen is the source of the radicals; and (3) inhibition of free radical reactions results in enhanced recovery of contractility (i.e., the radical reactions are necessary for postischemic dysfunction to occur).

Effect of oxygen radicals on cardiac function

Both *in vitro* and *in vivo* studies have demonstrated that oxygen metabolites depress myocardial function. Exposure of isolated rabbit interventricular septa [124], isolated rat [125] or rabbit papillary muscles, and isolated rat [126–128] or rabbit [129,130] hearts to free radical-generating solutions or pure H_2O_2 has uniformly resulted in decreased mechanical function and ATP levels, i.e., in changes similar to those observed in the stunned myocardium. In most of the studies in which an attempt was made to discern the relative roles of different oxygen species [124,125,128,129], it was found that the deleterious effects could be prevented by catalase or by ·OH scavengers, but not by SOD, suggesting that H_2O_2 or its byproduct, ·OH, were the oxygen metabolites responsible for the observed depression of contractile function. In one study [110], however, SOD was protective whereas catalase had no effect, implying that the major negative inotropic agent was $\cdot O_2^-$.

In summary, it is clear that reactive oxygen species depress myocardial contractility both *in vitro* and *in vivo*. There is substantial evidence that the detrimental effects of $\cdot O_2^-$ and H_2O_2 on cardiac function are mediated in part by generation of ·OH. This is in accordance with the results of *in vivo* studies [104–108], which suggest an important role of ·OH as a mediator of stunning. However, there is also evidence for a direct negative inotropic action of $\cdot O_2^-$. which is also congruent with observations *in vivo* [100]. The precise role of each species remains therefore to be defined.

Mechanism of oxyradical-mediated contractile dysfunction

The exact mechanism whereby oxygen metabolites depress contractile function remains speculative and represents one of the major unresolved issues pertaining to the pathogenesis of myocardial stunning. Free radicals are reactive species that can attack nonspecifically virtually all cellular components. Theoretically, every abnormality described thus far in the stunned myocardium (see above) could be caused by oxyradicals. At least two key cellular components, proteins and lipids, could be the key targets of free radical-initiated reactions, leading to protein denaturation and enzyme inactivation, as well as [131] peroxidation of the polyunsaturated fatty acids contained in cellular membranes [132]. The latter effect would impair selective membrane permeability and interfere with the function of various cellular organelles.

There is some evidence for the occurrence of lipid peroxidation in the stunned myocardium. Romaschin *et al.* [133] observed increased myocardial concentration of hydroxy conjugated dienes (which are products of free fatty acid oxidation) during and after a 45–min period of global normothermic ischemia in open-chest dogs. The maximal concentration of conjugated dienes was measured at 5 min of reflow. Importantly, the tissue examined after reperfusion was dysfunctional but not necrotic, thus representing stunned myocardium. Weisel *et al.* [134] subsequently reported that in patients undergoing cardioplegic arrest during coronary artery bypass surgery, there was myocardial release of conjugated dienes in the coronary sinus blood at 3 and 60 min of reperfusion, which was associated with a decrease in the myocardial concentration of the antioxidant, α-tocopherol. However, it is important to point out that evidence for the occurrence of lipid peroxidation in the stunned myocardium after a 15-min occlusion is still lacking.

Sarcoplasmic reticulum dysfunction may be an important mechanism whereby oxyradicals mediate the contractile abnormalities observed after reversible ischemia. As mentioned above, both calcium uptake and Ca^{2+}, Mg^{2+}-ATPase activity are significantly depressed in the stunned myocardium [94]. Exposure of isolated sarcoplasmic reticulum to oxygen radicals [132,135] results in a similar decrease in calcium uptake and Ca^{2+}, Mg^{2+}-ATPase activity, and oxyradical scavengers (particularly those that remove ·OH or prevent its generation) preserve sarcoplasmic reticulum function [132,135].

Other studies suggest that the sarcolemma may be a critical target of free radical-mediated damage, which interfere with its calcium transport and calcium-stimulated ATPase activity [136,137]. Oxygen radicals have also been shown to interfere with the Na^+-Ca^{2+} exchange [140] and to inhibit the Na^+-K^+-ATPase activity [138]. Impairment of the Na^+-K^+-ATPase activity results in Na^+ overload, with consequent activation of the Na^+-Ca^{2+} exchange activity [84,85]. This impairment is prevented by antioxidants [139]. All of these observations imply that excessive production of oxyradicals could result in increased transarcolemmal calcium influx and cellular calcium overload.

It is important to point out that the foregoing postulated mechanisms involve alterations in calcium homeostasis, and thus would reconcile the oxyradical hypothesis and the calcium overload hypothesis of stunning into one pathogenetic mechanism.

Sources of oxygen radicals in the stunned myocardium

Although there exist various potential mechanisms of oxyradical generation in the stunned myocardium, only two have been explored thus far, namely, the enzyme xanthine oxidase and the activated neutrophil. We found that the xanthine oxidase inhibitor allopurinol inhibited the increased cardiac production of urate observed in control dogs during ischemia and early reperfusion (indicating effective inhibition of xanthine oxidoreductase), and produced a marked improvement in the functional recovery of the stunned myocardium [140]. Attenuation of stunning has also been demonstrated with oxypurinol after 15 min [141] and 90 min [142] of ischemia and reperfusion. These data suggest that xanthine oxidase is one of the sources of the oxygen radicals that contribute to postischemic dysfunction in the dog. Whether this concept applies to humans remains controversial because reports regarding the myocardial content of the enzyme in the human heart are conflicting [143–147].

Contradicting these earlier reports [140–142] is a recent study [151] where oxypurinol and amflutizole (two xanthine oxidase inhibitors) failed to mitigate stunning after 15 min of ischemia in dogs. The reason(s) for the discrepancy is (are) presently unclear and could be due to different degrees of inhibition of xanthine oxidoreductase. In any case, the role of this enzyme in postischemic myocardial dysfunction does not seem to be critical because antioxidant therapy attenuates stunning in the rabbit [99,109], a species that apparently lacks myocardial xanthine oxidase activity; this indicates that there are other important sources of free radicals in the stunned myocardium besides xanthine oxidase.

Neutrophils are another potential source of oxygen metabolites [148,149]. However, no effect on myocardial stunning was demonstrated by depletion of neutrophils with antiserum [68,150] or with filtration [151], by administration of nafazatrom (which inhibits production of leukotrienes [152]), by administration of antibodies to the adhesion-promoting Mo1 glycoprotein [153], and by administration of dextran (which inhibits leukocyte adherence to the endothelium [154]). Recent studies have shown that the neutrophil content of the stunned myocardium after a 12-min period of ischemia is decreased [155] and that myeloperoxidase activity (a marker of neutrophils) in myocardium stunned by a 15-min occlusion is not different from nonischemic myocardium [153]. Furthermore, isolated heart preparations, which are devoid of circulating neutrophils, can exhibit myocardial stunning. Taken together, these results [68,150–155] suggest that granulocytes do not play a major role in the pathogenesis of stunning after brief, reversible ischemia, and indeed there is now a general consensus regarding this point [156].

In summary, in the canine model of myocardial stunning produced by a single, reversible ischemic episode, xanthine oxidase may be a source of free radicals (although the data are not entirely consistent), whereas neutrophils are relatively unimportant. Several other processes could lead to formation of $\cdot O_2^-$ and H_2O_2 during myocardial ischemia and reperfusion, including activation of the arachidonate cascade, autoxidation of catecholamines and other compounds, ischemia-induced damage of the electron transport chain in the mitochondria, and accumulation of reducing equivalents [132]. Identification of the sources of oxyradicals in the stunned myocardium represents another major unresolved issue, which is especially difficult to unravel in a complex system such as the intact animal.

Time course of free radical-induced damage in the stunned myocardium

We have observed that infusion of the antioxidant MPG attenuated postischemic dysfunction to a similar extent whether the infusion was started before ischemia or 1 min before reperfusion; however, infusion started 1 min after reflow was ineffective [105], suggesting that the critical radical-mediated injury occurs in the first few moments of reperfusion (Figure 1.6). We have subsequently obtained similar results with desferrioxamine [120]. Furthermore, the spin trap, PBN, enhances contractile recovery in open-chest animals even when the infusion is commenced 20 s before reflow; the magnitude of the protective effect is similar to that observed when the infusion is started before ischemia [118]. Captopril, an angiotensin converting enzyme inhibitor with free radical scavenging properties, has been reported to produce similar attenuation of postischemic dysfunction when the administration is started before ischemia and when it is started 2 min before reperfusion [157]. Antioxidant therapy started just before reperfusion has also been shown to reduce myocardial stunning in the rabbit [99].

That a substantial portion of the cellular damage responsible for stunning occurs immediately after reflow is further corroborated by direct measurements of free radicals [105,118,119] and lipid peroxidation products [133] in the stunned myocardium, both of which have shown a burst in the initial moments after reperfusion. Free radical inhibition during this initial burst, but not after the first 5 min of reperfusion (i.e., after the initial burst), will result in functional improvement [105] (Figure 1.7) These observations suggest that the free radicals important in causing myocardial stunning are those produced immediately after reflow.

In summary, myocardial stunning appears to be, in part, a form of oxyradical-mediated "reperfusion injury". This concept may have significant therapeutic implications, because it suggests that antioxidant therapies begun after the onset of ischemia could still be effective in preventing postischemic dysfunction; however, a delay in the implementation of such therapies until *after reperfusion* would result in loss of efficacy.

Role of oxygen radicals in other forms of myocardial stunning (*Table* 1.1)
The investigations reviewed thus far employed a single brief ($\leqslant$15 min) coronary occlusion. In recent studies in our laboratory we found that MPG (a ·OH scavenger) markedly improves contractile recovery after ten 5-min coronary occlusions separated by 10-min reflow periods in open-chest dogs [22]. Thus, oxyradicals also appear to contribute to the genesis of myocardial stunning after multiple brief ischemic episodes. Further, the surgical literature abounds with evidence for a pathogenetic role of oxygen radicals in postischemic dysfunction after global ischemia in *in vivo* models of cardioplegic arrest [4346]. Recent studies [158] suggest that oxyradicals also contribute to postoperative dysfunction in patients undergoing cardiac surgery. Finally, antioxidants consistently alleviate mechanical dysfunction after global ischemia in isolated hearts [33–39,42] but, as discussed above, the relevance of these *in vitro* preparations to myocardial stunning is often uncertain.

Whether oxygen radicals pay a role in myocardial stunning after a prolonged coronary occlusion (resulting in some degree of cell death) is still unclear. Three studies failed to detect improvement in functional recovery with SOD and catalase after coronary occlusions lasting 1 h [159], 90 min [160], and 2 h [161] in open-chest [161] or conscious dogs [159,160]. We [162] also observed that SOD fails to enhance recovery of contractility after a 2-h coronary occlusion in anesthetized dogs. These results suggest that short-term administration of antioxidant enzymes is not effective in mitigating myocardial stunning associated with subendocardial infarction, perhaps because the pathogenesis of postischemic dysfunction is different when this abnormality is caused by a prolonged period of ischemia. However, other studies [142,163,164] have shown that the cell-permeant antioxidants, oxypurinol, N-acetylcysteine and Trolox, attenuate myocardial stunning independently of infarct size limitation in closed-chest dogs subjected to 90 min of coronary occlusion and 24 h of reflow [142,163], and in open-chest pigs subjected to 45 min of coronary occlusion and 72 h of reperfusion [164].

Exercise-induced stunning is not alleviated by SOD and catalase [165].

In summary, there is strong evidence that oxyradicals contribute to postischemic dysfunction after global ischemia (*in vitro* as well as *in vivo* and after multiple episodes of regional ischemia. They do not appear to contribute to exercise-induced postischemic dysfunction. The role of oxygen radicals in myocardial stunning after a prolonged, partly irreversible ischemic insult remains uncertain and represents a major unresolved problem. Elucidation of this issue will be difficult because the dysfunction is due in part to the presence of infarction and in part to the presence of stunning – a situation that complicates the evaluation of therapy.

Integration of different hypotheses

As the data reviewed above suggest, myocardial stunning is probably a *multifactorial* process that involves complex sequences of cellular perturbations and the interaction of multiple pathogenetic mechanisms. Much remains to be learned regarding this phenomenon, as none of the theories discussed herein explains the entire cascade of events that culminates in postischemic contractile abnormalities. For example, the origin(s) of reactive oxygen species as well as the mechanism whereby they induce mechanical dysfunction remains uncertain. Integration of the various hypotheses is complicated by the fact that, for the most part, each hypothesis has been developed in a different experimental preparation (Table 1.1).

Nevertheless, it is important to emphasize that these hypotheses are not mutually exclusive and in fact may represent different parts of the same pathophysiological sequence. There is considerable evidence to suggest a link between generation of oxygen radicals and perturbed calcium homeostasis. For example, the damage associated with the 'calcium paradox' resembles that associated with the 'oxygen paradox' and probably has a similar pathogenetic mechanism [166]. Furthermore, as discussed above, oxyradicals generated upon reperfusion can cause dysfunction of the sarcoplasmic reticulum [132,135] and alter calcium flux across the sarcolemma [136–139,167]. These actions would result in excitation-contraction uncoupling and cellular calcium overload [132,136]. In this regard, it has been recently demonstrated that reoxygenation of cultured myocytes generates Ca^{2+} overload which can be greatly attenuated by antioxidant enzymes [82]. Oxygen radicals could also damage the contractile proteins so that their responsiveness to calcium is altered. On the other hand, calcium overload may exaggerate oxyradical production by promoting the conversion of xanthine dehydrogenase to xanthine oxidase, which appears to be mediated by a calcium-dependent protease [86], thereby leading to a vicious circle.

A unifying hypothesis for the pathogenesis of myocardial stunning is proposed in Figure 1.8 (a detailed description of the postulated mechanisms is provided in the figure legend). This paradigm is largely speculative, but nevertheless encompasses the evidence available at this time and discussed in this review. According to this conceptual diagram (Figure 1.8), oxyradical generation, calcium overload, and sarcoplasmic reticulum dysfunction can

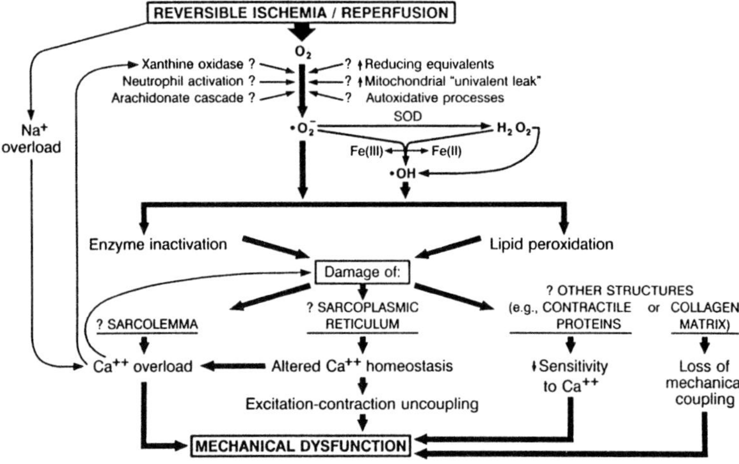

Figure 1.8. Illustration of the proposed pathogenesis of postischemic myocardial dysfunction. This proposal integrates and reconciles different mechanisms into a unifying pathogenetic hypothesis. Transient reversible ischemia followed by reperfusion could result in increased production of superoxide radicals ($\cdot O_2^-$) through several mechanisms, including (1) increased activity of xanthine oxidase; (2) activation of neutrophils; (3) activation of the arachidonate cascade; (4) accumulation of reducing equivalents during oxygen deprivation; (5) derangements of the intramitochondrial electron transport system resulting in increased univalent reduction of oxygen; and (6) autoxidation of catecholamines and other substances. Superoxide dismutase (SOD) dismutates $\cdot O_2^-$ to hydrogen peroxide (H_2O_2); in the presence of catalytic iron, $\cdot O_2^-$ and H_2O_2 interreact in a Haber-Weiss reaction to generate the hydroxyl radical ($\cdot OH$). H_2O_2 can also generate $\cdot OH$ in the absence of $\cdot O_2^-$ through a Fenton reaction provided that other substances (such as ascorbate) reduce Fe (III) to Fe (II). $\cdot O_2^-$ and $\cdot OH$ attack proteins and polyunsaturated fatty acids, causing enzyme inactivation and lipid peroxidation, respectively.

In the setting of reversible ischemia, the intensity of this damage is not sufficient to cause cell death, but is sufficient to produce dysfunction of key cellular organelles. Postulated targets of free radical damage include: (1) the sarcolemma, with consequent loss of selective permeability, impairment of calcium-stimulated ATPase activity and calcium transport out of the cell, and impairment of the Na^+-K^+-ATPase activity. The net result of these perturbations would be increased transarcolemmal calcium influx and cellular calcium overload. (2) The sarcoplasmic reticulum, with consequent impairment of calcium-stimulated ATPase activity and calcium transport. This would result in impaired calcium homeostasis: specifically, decreased calcium sequestration (which would contribute to increase free cytosolic calcium) and decreased calcium release during systole (which would cause excitation-contraction uncoupling). (3) Possibly other structures, such as the extracellular collagen matrix (with consequent loss of mechanical coupling) or the contractile proteins (with consequent decreased sensitivity to calcium). At the same time, reversible ischemia/reperfusion could cause cellular Na^+ overload due to (1) inhibition of sarcolemmal Na^+-K^+-ATPase, and (2) acidosis and Na^+-H^+ exchange. This could further exaggerate calcium overload via increased Na^+-Ca^{2+} exchange. An increase in free cytosolic calcium would activate phospholipases and other degradative enzymes and further exacerbate the injury to the aforementioned key subcellular structures (sarcolemma, sarcoplasmic reticulum, and contractile proteins). Thus, calcium overload could serve to amplify the damage initiated by oxygen radicals. In addition, calcium overload could in itself impair contractile performance and contribute to mechanical dysfunction. It is also possible that the increase in free cytosolic calcium could increase oxyradical production by promoting the conversion of xanthine dehydrogenase to xanthine oxidase. The ultimate consequence of this complex series of perturbations is a reversible depression of contractility. Reproduced with permission of the American Heart Association from Circulation 1990; 82: 723–38.

be viewed as different facets of the same pathogenetic mechanism, thereby reconciling the three major current hypotheses of myocardial stunning.

In summary, the pathogenesis of myocardial stunning has not been fully elucidated. Three abnormalities (oxyradical generation, calcium overload, and excitation-contraction uncoupling) have emerged as likely contributing factors (although in different experimental preparations), and *in vitro* evidence suggests that they are interrelated. It is now essential to clarify the precise interactions among these three factors *in vivo* and the role that each of them plays in the various experimental settings of myocardial stunning.

What is the clinical significance of myocardial stunning?

Despite the multiplicity of clinical situations in which myocardial stunning would be expected to occur, investigation of this phenomenon in humans has been hindered by several major problems, namely, the limited accuracy of the methods available to measure regional left ventricular function, the inability to quantify regional myocardial blood flow during acute ischemia, the difficulty in establishing with certainty the beginning and the end of an ischemic episode, and the uncontrolled influence of variables (such as preload, afterload, adrenergic tone, and inotropic therapy) that have a major impact on postischemic dysfunction [168]. Perhaps the major problem is to discern whether a reversible depression of contractile function is due to stunning, silent ischemia, or hibernation (i.e., chronic myocardial hypoperfusion) [168]. This differential diagnosis requires simultaneous measurement of regional myocardial function and flow, which thus far has not been generally possible.

Nevertheless, there is mounting evidence that myocardial stunning does occur in numerous clinical settings in which the myocardium is exposed to transient ischemia followed by reperfusion, including coronary angioplasty, exercise-induced angina, angina at rest (unstable or variant), acute myocardial infarction with early reperfusion (either spontaneous or induced by thrombolytic therapy), open-heart surgery with cardioplegic arrest, and cardiac transplantation [13,168]. Restoration of flow in these situations is associated with prolonged and sometimes profound mechanical abnormalities that resolve slowly over a period of hours or days [13,168]. Thus, it seems probable that stunning is a common occurrence in patients with coronary artery disease.

However, since stunning is by definition a reversible phenomenon, it may be argued that it is unimportant. Why are so much time and effort devoted to studying an abnormality that is transient and will resolve completely any way? In our view, several considerations suggest that postischemic dysfunction is clinically important despite its reversible nature [168]:

First, in patients with depressed baseline LV function, myocardial stunning may be an important factor precipitating LV failure with its attendant morbidity and mortality. Dramatic examples illustrating this point have been published [169–171]. In patients with unstable angina or acute myocardial infarction and early reperfusion who have a large amount of jeopardized myocardium (e.g., patients with proximal left anterior descending lesions), the development of postischemic LV abnormalities may cause hemodynamic instability requiring intensive monitoring, pharmacological and/or mechanical hemodynamic support, and urgent revascularization under less than ideal conditions. Furthermore, in those cases in which coronary bypass surgery carries a greater risk than normal (e.g., repeat surgery, prolonged aortic cross-clamping, unstable angina, concurrent valve replacement, etc.), the incidence and severity of postoperative complications may be significantly exacerbated by stunning.

Second, the concept of stunning is important because it implies that the postischemic contractile abnormalities observed in the aforementioned clinical settings can be effectively manipulated with appropriate therapy. As discussed above, experimental studies have clearly demonstrated that myocardial stunning can be reversed by inotropic agents [19,28,58–63] or prevented by various interventions such as antioxidant therapy [15].

Third, the appreciation of the phenomenon of stunning should allow the clinician to assess the efficacy of reperfusion therapy with greater accuracy. Such a situation arises, for example, in thrombolysis in the setting of myocardial infarction, where the extent of tissue salvage cannot be immediately appreciated because a portion of myocardium is stunned and the improvement in contractility may require several days, or possibly even longer. The notion that contractile function cannot be used as a measure of viability until myocardial stunning has fully dissipated poses frequent dilemmas to the clinician. Soon after thrombolytic therapy, a LV region may by akinetic either because it is necrotic or because it is viable but stunned, raising the question of whether mechanical revascularization with angioplasty or bypass surgery should be carried out. A similar problem is encountered when cardiogenic shock develops after thrombolytic therapy or cardiac surgery: how long should aggressive therapy be pursued? Is the LV failure due to infarction and scarring or to stunning? Obviously, the usefulness of maintaining pharmacological and/or mechanical circulatory support for extended periods of time will largely depend on whether the contractile dysfunction is reversible. There is clearly a need for techniques that can distinguish stunned from infarcted myocardium and that can be used to justify the termination of, or the exclusion of patients from, aggressive therapeutic approaches.

Fourth, the recognition of the phenomenon of myocardial stunning requires a reassessment of the criteria traditionally used to decide whether aggressive revascularization procedures are indicated in patients with coronary artery disease. Because the presence of hypokinesis or akinesis does not necessarily signify loss of viability, patients should not be denied mechanical revascularization solely because of an abnormal resting wall motion. Again, techniques for distinguishing stunned from necrotic myocardium are desirable in order to identify patients who could benefit from revascularization.

In our opinion, however, the most intriguing clinical implication of the concept of stunning is the possibility that this contractile abnormality may become persistent or chronic. Studies in experimental animals have shown that repeated brief episodes of ischemia have a cumulative effect on contractility, such that myocardial function remains depressed for periods of time much longer than with a single ischemic episode [17–23,172]. This has been demonstrated both after ischemia due to reduced oxygen supply (e.g., 5-min coronary occlusions [17,23]) and after ischemia due to increased oxygen demands (i.e., exercise-induced ischemia [172]). On the other hand, clinical studies have demonstrated that repetitive episodes of ischemia (mostly silent) occur in many patients with coronary artery disease, and recur at short intervals in the same territory [173]. In these patients the myocardial contractility may not be able to fully recover between the ischemic episodes and thus may remain reversibly depressed for prolonged periods of time, which perhaps could account for some cases of 'ischemic cardiomyopathy' [168]. Elucidation of this problem is one of the most fascinating and important areas for future research.

In summary, numerous clinical observations suggest that stunning does occur in various settings in which the myocardium is exposed to transient ischemia, including coronary angioplasty, exercise-induced angina, angina at rest (unstable or variant), acute myocardial infarction with early reperfusion, open-heart surgery, and cardiac transplantation. Recognition of this entity is important, amongst other reasons, because it is likely to cause significant morbidity that is potentially correctable (with inotropic therapy) or even preventable (e.g., with antioxidant therapy). In addition, the appreciation of the phenomenon of myocardial stunning should allow the clinician to make a more judicious selection of patients that will benefit from mechanical revascularization. Perhaps the most important clinical implication of the concept of stunning is the possibility that this contractile abnormality may become persistent or even chronic. Our understanding of myocardial stunning in humans is still relatively crude and will not significantly improve until studies are performed which measure *simultaneously* regional myocardial perfusion and function (so that stunning can be differentiated from silent ischemia and hibernation).

What potential therapies are available for myocardial stunning?

Postischemic dysfunction can be temporarily reversed with inotropic therapy [19,28,58–63], and indeed this form of therapy is the standard approach to the treatment of LV dysfunction in clinical situations where stunning is likely to be present. Given that inotropic agents are so effective, shouldn't one be content with this form of treatment?

Inotropic agents may unfortunately not be the optimal approach to the problem. There are several reasons why it is preferable to prevent stunning from occurring in the first place rather than to have to treat it with inotropic agents after it has developed: First, inotropic agents increase myocardial oxygen consumption, which is undesirable in patients with coronary artery disease; Second, most inotropic agents have the potential to cause arrhythmias; Third, inotropic therapy often requires invasive hemodynamic monitoring; Fourth, although brief inotropic therapy appears to be innocuous [60,61], it is unknown whether prolonged inotropic stimulation of stunned myocardium has deleterious effects; and finally, prevention of myocardial stunning might facilitate rapid weaning from bypass after cardiac surgery or transplantation and may shorten the duration of hemodynamic instability after thrombolysis.

Prophylaxis of myocardial stunning may soon become a clinical reality. As discussed above, there is strong experimental evidence that this contractile abnormality can be significantly attenuated by antioxidant therapy given before reflow [15,1741 or by calcium antagonists given before ischemia [93]. Some antioxidants (allopurinol, desferrioxamine, and mercaptopropionyl glycine) are already used clinically for other reasons, whereas other therapies (e.g., human recombinant superoxide dismutase) are being developed rapidly. Initial clinical trials are being (or will soon be) conducted to examine the effect of antioxidants (in particular, desferrioxamine and human superoxide dismutase) or calcium antagonists in patients undergoing myocardial reperfusion after open-heart surgery or after myocardial infarction. Compared with inotropic stimulation, therapy with antioxidants or calcium antagonists represents a novel approach because it could prevent rather than simply temporarily correct postischemic dysfunction. Evaluation of the clinical efficacy of antioxidants and calcium antagonists represents an important area of future research.

Summary

The concept of myocardial stunning represents one of the fastest growing and most challenging aspects of cardiology in the 90s. Its pathogenesis, however, has not been definitively determined. Among the numerous mechanisms proposed, three appear to be more plausible: (1) Generation of oxygen radicals, (2) calcium overload, and (3) excitation-contraction uncoupling. The evidence for a pathogenetic role of oxygen-derived free radicals in myocardial stunning is overwhelming. In the setting of a single 15-min coronary occlusion, mitigation of stunning by antioxidants has been reproducibly observed by several independent laboratories. Similar protection has been recently demonstrated in the conscious animal, i.e., in the most physiological experimental preparation available. Furthermore, generation of free radicals in the stunned myocardium has been directly demonstrated by spin trapping techniques, and attenuation of free radical generation has been repeatedly shown to result in attenuation of contractile dysfunction. Numerous observations suggest that oxyradicals also contribute to stunning in other settings: after global ischemia *in vitro*, after global ischemia during cardioplegic arrest *in vivo*, and after multiple brief episodes of regional ischemia *in vivo*. Compelling evidence indicates that the critical free radical damage occurs in the initial moments of reflow, so that myocardial stunning can be viewed, in part, as a sublethal form of oxyradical-mediated 'reperfusion injury'.

There is also considerable evidence that a transient calcium overload during early reperfusion contributes to postischemic dysfunction *in vitro*; however, the importance of this mechanism *in vivo* remains to be defined.

Finally, inadequate release of calcium by the sarcoplasmic reticulum, with consequent excitation-contraction uncoupling, may occur after multiple brief episodes of regional ischemia, but its role in other forms of postischemic dysfunction has not been explored.

It is probable that multiple mechanisms contribute to the pathogenesis of myocardial stunning. The three hypotheses outlined above are not mutually exclusive and in fact may represent different steps of the same pathophysiological cascade. Thus, generation of oxyradicals may cause sarcoplasmic reticulum dysfunction, and both of these processes may lead to calcium overload, which in turn could exacerbate the damage initiated by oxygen species. This speculation, however, is based entirely on *in vitro* evidence. It is now necessary to elucidate the precise interactions among oxyradical generation, sarcoplasmic reticulum dysfunction and calcium overload *in vivo* and the role that each of these abnormalities plays in the various experimental settings of postischemic dysfunction. Myocardial stunning is likely to occur commonly in patients with coronary artery disease and to contribute significantly to the morbidity associated with this disorder. It is hoped that the concepts discussed in this chapter will provide a conceptual framework for further investigation of the pathophysiology of reversible ischemia/reperfusion injury, as well as a rationale for developing clinically applicable interventions designed to prevent postischemic ventricular dysfunction.

Acknowledgements

The excellent secretarial assistance of Valerie R. Price is gratefully acknowledged. The work reported here was supported in part by NIH Grants HL43151 and by NIH SCOR Grant HL42267.

References

1. Bolli R. Oxygen-derived free radicals and myocardial reperfusion injury: An overview. Cardiovasc Drugs Ther 1991; 5: 249–68.
2. Weiner JM, Apstein CS, Arthur JH *et al.* Persistence of myocardial injury following brief periods of coronary occlusion. Cardiovasc Res 1976; 10: 678–86.
3. Theroux P, Ross J Jr, Franklin D *et al.* Coronary arterial reperfusion. III. Early and late effects on regional myocardial function and dimensions in conscious dogs. Am J Cardiol 1976; 38: 599–606.
4. Heyndrickx GR, Baig H, Nellens P *et al.* Depression of regional blood flow and wall thickening after brief coronary occlusions. Am J Physiol 1978; 234: H653–H659.
5. Kloner RA, Ellis SG, Lange R *et al.* Studies of experimental coronary artery reperfusion: effects on infarct size, myocardial function, biochemistry, ultrastructure and microvascular damage. Circulation 1983; 68(Suppl I): I-8–I-15.
6. Lavallee M, Cox D, Patrick TA *et al.* Salvage of myocardial function by coronary artery reperfusion 1, 2, and 3 hours after occlusion in conscious dogs. Circ Res 1983; 53: 235–47.
7. Bush LR, Buja LM, Samowitz W *et al.* Recovery of left ventricular segmental function after long-term reperfusion following temporary coronary occlusion in conscious dogs: comparison of 2- and 4-hour occlusions. Circ Res 1983; 53: 248–63.
8. Ellis SG, Henschke CI, Sandor T *et al.* Time course of functional and biochemical recovery of myocardium salvaged by reperfusion. J Am Coll Cardiol 1983; 1: 1047–55.
9. Matsuzaki M, Gallagher KP, Kemper WS *et al.* Sustained regional dysfunction produced by prolonged coronary stenosis: gradual recovery after reperfusion. Circulation 1983; 68: 170–82.
10. Bolli R, Zhu WX, Thornby JI *et al.* Time-course and determinants of recovery of function after reversible ischemia in conscious dogs. Am J Physiol 1988; 254: H102–H114.
11. Charlat ML, O'Neill PG, Hartley CJ *et al.* Prolonged abnormalities of left ventricular diastolic wall thinning in the "stunned" myocardium in conscious dogs: Time-course and relation to systolic function. J Am Coll Cardiol 1989; 13: 185–94.
12. Bolli R, Patel BS, Hartley CJ *et al.* Nonuniform transmural recovery of contractile function in the "stunned" myocardium Am J Physiol 1989; 257: H375–H385.
13. Heyndrickx GR, Millard RW, McRitchie RJ *et al.* Regional myocardial functional and electrophysiological alterations after brief coronary artery occlusion in conscious dogs. J Clin Invest 1975; 56: 978–85.
14. Braunwald E, Kloner RA. The stunned myocardium: prolonged, postischemic ventricular dysfunction. Circulation 1982; 66: 1146–49.
15. Bolli R. Mechanism of myocardial "stunning". Circulation 1990; 82: 723–38.
16. Jennings RB, Reimer KA. Factors involved in salvaging ischemic myocardium. Effects of reperfusion of arterial blood. Circulation 1983; 68(Supp I): I-25–I-36.
17. Nicklas JM, Becker LC, Bulkley BH. Effects of repeated brief coronary occlusion on regional left ventricular function and dimension in dogs. Am J Cardiol 1985; 56: 473–8.
18. Stahl LD, Aversano TR, Becker LC. Selective enhancement of function of stunned myocardium by increased flow. Circulation 1986; 74: 843–51.
19. Becker LC, Levine JH, DiPaula AF *et al.* Reversal of dysfunction in postischemic stunned myocardium by epinephrine and postextrasystolic potentiation. J Am Coll Cardiol 1986; 7: 580–9.
20. Schroder E, Kieso RA, Laughlin D *et al.* Altered response of reperfused myocardium to repeated coronary occlusion in dogs. J Am Coll Cardiol 1987; 10: 898–905.
21. Stahl LD, Weiss HR, Becker LC. Myocardial oxygen consumption, oxygen supply/demand heterogeneity, and microvascular patency in regionally stunned myocardium. Circulation 1988; 77: 865–72.
22. Triana JF, Jamaluddin U, Li XY *et al.* Oxygen free radicals cause myocardial stunning after repetitive ischemia. Circulation 1990; 82: III–36 (abstr.).

23. Cohen MV, Downey JM. Myocardial stunning in dogs: Preconditioning effect and influence of coronary collateral flow. Am Heart J 1990; 120: 282–91.
24. Taegtmeyer H, Roberts AFC, Raine AEG. Energy metabolism in reperfused heart muscle: metabolic correlates to return of function. J Am Coll Cardiol 1985; 6: 864–70.
25. Kusuoka H, Porterfield JK, Weisman HF *et al.* Pathophysiology and pathogenesis of stunned myocardium. Depressed Ca^{2+} activation of contraction as a consequence of reperfusion- induced cellular calcium overload in ferret hearts. J Clin Invest 1987; 79: 950–61.
26. Steenbergen C, Murphy E, Levy L *et al.* Elevation in cytosolic free calcium concentration early in myocardial ischemia in perfused rat heart. Circ Res 1987; 60: 700–7.
27. Porterfield JK, Kusuoka H, Weisman HF *et al.* Ryanodine prevents the changes in myocardial function and morphology induced by reperfusion after brief periods of ischemia. Clin Res 1987; 35: 315A (abstr.).
28. Ambrosio G, Jacobus WE, Bergman CA *et al.* Preserved high energy phosphate metabolic reserve in globally "stunned" hearts despite reduction of basal ATP content and contractility. J Mol Cell Cardiol 1987; 19: 953–64.
29. Kitakaze M, Weisfeldt ML, Marban E. Acidosis during early reperfusion prevents myocardial stunning in perfused ferret hearts. J Clin Invest 1988; 82: 920–7.
30. Ambrosio G, Jacobus WE, Mitchell MC *et al.* Effects of ATP precursors on ATP and free ADP content and functional recovery of postischemic hearts. J Physiol 1989; 256: H560–H566.
31. Marban E, Koretsune Y, Corretti M *et al.* Calcium and its role in myocardial cell injury during ischemia and reperfusion. Circulation 1989; 80(Suppl IV): IV-17–IV-22.
32. Kusuoka H, Koretsune Y, Chacko VP *et al.* Excitation-contraction coupling in postischemic myocardium: Does failure of activator Ca^{2+} transients underlie stunning? Circ Res 1990; 66: 1268–76.
33. Shlafer M, Kane PF, Kirsh MM. Superoxide dismutase plus catalase enhances the efficacy of hypothermic cardioplegia to protect the globally ischemic, reperfused heart. J Thorac Cardiovasc Surg 1982; 83: 830–9.
34. Shlafer M, Kane PF, Wiggins WY *et al.* Possible role for cytotoxic oxygen metabolites in the pathogenesis of cardiac ischemic injury. Circulation 1982; 66(Suppl 1): I-85–I-92.
35. Casale AS, Bulkley GB, Bulkley BH *et al.* Oxygen free radical scavengers protect the arrested globally ischemic heart upon reperfusion. Surg Forum 1983; 34: 313–6.
36. Menasche P, Grousset C, Gauduel Y *et al.* A comparative study of free radical scavengers in cardioplegic solutions. Improved protection with peroxidase. J Thorac Cardiovasc Surg 1986; 92: 264–71.
37. Myers CL, Weiss SJ, Kirsh MM *et al.* Effects of supplementing hypothermic crystalloid cardioplegic solution with catalase, superoxide dismutase, allopurinol, or deferoxamine on functional recovery of globally ischemic and reperfused isolated hearts. J Thorac Cardiovasc Surg 1986; 91: 281–9.
38. Ambrosio G, Weisfeldt ML, Jacobus WE *et al.* Evidence for a reversible oxygen radical-mediated component of reperfusion injury: Reduction by recombinant human superoxide dismutase administered at the time of reflow. Circulation 1987; 75: 282–91.
39. Ytrehus K, Gunnes S, Myklebust R *et al.* Protection by superoxide dismutase and catalase in the isolated rat heart reperfused after prolonged cardioplegia: A combined study of metabolic, functional and morphometric ultrastructural variables. Cardiovasc Res 1987; 21: 492–9.
40. Garlick PB, Davies MJ, Hearse DJ *et al.* Direct detection of free radicals in the reperfused rat heart using electron spin resonance spectroscopy. Circ Res 1987; 61: 757–60.
41. Kramer JH, Arroyo CM, Dickens BF *et al.* Spin-trapping evidence that graded myocardial ischemia alters postischemic superoxide production. Free Radical Biol Med 1987; 3: 153–9.
42. Ambrosio G, Zweier JL, Jacobus WE *et al.* Improvement of postischemic myocardial function and metabolism induced by administration of desferrioxamine at the time of

reflow: the role of iron in the pathogenesis of reperfusion injury. Circulation 1987; 76: 906–15.

43. Stewart JR, Blackwell WH, Crute SL *et al.* Inhibition of surgically induced ischemia/reperfusion injury by oxygen free radical scavengers. J Thorac Cardiovasc Surg 1983; 86: 262–72.
44. Johnson DL, Horneffer PJ, Dinatale JM Jr *et al.* Free radical scavengers improve functional recovery of stunned myocardium in a model of surgical coronary revascularization. Surgery 1987; 102: 334–40,
45. Gardner TJ. Oxygen radicals in cardiac surgery. Free Radical Biol Med 1988; 4: 45–50.
46. Illes RW, Silverman NA, Krukenkamp IB *et al.* Amelioration of postischemic stunning by deferoxamine-blood cardioplegia. Circulation 1989; 80(Suppl III): III-30–III-35.
47. Homans DC, Sublett E, Dai XZ *et al.* Persistence of regional left ventricular dysfunction after exercise-induced myocardial ischemia. J Clin Invest 1986; 77: 66–73.
48. O'Neill PG, Charlat ML Hartley CJ *et al.* Nonuniform transmural response of the "stunned" myocardium to inotropic stimulation. J Am Coll Cardiol 1987; 9: 145A (abstr.).
49. Preuss KC, Gross GJ, Brooks HL *et al.* Time course of recovery of "stunned" myocardium following variable periods of ischemia in conscious and anesthetized dogs. Am Heart J 1987; 114: 696–703.
50. DeBoer FWV, Ingwall JS, Kloner RA *et al.* Prolonged derangements of canine myocardial purine metabolism after a brief coronary artery occlusion not associated with anatomic evidence of necrosis. Proc Natl Acad Sci 1980; 77: 5471–5.
51. Reimer KA, Hill ML, Jennings RB. Prolonged depletion of ATP and of the adenine nucleotide pool due to delayed resynthesis of adenine nucleotides following reversible myocardial ischemic injury in dogs. J Mol Cell Cardiol 1981; 13: 229–39.
52. Swain JL, Sabina RL, McHale PA *et al.* Prolonged myocardial nucleotide depletion after brief ischemia in the open-chest dog. Am J Physiol 1982; 242: H818–H826.
53. Neely JR, Grotyohann LW. Role of glycolytic products in damage to ischemic myocardium: dissociation of adenosine triphosphate levels and recovery of function of reperfused ischemic hearts. Circ Res 1984; 55: 81: 6–24.
54. Przyklenk K, Kloner RA. Superoxide dismutase plus catalase improve contractile function in the canine model of the "stunned" myocardium. Circ Res 1986; 58: 148–56.
55. Glower DD, Spratt JA, Newton JR *et al.* Dissociation between early recovery of regional function and purine nucleotide content in postischemic myocardium in the conscious dog. Cardiovasc Res 1987; 21: 328–36.
56. Przyklenk K, Kloner RA. Effect of verapamil on postischemic "stunned" myocardium: Importance of the timing of treatment. J Am Coll Cardiol 1988; 11: 614–23.
57. Guth BD, Martin JF, Heusch G *et al.* Regional myocardial blood flow, function and metabolism using phosphorus-31 nuclear magnetic resonance spectroscopy during ischemia and reperfusion in dogs. J Am Coll Cardiol 1987; 10: 673–81.
58. Mercier JC, Lando U, Kanmatsuse K *et al.* Divergent effects of inotropic stimulation on the ischemic and severely depressed reperfused myocardium. Circulation 1982; 66: 397–400.
59. Ellis SE, Wynne J, Braunwald E *et al.* Response of reperfusion-salvaged, stunned myocardium to inotropic-stimulation. Am Heart J 1984; 107: 9–13.
60. Arnold JMO, Braunwald E, Sandor T *et al.* Inotropic stimulation of reperfused myocardium with dopamine: effects on infarct size and myocardial function. J Am Coll Cardiol 1985; 6: 1026–4.
61. Bolli R, Zhu WX, Myers ML *et al.* Beta-adrenergic stimulation reverses postischemic myocardial dysfunction without producing subsequent functional deterioration. Am J Cardiol 1985; 56: 964–8.
62. Ito BR, Tate H, Kobayashi M *et al.* Reversibly injured, postischemic canine myocardium retains normal contractile reserve. Circ Res 1987; 61: 834–6.
63. Heusch G, Schafer S, Kroger K. Recruitment of inotropic reserve in "stunned" myocardium by the cardiotonic agent AR-L 57. Basic Res Cardiol 1988; 83: 602–10.

64. Hoffmeister HM, Mauser M, Schaper W. Effect of adenosine and AICAriboside on ATP content and regional contractile function in reperfused canine myocardium. Basic Res Cardiol 1985; 80: 445–58.
65. Greenfield RA, Swain JL Disruption of myofibrillar energy use: dual mechanisms that may contribute to postischemic dysfunction in stunned myocardium. Circ Res 1987; 60: 283–9.
66. Ciuffo M, Ouyang P, Becker LC *et al.* Reduction of sympathetic inotropic response after ischemia in dogs: contributor to stunned myocardium. J Clin Invest 1985; 75: 1504–9.
67. Heusch G, Frehen D, Kroger K *et al.* Integrity of sympathetic neurotransmission in stunned myocardium. J Appl Cardiol 1988; 3: 259–72.
68. O'Neill PG, Charlat ML, Michael LH *et al.* Influence of neutrophil depletion on myocardial function and flow after reversible ischemia. Am J Physiol 1989; 256: H341–H351.
69. Bolli R, Triana JF, Jeroudi MO: Postischemic mechanical and vascular dysfunction (myocardial "stunning" and microvascular "stunning") and the effects of calcium channel blockers on ischemia/reperfusion injury. Clin Cardiol 1989; 12: III–16–III–25.
70. Bolli R, Triana JF, Jeroudi MO. Prolonged impairment of coronary vasodilation after reversible ischemia: Evidence for microvascular "stunning". Circ Res 1990; 67: 332–43.
71. Zhao M, Zhang H, Robinson TF *et al.* Profound structural alterations of the extracellular collagen matrix in postischemic dysfunctional ("stunned") but viable myocardium. J Am Coll Cardiol 1987; 10: 1322–34.
72. Charney RH, Takahashi S, Zhao M *et al.* Collagen loss in the stunned myocardium. Circulation 1989; 80(Suppl II): II-99 (abstr.).
73. Whittaker P, Przyklenk K, Boughner DR *et al.* Collagen damage in two different models of stunned myocardium. J Mol Cell Cardiol 1989; 21 (Suppl II): S163 (abstr.).
74. Guarnieri T: Direct measurement of $[Ca^{2+}]_i$ in early and late reperfused myocardium. Circulation 1989; 80(Suppl II): II-241 (abstr.).
75. Kitakaze M, Weisman HF, Marban E. Contractile dysfunction and ATP depletion after transient calcium overload in perfused ferret hearts. Circulation 1988; 77: 685–95.
76. Hori M, Kitakaze M, Sato H *et al.* Transient acidosis by staged reperfusion prevents myocardial stunning. Circulation 1989; 80(Suppl II): II-600 (abstr).
77. Marban E, Kitakaze M, Kusoka H *et al.* Intracellular free calcium concentration measured with ^{19}F NMR spectroscopy in intact ferret hearts. Proc Natl Acad Sci USA 1987; 84: 6005–9.
78. Lee H-C, Smith N, Mohabir R *et al.* Cytosolic calcium transients from the beating mammalian heart. Proc Natl Acad Sci USA 1987; 84: 7793–7.
79. Marban E, Kitakaze M, Koretsune Y *et al.* Quantification of $[Ca^{2+}]_i$ in perfused hearts: Critical evaluation of the 5F-BAPTA and nuclear magnetic resonance method as applied to the study of ischemia and reperfusion. Circ Res 1990; 66: 1255–67.
80. Krause SM, Hess ML. Characterization of cardiac sarcoplasmic reticulum dysfunction during short-term normothermic global ischemia. Circ Res 1985; 55: 176–84.
81. Lazdunski M, Frelin C, Vigue P. The sodium/hydrogen exchange system in cardiac cells: Its biochemical and pharmacological properties and its role in regulating internal concentrations of sodium and internal pH. J Mol Cell Cardiol 1985; 17: 1029–42.
82. Murphy JG, Smith TW, Marsh JD. Mechanisms of reoxygenation-induced calcium overload in cultured chick embryo heart cells. Am J Physiol 1988; 254: H1133–H1141.
83. Tani M, Neely JR. Role of intracellular Na^+ in Ca^{2+} overload and depressed recovery of ventricular function of reperfused ischemic rat hearts. Possible involvement of H^+-Na^+ and Na^+-Ca^{2+} exchange. Circ Res 1989; 65: 1045–56.
84. Grinwald PM. Calcium uptake during postischemic reperfusion in the isolated rat heart: influence of extracellular sodium. J Mol Cell Cardiol 1982; 14: 359–65.
85. Renlund DG, Gerstenblith G, Lakatta EG *et al.* Perfusate sodium during ischemia modifies postischemic functional and metabolic recovery in the rabbit heart. J Mol Cell Cardiol 1984; 16: 795–801.

86. McCord JM. Oxygen-derived free radicals in postischemic tissue injury. N Engl J Med 1985; 312: 159–63.
87. Opie LH. Reperfusion injury and its pharmacologic modification. Circulation 1989; 80: 1049–62.
88. Taylor AL, Golino P, Eckels R *et al.* Differential enhancement of postischemic segmental systolic thickening by diltiazem. J Am Coll Cardiol 1990; 15: 737–47.
89. Lamping KA, Gross GJ. Improved recovery of myocardial segment function following a short coronary occlusion in dogs by nicorandil, a potential new antianginal agent, and nifedipine. J Cardiovasc Pharmacol 1985; 7: 158–66.
90. Waritier DC, Gross GJ, Brooks HL *et al.* Improvement of postischemic, contractile function by the calcium channel blocking agent nitrendipine in conscious dogs. J Cardiovasc Pharmacol 1988; 12(Suppl 4): S120–S124.
91. Dunlap E, Millard RW. Amlodipine, a new long-acting calcium channel blocking agent, improves recovery of "stunned" myocardium. The Pharmacologist 1989; 31: 145 (abstr.).
92. Przyklenk K, Ghafari GB, Eitzman DT *et al.* Nifedipine administered after reperfusion ablates systolic contractile dysfunction of postischemic "stunned" myocardium. J Am Coll Cardiol 1989; 13: 1176–83.
93. Böhm M, Ehring T, Heusch G. Nisoldipine improves the functional recovery of stunned myocardium only when given before ischemia. Circulation 1991; 84(Suppl II): 656.
94. Krause SM, Jacobus WE, Becker LC. Alterations in cardiac sarcoplasmic reticulum calcium transport in the postischemic "stunned" myocardium. Circ Res 1989; 65: 526–30.
95. Zhu WX, Myers ML, Hartley CJ *et al.* Validation of a single crystal for measurement of transmural and epicardial thickening. Am J Physiol 1986; 251: H1045–H1055.
96. Myers ML, Bolli R, Lekich RF *et al.* Enhancement of recovery of myocardial function by oxygen free-radical scavengers after reversible regional ischemia. Circulation 1985; 72: 915–21.
97. Gross GJ, Farber NE, Hardman HF *et al.* Beneficial actions of superoxide dismutase and catalase in stunned myocardium of dogs. Am J Physiol 1986; 250: H372–H377.
98. Murry, CE, Richard VJ, Jennings RB *et al.* Free radicals do not cause myocardial stunning after four 5 minute coronary occlusions. Circulation 1989; 80(Suppl II): II-296 (abstr.).
99. Koerner JE, Anderson BA, Dage RC. Protection against postischemic myocardial dysfunction in anesthetized rabbits with scavengers of oxygen-derived free radicals: Superoxide dismutase plus catalase, N-2-mercaptopropionyl glycine and captopril. J Cardiovasc Pharmacol 1991; 17: 185–91.
100. Jeroudi MO, Triana FJ, Patel BS *et al.* Effect of superoxide dismutase and catalase, given separately, on myocardial "stunning". Am J Physiol 1990; 259: H889–H901.
101. Buchwald A, Klein HH, Lindert S *et al.* Effect of intracoronary superoxide dismutase on regional function in stunned myocardium. J Cardiovasc Pharmacol 1989; 13: 258–64.
102. Halliwell B, Gutteridge JMC. Oxygen toxicity, oxygen radicals, transition metals and disease. Biochem J 1984; 219: 1–14.
103. Fox RB. Prevention of granulocyte-mediated oxidant lung injury in rats by a hydroxyl radical scavenger, dimethylthiourea. J Clin Invest 1984; 74: 1456.
104. Bolli R, Zhu WX, Hartley CJ *et al.* Attenuation of dysfunction in the postischemic "stunned" myocardium by dimethylthiourea. Circulation 1987; 76: 458–68.
105. Bolli R, Jeroudi MO, Patel BS *et al.* Marked reduction of free radical generation and contractile dysfunction by antioxidant therapy begun at the time of reperfusion: evidence that myocardial "stunning" is a manifestation of reperfusion injury. Circ Res 1989; 65: 607–22.
106. Myers ML, Bolli R, Lekich RF *et al.* N-2-mercaptopropionylglycine improves recovery of myocardial function following reversible regional ischemia. J Am Coll Cardiol 1986; 8: 1161–8.
107. Bolli R, Patel BS, Zhu WX *et al.* The iron chelator desferrioxamine attenuates postischemic ventricular dysfunction. Am J Physiol 1987; 253: H1372–H1380.

108. Farber NE, Vercellotti GM, Jacob HS *et al.* Evidence for a role of iron-catalyzed oxidants in functional and metabolic stunning in the canine heart. Circ Res 1988; 63: 351–60.
109. Dage RC, Anderson BA, Mao SJT *et al.* Probucol reduces myocardial dysfunction during reperfusion after short-term ischemia in rabbit heart. J Cardiovasc Pharmacol 1991; 17: 158–65.
110. Schrier GM, Hess ML. Quantitative identification of superoxide anion as a negative inotropic species. Am J Physiol 1988; 24: H138–H143.
111. DiGuiseppi J, Fridovich I. Oxygen toxicity in streptococcus sanguis: The relative importance of superoxide and hydroxyl radicals. J Biol Chem 1982; 257: 4046–51.
112. Triana JF, Unisa A, Bolli R. Antioxidant enzymes attenuate myocardial "stunning" in the conscious dog. FASEB J 1990; 4: A622 (abstr.).
113. Sekili S, Li XY, Zughaib M *et al.* Evidence for a major pathogenetic role of hydroxyl radical in myocardial "stunning" in the conscious dog. Circulation 1991; 84(Supp II): 656.
114. Zweier JL Flaherty JT, Weisfeldt ML. Direct measurement of free radical generation following reperfusion of ischemic myocardium. Proc Natl Acad Sci USA 1987; 84: 1404–7.
115. Baker JE, Felix CC, Olinger GN *et al.* Myocardial ischemia and reperfusion: Direct evidence for free radical generation by electron spin resonance spectroscopy. Proc Natl Acad Sci USA 1988; 85: 2786–9.
116. Zweier JL. Measurement of superoxide-derived free radicals in the reperfused heart. J Biol Chem 1988; 263: 1353–7.
117. Bolli R, McCay PB. Use of spin traps in intact animals undergoing myocardial ischemia/reperfusion: A new approach to assessing the role of oxygen radicals in myocardial "stunning". Free Rad Res Comms 1990; 9: 169–80.
118. Bolli R, Patel BS, Jeroudi MO *et al.* Demonstration of free radical generation in "stunned" myocardium of intact dogs with the use of the spin trap α-phenyl N-tert-butyl nitrone. J Clin Invest 1988; 82: 476–85.
119. Bolli R, Jeroudi MO, Patel BS *et al.* Direct evidence that oxygen-derived free radicals contribute to postischemic myocardial dysfunction in the intact dog. Proc Natl Acad Sci USA 1989; 86: 4695–9.
120. Bolli R, Patel BS, Jeroudi MO *et al.* Iron-mediated radical reactions upon reperfusion contribute to myocardial "stunning". Am J Physiol 1990; 259: H1901–H1911.
121. Zughayb M, Sekili S, Li XY *et al.* Detection of free radical generation in the "stunned" myocardium in the conscious dog using spin trapping techniques. FASEB J 1991; 5: A704.
122. Leiboff RL, Arroyo CM, Schaer GL *et al.* Free radical generation in an *in vivo* model of regional myocardial stunning. FASEB J 1988; 2: A818 (abstr.).
123. Bolli R, Kaur H, Li XY *et al.* Demonstration of hydroyl radical generation in "stunned" myocardium of intact dogs using aromatic hydroxylation of phenylalanine. FASEB J 1991; 5: A704.
124. Burton KP, McCord JM, Ghai G. Myocardial alterations due to free-radical generation. Am J Physiol 1984; 246: H776–H783.
125. Blaustein AS, Schine L, Brooks WW *et al.* Influence of exogenously generated oxidant species on myocardial function. Am J Physiol 1986; 250: H595–H599.
126. Shattock MJ, Manning AS, Hearse DJ. Effects of hydrogen peroxide on cardiac function and postischemic functional recovery in the isolated "working" rat heart. Pharmacology 1982; 24: 118–22.
127. Ytrehus K, Myklebust R, Mjos OD. Influence of oxygen radicals generated by xanthine oxidase in the isolated perfused rat heart. Cardiovasc Res 1986; 20: 597–603.
128. Miki S, Ashraf M, Salka S *et al.* Myocardial dysfunction and ultrastructural alterations mediated by oxygen metabolites. J Mol Cell Cardiol 1988; 20: 1009–24.
129. Jackson CV, Mickelson JK, Pope TK *et al.* O_2 free radical-mediated myocardial and vascular dysfunction. Am J Physiol 1986; 251: H1225–H1231.
130. Goldhaber JI, Ji S, Lamp ST *et al.* Effects of exogenous free radicals on electromechanical

function and metabolism in isolated rabbit and guinea pig ventricle: Implications for ischemia and reperfusion injury. J Clin Invest 1988; 83: 1800–9.
131. Davies KJA. Protein damage and degradation by oxygen radicals. 1. General aspects. J Biol Chem 1987; 262: 9895–901.
132. Thompson JA, Hess ML. The oxygen free radical system: A fundamental mechanism in the production of myocardial necrosis. Prog Cardiovasc Dis 1986; 28: 449–62.
133. Romaschin AD, Rebeyka I, Wilson GJ *et al.* Conjugated dienes in ischemic and reperfused myocardium: an *in vivo* chemical signature of oxygen free radical mediated injury. J Mol Cell Cardiol 1987; 19: 289–302.
134. Weisel RD, Mickle DAG, Finkle CD *et al.* Myocardial free-radical injury after cardioplegia. Circulation 1989; 80(Suppl III): III-14–III-18.
135. Rowe GT, Manson NH, Caplan M *et al.* Hydrogen peroxide and hydroxyl radical mediation of activated leukocyte depression of cardiac sarcoplasmic reticulum: participation of the cyclooxygenase pathway. Circ Res 1983; 53: 584–91.
136. Kaneko M, Beamish RE, Dhalla NS. Depression of heart sarcolemmal Ca^{2+}-pump activity by oxygen free radicals. Am J Physiol 1989; 256: H368–H374.
137. Kaneko M, Elimban V, Dhalla NS. Mechanism for depression of heart sarcolemmal Ca^{2+} pump by oxygen free radicals. Am J Physiol 1989; 257: H804–H811.
138. Kramer JH, Mak IT, Weglicki WB. Differential sensitivity of canine cardiac sarcolemmal and microsomal enzymes to inhibition by free radical-induced lipid peroxidation. Circ Res 1984; 55: 120–4.
139. Kim M-S, Akera T. O_2 free radicals: cause of ischemia-reperfusion injury to cardiac Na^+-K^+-ATPase. Am J Physiol 1987; 252: H252–H257.
140. Charlat ML, O'Neill PG, Egan JM *et al.* Evidence for a pathogenetic role of xanthine oxidase in the "stunned" myocardium. Am J Physiol 1987; 252: H566–H577.
141. Holzgrefe HH, Gibson JK. Enhanced function recovery in the stunned canine myocardium by pretreatment with oxypurinol. J Am Coll Cardiol 1988; 11: 208A (abstr.).
142. Puen DW, Forman MB, Cates CU *et al.* Oxypurinol limits myocardial stunning but does not reduce infarct size after reperfusion. Circulation 1987; 76: 678–86.
143. Jarasch ED, Bruder G, Heid HW. Significance of xanthine oxidase in capillary endothelial cells. Acta Physiol Scand 1986; 548(Suppl): 39–46.
144. Eddy W, Stewart JR, Jones HP *et al.* Free radical-producing enzyme, xanthine oxidase, is undetectable in human hearts. Am J Physiol 1987; 253: H709–H711.
145. Muxfeldt M. Schaper W. The activity of xanthine oxidase in hearts of pigs, guinea pigs, rats, and humans. Basic Res Cardiol 1987; 82: 486–92.
146. Huizer T, de Jong JW, Nelson JA *et al.* Urate production by human heart. J Mol Cell Cardiol 1989; 21: 691–95.
147. Grum CM, Gallagher KP, Kirsh MM *et al.* Absence of detectable xanthine oxidase in human myocardium. J Mol Cell Cardiol 1989; 21: 263–7.
148. Lucchesi BR, Mullane KM. Leukocytes and ischemia-induced myocardial injury. Ann Rev Pharmacol Toxicol 1986; 26: 201–24.
149. Engler R. Granulocytes and oxidative injury in myocardial ischemia and reperfusion. Federation Proc 1987; 46: 2395–6.
150. Shea MJ, Simpson PJ, Werns SW *et al.* Effect of neutrophil depletion on recovery of "stunned" myocardium. Clin Res 1987; 35: 327A (abstr.).
151. Jeremy RW, Becker LC. Neutrophil depletion does not prevent myocardial dysfunction after brief coronary occlusion: J Am Coll Cardiol 1989; 13: 1155–63.
152. O'Neill PG, Charlat ML, Kim H-S *et al.* Lipoxygenase inhibitor nafazatrom fails to attenuate postischemic ventricular dysfunction. Cardiovasc Res 1987; 21: 755–60.
153. Schott RJ, Nao BS, McClanahan TB *et al.* $F(ab')_2$ Fragments of anti-mo1 (904) monoclonal antibodies do not prevent myocardial stunning. Circ Res 1989; 65: 1112–24.
154. Kerber RE, Shasby DM, Seabold J *et al.* Does reduction of leukocyte accumulation in reperfused myocardium affect stunning? Circulation 1989; 80(Supp II): II-401 (abstr.).
155. Go LO, Murry CE, Richard VJ *et al.* Myocardial neutrophil accumulation during reper-

fusion after reversible or irreversible ischemic injury. Am J Physiol 1988; 255: H1188–H1198.
156. Juneau CF, Ito BR, del Balzo U *et al.* Severe neutrophil depletion by leukocyte filters or cytotoxic drugs does not improve the recovery of contractile function in stunned myocardium. Circulation 1991; 85(Suppl II): II-655.
157. Westlin W, Mullane KM. Does captopril attenuate reperfusion-induced myocardial dysfunction by scavenging free radicals? Circulation 1988; 77(Suppl I): I-30–I-39.
158. Ferrari R, Alfieri O, Curello S *et al.* Occurrence of oxidative stress during reperfusion of the human heart. Circulation 1990; 81: 201–11.
159. Asinger RW, Peterson DA, Elsperger KJ *et al.* Long-term recovery of LV wall thickening after 1 hour of ischemia is not affected when superoxide dismutase and catalase are administered during the first 45 minutes of reperfusion. J Am Coll Cardiol 1988; 2: 163A (abstr.).
160. Nejima J, Knight DR, Fallon JT *et al.* Superoxide dismutase reduces reperfusion arrhythmias but fails to salvage regional myocardial function or myocardium at risk in conscious dogs. Circulation 1989; 78: 143–53.
161. Przyklenk K, Kloner RA. "Reperfusion injury" by oxygen-derived free radicals? Effect of superoxide dismutase plus catalase, given at the time of reperfusion, on myocardial infarct size, contractile function, coronary microvasculature, and regional myocardial blood flow. Circ Res 1989; 64: 86–96.
162. Patel BS, Jeroudi MO, O'Neill PG *et al.* Effect of human recombinant superoxide dismutase on canine myocardial infarction. Am J Physiol 1990; 258: H369–H380.
163. Forman MB, Puett DW, Cates CU *et al.* Glutathione redox pathway and reperfusion injury. Effect of N-acetylcysteine on infarct size and ventricular function. Circulation 1988; 78: 202–13.
164. Klein HH, Pich S, Schuff-Werner P *et al.* Trolox, a water-soluble vitamin E analogue, accelerates functional recovery but does not reduce infarct size in regionally ischemic, reperfused porcine hearts. Am Heart J (in press).
165. Homans DC, Sublett E, Asinger R *et al.* SOD + catalase does not attenuate regional left ventricular dysfunction following exercise induced ischemia. J Am Coll Cardiol 1988; 78: II-76 (abstr.).
166. Hearse DJ, Humphrey SM, Bullock GR. The oxygen paradox and the calcium paradox: two facets of the same problem? J Mol Cell Cardiol 1978; 10: 641–68.
167. Reeves JP, Bailey CA, Hale CC. Redox modification of sodium-calcium exchange activity in cardiac sarcolemmal vesicles. J Biol Chem 1986; 261: 4948–4955.
168. Bolli R, Hartley CJ, Rabinovitz RS. Clinical relevance of myocardial "stunning". Cardiovasc Drugs Ther 1991; 5: 877–90.
169. Mathias P, Kent NZ, Blevins RD *et al.* Coronary vasospasm as a cause of stunned myocardium. Am Heart J 1987; 113: 383–5.
170. Fine DG, Clements IP, Callahan MJ. Myocardial stunning in hypertrophic cardiomyopathy: Recovery predicted by single photon emission computed tomographic thallium-201 scintigraphy. J Am Coll Cardiol 1989; 13: 1415–8.
171. Luu M, Stevenson LW, Brunken RC *et al.* Delayed recovery of revascularized myocardium after referral for cardiac transplantation. Am Heart J 1990; 119: 668–70.
172. Homan DC, Laxson DD, Sublett E *et al.* Cumulative deterioration of myocardial function after repeated episodes of exercise-induced ischemia. Am Physiol Soc 1989; 256: H1463–H1471.
173. Cohn PF. Silent myocardial ischemia: classification, prevalence, and prognosis. Am J Med 1985; 79(Suppl 3A): 2–12.
174. Bolli R. Oxygen-derived free radicals and postischemic myocardial dysfunction ("stunned myocardium"). J Am Coll Cardiol 1988; 12: 239–49.

2. Severe ischemic injury and the oxygen paradox

HANS MICHAEL PIPER, BERTHOLD SIEGMUND and KLAUS-DIETER SCHLÜTER

Introduction

If the blood supply to the myocardium is interrupted or greatly reduced in the course of a surgical operation on the heart, the myocardial cells develop an energetic deficit. This is because they are unable to cover their demands of energy satisfactorily by means other than oxidative energy production. Caused by the progressive loss of cellular energy reserves, the oxygen-deprived myocardial cell first fails functionally and then becomes increasingly injured, metabolically as well as structurally. If the loss of energy reserves and the cellular injury has not progressed too far, a restoration of normal supply conditions leads to a full structural, metabolic and functional recovery (Figure 2.1). Full recovery of function may, however, occur only after some delay. The state of transiently reduced function has been termed 'stunning' [1]. If conditions of oxygen deprivation have persisted for too long, full recovery is no longer possible, i.e. the myocardium has become irreversibly injured. It would obviously be very helpful for the cardiac surgeon if he could monitor the progression of myocardial injury towards the borderline of irreversible cell injury, but at present this is not feasible. The reason for this limitation seems not a technical one. Instead, the present knowledge on the causal key events in the progression of injury towards irreversibility is too limited.

The most important test whether a certain state of ischemic or hypoxic myocardial cell injury is still reversible, consists in re-supplying the myocardium with oxygen and substrates and removing the waste products of anaerobic metabolism from the tissue. Failure of the myocardium to recover can have different causes, however. After a very long period of oxygen deprivation, cellular injury can have reached a state so severe that reoxygenation has no longer an effect. Between the extremes of full recovery (that may take some time) and non-responsive manifest injury yet another possibility exists. Prior to the state where the tissue becomes non-responsive, the energy-depleted myocardial cell is in a state in which reoxygenation leads to a rapid exacerbation of the injury developed so far. This phenomenon of acute reoxygenation-associated myocardial injury has been termed 'oxygen paradox' [2]. It seems to occur at the edge between reversibility and irreversibility.

In this chapter we will concentrate on the mechanism of the acute reoxyge-

H.M. Piper and C.J. Preusse (eds): Ischemia-reperfusion in cardiac surgery, 41–66.

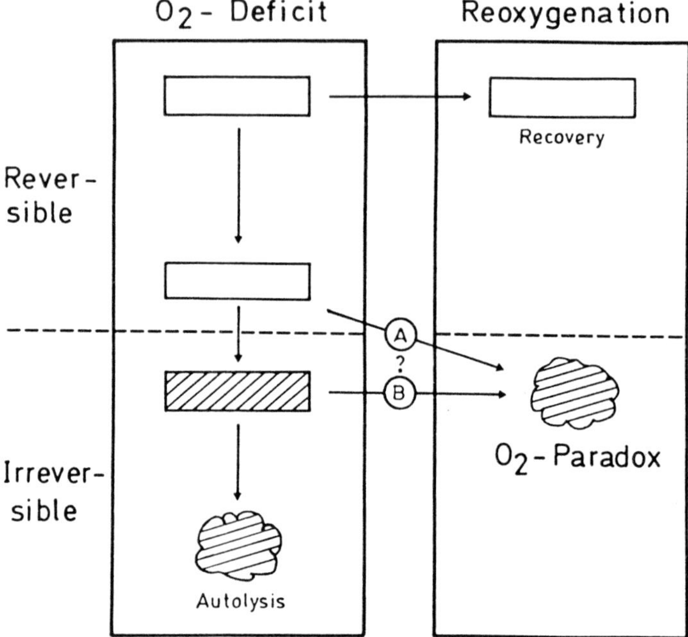

Figure 2.1. on the development of myocardial cell injury in hyoxia/ischemia and reoxygenation. In the presence of an oxygen deficit, the cells progressively develop cellular injury, which is still reversible when they are reoxygenated, but later becomes irreversible. Lack of oxygen eventually leads to cellular self-decomposition (autolysis). Reoxygenation at the supposed borderline between reversible and irreversible injury acutely exacerbates cell injury (oxygen paradox). For long, it has been an open question whether cell the oxygen paradox leads from still reversible to irreversible cell injury (A) or represents only an epiphenomenon of already irreversible cell injury (B).

nation-associated injury, i.e. the oxygen paradox. The most frequent, naturally occurring situation of a myocardial oxygen deficiency is a reduction or cessation of blood flow, i.e. ischemia, due to occlusion of the supplying coronary artery. In cardiac surgery, many operations require artificial ischemia, to prevent extensive bleeding. When ischemic tissue is reperfused with normal blood it is also reoxygenated and may therefore suffer from oxygen paradox injury. But reperfusion of previously ischemic tissue can aggravate its injury also by other than this mechanism. Thus, abrupt changes in pH [3–5] and tissue osmolality [6–8] may have negative effects. Furthermore, the cellular elements of the blood may also influence the result, since reperfusion of ischemically injured myocardium may lead to the activation of circulating neutrophils and their chemo-attraction by factors released from the injured tissue. This can initiate an inflammatory process that may further aggravate the state of injury [9]. Many of these additional aspects of reperfusion of ischemic tissue are discussed in other chapters of this book.

The oxygen paradox is characterized by an abrupt release of intracellular constituents due to the sudden rupture of cell membranes and the unique phenomenon of contraction band formation [10]. Whether this reoxygenation-associated injury is a secondary manifestation of cell damage, that has been present in a less apparent manner already in the hypoxic cell, or whether it originates directly from the reintroduction of oxygen, has been a matter of discussion for a long time. If this injury directly originated from reoxygenation, it would not only be reoxygenation-associated but reoxygenation-induced injury. In other words, it would represent 'reperfusion injury' in the sense of Rosenkranz and Buckberg [11] who defined this as "those metabolic, functional, and structural consequences of restoring coronary arterial flow . . . that can be avoided or reversed by modification of the conditions of reperfusion". This definition limits the use of the term 'reperfusion injury' to damage caused by events, which may take place when ischemic tissue is reperfused/reoxygenated without any specific precautions, but which are not inevitable consequences of ischemia. If the oxygen paradox represents a case of reperfusion injury, with the outcome of irreversibility, it must be possible to perform reperfusion in some way avoiding irreversibility.

Recent studies, discussed in greater detail in this chapter, have shown that oxygen paradox injury represents indeed genuine 'reperfusion injury', one that is lethal for the myocardial cells. When the re-supply of the energy-depleted myocardial cells with oxygen is performed by a simple restoration of blood flow, this mechanism of reperfusion injury represents the practical limit of reversibility in ischemia-reperfusion. It is now known that there are ways to avoid such a deleterious outcome of reperfusion. From this it follows that the absolute limit of reversibility in ischemia-reperfusion must be at a later stage than the one normally provoking oxygen paradox injury.

The oxygen paradox represents only one of many possible kinds of 'reperfusion injury'. Possible other candidates for genuine reperfusion injury include the reversible phenomena of 'stunning' [1] and 'reperfusion arrhythmias' [12], observed after relatively brief periods of ischemia. The above-mentioned postischemic attack of injured myocardium by activated neutrophils represents another case of 'reperfusion injury' that may result in irreversible cell injury.

Some clinicians may doubt whether reperfusion injury with a lethal outcome for myocardial cells exists at all, impressed by the largely positive results of reperfusing ischemic myocardium within the first 12 h of an acute coronary occlusion [13]. It has to be admitted that a clear proof for the existence of reperfusion injury in humans is still lacking, both for cases of reversible and irreversible reperfusion injury. This is in contrast to the experiences with animal studies and may primarily be due to the practical limitations to explore in detail the process of ischemia-reperfusion in humans. The clinical experiences to date certainly do not disprove the existence of reperfusion injury in the human heart, as yet untested modifications of reperfusion conditions may lead to even better tissue preservation.

In this chapter, the present understanding of how reoxygenation after a prolonged period of oxygen depletion may cause acute lethal cellular injury (oxygen paradox) is reviewed. In the analysis of this phenomenon much has been achieved by using experimental models of reduced complexity. It has been demonstrated that the basic elements of the oxygen paradox can also be identified in single isolated cardiomyocytes subjected to anoxia and reoxygenation. Such simple experimental models have permitted a far more detailed causal analysis of the pathomechanism of the oxygen paradox than possible before using whole heart preparations and gave rise to new approaches toward protection against this type of reperfusion injury.

The cardiomyocyte in the oxygen-deprived state

Loss of cellular energy reserves

In the heart as a whole large gradients for oxygen exist that render impossible a detailed analysis of the metabolic response of the myocardial cell to its immediate supply with oxygen. Such an analysis has become feasible, however, using isolated heart muscle cells for which the ambient oxygen pressure can be experimentally controlled [14,15]. It was demonstrated for isolated cardiomyocytes (Figure 2.2) that mitochondrial respiration does not cease and glycolytic flux is not stimulated unless exogenous pO_2 has dropped below 1 torr. Above 3 torr, the oxygen consumption of the cardiomyocytes is constant. Below 3 torr, the rate of oxygen consumption declines. The half-maximal rate is observed at a PO_2 of about 1 torr, only below this level the lactate production increases.

These results show that the respiratory machinery in the cardiomyocytes as a whole cell is almost as sensitive to low oxygen pressure as the oxygen uptake of the isolated mitochondrion. In fact, a comparison of the pO_2 at half-maximal oxygen uptake with the K_m of cytochrome c oxidase (≤ 0.2 torr; [16,17]) indicates that the oxygen gradient across the sarcolemma toward the mitochondria amounts to only 0.8 torr on average. Other investigators came to similar conclusions [18,19]. It has been attributed to the presence of myoglobin as an oxygen binding capacity in the cytosol of these large cells that the cytosolic gradient for oxygen is not more pronounced [18]. Unlike single isolated cardiomyocytes, the perfused heart responds metabolically in a gradual fashion to lowering of the oxygen tension. This can be explained as a statistical phenomenon: The lower the total amount of oxygen supplied to the heart per unit of time, the fewer cells along the perfusion path can satisfy their oxygen demand. 'Mild' or 'partial' ischemia and hypoxia of myocardial tissue must be envisaged as a patchwork of cardiomyocytes containing more or less cells either being still on the aerobic or already on the anaerobic side of metabolism. It is highly unlikely that in 'mild ischemia'

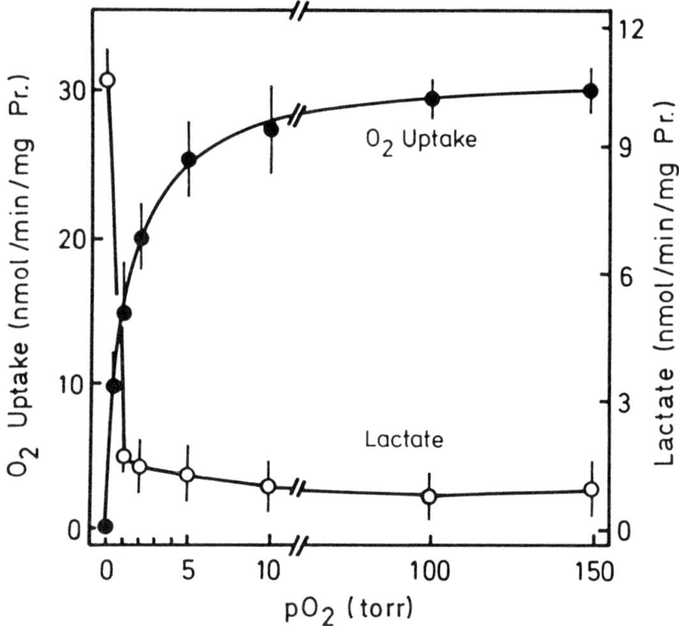

Figure 2.2. Oxygen sensitivity of respiration and anaerobic glycolysis in isolated cardiomyocytes (ventricular, from adult rat). Rates of oxygen consumption (closed circles) and lactate production (open circles) are shown for different pO_2 levels. Rate of lactate production was determined as the mean rate during the initial 15 min after establishing the indicated pO_2. Means ± S.D., n = 4 separate cell preparations. [From Ref. 15, reprinted with permission]

many cells are in the intermediate state around 1 torr ambient oxygen pressure.

When the myocardial cell becomes sufficiently deprived of oxygen, by a stop of perfusion (ischemia) or lack of oxygen in the perfusate (hypoxia), respiratory generation of ATP is slowed down or may even cease. Even though the cardiomyocytes exhibit a pronounced Pasteur effect, glycolytic energy production is insufficient to fully compensate for the loss of respiratory ATP in the working myocardium [20]. Therefore, the energy balance soon becomes negative and the cellular stores of high-energy phosphates are progressively depleted. Concomitantly with the onset of a negative energy balance, the heart loses its ability to develop contractile force. But even though this greatly reduces the energy demand of the myocardium, the energy balance normally remains negative and the loss of energy reserves progresses. (Exceptionally, it may reach a new balance at a lower metabolic level, termed 'hibernation' [21].) The reasons why the myocardium does not normally reach a new balance between energy production and demand are only partly understood. In ischemic tissue, the accumulating endproducts of anaerobic metabolism, protons and lactate, can inhibit glycolytic flux. But progressive energy depletion is also observed in experimental models of the hypoxically perfused heart [20] and of hypoxic isolated cardiomyocytes [22], i.e. in models in which these factors do not greatly accumulate. The failure of oxygen-depleted myocardial cells to reach a new metabolic steady state leads to the question whether their progressive loss of energy is only due to a deficit on the supply side or whether it also involves a stimulation of energy-consuming reactions not normally active in well-energized cells.

One possible energy-wasting mechanism of this kind has been identified in studies by Rouslin and collaborators [23,24]. They found that in ischemic and autolyzing canine heart muscle mitochondrial ATP hydrolysis can contribute to the progressive loss of ATP. The mitochondrial site of ATP hydrolysis was identified to be the oligomycin-sensitive F_1,F_0-proton ATPase. The presumed mechanism of the activation of mitochondrial ATP hydrolysis is the following [23,24]: when blood flow to cardiac muscle is interrupted, there is a rapid depletion of tissue oxygen and consequent cessation of mitochondrial electron flow. Dissipation of the mitochondrial trans-membrane electrochemical gradient activates mitochondrial ATPase hydrolytic activity, as well known from studies in isolated mitochondria [25]. In the cited studies [23,24], the decline of high-energy phosphates and the stimulation of glycolysis were taken to indicate an aerobic-anaerobic metabolic transition within the tissue preparations. It was not established, however, that these signs of an aerobic-anaerobic metabolic transition occur only in response to the *cessation* of mitochondrial electron flow and the consequent dissipation of the mitochondrial electrochemical gradient.

We recently investigated this hypothesis in greater detail [15]. Isolated cardiomyocytes were exposed to a one thousand-fold reduction of the extracellular oxygen pressure below the normal arterial level, i.e. $pO_2 \leq 0.1$ torr. Such an extreme reduction of oxygen is likely to be present also in large parts of regionally ischemic myocardium. In the described experiments it led to an aerobic-anaerobic metabolic transition with the signs of a maximal stimulation of glycolysis and a progressive decline of the cellular contents of high-energy phosphates. Oligomycin, however, did not decelerate but rather slightly accelerated the decline of cellular ATP contents. This demonstrated that at this very low level of ambient oxygen still some net synthesis of ATP occurred. Since oligomycin is a specific inhibitor of mitochondrial ATP synthesis or hydrolysis at the F_1,F_0-proton ATPase [26] and this complex catalyses net ATP synthesis only in polarised mitochondria [25], it can be concluded that the mitochondrial membranes were not depolarised in these hypoxic cells. As demonstrated by LaNoue *et al.* [27] it needs only a partial depolarisation of mitochondria to shift them from a net synthesis to a net hydrolysis of ATP. These results have the implication that activation of glycolysis and the development of an energetic deficit *per se* (aerobic-anaerobic metabolic transition) does not necessarily go along with mitochondrial depolarisation and an activation of mitochondrial ATPase hydrolytic activity.

The cited study provided also evidence that at oxygen levels as low as

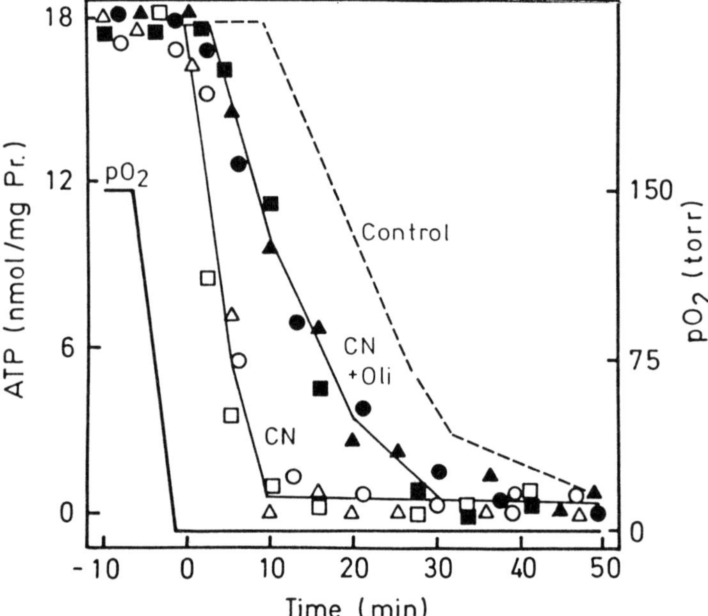

Figure 2.3. Progression of the loss of ATP in hypoxic cardiomyocytes (from adult rat). The pO_2 was reduced initially from normoxic values (150 torr) to ≤0.1 torr. The broken line (Control) indicates ATP depletion, in response to deep hypoxia alone. Data points are shown for the effects of NaCN (CN, 5 mM) ± oligomycin (Oli, 20 μM) on ATP depletion of hypoxic cardiomyocytes. Oli and CN were added at time zero, i.e. 1 min after a $pO_2 \leq 0.1$ torr was reached. Open symbols: experiments in the absence of Oli; closed symbols: experiments in the presence of Oli. Data of 3 experiments of separate cell preparations. The oligomycin-inhibitable mitochondrial ATP hydrolysis is only activated in deep hypoxia if residual electron flux is inhibited additionally by a chemical blocker (cyanide). [From Ref. 15, reprinted with permission]

$pO_2 \leq 0.1$ torr preservation of a polarised mitochondrial state depends on flux of electrons through at least parts of the electron chain since it could be abolished by the specific blocker of electron flux, cyanide (Figure 2.3). In presence of cyanide the decline of ATP was greatly accelerated. The acceleration could be inhibited, however, by oligomycin and could thus be identified as being due to an activation of mitochondrial ATPase hydrolytic activity and, therefore, also mitochondrial depolarisation. The effects of cyanide on the hypoxic cardiomyocyte were comparable to those of an uncoupler.

It was demonstrated by this study that hypoxic states of the heart muscle cell are possible in which it exhibits the signs of an aerobic-anaerobic metabolic transition and yet retains a low level of mitochondrial ATP synthesis which indicates a polarised state of its mitochondria. This has the implication that in states of deep tissue hypoxia mitochondria do not necessarily turn into a major sink for cellular ATP (and not because [28] binding of the natural inhibitor protein or serious damage to the F_1,F_0-proton ATPase complex would prevent ATP hydrolytic activity).

In human myocardial pathology, where regional ischemia is the most frequent natural case of myocardial oxygen deficiency, collateral flow can prevent very deep levels of hypoxia to a variable degree. The distribution of residual flow and, thereby, of residual oxygenation is known to be inhomogeneous in regionally ischemic myocardium. It is not known whether factors accumulating in cardiomyocytes in ischemic tissue more than in hypoxic isolated cardiomyocytes, e.g. lipid metabolites [29], could interfere with the stability of mitochondrial polarisation at very low rates of electron flux, thus increasing the leak conductivity of the inner mitochondrial membrane and the propensity of the mitochondria to depolarise. The finding by Rouslin and collaborators that mitochondrial ATP hydrolysis can be activated in the myocardium under certain ischemic conditions is of potential therapeutic interest since an inhibition of this energy-wasting might improve myocardial preservation during ischemia. Theoretically, the use of a blocker of the F_1,F_0-proton ATPase on the ischemic heart may be beneficial as an inhibition of wasting of ATP in depolarised mitochondria may outweigh the disadvantage from inhibiting some residual ATP synthesis. But such blockers are, of course, extremely dangerous when a washout into the circulation can occur, as they inhibit oxidative phosphorylation everywhere.

Another hypothetical mechanism that might contribute to the breakdown of ATP specifically in the hypoxic cell is the activation of the myosin ATPase by the formation of rigor complexes [30,31]. Since the formation of rigor complexes itself is already a result of a substantial loss of cellular energy reserves, this mechanism could be understood as one leading to a final critical drop of cellular ATP reserves. Direct evidence for the existence of this mechanism in the energy-depleted myocardial cell has recently been provided by experiments in which the cytosolic ATP levels in single cardiomyocytes were monitored in a qualitative manner through the luminescence of the ATP-indicator reaction of luciferase directly injected into the cells [32]. In these experiments the ATP signal dropped sharply at the time when rigor tension started developing. These results suggest that it could be therapeutically useful to inhibit rigor bond formation in the myocardium developing a progressive energetic deficit. Specific cell-permeable inhibitors of rigor bond formation are not yet available, however.

It is at present time unclear, at which cytosolic concentration of ATP rigor complexes start forming. In isolated preparations of myofibrillar proteins and in permeabilised myocardial cells a reduction of the free concentration of ATP to between 1 and 100 μM was necessary for rigor complexes to form [30–35]. These results are in apparent contrast to observations that rigor tension develops in non-permeabilised hypoxic cardiomyocytes already at average cytosolic ATP concentrations of about 1 mM [36]. It may be that this difference can be accounted for by the fact that in myofibrillar preparations and permeabilised isolated cells the influence of factors other than the pure concentration of free ATP has not been sufficiently investigated and that such additional factors may lead to rigor complexes at a much less pronounced reduction of cytosolic ATP concentration. Alternatively, a cytosolic sub-compartmentalisation of ATP has been discussed [37].

Tissue acidification, which occurs in ischemic myocardium as a consequence of lactic acid production and the breakdown of ATP, has also effects on the rapidity of high-energy phosphate depletion. In the whole cell, the consequences of acidification are not totally negative, in contrast to what one might expect from the known inhibition of glycolytic energy production by acidosis. Severe acidosis (tissue $pH \leqslant 6.6$) clearly aggravates tissue injury caused by oxygen and substrate deprivation [38–40], but the effect of mild acidosis ($6.6 < pH < 7.4$), developing in the early stage of ischemia or in partial ischemia with some residual flow, is less clear. In the hypoxic perfused heart [38] or papillary muscle incubated under hypoxic conditions [41], mild acidosis of the perfusate or the incubation medium, respectively, have been shown to exert a protective effect. In these models the protection by acidosis was mainly attributed to a conservation of energy through a reduction of contractile force.

It was recently investigated [42] whether mild acidosis can provide energetic protection of the hypoxic myocardial cell also by mechanisms *other* than negative inotropy. Ventricular cardiomyocytes from adult animals were used as experimental model since these are mechanically quiescent and inotropic effects are therefore excluded. Mild acidosis was found to conserve energy under oxygen deprivation. The optimum of the energy-saving occurred when cells were incubated at pH 7.0; at pH 7.4 and 6.6 the depletion of cellular energy reserves progressed more rapidly. The energy-conserving effect of mild acidosis was not caused by a better supply of energy at that pH, but by a smaller energy demand. It was striking that the optimum pH of about 7.0 coincided with the point of intra-extracellular pH-identity. This may suggest that the observed energy-conserving effect is due to a reduction of the energetic expense for the transsarcolemmal pH gradient. The explanation remains speculative, however, since the total costs of energy for the transsarcolemmal pH gradient do also depend on the transsarcolemmal distribution of other ions [43,44]. The latter consideration also leads to caution in extrapolating the optimum pH from the hypoxic cardiomyocytes used in this study, in which the extracellular medium had a physiological saline composition, to cardiomyocytes arrested by use of specific cardioplegic solutions, which differ greatly in their composition.

Loss of Ca^{2+} control in the energy depleted cardiomyocyte

The development of cell injury in ischemic tissue starts with a deficit in the cellular balance of energy. The energetic deficit leads to the slowdown or cessation of important metabolic functions, among these the control of the cellular control of Ca^{2+} ions. The loss of cellular Ca^{2+} homeostasis is a sign of advanced, but not necessarily irreversible cell injury. In the energy-depleted cell, Ca^{2+} gradually accumulates, but not due to large wholes that would form in the plasmalemma [45]. The routes by which Ca^{2+} enters the cell are not yet known in detail. A major share of the amount of Ca^{2+} which accumulates in energy-depleted myocardial cells seems to intrude from the exterior space [45]. Several lines of experiments suggest that this influx of Ca^{2+} is secondary to a loss of the cytosolic sodium balance. Thus, a reduction in extracellular sodium activity postpones a rise of cytosolic Ca^{2+} in energy-depleted cardiomyocytes [46]. In energy-depleted cardiomyocytes the free Na^{+} activity indeed increases [47].

The source of the leak for sodium in the sarcolemma has not yet been identified. Suggestions are, e.g., the opening of non-selective cation-channels [48] or activation of the Na^{+}/H^{+} exchanger by a fall of the cytosolic pH in the anoxic, and even more the ischemic cell [49]. The latter mechanism may only be of minor importance, however, in isolated cardiomyocytes incubated in well-buffered anoxic medium as in this system the intracellular pH does not change very much [42]. Simple diffusion may also account for part of the sodium uptake since the lipid bilayer of biological membranes is always somewhat permeable to ions. One of the main causes contributing to an early rise of cytosolic Na^{+} in energy-depleted myocardial cells seems to be a reduced activity of Na^{+}/K^{+} ATPase which requires a high energy level for ATP hydrolysis for normal function [37].

Ca^{2+} does not enter the cells through the slow Ca^{2+} channels [50]. The Na^{+}/Ca^{2+} exchanger seems to represents the mechanism by which most Ca^{2+} enters the energy-depleted cell [51]. This sodium-dependent mechanism is not the only route, however, by which Ca^{2+} enters the energy-depleted cell. We recently found that Ca^{2+} does eventually also rise progressively in cardiomyocytes which had been first depleted from endogenous sodium and where then submitted to anoxia in a sodium-free medium (unpublished).

An early rise in intracellular Ca^{2+} has also been demonstrated for ischemic whole myocardium [49,52,53]. This finding must be distinguished from earlier reports on a rise of total tissue Ca^{2+} in the post-ischemic period [54,55], for which the causes could be completely different ones, including a filling with interstitial fluid of spaces left from disintegrating cells.

Mechanical fragility of energy-depleted cardiomocytes

Energy-depleted cardiomyocytes become increasingly mechanically fragile [56]. This may be partly due to the hydrolysis of phospholipids in the sarcolemma [57]. A major cause for an increased mechanical fragility seems to be injury to the cytoskeleton and the cytoskeleton-membrane connections. Detachment of the sarcolemma from the underlying cytoskeletal skaffold becomes apparent early in energy-depleted cardiomyocytes, by the protrusion of sarcolemmal blebbs [58]. In anoxic isolated cardiomyocytes [59] and anoxic and ischemic tissue [60,61] a progressive decline of cytoskeletal immunreactivity for vinculin, α-actinin and tubulin has been documented. The stability of cytoskeletal structures can be prolonged by phosphatase inhibitors, indicating that lack of ATP destabilizes the cytoskeleton by causing a reduction in the net-level of protein phosphorylation [62].

Ongoing phospholipolysis and progressive destabilization of the cytoskeleton need not lead to cell deterioration for a long time. It has been learned from the reaction of isolated cardiomyocytes exposed to anoxia-reoxygenation in the absence of external forces, that the metabolic derangements remain reversible and this seems to be the cause for a rapid repair of the subtle initial structural damage [58]. In tissue, increased mechanical fragility can make a big difference, however, since forces are exchanged among adjacent cells. Intramyocardial forces that would not injure an intact aerobic cell may disrupt cells that have been energy-depleted. This is one of the reasons why it might be helpful to allow ischemic myocardium to recover from energy-depletion in a first period of reperfusion with all mechanical activity being inhibited. In heart surgery, this would mean that the ischemic heart is first selectively reperfused under artificial mechanical arrest while extracorporeal circulation is continued (reperfusion cardioplegia).

Reoxygenation of the oxygen depleted myocardial cell

Reoxygenation-induced hypercontracture

In myocardial tissue, reoxygenation after prolonged hypoxia can lead to an abrupt aggravation of tissue injury, i.e. the oxygen paradox, characterized by a sudden onset of contracture and massive enzyme release. The oxygen paradox is a genuine pathomechanism of the myocardial cells in the heart, vascular cells seem not primarily involved [63]. Interestingly, this mechanism of tissue injury is an energy-dependent process; it does not occur or is attenuated when the ability to generate oxidative energy is abolished [9,64]. We hypothesized [37] that the primary cause for the deterioration of reoxygenated cardiomyocytes by the oxygen paradox is the development of hypercontracture and this in turn is caused by the re-supply of energy (from oxidative phosphorylation) to myofibrils which are potentially highly activated under this condition, by an elevated cytosolic Ca^{2+} concentration (a consequence of hypoxic energy-depletion).

When the oxygen paradox develops in reoxygenated myocardial tissue, disruption of the sarcolemma and massive influx of Ca^{2+} into disrupted myocardial cells soon terminate mitochondrial ATP production. Isolated cardiomyocytes, subjected to prolonged hypoxia and subsequent reoxygenation, do not lyse when hypercontracting even though they become extremely distorted in their structure [36] apparently because they do not mutually exchange forces. The incompleteness of the oxygen paradox injury in isolated cardiomyoctes has been exploited in several studies designed to analyse the early phase of reoxygenation in respect to cellular metabolism and Ca^{2+} homeostasis (see below).

Mitochondrial competence

Recovery of the myocardium from a period of oxygen depletion requires sufficient preservation of the mitochondrial capability for oxidative phosphorylation. Since the possibilities to analyse mitochondrial functions in experiments with intact cells or tissue are limited, many of the current concepts about mitochondrial injury are derived from studies on mitochondria isolated from injured hearts. In most of these studies, mitochondrial functions were found progressively impaired in the course of ischemic or anoxic tissue injury [65]. A point in time at which mitochondrial respiratory functions would suddenly and markedly deteriorate has not been identified, however.

Studies on mitochondria isolated from injured tissue have to be interpreted with some caution. They certainly provide detailed biochemical results, but their relevance remains in many cases unclear. One of the reasons is that the fraction of mitochondria isolated from injured hearts may not be the same as that isolated from control hearts, due to differences in the physical consistency of the tissue and its influence of the isolation protocol. Another reason is that soluble factors acting on the mitochondria in the living cell are lost during the isolation procedure. A third one is that reduction of mitochondrial function in an *in vitro* assay, designed to measure a functional maximum, may not represent a relevant functional impairment within the living cell. As an example for this point, the following may be considered: We found that the mitochondrial capability for oxidative phosphorylation is reduced by 40% at a time when tissue ATP has dropped from 24 to 17 μmol/g dry weight in the ischemic guinea pig heart [66]. Can this deficit be now regarded responsible for the functional inability of the heart reperfused after such a loss of ATP? One might doubt this, since in a working heart at normal work load only part of the total respiratory capacity of normal mitochondria is used; after an ischemic or hypoxic period, however, functional insufficiency becomes apparent already at a low energy demand.

In contrast to the reports on various functional deficits in mitochondria isolated from ischemic-reperfused or anoxic-reoxygenated hearts, studies on whole hearts and isolated cardiomyocytes prone to undergo oxygen paradox-injury have shown that mitochondria retain sufficient functional competence at times when other crucial cell functions are already failing. As mentioned before, the oxygen paradox can only be provoked in cells in which oxidative phosphorylation has not been abolished. In isolated cardiomyocytes, mitochondrial function was found to survive severe hypoxic cytosolic Ca^{2+} overload and the deterioration of large parts of the cytoskeletal ultrastructure [36].

In the reoxygenated cardiomyocyte a useful indicator of mitochondrial functional recovery is the rise in the cytosolic free energy of ATP hydrolysis,

$$\Delta G_{ATP} = \Delta G^{\circ}_{ATP} + R \cdot T \ln([ATP]/[ADP] \cdot [P_i]),$$

where [ATP], [ADP] and $[P_i]$ represent cytosolic concentrations, ΔG°_{ATP} the absolute value of the standard free energy, R the universal gas constant, and T the absolute temperature [67]. ΔG_{ATP} is a measure of how much energy is available from ATP hydrolysis within the cytosol for energy-dependent reactions. The ratio $([ATP]/[ADP] \cdot [P_i])$ is determined by oxidative phosphorylation as respiring mitochondria import ADP and P_i, phosphorylate ADP to ATP and export this ATP into the cytosol. It is important to understand that the recovery of ΔG_{ATP} does not presuppose that ATP concentrations do recover (as it is a ratio). Once the purine pool of the myocardial cell is largely exhausted (as after an extended period of oxygen-depletion), cellular ATP contents remain depressed for a long time in the myocardial cell, due to the very low rate of de-novo synthesis [68].

It was found that ΔG_{ATP} rapidly recovers in anoxic-reoxygenated cardiomyocytes, which hypercontract but do not lyse upon reoxygenation (Figure 2.4). Most ATP-dependent reactions are directly determined by ΔG_{ATP}. A normal ΔG_{ATP} indicates, therefore, that such ATP-dependent reactions can proceed. A ΔG_{ATP} level of 50 kJ/mol ATP which is found in reoxygenated cardiomyocytes is sufficient for driving the major cation pump systems of the cell, i.e. the Ca^{2+}-ATPase of the sarcoplasmic reticulum and the Ca^{2+}- and Na^{+}/K^{+}-ATPases of the sarcolemma [69]. Recovery of ΔG_{ATP} does not guarantee, however, that processes depending on the energy of ATP hydrolysis can proceed at a high rate. This is because in presence of only a small 'buffer' of ATP even hydrolysis of a small amount of ATP leads to a depression of ΔG_{ATP}. It may then need some time for 'recharging' ΔG_{ATP} by the respiring mitochondria. In cardiomyocytes which have lost their purine reserves to a large extent it seems therefore advisable to prevent energy expenditure for non-vital cell functions, such as contractile activity. They may then be better capable to struggle for recovery of the control on cellular ion homeostasis and repair of structural injury. That is to say, severely ischemic myocardium should be reperfused first in contractile arrest.

Cellular calcium homeostasis

The finding that the free energy of ATP hydrolysis recovers quickly in reoxygenated cardiomyocytes gave rise to the question whether reoxygenated cardiomyocytes would indeed be capable to recover from severe hypoxic disturbances of their Ca^{2+} homeostasis. This question was investigated in a recent study [70] in which cardiomyocytes were first allowed to accumulate cytosolic Ca^{2+} up to a level of 10^{-5} M and then reoxygenated (Figure 2.5). Reoxygenation of cardiomyocytes led to a rapid fall of the cytosolic Ca^{2+}

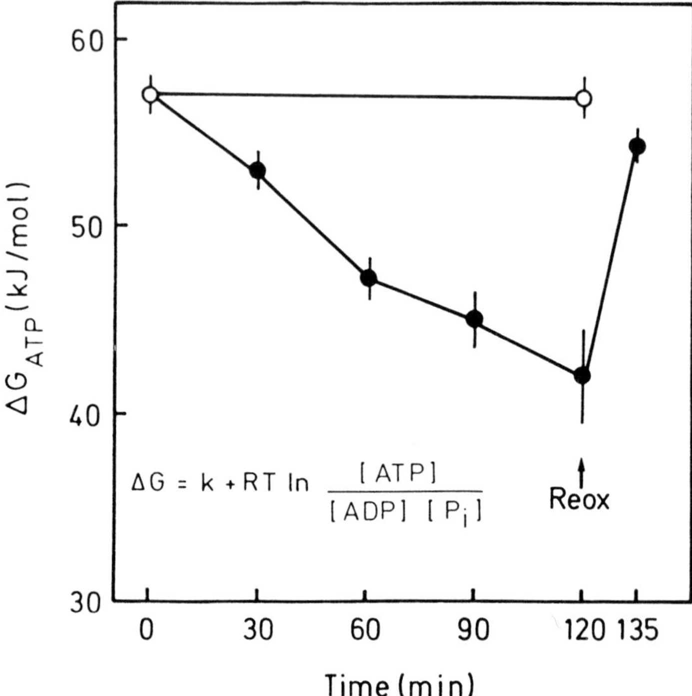

Figure 2.4. Free energy of ATP hydrolysis (ΔG_{ATP}) in cardiomyocyte (ventricular, from adult rat) exposed to anoxia-reoxygenation. Values were determined under normoxic control conditions (open circles) and under 120 min anoxia followed by 15 min reoxygenation (closed circles) in glucose-free medium. Means ± S.D., n = 4 culture preparations. The anoxically depressed ΔG_{ATP} rapidly recovers upon reoxygenation, even though at this time the cells develop extreme hypercontracture. [Data from Ref. 36]

level, followed by a period of Ca^{2+} oscillations, due to uptake and release of Ca^{2+} into the sarcoplasmic reticulum.

The role of the sarcoplasmic reticulum in the process of re-establishing a normal cytosolic Ca^{2+} control was investigated further by impairing the ability of the sarcoplasmic reticulum to sequester Ca^{2+} [70]. The cells were treated before and during reoxygenation with thapsigargin which inhibits irreversibly the Ca^{2+} ATPase of the sarcoplasmic reticulum and thus the storage of Ca^{2+} within this organelle [71]. In contrast to control conditions, the initially achieved reduction of the cytosolic Ca^{2+} concentration could not be preserved in thapsigargin-treated cardiomyocytes. Cytosolic Ca^{2+} did no longer recover in cardiomyocytes reoxygenated in the presence of thapsigargin. The results demonstrated that Ca^{2+} sequestration in the sarcoplasmic reticulum is of crucial importance for the recovery from hypoxic cytosolic Ca^{2+} overload.

Interestingly, the deleterious consequences of impairing the function of

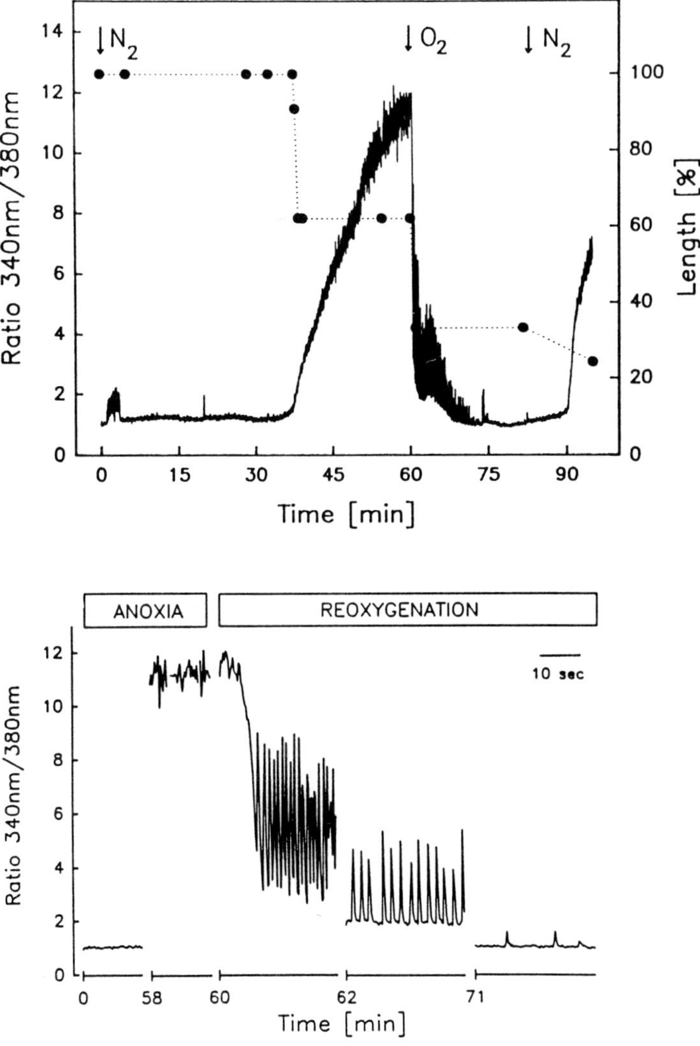

Figure 2.5. Single isolated adult cardiomyocyte from rat subjected to anoxia-reoxygenation (N_2, O_2) Top: Cell length and free cytosolic Ca^{2+}. The ordinate shows the ratio of fura-2 fluorescence at 340 and 380 nm excitation, as a relative measure for cytosolic Ca^{2+}. Media were glucose-free. Below: Parts of the Ca^{2+} tracing at higher temporal resolution. Anoxia causes a partial rigor-shortening, but extreme hypercontracture is provoked by reoxygenation. Reoxygenation nevertheless leads to reversion of the anoxic Ca^{2+} overload, with decelerating oscillatory Ca^{2+} movements during the early phase. [From Ref. 70, reprinted with permission]

the sarcoplasmic reticulum could be antagonized by ruthenium red. This polycationic dye is an inhibitor of mitochondrial Ca^{2+} uptake, both in preparations of isolated mitochondria and in the living cell [72–75]. The results suggested that the protective effect of ruthenium red under conditions of a functional impairment of the sarcoplasmic reticulum is due to the prevention of mitochondrial Ca^{2+} overload. The beneficial effect of inhibition of mitochondrial Ca^{2+} uptake by ruthenium red for the recovery of Ca^{2+} control in the reoxygenated cardiomyocyte with inhibited function of the sarcoplasmic reticulum may be explained as follows: when the rapid intracellular buffer for cytosolic Ca^{2+}, the sarcoplasmic reticulum, is functionally impaired, the cytosolic Ca^{2+} concentration stays high during the early phase of reoxygenation. Sustained elevation of extramitochondrial Ca^{2+} concentration, however, creates a dangerous situation for respiring mitochondria. These are forced to take up Ca^{2+} at the expense of respiratory energy [76]. Mitochondria with a manifest Ca^{2+} overload become increasingly incompetent to produce ATP [65]. Consequently, the energy supply for extramitochondrial pump systems controlling the cytosolic Ca^{2+} homeostasis would decline.

The foregoing considerations indicate that ruthenium red prevents the deleterious consequences of a functional failure of the sarcoplasmic reticulum because it prevents Ca^{2+} overload and the consecutive functional deterioration of mitochondria. In reoxygenated cardiomyocytes under control conditions a specific protection of the mitochondria seems not necessary since the sarcoplasmic reticulum can serve transiently as a large and rapid storage capacity for excess Ca^{2+}. The fact, that a normal Ca^2 control can be reestablished in presence of ruthenium red even when the function of the sarcoplasmic reticulum is impaired, indicates that the Ca^{2+} transport systems of the sarcolemma alone are sufficient for a complete recovery from Ca^{2+} overload as long as respiring mitochondria continue to provide sufficient energy to drive the sarcolemmal extrusion process.

In the ischemic myocardium pronounced damage of the sarcoplasmic reticulum seems to develop earlier than in the model of hypoxic isolated cardiomyocytes [77]. Protection of the mitochondria from Ca^{2+} overload may therefore be even more desirable as an adjunct to other protective interventions for the early phase of reperfusion. Some previous studies on ischemic-reperfused hearts have indeed already demonstrated a beneficial effect of ruthenium red [78–80]. Unfortunately, to date inhibitors of mitochondrial Ca^{2+} uptake with higher specificity and better cell permeability than ruthenium red are not available.

Causal analysis of the oxygen paradox

Prevention of the oxygen paradox by temporary contractile blockade

It has been hypothesized previously [37,55,81] that in whole myocardial tissue the development of hypercontracture of the myofibrils is the key event in producing the oxygen paradox and that cytolysis, indicated by a massive loss of macromolecules from the tissue, represents a secondary event. The secondary nature of cytolysis is elucidated by the finding that reoxygenation following extensive hypoxic energy depletion causes extreme hypercontracture but not cytolysis in isolated cardiomyocytes which are unable to exchange mutually mechanical forces [36]. The question whether hypercontracture represents the primary key event for the oxygen paradox was investigated by the attempt to prevent it with a blockade of the contractile apparatus.

In a first series of experiments [82], isolated cardiomyocytes, submitted to anoxia-reoxygenation which would normally lead instantaneously to their hypercontracture, were reoxygenated in the presence of the contractile blocker 2,3-butanedione monoxime (BDM). BDM is known to reduce the myofibrillar sensitivity to Ca^2 and also to directly interfere with the formation of cross-bridges [83–86]. It has a rapid onset of action and can also be quickly removed (within 1 min) from a muscle preparation. In a second series [87], hypoxically perfused or ischemic hearts were reperfused with normoxic medium, which normally provoked severe oxygen paradox injury, again in the presence of BDM. In both experimental *in vitro* models reoxygenation-induced hypercontracture remained absent. In whole hearts, the massive loss of enzymes, characteristic for the full picture of the oxygen paradox, was also prevented (Figure 2.6 and 2.7). The most important finding was that the presence of BDM was needed only for a limited initial time of reoxygenation, in order to prevent oxygen paradox injury. A later removal of BDM did not provoke a delayed contracture. This indicated that this mechanism of severe cell injury depends on a critical 'vulnerable phase' at the onset of reoxygenation.

The protection against the oxygen paradox by a temporary contractile blockade during the initial phase of reoxygenation was also found effective in the pig heart *in vivo*. A recent study by Garcia-Dorado *et al.* [88] has demonstrated that reoxygenation-induced tissue necrosis in the regionally ischemic heart of open-chest pigs is also greatly attenuated when reperfusion is performed with BDM being present for the first hour.

The causal mechanism of the oxygen paradox can now be explained as follows (Figure 2.8): After extensive energy depletion cardiomyocytes have developed a pronounced cytosolic Ca^{2+} overload. At the myofibrils this creates a state of activation, which does not lead to mechanical activity, however, as long as the energy of ATP hydrolysis is too low to drive the cross bridge cycle. When oxidative phosphorylation is resumed with the

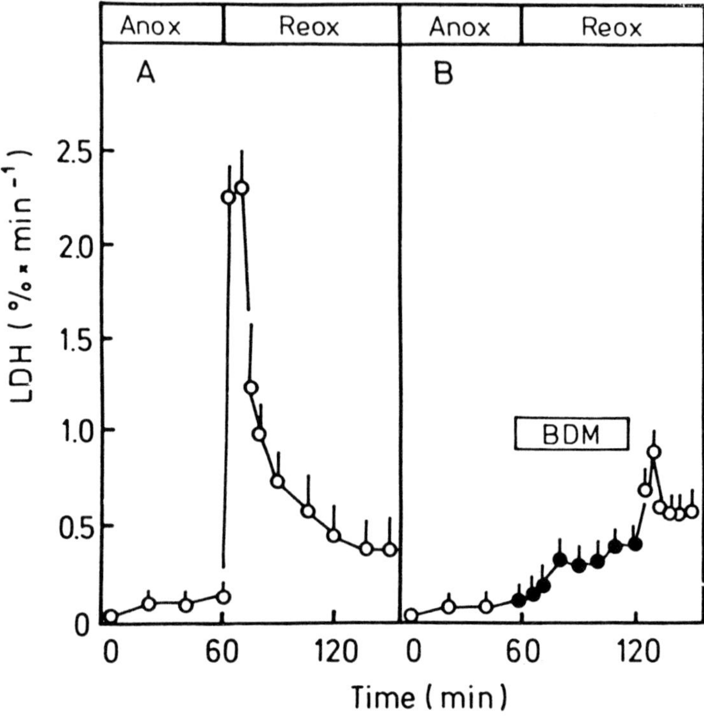

Figure 2.6. Release of lactate dehydrogenase (LDH) from perfused rat hearts during 60 min anoxia (Anox) and subsequent reoxygenation (Reox), expressed as a percentage of initial total tissue enzyme activities. A: Reoxygenation without BDM. B: Reoxygenation in presence of BDM (20 mM) during the first 60 min (closed circles). Means ± S.E.M, n = 8 hearts. [Data from Ref. 87]

resupply of oxygen, the fuel for the contractile machinery becomes available to myofibrils which are highly activated by the (still) high cytosolic concentration of Ca^{2+}. This causes a very forceful, uncontrolled contraction, leading to disruptions in the cytoskeleton, i.e. the structural damage of 'hypercontracture'. The onset of mitochondrial energy production, therefore, creates a 'suicide' situation for the reoxygenated cardiomyocyte. One of the apparently paradoxical aspects of the oxygen paradox is, therefore, that during the antecedent hypoxic state the cells were much less in acute jeopardy.

In accordance with this explanation of the oxygen paradox are the findings that reoxygenation-induced hypercontracture presupposes that cardiomyocytes are able to resume oxidative phosphorylation and that they indeed rapidly do so at the time they hypercontract. The effect of BDM has been analysed on cellular level. It was shown, firstly, that presence of BDM during the early phase of reoxygenation does not alter the rapid recovery of ΔG_{ATP} [82]. In cardiomyocytes arrested in their prereoxygenation cell length by the

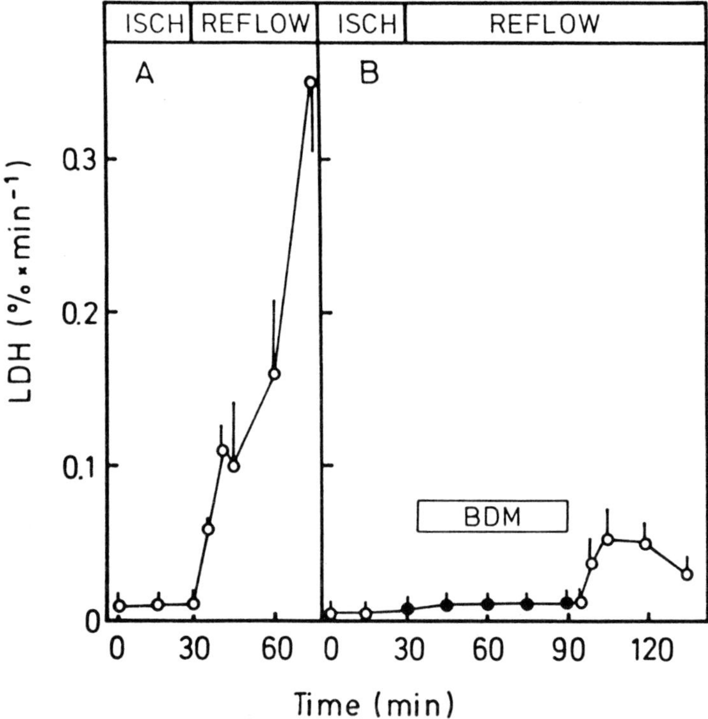

Figure 2.7. Release of lactate dehydrogenase (LDH) from perfused rat hearts during 30 min low-flow ischemia (Isch) and subsequent reperfusion (Reflow), expressed as a percentage of initial total tissue enzyme activities. A: Reperfusion without BDM. B: Reperfusion in presence of BDM (20 mM) during the first 60 min (closed circles). Means ± S.E.M, n = 4 hearts.

presence of BDM, the cytosolic Ca^{2+} concentration recovers to resting levels. It was found, secondly, that the contractile blockade can be removed without the danger of hypercontracture, once the cytosolic Ca^{2+} level is sufficiently reduced (Figure 2.9). Based on this body of evidence, the above hypothesis on the causal mechanism of the oxygen paradox seems well-established.

In summary, reoxygenation-induced hypercontracture can be abolished if the contractile apparatus is blocked for the time needed to re-establish a normal cytosolic control of Ca^{2+}. Contractile blockade must be achieved prior to the re-supply of energy, caused by the re-introduction of oxygen.

Alternative routes to prevent the oxygen paradox

Blockers of the myofibrillar machinery can be used on the heart *in vivo* only with caution. To date BDM is the only known permeable substance which effectively and reversibly inhibits muscular contraction. It is not completely specific for this intracellular effect, though, and high concentrations are

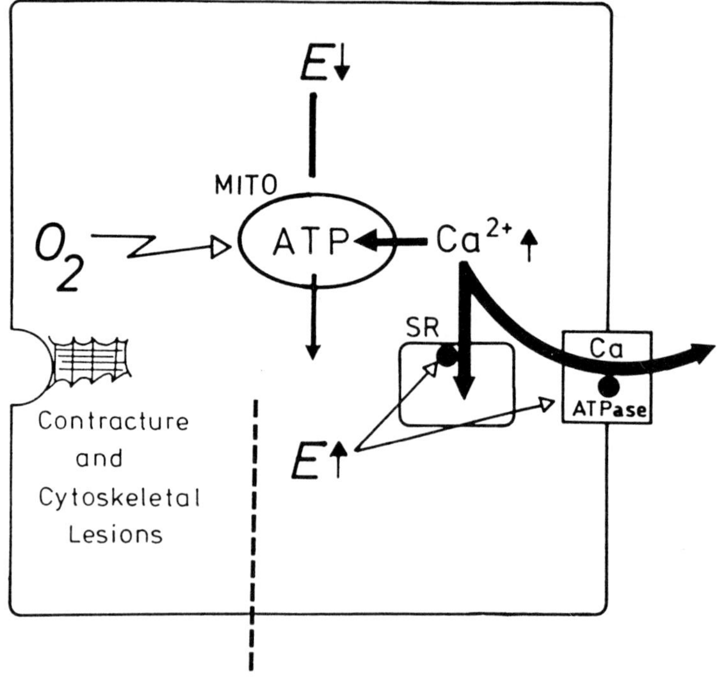

Figure 2.8. Reoxygenation of an anoxic cardiomyocyte at an elevated cytosolic free Ca^{2+} concentration. Scheme of changes in energy metabolism and Ca^{2+} control. Reoxygenation leads to a rapid restoration of oxidative phosphorylation by the mitochondria (MITO). The recovery of the cytosolic energetic state (E) reactivates the Ca^{2+} pumps of sarcoplasmic reticulum (SR) and sarcolemma thereby reducing the concentration of cytosolic Ca^{2+}. Activation of myofibrils by high Ca^{2+} and restored energy supply can lead to contracture. BDM prevents contractile activation by these factors (dashed line), while allowing a recovery of the energetic state and cytosolic Ca^{2+} control.

needed to achieve complete protection against hypercontracture (e.g., 20 mM). Research on more effective and specific agents is highly desirable. Nevertheless, BDM can be used very beneficially if administered during reperfusion only to the previously ischemic area, as demonstrated by experiments carried out on ischemic-reperfused myocardium *in vivo* [88]. These experiments have clearly demonstrated, therefore, the great potential of this novel therapeutic approach.

One may wonder whether the knowledge on the causal mechanism of the oxygen paradox would not allow also for other routes of protection against the oxygen paradox. The three key factors involved are Ca^{2+} overload, recovery of energy supply and, as a consequence of the co-presence of these first two factors, myofibrillar activation. Use of BDM inhibits myofibrillar activation. Could one, alternatively, change the impact of one of the other two factors?

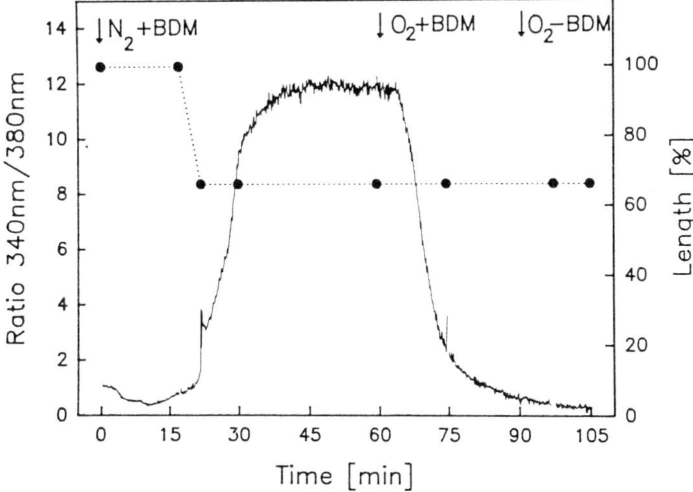

Figure 2.9. Single isolated adult cardiomyocyte from rat subjected to anoxia-reoxygenation (N_2, O_2) in the presence of 2,3–butanedione monoxime (BDM, 20 mM). Cell length and free cytosolic Ca^{2+}. The ordinate shows the ratio of fura-2 fluorescence at 340 and 380 nm excitation. Media were glucose-free. Reoxygenation leads to reversion of the anoxic Ca^{2+} overload. Removal of BDM after reestablishment of a normal (resting) cytosolic Ca^{2+} concentration leaves the cell without hypercontracture.

Firstly, it has been shown that the inhibition of mitochondrial ATP generation at the onset of reoxygenation (by blockade or uncoupling of mitochondrial respiration) prevents indeed the sudden exacerbation of tissue injury in reoxygenated myocardium [9,64]. For a therapeutic purpose, however, metabolic inhibition cannot be used since it would never allow to reverse the state of injury due to oxygen deprivation. It has been an interesting corollary of the cited experimental results that the mere presence of oxygen, e.g. by spontaneous generation of oxygen radicals, is not the immediate cause for the oxygen paradox injury. This conclusion is supported by more direct evidence [89].

Secondly, it may be tried to reduce the cytosolic Ca^{2+} concentration passively before oxidative phosphorylation becomes re-activated. This would require a Ca^{2+} gradient driving Ca^{2+} out of the cells. In order to allow a lowering of the cytosolic Ca^{2+} concentration to resting levels, the extracellular Ca^{2+} concentration would have to be of the order of 0.1 μM or lower and therefore create a Ca^{2+} paradox [90,91]. This approach is thus not feasible. One may speculate whether it would be possible to load the hypoxic cells immediately prior to reoxygenation with intracellular Ca^{2+} buffers (e.g., by performing a first phase of reperfusion anoxically with additions of agents like Quin-2 or BAPTA) and thus chelate the excess Ca^{2+} in the cytosol prior to the aerobic re-ernergetization of the cells. As with BDM this also requires a local access to the injured piece of myocardium. So far, this possibility has not been investigated.

Conclusions

It has been demonstrated that the characteristic sudden and, in tissue, lethal cell injury of the oxygen paradox can be prevented when the myocardial cells are allowed to recover under the initial protection of a paralysis of the myofibrils. Consequently, there is no reason to believe that the state of hypoxic injury in which the oxygen paradox can be provoked is already irreversible. In the past, the oxygen paradox represented the practical limit of reversibility in the course of ischemia-reperfusion. Now that a better understanding of its causal mechanism has led to a strategy to prevent it, the absolute limit of reversibility must be searched for in a yet later stage of ischemic injury. Myocardium saved from oxygen paradox injury must be regarded as extremely ‘stunned’. It is a challenge for future research to investigate the possible extent of and the optimal conditions for recovery.

The cardiac surgeon may wonder how relevant strategies to protect myocardium at the far edge of reversibility are for his clinical problems of resuscitating hearts made ischemic for surgical necessities. In most cases, the slow-down of the progression of ischemic injury by cardioplegia is sufficient to prevent that the myocardium would become susceptible to oxygen paradox injury. With pre-damaged myocardium one cannot be so sure, however. The analysis of the recovery of myocardial cells from severe derangements of metabolism and ion homeostasis has suggested a general benefit from the use of contractile arrest during the early phase of reoxygenation for the recovery process. That is because contractile arrest would allow to spend energy first for the processes of recovery and repair before sharing it with the contractile mechanism. Protection from oxygen paradox injury together with this general benefit can best be obtained when cardiac arrest is achieved directly at the myofibrils. Means to interrupt electromechanical coupling at other sites, as used in standard protocols for cardioplegia (e.g., high K^+, low Ca^{2+}), may be helpful for the recovery from early stages of ischemic injury but not when this has already led to severe cytosolic Ca^{2+} overload. A transient reperfusion of ischemic myocardium under direct contractile blockade, therefore, seems to be in general a valuable adjunct to the present strategies for myocardial preservation in cardiac surgery.

Acknowledgement

This work was supported by the Deutsche Forgchungsgemeinschaft, SFB 242, project C 6.

References

1. Braunwald E, Kloner RA. The stunned myocardium: prolonged, postischemic ventricular dysfunction. Circulation 1982; 66: 1146–9.
2. Hearse DJ, Humphrey SM, Chain EB. Abrupt reoxygenation of the anoxic potassium-arrested perfused rat heart: A study of myocardial enzyme release. J Mol Cell Cardiol 1973; 5: 395–407.
3. Bhatti S, Zimmer G, Bereiter-Hahn J. Enzyme release from chick myocytes during hypoxia and reoxygenation. Dependence on pH. J Mol Cell Cardiol 1989; 21: 995–1008.
4. Panagiotopoulos S, Daily MJ, Nayler WG. Effect of acidosis and alkalosis on postischemic Ca gain in isolated rat heart. Am J Physiol 1990; 258: H821–H828.
5. Bond J, Herman B, Lemasters JJ. Protection by acidotic pH against anoxia/reoxygenation injury to rat neonatal cardiac myocytes. Biochem Biophys Res Commun 1991; 179: 798–803.
6. Tranum-Jensen J, Janse M, Fiolet JW *et al.* Tissue osmolality, cell swelling and reperfusion in acute regional myocardial ischemia in the isolated porcine heart. Circ Res 1987; 49: 364–81.
7. Kloner RA, Reimer KA, Willerson JT *et al.* Reduction of experimental infarct size with hyperosmotic mannitol. Proc Soc Exp Biol Med 1976; 151: 677–3.
8. Garcia-Dorado D, Theroux P, Munoz R *et al.* Favorable effects of hyperosmotic reperfusion on myocardial edema and infarct size. Am J Physiol 1992; 262: H17–H22.
9. Mullane KM, Smith CW. The role of leukocytes in ischemic damage, reperfusion injury and repair of the myocardium. In Piper HM (ed): Pathophysiology of severe ischemic myocardial injury. Dordrecht: Kluwer 1990; 239–68.
10. Ganote CE. Contraction band necrosis and irreversible myocardial injury. J Mol Cell Cardiol 1983; 15: 67–73.
11. Rosenkranz ER, Buckberg GD. Myocardial protection during surgical coronary reperfusion. J Am Coll Cardiol 1983; 1: 1235–46.
12. Manning AS, Hearse D. Reperfusion-induced arrhythmias: mechanisms and prevention. J Mol Cell Cardiol 1984; 16: 497–518.
13. Fox KAA. Reperfusion injury: a clinical perspective. In Yellon DM, Jennings RB (eds): Myocardial protection. New York: Raven Press, 1992; 151–64.
14. Noll T, de Groot H, Wissemann P. A computer-supported oxystat system maintaining steady-state O_2 partial pressures and simultaneously monitoring O_2 uptake in biological systems. Biochem J 1986; 236: 765–9.
15. Noll T, Koop A, Piper HM. Mitochondrial ATP-synthase activity in cardiomyocytes after aerobic-anaerobic metabolic transition. Am J Physiol 1992; 262: C1297–C1303.
16. Chance B. Reaction of oxygen with the respiratory chain in cells and tissue. J Gen Physiol 1965; 49: 163–88.
17. de Groot H, Noll T, Sies H. Oxygen dependence and subcellular partitioning of hepatic menadione-mediated oxygen uptake. Arch Biochem Biophys 1987; 243: 556–62.
18. Wittenberg BA, Wittenberg JB. Oxygen pressure gradients in isolated cardiac myocytes. J Biol Chem 1985; 260: 6548–54.
19. Rumsey WL, Schlosser C, Matti Nuutinen E *et al.* Cellular energetics and the oxygen dependence of respiration in cardiac myocytes isolated from adult rat. J Biol Chem 1990; 265: 15392–9.
20. Kübler W, Spieckermann PG. Regulation of glycolysis in the ischemic and the anoxic myocardium. J Mol Cell Cardiol 1970; 1: 351–77.
21. Rahimtoola SH. The hibernating myocardium. Am Heart J 1989; 117: 211–21.
22. Piper HM, Schwartz P, Hütter JF *et al.* Energy metabolism and enzyme release of cultured adult rat heart muscle cells during anoxia. J Mol Cell Cardiol 1984; 16: 995–1007.
23. Rouslin W, Erickson JL, Solaro RJ. Effects of oligomycin and acidosis on rates of ATP depletion in ischemic heart muscle. Am J Physiol 1986; 250: H503–H508.

24. Rouslin W, Broge CW, Grupp IL. ATP depletion and functional loss during ischemia in slow and fast heart-rate hearts. Am J Physiol 1990; 259: H1759–H1766.
25. Schwerzmann K, Pedersen P. Regulation of the mitochondrial ATP synthase/ATPase complex. Arch Biochem Biophys 1986; 250: 1–18.
26. Lardy HA. Antibiotic inhibitors of mitochondrial energy transfer. In Erecinska M, Wilson DF (eds): Inhibitors of Mitochondrial Function. Oxford: Pergamon Press 1981; 187–98.
27. LaNoue KF, Jeffries FMH, Radda GK. Kinetic control of mitochondrial ATP synthesis. Biochemistry 1986; 25: 7667–75.
28. Rouslin W. Protonic inhibition of the mitochondrial oligomycin-sensitive adenosine 5'-triphosphatase in ischemic and autolyzing cardiac muscle. J Biol Chem 1983; 258: 19657–61.
29. Piper HM, Das A. Detrimental actions of endogenous fatty acids and their derivatives: A study of ischaemic mitochondrial injury. Basic Res Cardiol 1987; 82 (Suppl. 1): 187–91.
30. Bremel RD, Weber A. Cooperation within actin filament in vertebrate skeletal muscle. Nature New Biol 1972; 238: 97–101.
31. Murray JM, Knox KM, Trueblood CE *et al.* Potentiated state of the tropomyosin actin filament and nucleotide-containing myosin subfragment 1. Biochemistry 1982; 21: 906–15.
32. Bowers K, Allshire AP, Cobbold PH. Bioluminescent measurement in single cardiomyocytes of sudden cytosolic ATP depletion coincident with rigor. J Mol Cell Cardiol 1992; 24: 211–6.
33. Fabiato A, Fabiato F. Effects of magnesium on contractile activation of skinned cardiac cells. J Physiol (London) 1975; 249: 497–517.
34. Altschuld RA, Wenger WC, Lamka KG *et al.* Structural and functional properties of adult rat heart myocytes lysed with digitonin. J Biol Chem 1985; 260: 14325–35.
35. Nichols CG, Lederer WJ. The role of ATP in energy-deprivation contractures in unloaded rat ventricular myocytes. Can J Physiol Pharmacol 1990; 68: 183–94.
36. Siegmund B, Koop A, Klietz T *et al.* Sarcolemmal integrity and metabolic competence of cardiomyocytes under anoxia-reoxygenation. Am J Physiol 1990; 258: H285–H291.
37. Piper HM. Energy deficiency, calcium overload or oxidative stress: possible causes of irreversible ischemic myocardial injury. Klin Wschr 1989; 67: 465–76.
38. Nayler WG, Ferrari R, Poole-Wilson PA *et al.* A protective effect of mild acidosis on hypoxic heart muscle. J Mol Cell Cardiol 1979; 11: 1053–71.
39. Acosta D, Li CP. Actions of extracellular acidosis on primary cultures of rat myocardial cells deprived of oxygen and glucose. J Mol Cell Cardiol 1980; 12: 1459–63.
40. Preusse CJ, Gebhard MM, Bretschneider HJ. Interstitial pH value in the myocardium as indicator of ischemic stress of cardioplegically arrested hearts. Basic Res Cardiol 1982; 77: 1372–87.
41. Bing OHL, Brooks WW, Messer JV. Heart muscle viability following hypoxia: Protective effect of acidosis. Science 1973; 180: 1297–8.
42. Koop A, Piper HM. Protection of energy status of hypoxic cardiomyocytes by mild acidosis. J Mol Cell Cardiol 1992; 24: 55–65.
43. Frelin C, Vigne P, Ladoux A *et al.* The regulation of the intracellular pH in cells from vertebrates. Eur J Biochem 1988; 174: 3–14.
44. Madshus IH. Regulation of intracellular pH in eukaryotic cells. Biochem J 1988; 250: 1–8.
45. Allshire A, Piper HM, Cuthbertson KSR *et al.* Cytosolic free Ca^{2+} in single rat heart cells during anoxia and reoxygenation. Biochem J 1987; 244: 381–5.
46. Li Q, Altschuld RA, Stokes BT. Myocyte deenergization and intracellular free calcium dynamics. Am J Physiol 1988; 255: C162–C168.
47. Donoso P, Mill JG, O'Neill SC *et al.* Fluorescence measurement of cytoplasmatic and mitochondrial sodium concentration. J Physiol (London) 1992; 448: 493–509.
48. Hess P, Tsien RW. Mechanisms of ion permeability through calcium channels. Nature 1984; 309: 453–6.
49. Mohabir R, Lee HC, Kurz RW *et al.* Effects of ischemia and hypercarbic acidosis on

myocyte calcium transients, contraction, and pH_i in perfused rabbit hearts. Circ Res 1991; 69: 1525–37.
50. Allshire A, Cobbold P. Ca^{2+} flux into metabolically deprived cardiomyocytes. Biochem Soc Transact 1987; 15: 960.
51. Ziegelstein R, Zweier JL, Mellitis ED *et al.* Dimethylurea, an oxygen radical scavanger, protects isolated cardiac myocytes from hypoxic injury by inhibition of Na^+-Ca^{2+} exchange and not by its antioxidant effects. Circ Res 1992; 70: 804–11.
52. Marban E, Kitakaze M, Kusuoka HJ *et al.* Intracellular free calcium concentration measured with ^{19}F NMR spectroscopy in intact ferret hearts. Proc Natl Acad Sci USA 1987; 84: 6005–9.
53. Steenbergen C, Murphy E, Levy L *et al.* Elevation in cytosolic free calcium concentration early in myocardial ischemia in perfused rat heart. Circ Res 1987; 60: 700–7.
54. Grinwald PM. Calcium uptake during post-ischemic reperfusion in the isolated rat heart: Influence of extracellular sodium. J Mol Cell Cardiol 1982; 14: 359–65.
55. Elz J, Nayler WG. Contractile activity and reperfusion-induced calcium gain after ischemia in the isolated rat heart. Lab Invest 1988; 58: 653–9.
56. Ganote CE, Vander Heide RS. Irreversible injury of isolated adult rat myocytes. Osmotic fragility during metabolic inhibition. Am J Pathol 1988; 132: 212–22.
57. Van der Vusse GJ, van Bilsen M, Sonderkamp T *et al.* Hydrolysis of phospholipids and cellular integrity. In Piper HM (ed): Pathophysiology of Severe Ischemic Myocardial Injury. Dordrecht: Kluwer 1990; 167–93.
58. Schwartz P, Piper HM, Spahr R *et al.* Ultrastructure of adult myocardial cells during anoxia and reoxygenation. Am J Pathol 1984; 115: 349–61.
59. Ganote CE, Vander Heide RS. Cytoskeletal lesions in anoxic myocardial injury. Am J Pathol 1987; 129: 327–44.
60. Steenbergen CJ, Hill ML, Jennings RB. Cytoskeletal damage during myocardial ischemia: changes in vinculin immunofluorescence staining during total *in vitro* ischemia and in canine heart. Circ Res 1987; 69: 478–86
61. Armstrong SC, Ganote CE. Flow cytometric analysis of isolated cardiomyocytes: vinculin and tubulin fluorescence during metabolic inhibition and ischemia. J Mol Cell Cardiol 1992; 24: 149–62.
62. Ganote CE, Armstrong SC. Cytoskeletal lesions in anoxic myocardial injury. J Mol Cell Cardiol 1992; 24 (Suppl I): 26 (abstr.).
63. Buderus S, Siegmund B, Spahr R *et al.* Resistance of coronary endothelial cells to anoxia-reoxygenation in isolated perfused guinea pig hearts. Am J Physiol 1989; 257: H488–H493.
64. Vander Heide RS, Angelo JP, Altschuld RA *et al.* Energy dependence of contraction band formation in perfused hearts and isolated adult cardiomyocytes. Am J Pathol 1986; 125: 55–68.
65. Piper HM. Mitochondrial injury in the oxygen-depleted and reoxygenated myocardial cell. In Piper HM (ed): Pathophysiology of Severe Ischemic Myocardial Injury. Dordrecht: Kluwer 1990; 91–114.
66. Piper HM, Sezer O, Schleyer M *et al.* Development of ischemia-induced damage in defined mitochondrial subpopulations. J Mol Cell Cardiol 1985; 17: 186–98.
67. Siegmund B, Koop A, Piper HM. The use of the creatine kinase reaction to determine free energy change of ATP hydrolysis in anoxic cardiomyocytes. Pflügers Arch 1989; 413: 435–7.
68. Zimmer HG, Trendelenburg C, Kammermeier H *et al.* De novo synthesis of myocardial adenine nucleotides in the rat. Circ Res 1973; 32: 635–42.
69. Kammermeier H. High energy phosphate of the myocardium: Concentration versus free energy change. Basic Res Cardiol 1987; 82 (suppl. 2): 31–6.
70. Siegmund B, Zude R, Piper HM. Recovery of anoxic-reoxygenated cardiomyocytes from severe Ca^{2+}-overload. Am J Physiol 1992; 263: H1262–9.
71. Sagara Y, Wade JB, Inesi G. A conformational mechanism for formation of a dead-end

complex by the sarcoplasmic reticulum ATPase with thapsigargin. J Biol Chem 1992; 1267: 1286–92.

72. Reed KC, Bygrave FL. The inhibition of mitochondrial calcium transport by lanthanides and ruthenium red. Biochem J 1974; 140: 143–55.
73. McCormack JG, England PJ. Ruthenium red inhibits the activation of pyruvate dehydrogenase caused by positive inotropic agents in the perfused rat heart. Biochem J 1983; 214: 581–5.
74. Hansford RG. Relation between cytosolic free Ca^{2+} concentration and the control of pyruvate dehydrogenase in isolated cardiac myocytes. Biochem J 1987; 241: 145–51.
75. Gupta MP, Innes IR, Dhalla NS. Response of contractile function to ruthenium red in rat heart. Am J Physiol 1988; 255: H1413–20.
76. Carafoli E. Intracellular calcium homeostasis. Ann Rev Biochem 1987; 56: 395–433.
77. Krause SM, Jacobus WE, Becker LC. Alterations in cardiac sarcoplasmic reticulum calcium transport in the postischemic 'stunned' myocardium. Circ Res 1989; 65: 526–30.
78. Peng CF, Kane JJ, Straub KD *et al.* Improvement of mitochondrial energy production in ischemic myocardium by *in vivo* infusion of ruthenium red. J Cardiovasc Pharmacol 1980; 2: 45–54.
79. Ferrari R, di Lisa F, Raddino R *et al.* The effects of ruthenium red on mitochondrial function during post-ischemic reperfusion. J Mol Cell Cardiol 1982; 14: 737–40.
80. Benzi RH, Lerch R. Dissociation between contractile function and oxidative metabolism in postischemic myocardium. Attenuation by ruthenium red administered during reperfusion. Circ Res 1992; 71: 567–76.
81. Ganote CE, Sims MD, Safavi S. Effects of dimethylsulfoxide (DMSO) on the oxygen paradox in perfused rat hearts. Am J Physiol 1982; 109: 270–6.
82. Siegmund B, Klietz T, Schwartz P *et al.* Temporary contractile blockade prevents hypercontracture in anoxic-reoxygenated cardiomyocytes. Am J Physiol 1991; 260: H426–H435.
83. Li T, Sperelakis N, Teneick RE *et al.* Effects of diacetyl monoxime on cardiac excitation-contraction coupling. J Pharmacol Exp Therap 1985; 232: 688–95.
84. Fryer MF, Neering IR, Stephenson DG. Effects of 2,3–butanedione monoxime on the contractile activation of fast- and slow-twitch rat muscle fibres. J Physiol (London) 1988; 407: 53–75.
85. West JM, Stephenson DG. Contractile activation and the effects of 2,3–butanedione monoxime (BDM) in skinned cardiac preparations from normal and dystrophic mice (129/ReJ). Pflügers Arch 1989; 413: 546–52.
86. Gwathmey JK, Hajjar RJ, Solaro RJ. Contractile deactivation and uncoupling of crossbridges. Effects of 2,3–butanedione monoxime on mammalian myocardium. Circ Res 1991; 69: 1280–92.
87. Schlüter KD, Schwartz P, Siegmund B *et al.* Prevention of the oxygen paradox in anoxic-reoxygenated hearts. Am J Physiol 1991; 261: H416–23.
88. Garcia-Dorado D, Theroux P, Duran JM *et al.* Selective inhibition of the contractile apparatus. A new approach to modification of infarct size, infarct composition, and infarct geometry during coronary artery occlusion and reperfusion. Circulation 1992; 85: 1160–74.
89. Kehrer JP, Piper HM, Sies H. Xanthine oxidase is not responsible for reoxygenation injury in isolated-perfused rat heart. Free Rad Res Comms 1987; 3: 69–78.
90. Rich TL, Langer GA. Calcium depletion in rabbit myocardium. Calcium paradox protection by hypothermia and cation substitution. Circ Res 1982; 51: 131–41.
91. Altschuld RA, Ganote CE, Nayler WG *et al.* What constitutes the calcium paradox? J Mol Cell Cardiol 1991; 23: 765–7.

3. Role of leukocytes in reperfusion injury

SHARON L. HALE and ROBERT A. KLONER

Introduction

Reperfusion represents a paradoxical situation with both beneficial and potentially detrimental consequences to the ischemic myocardium. Reperfusion is essential for the survival of myocytes subjected to severe ischemia; without reperfusion, viable cells undergo irreversible changes and die. However some investigators believe that cells, still viable at the time of reperfusion, may undergo further injury due to the re-establishment of coronary perfusion. Thus reperfusion injury refers to damage caused by the reinstitution of blood flow, in contrast to cell death caused by the preceding ischemic episode. This cellular damage may be reflected as structural, functional or metabolic derangements.

The clinical implications of reperfusion injury include patients that receive thrombolytic therapy, angioplasty or coronary artery bypass surgery for acute myocardial infarction or unstable angina. Reperfusion injury may also be important to myocardium during cardiac transplantation, when the newly transplanted heart is reperfused after a prolonged period of hypothermic global ischemia. In addition, it may play a role following prolonged cardioplegic arrest in patients undergoing cardiac surgery, who are exposed to ischemia and then to reperfusion when the aortic crossclamp is removed.

Coronary artery reperfusion has been the most effective therapy for reducing the extent of necrosis and improving ventricular function and prognosis in patients with acute myocardial infarction. However in the late 1970s Hearse suggested that reperfusion *per se* may lead to deleterious effects on the myocardium [1], and as Braunwald and Kloner have stated, reperfusion is potentially a 'double-edged sword' [2]. The concept of reperfusion injury is controversial. The most direct evidence for its existence is in animal models in which the final extent of the infarct is reduced by therapeutic manipulation administered at the time of reperfusion.

Reperfusion injury may have several manifestations. Indeed the term 'reperfusion injury' itself has come to reflect various meanings, and it is important to note that the pathogenesis (and thus potential treatment) of these various aspects may be different. These aspects include: (1) functional abnormalities associated with nonlethal cell damage, so called 'stunning' of myocardial tissue; (2) accelerated necrosis of irreversibly injured cells; (3) lethal

H.M. Piper and C.J. Preusse (eds): Ischemia-reperfusion in cardiac surgery, 67–80.

reperfusion injury-cell death due to reperfusion *per se* rather than from the preexisting ischemia; and (4) reperfusion-associated arrhythmias.

When acute myocardial infarction is followed by reperfusion, there is an associated rapid influx of neutrophils. That neutrophils may participate in reperfusion injury is suggested by the fact that neutrophils accumulate rapidly after reperfusion, the influx occurs specifically in regions of the heart subjected to ischemia and reperfusion, and the quantity of neutrophils is directly related to the severity of ischemia. It is well known that neutrophils have the ability to release many toxic mediators, such as free radicals, proteolytic enzymes, and active metabolites of arachidonic acid, all of which could cause the destruction of otherwise viable myocardial cells. Thus the neutrophil has been implicated as one factor that might contribute to reperfusion injury.

The purpose of the following review will be to discuss: (1) the time course of neutrophil infiltration following myocardial infarction; (2) the role of endogenous leukocytes; (3) neutrophils as a source of oxygen free radicals; (4) the question of whether neutrophils contribute to myocyte death; (5) the role of neutrophils in no-reflow; (6) the role of neutrophils in myocardial stunning; and (7) their role in reperfusion arrhythmias.

Time course of neutrophil infiltration

Adhesion of neutrophils to the vascular endothelium is the first step in the inflammatory process and is a necessary prerequisite for activation, diapedesis and migration of neutrophils into subendocardial layers. Normally the endothelium repels neutrophils. Surface charges on the cells cause electrostatic repulsion. Also the endothelium produces substances that both promote and inhibit adherence. Substances produced by endothelial cells that increase neutrophil adhesiveness include monokines, interleukin 1 and platelet activating factor (PAF); substances that inhibit adherence include adenosine, prostacyclin and cyclic AMP.

Neutrophil localization occurs rapidly after injury. Reperfusion is accompanied by an expression of chemotactic activity that peaks within the first hour of reperfusion and has been found in cardiac lymph [3]. This localized production of chemotactic activity is thought to represent a means by which neutrophils are stimulated during ischemia and reperfusion.

It was long ago observed that neutrophils are associated with myocardial infarction as a part of the early inflammatory response [4]. In patients, neutrophils were known to accumulate in infarcted myocardium 12–24 hours after acute myocardial infarction, to peak 3–4 days after infarction and to decline after about 1 week. Tennant and associates showed leukocyte infiltration 28 hours after coronary occlusion and also demonstrated some infiltration after 2 hours of ischemia when followed by reperfusion [5]. Histologic studies by Sommers and Jennings [6] showed that leukocyte margination occurred in the periphery of the infarct as early as 4 hours after non-reperfused coronary artery occlusion.

In response to acute myocardial infarction, the inflammatory reaction, observed histologically, is apparent 12–24 hours after permanent coronary artery occlusion. Neutrophil margination of venules has been observed in the periphery of the necrotic zone as early as 4 hours in non-reperfused experimental infarcts [6]. In humans, granulocyte infiltration has been observed as early as 6 hours after infarction [7]. Leukocytes accumulate at the margin of the necrotic area. Over several days, the infiltration covers the entire necrotic area. These cells remove the necrotic debris. This response peaks at 3–4 days and declines after about 1 week [4].

With reperfusion however, the time course of leukocyte infiltration is altered. Recent studies of neutrophil influx, employing techniques such as ^{111}indium-labeling of neutrophils, indicate that neutrophil infiltration begins earlier than was originally believed and that reperfusion accelerates the influx. Many investigators have found neutrophils to be present in increased numbers after short periods of ischemia. Engler and others [8] measured neutrophil influx in dogs using ^{111}indium-labeled autologous granulocytes. After 3 hours of coronary artery occlusion, all hearts in the permanent occlusion group showed an approximate 50% increase in accumulation of white cells in the ischemic tissue. Leukocytes appeared to be trapped during occlusion and further accumulation may have occurred during ischemia via collateral blood flow. The increase was greatest in the more severely ischemic subendocardium. After only 5 minutes of reperfusion, the subendocardial granulocyte content was increased by an additional 25%.

In our laboratory, we studied the time course of infiltration of neutrophils in rat hearts after coronary artery occlusion. Findings from our study showed that the number of neutrophils increased after the onset of ischemia, even in the absence of reperfusion, since more neutrophils were present in the myocardium of animals subjected to permanent occlusion than in that of sham operated animals. We also observed an increase in neutrophils with ischemia alone (2 hours) in the nonreperfused ischemic zone, with a greater number of neutrophils present after 3 hours of ischemia. With reperfusion we observed dramatically enhanced accumulation after 2 hours of reperfusion [9].

Mullane and others studied dogs after 1 hour of coronary artery occlusion, followed by 30 minutes to 5 hours of reperfusion. At the end of the ischemic period they observed neutrophils adhering to the endothelium of vessels in the ischemic region. A few leukocytes were observed in the myocardium after 30 minutes of reperfusion. However with increased duration of reperfusion the number of leukocytes increased and after 5 hours the accumulation was extensive [10].

Dreyer and coworkers, using ^{99m}Tc-labeled neutrophils, have recently shown that the rate of neutrophil influx is greatest during the first hour of reperfusion. After 1 hour of ischemia and 1 hour of reperfusion, neutrophil accumulation was inversely related to regional blood flow and occurred preferentially in the subendocardium. The rate of influx was attenuated by 4 hours of reperfusion, but the cumulative influx proceeded for more than 24 hours [11].

The distribution of neutrophils also changes over time. We observed that after 1 hour of reperfusion, approximately 74% of the accumulated neutrophils were located within the lumen of or marginating vessel walls. But by 2 hours of reperfusion only about 30% of the accumulated neutrophils were located in vessels, with most neutrophils now located in the interstitium and in myocytes [9]. Mullane and coinvestigators [10] also noted the transition from the vasculature to the tissue. After 30 minute of reperfusion they saw neutrophils adhering to the vascular endothelium but very few in the myocardium. After 3 hours of reperfusion neutrophil presence in myocardial tissue was extensive.

Neutrophils also tend to distribute in proportion to the severity of the ischemic insult. Go and coworkers found that with reperfusion after a short ischemic period (12 minutes) the number of neutrophils present was actually fewer than in nonischemic tissue. After a 40 minute period of ischemia or a 90 minute period there was a 2 to 6 times increase in the ischemic versus nonischemic tissue. The influx was greater with increased duration of ischemia as the influx was greater after 90 minutes of occlusion than after 40 minutes [12]. They also observed a transmural gradient, with the greater accumulation in the more ischemic endocardium. Dreyer [11] also noted a greater accumulation in the subendocardium and mid-myocardium than subepicardium. This accumulation was inversely related to blood flow during ischemia.

Role of endogenous white cells

Keller and coworkers [13] studied the resident leukocyte population in isolated rat hearts. They found numerous resident cardiac mast cells, macrophages and some lymphocytes, but no neutrophils were observed. This suggests that neutrophils are primarily recruited after the onset of ischemia, either from blood being trapped during the occlusion or by delivery through collateral circulation.

They demonstrated that in an isolated, perfused heart, these resident cells have the ability to produce significant amounts of peroxidase during reoxygenation. The extent of tissue injury as measured by creatine kinase release was related to the amount of peroxidase released. When degranulation of mast cells was prevented using Lodoximide, peroxidase release was reduced as was tissue injury.

Neutrophils as a source of oxygen-free radicals

One theory of the cause of reperfusion injury is the oxygen-free radical hypothesis. On one hand, the reinstitution of flow is crucial to rescue cells that are perhaps damaged, but still alive at the time of reperfusion; however the reintroduction of oxygen with concomitant production of oxygen free-radicals could result in damage that kills otherwise reversibly injured cells. It has been proposed that oxygen-derived free radicals released at the time of reperfusion may contribute to the functional aberration known as 'stunning', after relatively short duration of ischemia, or cause cell death after more prolonged ischemia.

Free radicals are highly reactive molecules that have unpaired electrons in their outer shell. The primary oxygen free radicals are the superoxide radical ($\cdot O^{2-}$), the hydroxyl radical ($-OH$), and hydrogen peroxide (H_2O_2). Oxygen free radicals have the ability to damage cells. For example, they can attack membrane phospholipids and act upon unsaturated fatty acids to produce lipid peroxidation, which results in increased membrane fluidity, permeability and loss of membrane integrity [14].

Many metabolic pathways generate free radicals and have been proposed as potential sources of free radicals in the setting of ischemia and reperfusion. One potential source is the oxidation of catecholamines that are released during ischemia. A second potential source is the metabolism of arachidonic acid [15].

The xanthine oxidase pathway is another possible basis for free radical generation [16]. During ischemia ATP is degraded to hypoxanthine, which accumulates. At reperfusion, with the reintroduction of molecular oxygen, xanthine oxidase produces O^{2-}, the superoxide radical, as a byproduct of the oxidation of hypoxanthine to uric acid. While the xanthine oxidase pathway may be important in canine myocardium, some species appear to be lacking this enzyme. Rabbits, pigs and humans have little or no detectable xanthine oxidase.

Many investigators have suggested that neutrophils are a source of free radicals, produced via the NADPH-oxidase reaction. When activated, neutrophils release superoxide and the hypochlorous anion (OCl^-). Seventy percent of the oxygen used by activated neutrophils is initially converted to superoxide [17], and this is a fundamental mechanism for their attack on bacteria and damaged cells. Studies have shown that activation of the neutrophil system *in vitro* results in the generation of free radicals that are capable of producing cardiac dysfunction [18].

It has been shown experimentally that a burst of free radicals occurs at reperfusion and levels can remain elevated for several hours [19]. Also it is known that exogenous free radicals can damage myocytes [20]. However whether there is sufficient free radical production from neutrophils to contribute to myocardial cell death after ischemia and reperfusion remains to be determined. When ischemia is extended for longer periods, and is accompanied by reperfusion, the adhering activated neutrophils could generate the cytotoxic metabolites of oxygen, and theoretically kill otherwise viable myocytes.

The most convincing evidence that free radicals augment cell death comes from studies showing a reduction in experimental infarct size when free radical scavengers are given as therapy. The heart has normal protective mechanisms against free radicals such as endogenous superoxide dismutase and glutathione peroxidase, but these cellular systems may be depleted during ischemia or reperfusion. Work by Jolly and others in 1984 provided the first *in vivo* evidence for the participation of free radicals in myocardial injury [21]. They found that the administration before reperfusion of the free radical scavengers superoxide dismutase and catalase significantly reduced infarct size. Other investigators later confirmed these observations [22]. These data suggested that free radicals play a role in reperfusion injury. However not all studies using these agents have been positive [23,24], and the contribution of oxygen radicals to myocyte death is still unresolved.

Do neutrophils contribute to an increase in infarct size after coronary artery occlusion and reperfusion?

The role of neutrophils as potential contributors to myocardial cellular injury in response to ischemia was suggested by Hill and Ward in 1971 [25], and their possible contribution to reperfusion injury was suggested by other studies. In 1983 it was shown that ultimate infarct size after 90 minutes of ischemia followed by reperfusion for 6 hours was reduced in canine hearts made neutropenic [26]. This observation has been corroborated by other investigators using alternative means of inducing neutropenia [27,28]. Especially suggestive that neutrophils might enhance or accelerate myocyte death during reperfusion was the study performed by Litt and associates [28] showing that neutrophil depletion limited to reperfusion only, produced a significant reduction in infarct size. Further evidence for the detrimental effect of neutrophils during reperfusion was supplied by studies that reduced infarct size by altering neutrophil function [10,29].

Evidence that neutrophils may affect infarct size is provided by experimental studies in which ultimate infarct size is reduced by neutropenia or by altering neutrophil function. In the early 1980s, Romson and coworkers noted that ibuprofen, a nonsteroidal anti-inflammatory drug, reduced experimental infarct size [30]. They noted in particular that the infarct size reduction was associated with a significant decrease in leukocyte infiltration. This data suggested a possible role of leukocytes in the process of tissue injury. To investigate this phenomenon, a study was performed by this group examining the role of neutrophils after ischemia and reperfusion in dogs made neutropenic using rabbit antiserum to canine neutrophils [26]. After 90 minutes of occlusion and 6 hours of reperfusion, infarct size was measured and the hearts were examined by histology. Neutrophil infiltrate was absent in the infarcted myocardium of the neutropenic dogs, and although all animals had necrotic injury, infarct size was reduced an average of 43% in the neutropenic group. Other investigators found similar beneficial effects [27,31].

Some studies have failed to find a reduction in infarct size with leukopenia [32]. Chatelain and coworkers studied dogs after permanent coronary occlusion and compared these animals with a second group that received 3 hours of occlusion and 21 hours of reperfusion and a third group that was subjected to a similar reperfusion protocol except that the dogs were made leukopenic. Non-neutropenic, control animals that received reperfusion had an 80% increase in the number of neutrophils in the ischemic/reperfused region compared with animals permanently occluded. However infarct size in all three groups was similar. These data suggested that neutrophil accumulation did not have an adverse effect on infarct size. The discrepancy between this study and others is not clear, although perhaps the modification of infarct size after a relatively long period (3 hours) of ischemia was too small to quantify.

Since leukocyte depletion before ischemia is not a clinical possibility, an interesting approach to the problem is to find compounds that modify neutrophil behavior without affecting cell count. A reduction in infarct size was shown to occur in animals with normal neutrophil populations in which neutrophil function was altered. BW755C, a drug that inhibits lipoxygenase and cyclooxygenase pathways of arachidonic metabolism, thus attenuating leukocyte infiltration into infarcted myocardium, reduced infarct size in pigs, a model of low collateral flow [33] and in dogs [10]. Hydroxyurea, which reduces circulating leukocytes also reduced infarct size in this second study. In contrast, indomethacin and dexamethasone, which do not affect migration of neutrophils, did not reduce infarct size. Infarct size reduction was also noted when animals were treated with Fluosol, a perfluorochemical known to reduce neutrophil demargination and infiltration [34], and when animals were administered a monoclonal antibody that inhibits neutrophil adhesion [35].

A recent study by deLongreil and coworkers [36] also suggested that neutrophil infiltration may augment myocardial necrosis. Infarct size was assessed in dogs subjected to 2 hours of coronary artery occlusion followed by various reperfusion periods of 0 to 24 hours. In this study infarct size was significantly smaller in the group of animals with 3 hours of reperfusion compared with 6 or 24 hours of reperfusion. Neutrophil accumulation, assessed by scintigraphy of ^{111}indium-labeled neutrophils was greatest between 3 hours and 6 hours; during this time period, infarct size on average increased by 40%.

Further evidence that neutrophils might increase or accelerate myocyte death during reperfusion was provided by the study performed by Litt and associates showing that neutrophil depletion limited to reperfusion only, produced a significant reduction in infarct size [28].

Data from the above studies provide indirect evidence that neutrophils are implicated in the extension of cell death in the setting of ischemia and reperfusion. However in order to prove directly the existence of neutrophil-induced reperfusion injury it would be necessary to prove that cells, viable before reperfusion, are indeed killed by this aspect of reperfusion. To date, this evidence has not come to light. Thus many investigators feel that reperfusion does not cause lethal damage, but merely hastens the death of myocytes already doomed by ischemia [37].

Neutrophils and the no-reflow phenomenon

In early studies of ischemia and reperfusion in canine hearts, Kloner and coworkers observed that a dye marker, injected after reperfusion of myocardium ischemic for 90 minutes, failed to penetrate some areas [38]. This was termed the 'no-reflow' phenomenon and has been defined as "the inability to perfuse previously ischemic myocardium, even when blood flow has been restored to the large arteries supplying the tissue" [39].

Several possible mechanisms for this phenomenon have been described. One theory is that localized areas of endothelial swelling (blebs) plug the lumen on the vessel. A second theory of the cause of no-reflow is that capillaries are compressed by myocyte swelling; however this has not been confirmed by histologic observation [38]. Another potential cause is functional abnormalities of endothelial cells. Endothelial cells regulate vascular reactivity by release of factors such as endothelial-derived relaxing factor (EDRF), adenosine and prostacyclin. After ischemia and reperfusion there may be impaired production of these substances or a washout at reperfusion. When endothelial cells are unable to release relaxing factors into a vasoconstricted bed, it may cause a progressive decline in blood flow after reperfusion.

While microthrombi were once thought to be a potential cause of no-reflow, administration of streptokinase [40] failed to prevent this phenomenon. Rouleaux formation (red cell packing) is seen in areas of no-reflow, however this is probably due to sluggish blood flow due to other causes.

Neutrophils plugging of blood vessels was implicated as a cause of the no-reflow phenomenon. In addition, neutrophils are capable of releasing mediators that cause vasoconstriction such as thromboxanes and leukotrienes. Several investigators have suggested that the failure to achieve uniform reperfusion in postischemic myocardium is due to mechanical capillary plugging by neutrophils. Neutrophils blocking capillaries during ischemia could cause a decrease in collateral blood flow; blockage during reperfusion could then lead to a myocardial perfusion defect. Engler and associates [41] showed that neutrophils are trapped during coronary artery occlusion and that the further accumulation during reperfusion results in capillary plugging. This may lead to a further deterioration in regional perfusion. When hearts were reperfused with leukocyte-depleted blood [42], the progressive decline in flow in the ischemic area was decreased in the subendocardium. When the tissue was examined histologically, hearts perfused with whole blood exhibited blockage of 27% of the capillaries in the previously ischemic subendocardium compared with 1% in leukocyte-depleted animals. Blockage of capillaries was associated with a significant reduction in subendocardial blood flow.

No-reflow has been considered a consequence of microvascular damage occurring during the ischemic phase and thus established at the time of reperfusion. However Ambrosio and coworkers [43] have shown that no reflow is progressive and is associated with an increase in neutrophil accumulation. When a dye marker was injected 2 minutes after reperfusion, the perfusion defect in the previously ischemic myocardium was very small, but after 3.5 hours of reperfusion it was significantly larger. Regional blood flow measurements at 2 minutes showed hyperemic flow in this area; after 30 minutes flow was still adequate, but by 3.5 hours there was negligible flow. Intravascular neutrophil accumulation was negligible after 2 minutes of reperfusion, but there was a 20-fold increase after 3.5 hours. This delayed progressive decline in flow suggests a dynamic process of microvascular deterioration associated with neutrophil accumulation.

Other investigations have found contradicting results regarding the role of the neutrophil in no-reflow. Carlson and others [48] showed a reduction in infarct size in leukopenic dogs compared with controls. However neutrophil depletion failed to modify the no-reflow region, and there were no differences between groups in regional blood flow in either early or late reperfusion. Others [44] have found that leukocytes are not required for the development of no-reflow, but their presence exacerbates the effect.

No-reflow is a capillary phenomenon and its contribution to additional myocardial injury at reperfusion is unclear. In a normally functioning heart, only 50–60% of capillaries are perfused [45]. Therefore substantial capillary reserve exists, and a decrease in flow would occur only when this reserve was exhausted. No-reflow may be relatively unimportant, since it occurs in regions that are already extensively damaged [38,43].

On the arteriolar level, margination of neutrophils may contribute to stenosis of the vessel by reduction of the lumen diameter with a significant increase in microvascular resistance. Another potential source of neutrophil damage to coronary vasculature was described by Kloner and coworkers [46]. In a series of studies, these investigators studied neutrophil infiltration into the walls of large epicardial coronary arteries after ischemia (induced with a proximal and distal coronary artery clamp) and reperfusion. They observed that in addition to the influx of neutrophils into the microvasculature, neutrophils also migrate into the walls of the large coronary arteries. This was associated with reduced endothelial-dependent and endothelial-independent coronary vasodilator reserve.

Do neutrophils contribute to post-ischemic myocardial 'stunning'?

Myocardial 'stunning' is a type of functional reperfusion injury that occurs after ischemia of relatively short duration, i.e. when the cells are still in the phase of reversible injury. Contractile function of myocardium subjected to brief episodes of ischemia followed by reperfusion can remain depressed or 'stunned' for hours to days [47]. Stunning has been shown to occur in humans after thrombolytic therapy and after exercise testing [48]. Several mechanisms have been proposed to cause myocardial stunning, the most pervasive of which is oxygen free radical damage. Some investigators have suggested that stunning may result, at least in part, from free radicals produced by neutrophils, and studies have been reported in which the depletion of neutrophils prior to 15 minutes of ischemia prevents [49] or alleviates [50] ventricular dysfunction. Other studies have failed to show an attenuation of postischemic dysfunction with neutropenia [51,52]. For example, Jeremy and associates reperfused myocardium subjected to 10 minutes of ischemia with neutrophil-free blood. Although neutrophils were virtually absent from this region, myocardial dysfunction, assessed by segment-shortening, was similar to that in control animals whose myocardium was perfused with whole blood [52].

Critical to this hypothesis is that neutrophils are present in large enough numbers to cause damage during the relatively short ischemic period. In fact, their presence has not been documented during brief ischemia. Go and associates reported that after 12 minutes of ischemia the number of ^{111}indium-labeled neutrophils in the reperfused region was actually lower than in the nonischemic control areas [12]. Also reported was that myeloperoxidase activity, a marker of leukocytes, was not different in ischemic and non-ischemic tissue following 15 minutes of ischemia and reperfusion [53]. These studies provide evidence that neutrophils probably do not play and important role in myocardial stunning.

Neutrophils and reperfusion arrhythmias

A negative consequence of reperfusion after regional ischemia is the occurrence of reperfusion-induced arrhythmias. These arrhythmias, including ventricular tachycardia and ventricular fibrillation are notable in experimental models of ischemia and reperfusion, and appear to be more pronounced with reperfusion after short periods of ischemia, for example 5 minutes of ischemia in rats and up to 30 minutes of ischemia in dogs. Since reflow arrhythmias occur within seconds of reflow this may be considered a form of reperfusion injury. However this injury is probably due to other aspects of reperfusion than neutrophils, since neutrophil accumulation does not occur with brief periods of ischemia and reperfusion [12]. The contribution of resident neutrophils to arrhythmias at this early time has yet to be established.

In early experimental studies examining neutrophil depletion, Engler and coworkers noted that leukocyte depletion had a beneficial effect on the incidence of ventricular fibrillation during 60 minutes of ischemia. Premature ventricular contractions were also reduced [43]. It was also noted that administration of BW755C, a drug that reduces leukocyte infiltration, showed striking antiarrhythmic effects in an experimental ischemia/reperfusion protocol. Given at 30 minutes of reperfusion this drug produced an immediate and pronounced decline in ventricular arrhythmias when compared with control animals [10]. However this apparent beneficial effect may have resulted from a smaller infarct in the treated group or from some other antiarrhythmic properties of the drug.

Although ventricular arrhythmias occur in patients after reflow, the incidence is less common and of less severity than is observed in the experimental setting, perhaps because the duration of ischemia is normally longer and reflow more gradual in patients. Kuzuya and associates [54] studied 21 patients with acute myocardial infarction, dividing them into 3 groups based on the incidence and severity of their ventricular arrhythmias as measured on Holter monitor. They found that the neutrophil count and leukotriene B4 production were increased with increased severity of ventricular arrhythmias. They concluded that a positive association existed between neutrophils and the incidence and severity of ventricular arrhythmias in patients after acute myocardial infarction but that the causal relationship remains to be determined.

Neutrophil reduction and healing

While it is possible that selective inhibition of the acute phase of the accumulation of neutrophils may protect myocardium during early reperfusion, the primary role of neutrophils is to remove cellular debris as the first step in the healing process. The migration of neutrophils into necrotic myocardium represents the initial phase of a process that leads to reorganization of injured tissue and its replacement by scar. Therefore, interventions that suppress the influx of neutrophils or their functions could interfere with the healing process. For example, the administration of anti-inflammatory agents, such as methylprednisolone and ibuprofen, has been shown to cause marked scar thinning and a reduction in regional function after coronary artery occlusion in dogs [55,56].

If anti-inflammatory agents impair the healing process, they will be of limited use in the clinical setting. However there may be an acute phase of the inflammatory response that differs from the chronic phase, and future studies may show that it is possible and desirable to alter early neutrophil response without subsequent impairment of healing.

Summary

Overwhelming evidence indicates that early reperfusion reduces cardiac mortality. In the presence of infarction, early reperfusion is so beneficial that coronary artery reperfusion via balloon angioplasty or thrombolysis has become the therapy of choice. Reperfusion is a prerequisite for the survival of the ischemic myocardium, but experimental studies have provided evidence that reperfusion *per se* may have deleterious effects, such as have been reviewed in this chapter. The causal relationship between neutrophil accumulation and such factors as reperfusion arrhythmias, no-reflow and infarct extension have yet to be firmly established. Understanding these associations may provide practical value for therapeutic approaches in the future.

References

1. Hearse DJ. Reperfusion of the ischemic myocardium. J Mol Cell Cardiol 1977; 9: 605–16.
2. Braunwald E, Kloner RA. Myocardial reperfusion: a double-edged sword? J Clin Invest 1985; 76: 713–9.
3. Dreyer WJ, Smith CW, Michael LH *et al.* Canine neutrophil activation by cardiac lymph obtained during reperfusion of ischemic myocardium. Circ Res 1989; 65: 1751–62.
4. Mallory GK, White PD, Salcedo-Salgar J. The speed of healing of myocardial infarction: a study of the pathologic anatomy in 72 cases. Am Heart J 1939; 18: 647–71.
5. Tennant R, Grayzel DM, Sutherland FA *et al.* Studies on experimental coronary occlusion. Chemical and anatomical changes In the myocardium after coronary ligation. Am Heart J 1936; 12: 168–73.
6. Sommers HM, Jennings RB. Experimental acute myocardial infarction: histologic and histochemical studies of early myocardial infarcts induced by temporary or permanent occlusion of a coronary artery. Lab Invest 1964; 13: 1491; 1502.
7. Fishbein MC, Maclean D, Maroko PR. The histopathologic evolution of myocardial infarction. Chest 1978; 73: 843–9.
8. Engler RL, Dahlgren MD, Peterson MA *et al.* Accumulation of polymorphonuclear leukocytes during 3-h experimental myocardial ischemia. Am J Physiol 1986; 251: H93–H100.
9. Hale SL, Kloner RA. Time course of infiltration and distribution of neutrophils following coronary artery reperfusion in the rat. Coronary Artery Dis 1991; 2: 373–8.
10. Mullane KM, Read N, Salmon JA *et al.* Role of leukocytes in acute myocardial infarction in anesthetized dogs: relationship to myocardial salvage by anti-inflammatory drugs. J Pharmacol Exptl Therap 1984; 228: 510–22.
11. Dreyer WJ, Michael LH, West MS *et al.* Neutrophil accumulation in ischemic canine myocardium: insights into time course, distribution, and mechanism of localization during early reperfusion. Circulation 1991: 84: 400–11.
12. Go LO, Murry CE, Richard VJ *et al.* Myocardial neutrophil accumulation during reperfusion after reversible or irreversible ischemic injury. Am J Physiol 1988; 255: H1188–H1198.
13. Keller AM, Clancy RM, Barr ML *et al.* Acute reoxygenation injury in the isolated rat heart: role of resident cardiac mast cells. Circ Res 1988; 63: 1044–52.
14. Mead JF. Free radical mechanisms of lipid damage and consequences for cellular membranes. In Pryor WA (ed): Free radicals in biology. New York: Academic Press 1976; 51–68.
15. Hammond B, Kontos HA, Hess ML. Oxygen radicals in the adult respiratory distress

syndrome, in myocardial ischemia and reperfusion injury, and in cerebral vascular damage. Can J Physiol Pharmacol 1985; 63: 173–87.

16. McCord JM. Oxygen-derived radicals in postischemic tissue injury. N Engl J Med 1985; 312: 159–63.
17. Babior BM. The respiratory burst of phagocytes. J Clin Invest 1984; 73: 599–601.
18. Rowe GT, Eaton LR, Hess ML. Neutrophil-derived, oxygen free radical-mediated cardiovascular dysfunction. J Mol Cell Cardiol 1984; 16: 1075–9.
19. Bolli R, Patel BS, Jerroudi MO *et al.* Demonstration of free radical generation in "stunned" myocardium of intact dogs with the use of the spin trap L-Phenyl N-Tret-Butyl-Nitrone. J Clin Invest 1988; 82: 476–85.
20. Burton KP, McCord JM, Ghai G. Myocardial alterations due to free radical generation. Am J Physiol 1984; 246: H776–H783.
21. Jolly SR, Kane WJ, Bailie MB *et al.* Canine myocardial reperfusion injury: its reduction by the combined administration of superoxide dismutase and catalase. Circ Res 1984; 54: 277–85.
22. Chambers DE, Parks DA, Patterson G *et al.* Xanthine oxidase as a source of free radical damage in myocardial ischemia. J Mol Cell Cardiol 1985; 17: 145–52.
23. Przyklenk K, Kloner RA. Reperfusion injury by oxygen free radicals? Effect of superoxide dismutase plus catalase, given at the time of reperfusion, on myocardial infarct size, contractile function, coronary microvasculature. Circ Res 1989; 64: 86–96.
24. Uraizee A, Reimer KA, Murry CE *et al.* Failure of superoxide dismutase to limit infarct size of myocardial infarction after 40 minutes of ischemia and 4 days of reperfusion in dogs. Circulation 1987; 75: 1237–48.
25. Hill JH, Ward PA. The phlogistic role of C3 leukotactic fragments in myocardial infarcts of rats. J Exp Med 1971; 133: 885–900.
26. Romson JL, Hook BB, Kunkel SL *et al.* Reduction of the extent of ischemic reperfusion injury by neutrophil depletion in the dog. Circulation 1983; 67: 1016–23.
27. deLorgeil M, Basmadjian A, Lavallée M *et al.* Influence of leukopenia on collateral flow, reperfusion flow, reflow ventricular fibrillation and infarct size in dogs. Am Heart J 1989; 117: 523–32.
28. Litt MR, Jeremy RW, Weisman HF *et al.* Neutrophil depletion limited to reperfusion reduces myocardial infarct size after 90 minutes of ischemia. Evidence for neutrophil-mediated reperfusion injury. Circulation 1989; 80: 1816–27.
29. Simpson PJ, Fantone JC, Mickelson JK *et al.* Identification of a time window for therapy to reduce experimental canine myocardial injury: suppression of neutrophil activation during 72 hours of reperfusion. Circ Res 1988; 63: 1070–9.
30. Romson JL, Hook B, Rigot VH *et al.* The effect of ibuprofen on accumulation of indium-111-labeled platelets and leukocytes in experimental myocardial infarction. Circulation 1982; 66: 1002–11.
31. Carlson RE, Schott RJ, Buda AJ. Neutrophil depletion fails to modify myocardial no-reflow and functional recovery after coronary reperfusion. Am J Cardiol 1989; 14: 1803–13.
32. Chatelain P, Latour J-G, Tran D *et al.* Neutrophil accumulation in experimental infarcts: relation with extent of injury and effect of reperfusion. Circulation 1987; 75: 1083–92.
33. Klein HH, Pich S, Bohle RM *et al.* Antiinflammatory agent BW 755 C in ischemic reperfused porcine hearts. J Cardiovasc Pharmacol 1988; 12: 338–44.
34. Forman MB, Bingham S, Kopelman HA *et al.* Reduction of infarct size with intracoronary perfluorochemical in a canine preparation of reperfusion. Circulation 1985; 71: 1060–88.
35. Simpson DJ, Todd RF, Fantone JC *et al.* Reduction of experimental canine myocardial reperfusion injury by a monoclonal antibody (anti-Mol, anti-CD 116) that inhibits leukocyte adhesion. J Clin Invest 1988; 81: 624–9.
36. deLorgeril M, Rousseau G, Basmadjian A *et al.* Spacial and temporal profiles of neutrophil accumulation in the reperfused ischemic myocardium. Am J Cardiovasc Pathol 1990; 3: 143–54.

37. Hearse DJ, Bolli R. Reperfusion induced injury: manifestations, mechanisms, and clinical relevance. Cardiovasc Res 1992; 26: 101–8.
38. Kloner RA, Ganote CE, Jennings RB. The "no-reflow" phenomenon after temporary coronary occlusion in the dog. J Clin Invest 1974; 54: 1496–508.
39. Kloner RA, Przyklenk K. Consequences of ischemia-reperfusion on the coronary microvasculature. In Yellon DM, Jennings RB (eds): Myocardial protection: the pathophysiology of reperfusion and reperfusion injury. New York: Raven Press 1992; 85–103.
40. Kloner RA, Alker KJ. The effect of streptokinase on intramyocardial hemorrhage, infarct size, and the no-reflow phenomenon during coronary reperfusion. Circulation 1984; 70: 513–21.
41. Engler R, Schmid-Schonbein GW, Pavelec RS. Leukocyte capillary plugging in myocardial ischemia and reperfusion in the dog. Am J Pathol 1983; 111: 98–111.
42. Engler RL, Dahlgren MD, Morris DD *et al.* Role of leukocytes in response to acute myocardial ischemia and reflow in dogs. Am J Physiol 1986; 251: H314–H322.
43. Ambrosio G, Weisman HF, Mannisi JA *et al.* Progressive impairment of regional myocardial perfusion after initial restoration of postischemic blood flow. Circulation 1989; 80: 1846–61.
44. Reynolds JM, McDonagh PF. Early in reperfusion, leukocytes alter perfused coronary capillarity and vascular resistance. Am J Physiol 1989; 256: H982–H989.
45. Duran WN, Marsicano TH, Anderson RW. Capillary reserve in isometrically contracting dog hearts. Am J Physiol 1977; 232: H276–H281.
46. Kloner RA, Giacomelli F, Alker KJ *et al.* Influx of neutrophils into the walls of large epicardial coronary arteries in response to ischemia/reperfusion. Circulation 1991; 84: 1758–71.
47. Braunwald E, Kloner RA. The stunned myocardium: prolonged postischemic ventricular dysfunction. Circulation 1982; 66: 1146–9.
48. Patel B, Kloner RA, Przyklenk K *et al.* Postischemic myocardial "stunning": a clinically relevant phenomenon. Ann Intern Med 1988; 108: 6627–9.
49. Engler R, Covell JW. Granulocytes cause reperfusion ventricular dysfunction after 15-minute ischemia in the dog. Circ Res 1987; 61: 20–8.
50. Westlin W, Mullane KM. Alleviation of myocardial stunning by leukocyte and platelet depletion. Circulation 1989; 80: 1828–36.
51. O'Neill PG, Charlat ML, Michael LH *et al.* Influence of neutrophil depletion on myocardial function and flow after reversible ischemia. Am J Physiol 1989; 256: H341–H351.
52. Jeremy RW, Becker LC. Neutrophil depletion does not prevent myocardial dysfunction after brief coronary occlusion. J Am Coll Cardiol 1989; 13: 1155–63.
53. Schott RJ, Nao BS, McClanahan TB *et al.* F(ab')2 Fragments of anti-mol (904) monoclonal antibodies do not prevent myocardial stunning. Circ Res 1989; 65: 1112–24.
54. Kuzuya T, Hoshida S, Suzuki K *et al.* Polymorphonuclear leukocyte activity and ventricular arrhythmia in acute myocardial infarction. Am J Cardiol 1988; 62: 868–72.
55. Hammerman H, Kloner RA, Hale SL *et al.* Dose-dependent effects of short term methylprednisolone on myocardial infarct extent, scar formation and ventricular function. Circulation 1983; 68: 446–52.
56. Brown EJ, Kloner RA, Schoen FJ *et al.* Scar thinning due to ibuprofen administration following experimental myocardial infarction. Am J Cardiol 1983; 51: 877–83.

4. Ischemia of the neonatal heart

FLAVIAN M. LUPINETTI

Introduction

In the forty years during which corrective surgical treatment of congenital intracardiac defects has become established, a gradual appreciation has developed for the distinct properties of the neonatal myocardium. Although the dividing lines between 'neonate', 'infant' and 'adult' are necessarily vague, it is clear that from a practical standpoint, profound developmental differences in cardiac physiology and metabolism require particular attention. It is inappropriate for the cardiac surgeon to approach the heart of the neonate as if it is the heart of a small adult. In order to plan appropriate methods of protection, it is first necessary to consider the unique characteristics of the neonatal myocardium both under normal conditions and in the context of global ischemia.

Structural, metabolic and functional characteristics of the neonatal myocardium

Structural and ultrastructural characteristics of the neonatal myocardium

Some of the important characteristics of the neonatal myocardium are very much apparent. The small size of the neonatal heart makes the ratio of surface area to wall thickness far greater than that of the adult heart. This geometry predisposes the neonatal heart to nonuniform rewarming from ambient sources of heat. Histologically, the myocardial cells of the newborn are smaller and contain a greater proportion of noncontractile elements such as nuclei, mitochondria, and membranes, compared to those of the adult [1].

Metabolic characteristics of the neonatal myocardium

Although the mitochondria of the immature heart are smaller and fewer per cell than those of the adult, they have increased activity of cytochrome c oxidase and a higher aerobic capacity. The neonate also has a greater capacity for anerobic glycolysis, and is therefore less dependent on fatty acids as a substrate for energy production. The neonatal myocardium consequently

H.M. Piper and C.J. Preusse (eds): Ischemia-reperfusion in cardiac surgery, 81–103.

displays more abundant glycogen stores than does the mature myocardium. Furthermore, under normal conditions, the neonatal myocardium is able to perform work more efficiently for the volume of oxygen consumed [2].

Jarmakani and colleagues first showed that, compared to older hearts, the neonatal myocardium exhibits greater metabolic tolerance for *hypoxia* – perfusion with nonoxygenated media – as distinguished from *ischemia* – the absence of perfusion [3].These investigators subjected rabbit hearts to isolated perfusion with solutions containing 95% oxygen or 95% nitrogen and studied adenosine triphosphate (ATP) and creatine phosphate (CP) concentrations. The neonate exhibited control levels of ATP even after 30 min of hypoxia, with ATP levels remaining at 74% of control after one hour. ATP in adult myocardium fell to 68% of baseline levels within two minutes of hypoxic perfusion, with a further decline to 39% of control concentrations by one hour. CP content showed parallel changes, with two minutes of hypoxia causing a fall to 55% of control in the neonate and 10% of control in the adult. These data suggest that the metabolism of the neonatal myocardium may allow more tolerance of unfavorable conditions, which may in turn result in more well preserved mechanical function.

Calcium metabolism

Calcium metabolism of the neonatal heart differs in important ways from that of the adult [4]. This is at least partly mediated by the differences in calcium-related organelles. In the neonate, the sarcolemma is the sole regulator of calcium activation of contraction because there is very little sarcoplasmic reticulum, and T-tubules are absent [5]. Evidence of the importance of these organelles is provided by experiments using ryanodine, a substance that interferes with calcium uptake and release by the sarcoplasmic reticulum. In voltage clamp studies, stimulation of adult papillary muscles in the absence of ryanodine leads to an early peak of tension (phasic tension) followed by a plateau (tonic tension). Neonatal papillary muscles demonstrate almost exclusively tonic tension with very little phasic tension. With increasing age, the ratio of phasic to tonic tension rises. Ryanodine causes a profound fall in the phasic tension in the adult papillary muscle, and also a small but significant decrease in phasic tension in newborn papillary muscle. These findings indicate that the excitation-contraction coupling in the neonate is almost completely dependent on membrane depolarization, which directly controls calcium flux across the sarcolemma. With aging, there is increasing dependence on the developing sarcoplasmic reticulum, which in turn accounts for many of the observed differences in neonatal and mature calcium physiology.

This dependence on extracellular calcium also makes the neonatal myocardium more sensitive to changes in the extracellular calcium concentration. The neonatal heart displays a much greater response to exogenously administered calcium than does the adult heart. On the other hand, the magnitude of calcium influx in the presence of a given extracellular calcium concentration is less variable in the neonatal myocardium than it is in older hearts. Because the actions of inotropic agents are mediated largely by their effect on calcium influx, the newborn heart is less sensitive to inotropes. Furthermore, the neonatal heart exhibits a more marked negative inotropic response to calcium channel blockade [6]. The difference in calcium metabolism may also explain the disparate response to stresses. Unlike the adult myocardium which has the capacity for greater functional reserve, the neonatal heart is operating at near maximum levels at all times [1].

The critical nature of calcium concentration may be magnified in the typical isolated heart preparation that is the basis for so many of the observations discussed in this chapter. Most such preparations use a cardiac perfusate based on Krebs-Henseleit bicarbonate buffer with a calcium content of 2.4 mmol/L. This value is based on normal whole blood, however, which contains a number of proteins that bind calcium. As a result of this calcium binding, blood typically has an ionized calcium content of 1.2–1.4 mmol/L. Thus, some crystalloid perfusates used in isolated heart preparations may actually have an ionized calcium concentration that is about twice the true normal value. Calcium adjustment in this experimental model is delicate, as too low a calcium concentration may lead to contractile dysfunction and instability. Contractile function in the isolated neonatal rat heart is optimal with a perfusate that has an ionized calcium concentration of 1.8–2.5 mmol/L [7].

Buffering capacity

It is possible that the neonatal myocardium has a greater buffering capacity proportional to its mass than does the adult myocardium. Although acidosis, either metabolic or respiratory, impairs contractile function in the neonatal myocardium, this reduction is less than that seen in adult myocardium [8].

Functional characteristics of the neonatal myocardium

Some of the aforementioned metabolic features of the neonatal myocardium can predict functional characteristics. Compared to the adult heart, the neonatal myocardium is less compliant. It develops tension more slowly, and exhibits greater coupling of the right and left ventricles. Immature hearts have been shown in clinical studies to have a variable response to expansion of intravascular volume following global ischemia. Burrows and coworkers demonstrated that volume loading of hearts with certain pathologic features may be associated with reduced cardiac index and stroke work index and deterioration of cardiac performance [9]. These changes appeared to be maximal between four and 12 hours after cardiopulmonary bypass, and gradually resolved within 24 hours of operation. The mechanism of this deterioration is unknown, and may be related to changes in compliance, contractility, or both.

As the preceding discussion suggests, most studies addressing developmental differences in cardiac physiology have focused on the ventricles. Differences exist as well, however, between immature and mature hearts with respect to atrial vulnerability. In newborn puppies, the atrium responds to premature extrasystolic stimulation with significantly more repetitive responses than does that of adult dogs or even that of older puppies [10]. This observation may be relevant to the phenomenon of primary reentrant atrial arrhythmias in children, which occur with a much higher frequency than in adults.

Pharmacologic response of the neonatal myocardium

Of particular relevance to considerations of surgical management is the response of the immature heart to a variety of pharmacologic agents. The neonatal response may differ in important ways from that of adult hearts. The effect of anesthetic agents on myocardial performance is one area. In adult hearts, the negative inotropic effect of many inhalational anesthetics is balanced by peripheral vasodilatation, and the net effect on cardiac output is minimal. In neonatal hearts, in contrast, the negative inotropic effect is predominant [11]. This response is not caused by depression of oxidative phosphorylation [12], nor does it appear to be mediated by depression of calcium dependent contractile proteins [13]. The neonatal myocardium does not respond to inotropic agents as does the mature heart muscle. Neonatal hearts stimulated by epinephrine not only exhibit less inotropic response, they also display a degree of epinephrine-induced cardiotoxicity that is seldom observed in the adult myocardium [14]. Digitalis preparations may also elicit unexpected responses in the newborn heart. Especially in the period after global ischemia, digitalis may cause impairment of both systolic and diastolic function [15].

Response of the neonatal myocardium to ischemia

As is true of the mature myocardium, the initiation of global ischemia results in the almost immediate termination of all oxygen-dependent processes. The rapidity with which metabolic events are discontinued is a reflection of the lack of an intracellular oxygen reserve [16]. The minimal quantity of myocardial perfusion contributed by the noncoronary collaterals is entirely inadequate for the continuation of ordinary physiologic processes. The limited noncoronary collateral flow may actually be harmful, in that it may contribute to myocardial rewarming and thereby increase ischemic injury. Although the neonatal heart is capable of anerobic glycolysis to a far greater degree than the adult heart, this may result only in a more rapid accumulation of lactate, a more acidic milieu, and a termination of ATP production that may be as rapid as that observed in the adult [17]. ATP content of the immature myocardium may show a closer correlation to functional status than is observed in adults. Decline of myocardial ATP content to levels less than 40% of pre-ischemic levels has been shown to be associated with impaired ventricular function and an increased risk of death in children undergoing open heart operations [18]. In addition, ischemia causes a buildup of pyruvate. Because pyruvate cannot enter the tricarboxylic acid cycle in the absence of oxygen, it also is converted to lactate. The ability of the cell membranes to maintain ionic gradients is abolished as the cells become rapidly depleted of their high-energy phosphate stores. In turn, there is intracellular calcium influx, cellular edema, and eventually cell lysis.

A number of experimental studies have now established certain principles regarding the ability of the neonatal myocardium to tolerate global ischemia, reperfusion, and the demands of postischemic functional recovery. Perhaps the most important principle is that, in the absence of any protective measures, the neonatal myocardium tolerates ischemia better than the adult myocardium. Yano and associates have shown that this difference persists across a broad spectrum of ischemic durations and over a wide range of ages. Using isolated perfused rat hearts maintained at 37°C, these investigators found that functional recovery was significantly better in neonatal hearts than in either adult or older infant hearts. Furthermore, creatine kinase leakage from the neonatal myocardium was considerably less than that from adult or older infant myocardium [19]. Grice and colleagues, using rabbit hearts, also showed that recovery of left ventricular pressure and developed pressure was much better in neonatal than in adult hearts. Furthermore, they demonstrated that this superiority in recovery of contractile function by the neonatal heart occurred not only with normothermic ischemia and reperfusion, but with hypothermic arrest and warm or cool reperfusion as well [20]. Magovern and colleagues have shown that under normothermic conditions with an equivalent duration of global ischemia in immature and adult isolated rabbit hearts, the younger hearts exhibited significantly greater recovery of cardiac output, arterial pressure, ATP content, and glycogen content [21]. Bove and associates studied the effects of ischemia on the response to volume loading in neonatal and adult hearts. They measured the slope of the curve describing the relationship between left ventricular end-diastolic pressure and percent recovery of left ventricular systolic pressure. They discovered that the slope of this curve in the neonate was not significantly different from zero, indicating an excellent preservation of preload reserve. In the adult heart, however, the slope of this curve did rise significantly above zero, indicating worse recovery [22].

Although the above studies are based on isolated heart models, similar observations have made in intact animals. Julia and coworkers performed a comparison between 10 adult dogs and 10 six- to ten-week-old puppies [23]. Each animal was placed on cardiopulmonary bypass and subjected to 45 minutes of normothermic ischemia. Puppies demonstrated superior functional recovery (85% of stroke-work index vs. 33% in adults) and survival (ten of ten vs. seven of ten in adults). Puppy hearts also had significantly less edema (0.4% weight gain vs. 2% in adults).

Not all investigators agree, however, that the neonatal myocardium shows better tolerance of global ischemia. Wittnich and associates have concluded that the neonatal heart tolerates ischemia less well than does the adult heart. This conclusion was based on subjecting neonatal and adult pig hearts to global ischemia and comparing the duration of ischemia required to achieve ischemic contracture. In this study, neonatal hearts required significantly less time to exhibit ischemic contracture, and also showed more rapid lactate accumulation. Glycogen depletion and decline in ATP content were not significantly different between the two groups, however [24].

In comparing these conflicting views, it seems that the functional studies evaluating recovery after ischemia should be more convincing than those based on the time to ischemic contracture, in essence a measurement of the development of irreversible damage. Therefore, the weight of evidence appears to support the hypothesis that neonatal hearts tolerate ischemia better. This also has the intuitive support of many, if not most, surgeons working in this area, who are familiar with the great latitude that they have in extending ischemic periods in the neonate far beyond those that would be acceptable in adults. There may, however, be a better explanation that reconciles these apparently divergent results. Chiu and Bindon also observed a more rapid time to ischemic contracture in newborn hearts. They sacrificed rats and maintained them at normothermia for varying periods of time before excision of the hearts. They then measured lactate concentration of the excised hearts and found that neonatal hearts had significantly more lactate than adult hearts. They hypothesized that the greater glycolytic capacity of the neonatal myocardium may lead to greater lactate accumulation and a consequently more rapid onset of irreversible tissue damage. The results of this study suggested that providing adequate washout to the ischemic neonatal myocardium could prevent lactate accumulation and thereby negate any disadvantage resulting from increased glycolytic activity [25].

The second generally accepted principle regarding ischemia in the neonatal heart is that under hypothermic conditions, the greater tolerance of ischemia by the neonatal myocardium is further demonstrated. Grice and associates have studied both neonatal and adult rabbit hearts that were given the protective benefits of hypothermia, as is typically the case for cardiac surgery. In this preparation the greater functional recovery of the neonatal myocardium was even more pronounced. The neonatal heart also demonstrates better coronary blood flow than the adult heart under these conditions [20]. Bove and Stammers demonstrated that not only did adult hearts have poorer recovery of postischemic function than did neonatal hearts, but also had significant creatine kinase release which the neonatal hearts did not. This indicated that the adult hearts had greater myocardial injury than the neonatal hearts for the identical duration of ischemia [26].

This superior tolerance of global ischemia by the neonatal myocardium is observed in multiple mammalian species. Although most of the above studies used rat and rabbit hearts, other investigators studying guinea pigs [27], pigs [28], and dogs [23] have made similar observations.

The neonatal heart appears to be more tolerant of variations in pH compared to adult hearts. In adult hearts, it is generally recognized that pH may have a considerable influence on postischemic functional recovery. Indeed, one of the major advances in recent years in the protection of the adult myocardium was the recognition of the importance of an alkalotic pH during hypothermic arrest. The previously standard method of pH control, the alpha stat method, maintained a pH at neutrality during hypothermia. This strategy in effect neglected the change in the ionization constant of water (K_W), which falls during hypothermia. The pH stat approach, on the other hand, uses a more alkalotic pH, typically 7.8, during hypothermia. The pH stat strategy thereby maintains equal concentrations of hydrogen and hydroxide ions. Use of pH stat management, keeping the perfusate pH more alkalotic, has been shown in the adult myocardium to result in better recovery following global ischemia. The neonatal heart, however, can tolerate a wide range of pH during hypothermic perfusion and ischemia with little difference in functional recovery. Eton and colleagues studied isolated neonatal pig hearts subjected to a temperature of 10°C with a pH of 7.0, 7.4, or 7.9. Another group of hearts perfused at a pH of 7.0 was subjected to one hour of ischemia at 10°C. After rewarming to 37°C, all four groups had nearly identical functional recovery, with cardiac outputs 92–95% of baseline measurements. These results suggest that the neonatal myocardium is relatively resistant to tissue damage resulting from extreme changes in pH, at least under hypothermic conditions [29].

The reasons for this greater inherent tolerance of global ischemia have not been completely elucidated. One possible mechanism for increased tolerance of global ischemia by the immature heart is the superior conservation of high-energy phosphate compounds and their precursors. In man, as well as in animals, the immature myocardium exhibits reduced loss of high-energy phosphates for a given degree of global ischemic insult [30,31]. Ischemia result in the breakdown of ATP to adenosine diphosphate (ADP) and adenosine monophosphate (AMP). AMP is further broken down to adenosine, a process that is mediated by 5′-nucleotidase. This last step is of great importance, because adenosine, unlike the phosphated moieties, is freely diffusible and can be rapidly lost from the cell. It is likely that this loss of adenosine delays the repletion of high-energy phosphates following reperfusion, and it is this reduced ability to restore the normal levels of these compounds that may explain impaired functional recovery. Grosso and coworkers have recently shown that the neonatal myocardium has significantly lower 5′-nucleotidase activity than does the adult heart. They also showed that this lower enzymatic activity in the neonate correlated with improved post-ischemic recovery in the isolated perfused heart [32].

The breakdown of nondiffusible nucleosides to diffusible nucleosides may have additional deleterious effect beyond the impairment of replenishing ATP stores. Adenosine is further degraded to hypoxanthine, which is converted by xanthine oxidase into xanthine. A byproduct of this latter reaction is superoxide, a very damaging free radical.

Another possibly protective mechanism in the neonatal heart is its resistance to increased water content following ischemia and reperfusion [26], although other investigators have found that hemodilution in immature hearts is associated with greater edema and a marked decrease in compliance [33].

Response of the neonatal myocardium to reperfusion

In recent years, greater attention has been paid to the conditions of early myocardial reperfusion and the importance of reperfusion injury. Many of the manifestations of cellular injury are unseen in myocardium that has been made ischemic but which has not been reperfused. Only after reperfusion is there clear evidence of cellular swelling and mitochondrial damage [34] and increased intracellular calcium [35]. Reperfusion of the neonatal myocardium with blood that has a normal calcium content may be damaging, especially when the reperfusate is normothermic. Under these conditions, reperfusion is associated with increased cellular injury, as assessed by creatine kinase levels, and worse functional recovery [36].

Reperfusion injury may in large part be mediated by free oxygen radicals that lead to peroxidation of the lipid component of cell membranes and result in damage to myocardial cells already compromised by ischemia. Kohman and Veit measured myocardial malondialdehyde (MDA), which is produced by peroxidation of fatty acids containing three or more double bonds, as a marker of lipid peroxidation. They demonstrated that following global ischemia and reperfusion, adult hearts had significantly higher MDA levels than did neonatal hearts. Reperfusion with the addition of free radical scavengers resulted in a significant decrease in the MDA levels in adult hearts, but did not affect the already low levels in the immature myocardium [37]. Other investigators have reached a diametrically opposite conclusion. It was observed by del Nido and coworkers that neonatal hearts had greater quantities of conjugated dienes after normothermic ischemia and reperfusion than did adult hearts. Conjugated dienes constitute evidence of free radical peroxidation of lipids, including that of the phospholipids that make up the myocyte membranes. This finding indicates that the neonatal myocardium in fact generates more free radicals than adult hearts [38]. These same investigators have demonstrated that conjugated dienes are detectable in the myocardium of children undergoing open heart operations prior to the onset of ischemia, as well as during and after ischemia [39].

If it is the case that free radicals are important mediators of post-reperfusion myocardial damage in the neonate, depletion of leukocytes from the reperfusate blood may ameliorate this damage. This is because leukocytes are thought to be some of the most important producers of superoxide radicals. In some recent animal studies, leukocyte depletion of blood used to reperfuse neonatal hearts subjected to global ischemia resulted in better functional recovery, less ultrastructural damage, and reduced myocardial edema [40].

Characteristics of congenital heart anomalies

From the foregoing, it seems quite logical to expect that the demonstrated tolerance of the immature myocardium for global ischemia in most experimental studies would be paralleled by similar findings in clinical cardiac surgery. In fact, following neonatal open heart procedures there is probably a higher frequency of low cardiac output than there is following cardiac operations on adult patients. The study of Bull and associates found a high frequency of inadequate preservation of the pediatric myocardium, and this was not improved by the methods of myocardial protection available at that time [41].

Some of the characteristics of myocardial ischemia in the neonate arise from the nature of the disorders that require operative correction. Although the *normal* neonatal heart may have excellent functional recovery following moderate periods of ischemia, it does not necessarily follow that the congenitally abnormal heart is equally resistant to ischemic injury. Congenital heart defects may result in pressure and/or volume overload, coronary artery insufficiency, and hypoxemia. These problems may be important in contributing to secondary manifestations such as hypertrophy, chamber dilatation, ischemia, fibrosis, polycythemia, and other results of the primary defect that have their own injurious consequences for the heart. Boucek and associates found abnormal elevations of the creatine kinase MB isoenzyme (CK MB) at the time of cardiac catheterization in patients with a variety of cardiac defects, suggesting the presence of ongoing myocardial injury prior to operative intervention. They found that among patients with left-to-right shunts, the size of the shunt and severity of the symptoms correlated with the magnitude of CK MB. Symptomatic patients with left ventricular pressure overload lesions also had significant elevations of CK MB. Some of the highest CK MB levels were observed in patients with cyanotic heart disease [42].

Operations for congenital heart defects commonly require incision or excision of cardiac muscle, further contributing to myocardial dysfunction. It is evident that studies of ischemia in the normal neonatal heart may be helpful in predicting the myocardial response of patients with congenital heart disease. It must be remembered, however, that the hearts of patients with congenital anomalies often exhibit deranged physiology prior to operation. Present efforts to simulate congenital heart defects with experimental animal models must be considered rather crude and of unproven relevance to clinical abnormalities. Nonetheless, these models appear to provide some useful data that may be far more informative than findings obtained in studies of normal hearts.

Myocardial hypertrophy

Ventricular hypertrophy is a frequent consequence of congenital anomalies in the neonatal heart and may have significant direct and indirect effects that contribute to myocardial injury. Normal hearts, for example, exhibit greater subendocardial than subepicardial blood flow. In animal models of left ventricular hypertrophy, subendocardial flow is not significantly greater than subepicardial flow. This difference is magnified under conditions of heavy exercise. Bache and colleagues subjected to puppies to aortic banding, resulting in left ventricular to body weight ratios 80% greater than that of control animals. At rest, normal dogs exhibited significantly greater subendocardial than subepicardial blood flow, whereas hypertrophied animals' subendocardial flow was not significantly greater than that of the subepicardium. At increasing levels of exercise, the myocardium of control dogs exhibited a slight fall in the ratio of subendocardial to subepicardial flow. In hypertrophied ventricles, exercise caused a significantly lower endo/epi ratio, and subendocardial flow actually fell below that of the subepicardium [43]. This same group demonstrated that rapid cardiac pacing produced an even more profound redistribution of blood away from the subendocardium in the presence of left ventricular hypertrophy, although subendocardial flow is maintained in normal ventricles subjected to rapid pacing [44].

Perhaps in part as a response to this maldistribution of coronary blood flow, chronically hypertrophied left ventricles may have significantly lower ATP and CP content than normal hearts [45–47]. This lower content of high-energy phosphates has been correlated with decreased time to ischemic contracture, indicating a greater susceptibility to ischemic injury [48]. Diminished high energy phosphate content prior to ischemia has been demonstrated in humans with left ventricular hypertrophy as well [49]. Methods of myocardial protection during global ischemia may be less efficacious in the presence of hypertrophy. Hypertrophied ventricles cool more slowly, are depleted of ATP and CP more rapidly, and produce more lactate during ischemia [50].

Hypertrophy of the right ventricle may also have important implications for the neonatal heart. Isolated right ventricular hypertrophy following placement of a pulmonary artery band has been shown to cause secondary changes in the left ventricle, including diminished left ventricular compliance and increased left ventricular mass [51]. Under resting conditions, left ventricular function in the presence of right ventricular hypertrophy may be normal. During exercise, however, a reduced contribution of the ventricular septum may cause regional abnormalities of left ventricular contraction [52]. Right ventricular hypertrophy is also associated with more profound injury to the left ventricle following global ischemia, a phenomenon that may be related to a more accelerated decline in myocardial ATP content [53]. It is controversial, however, whether right ventricular hypertrophy is associated with maldistribution of coronary blood flow, loss of coronary reserve, or myocardial ischemia. Merrill and coinvestigators studied dogs subjected to pulmonary artery banding. They found that total right ventricle perfusion and transmural distribution remained normal both at rest and during stress caused by pacing, left-to-right shunting, and acute aortic constriction [54]. These investigators suggested that a fall in coronary vascular resistance perhaps was important in maintaining adequate myocardial perfusion despite the hypertrophy. This is supported by the study of Archie and colleagues, who observed vasodilatation of the coronary arterial supply of the right ventricle in the presence of hypertrophy [55]. Manohar and coworkers showed that with isoproterenol infusion, however, the right ventricular endo/epi ratio fell to very low levels, whereas this did not occur in the left ventricle of these animals or the right or left ventricles of normal animals [56]. These findings indicate that although the hypertrophied right ventricle can maintain coronary blood flow under resting conditions and under some conditions of stress, this maintenance of coronary perfusion does occur at some cost, and that cost is a loss of coronary reserve that may be manifest by a strong stimulus of vasodilatation.

Cyanosis

Cyanosis is another characteristic of some forms of congenital heart disease that may cause adverse consequences in the neonatal heart subjected to global ischemia. Cyanosis may cause impairment of function even prior to the additional insult of ischemia. Graham and coworkers have observed significant functional impairment in left ventricles of patients with a variety of cyanotic defects. This dysfunction appears to be correlated with the duration of the cyanosis and the degree of left ventricular dilatation that has occurred [57]. Experimental studies of hearts subjected to chronic cyanosis have observed diminished contractile reserve and reduced compliance [58]. Long-term cyanosis also leads to profound abnormalities in the geometric pattern of ventricular contraction [59]. Measurements of lactate production or extraction across the coronary bed have been performed to study the effects of cyanosis at rest and during stress. These studies have found that normal hearts exhibit the same arteriovenous lactate differences at rest or during isoprenaline infusions. In chronic cyanosis, however, an isoprenaline infusion is associated with a physiologic change to net production of lactate, indicating a change to anerobic metabolism under moderate degrees of stress

[60]. Cyanosis has been shown to result in a diminished density of β-adrenergic receptors and concurrent increase in circulating epinephrine [61]. Rabbits raised from birth in a hypoxic environment have exhibited abnormal cardiac rhythm, including tachyarrhythmias, bradyarrhythmias, and conduction defects [62].

Patients with cyanosis typically exhibit myocardial oxygen consumption similar to that of normal individuals. In order to achieve this, the myocardium must become a more efficient extractor of oxygen. This may be limited by coronary blood flow, which may be subject to impairment by additional stresses of inotropic stimulation or exercise [63]. Qualitatively, however, metabolism of myocytes in a cyanotic milieu is normal. When the myocardium of cyanotic individuals is provided with adequate substrate and oxygen, it can demonstrate normal physiologic processes [64].

In neonatal lambs made cyanotic by a pulmonary artery to left atrial shunt, global myocardial ischemia at 15°C was shown to be associated with a significant impairment of recovery of maximum developed pressure in the postischemic period [65]. This study was performed using isolated heart preparations, however. Other studies of *in situ* myocardial function in cyanotic dogs have observed similar impairments in recovery after global ischemia [66, 67]. However, the explanations for the poor recovery in these *in situ* studies were diametrically opposed. Silverman and associates, using a pulmonary artery to left atrium preparation with pulmonary artery banding, found that global ischemia in their cyanotic animals led to a profound depletion of ATP stores, which was not observed in acyanotic animals [66]. Lupinetti and coworkers, in contrast, found that ATP content before, during, and after ischemia were virtually identical in the cyanotic and the control animals [67]. To establish a chronic model of cyanosis, the latter study employed an inferior vena cava to left atrium anastomosis, a preparation that did not lead to ventricular hypertrophy and therefore may not have had the effect on ATP metabolism observed by Silverman's group. It is also possible that abnormalities of myocardial blood flow distribution influenced contractile dysfunction in the inferior vena cava-left atrium preparation.

Polycythemia

Polycythemia, often a secondary effect of cyanosis, may also affect myocardial performance. In part, this may be mediated by the decline in cardiac output that results. Although polycythemia increases blood oxygen carrying capacity, this change is insufficient to balance the fall in blood flow, and systemic oxygen delivery is therefore decreased. Polycythemia causes increased blood viscosity, and although coronary vascular resistance tends to fall, total myocardial blood flow declines significantly. Transmural blood flow distribution tends to be preserved, but subendocardial ischemia occurs during higher perfusion pressures in the polycythemic than in normocythemic states.

It is also possible for polycythemia to have even more adverse affects on myocardial perfusion in the setting of maximal coronary vasodilation [68].

Aortopulmonary shunting

The neonatal circulation may be affected by aortopulmonary shunting arising either as a result of congenital malformations or following surgical creation of a shunt for palliation of structural defects. Such shunting may create additional stresses both by increasing the volume load to the left ventricle and by reducing aortic root pressure, thereby diminishing coronary perfusion. Myocardial oxygen consumption in the presence of an aortopulmonary shunt in awake lambs was shown by Toorop and associates to be approximately twice as much as in the absence of a shunt [69]. This was achieved by a proportional increase in coronary blood flow, because arteriovenous oxygen extraction was similar in shunted and control animals. Experimental work by Fixler and coinvestigators has shown that underperfusion of the subendocardium of the left ventricle by aortopulmonary shunting was primarily mediated by the diminution of diastolic pressure and that the magnitude of the shunt in itself did not affect subendocardial perfusion [70].

Implications for protection of the neonatal myocardium

In the earlier days of cardiac surgery, neonates were candidates only for palliative operations without cardiopulmonary bypass or global ischemia. A thorough understanding of the particular characteristics of the neonatal myocardium has made it possible to undertake corrective surgical treatment, rather than palliation, in this vulnerable group of patients. Palliative operations for some congenital heart defects necessarily expose patients to the risks of two operations rather than one, long term problems related to the palliative procedure itself, and the possibility of patients being lost to follow-up or reevaluation. As a result, the apparently lower risk of a strategy of palliation may actually be be similar to or higher than the risk of primary repair. Aberdeen has calculated that a corrective operation is to be preferred unless a palliative operation offers at least a 10% better survival in that patient at that time [71]. Current methods of management have enabled many corrective operations in the neonate with considerable safety.

Hypothermia

The use of hypothermia is clearly the most protective measure in avoidance of ischemic injury to the neonatal myocardium. In general, the metabolic demands of biological tissues decline by approximately 50% for every 10°C decline in temperature. Hypothermia thus results in improved tolerance of limited oxygen and substrate and greater accumulations of metabolic waste products. Hypothermia may be maintained by combination of systemic cooling, topical use of ice or cold crystalloid solutions, and perfusion of the myocardium with cold cardioplegia solutions. Systemic hypothermia is established with the cardiopulmonary bypass circuit and/or with external sources of cooling such as ice packs or circulating water-filled cooling devices placed on the body. This helps to reduce temperature gradients between the heart and the rest of the body and prevents rewarming of the heart. Topical hypothermia by itself is highly effective in preserving postischemic function in the neonate [72–74]. Chemical arrest with cardioplegia is clearly more effective when given at extremely low temperatures [75]. It is not known what is the optimum temperature for the neonatal myocardium during ischemia. There is evidence that both very low myocardial temperatures (6–10°C) and higher temperatures (exceeding 18°C) are associated with greater ischemic injury to the neonatal heart [76]. There are differences of opinion regarding what is the optimal rate of myocardial cooling prior to arrest. It has been asserted that rapid cooling is potentially harmful and may induce contracture. Hosseinzadeh and associates studied isolated neonatal piglet hearts subjected to global ischemia preceded by rapid or slow cooling to 15°C, both with and without cardioplegic arrest. They found that functional recovery and ATP recovery both were superior with rapid cooling. Furthermore, the detrimental effect of cooling appeared to be related to the duration of cooling rather than the rate [77].

Cardioplegia

Among the controversial areas regarding global ischemia in the neonate is the question of whether cardioplegic solutions provide additional protection. Fujiwara and associates studied isolated neonatal lamb hearts protected with topical hypothermia alone, cold crystalloid cardioplegia, or cold blood cardioplegia. The three groups did not differ with respect to systolic function or diastolic function. These data were interpreted as indicating that hypothermia alone was the dominant factor in post-ischemic recovery, and that cardioplegia, regardless of formulation, was of little or no additional benefit [73]. Ultrastructural studies of the hearts of very young and somewhat older children compared to adults have reached conflicting conclusions regarding the quality of preservation provided by cardioplegia [78,79]. Watanabe and colleagues have gone even further, suggesting that cardioplegia may be deleterious in the neonate. This harmful effect of cardioplegia in the neonatal myocardium may result from the development of contracture following the administration of cardioplegia [27].

This lack of clarity regarding the attributes of cardioplegia is markedly different from the findings in the adult myocardium, which in virtually all studies has shown superior post-ischemic recovery when cardioplegic solutions are administered. Both clinical and experimental studies for the most part support the use of cardioplegia as an adjunct to hypothermia in the protection of the neonatal heart [72, 80–83].

It is possible that the formulation of cardioplegic solutions is more critical in the neonatal heart than it is in the adult. Kempsford and Hearse have shown that St. Thomas' and Tyers solutions contributed to good protection of the neonatal myocardium. Bretschneider and Roe solutions, however, resulted in much less effective protection [84]. Baker and associates, on the other hand, demonstrated that simple Krebs-Henseleit buffer may provide very good myocardial protection and that St. Thomas' solution may be harmful to the neonatal myocardium [74]. In another study, Baker and associates showed that the superior preservation of Krebs solution compared to St. Thomas' solution was not related to differences in oxygen-carrying capacity between the two [85]. It is possible that differences in calcium concentration among these solutions may explain part of the difference in their protective abilities. Zweng and colleagues observed a marked difference in the protective effects of St. Thomas' solution when the calcium concentration was altered. They found that acalcemic solutions were extremely damaging to neonatal hearts, and that the best recovery of function was achieved with a calcium concentration of 1.2 mmol/L [86]. This explanation is disputed by the work of Diaco and colleagues, who found that alterations in sodium and calcium content of cardioplegia have little or no affect on post-ischemic functional recovery [83]. Baker and coinvestigators, on the other hand, have shown that the recovery of neonatal hearts subjected to hypothermic cardioplegic arrest is highly dependent on the calcium content of the perfusate solution. This study demonstrated that optimum functional recovery was obtained with a calcium concentration of 0.3 mmol/L with a gradual decline in functional recovery at higher or lower calcium contents [87].

Some evidence exists that the immature myocardium may be better protected from ischemic injury by the addition of certain other substances to cardioplegic solutions. The addition of red blood cells to crystalloid solutions may permit more oxygen delivery and provide additional buffering capacity. Some evidence exists that the neonatal myocardium does have less ischemic injury when protected by a cardioplegic solution that contains red blood cells than after protection with asanguinous cardioplegia [72]. Appropriate buffering of cardioplegic solutions may result in superior preservation of ATP, better functional recovery, and reduced myocyte necrosis [88]. Buffering with bicarbonate, THAM, and histidine have been described. Calcium channel blockers have been used in both experimental [89] and clinical studies [90] to augment conventional cardioplegic solutions. Calcium channel blockers may provide some benefits in terms of functional recovery and enzymatic assays of myocardial damage. The addition of oxygen to crystalloid cardioplegia appears to have few or no benefits in ameliorating ischemic injury [91]. The efficacy of any of these manipulations of cardioplegic formulations remains unproven at this time.

The importance of methods and frequency of delivery of cardioplegia to the neonatal heart should also be appreciated. Unlike adult hearts subjected to longer periods of ischemia, which appear to be protected better by periodic readministration of cardioplegia, the neonatal myocardium is not protected better by multiple doses of cardioplegia. A recent study in a relatively homogeneous group of patients with long periods of global ischemia failed to show any benefit of readministration of cardioplegia [92]. Other studies have found that multiple dose cardioplegia in the neonate may actually lead to worse structural and functional recovery [93–95]. This phenomenon does not appear to reflect differences in preservation of myocardial ATP content, which is as well maintained by multidose cardioplegia in the neonate as it is in the adult [96]. It has been proposed that this worsened ischemic injury may be an effect of increased permeability of the immature microvasculature and resulting myocardial edema [97]. Another possibility is that temperature differences play a role in this physiology, with multidose cardioplegia more likely to cause damage at very low temperatures [98].

Although cardioplegia is most commonly administered to neonates in an antegrade fashion via aortic root infusion, the capacity for retrograde administration of cardioplegia via the coronary sinus also exists. In the usual course of performing open heart operations in the neonate the right atrium often must be opened. This makes direct cannulation of the coronary sinus quite convenient and free of the complications that are sometimes associated with blind methods of coronary sinus cannulation. This route of cardioplegia administration has been described by Yonenaga and associates in a series of infants undergoing arterial switch repair of transposition of the great arteries.

In this series, coronary sinus cardioplegia was associated with no differences in enzyme indices of myocardial injury or postoperative hemodynamics. These authors suggested that retrograde cardioplegia simplified the operative procedure and provided myocardial protection equal to that of standard methods [99]. Combined antegrade/retrograde cardioplegia has been reported as well [100]. It is as yet unknown whether retrograde cardioplegia has any advantages over antegrade administration in protection of the neonatal myocardium.

Inflow occlusion

Occlusion of the venae cavae to allow the heart to be emptied of blood can be performed to permit very quick intracardiac procedures. This technique is most applicable to aortic or pulmonary valvotomy and is rarely employed beyond the neonatal period. It may in fact be thought of as the closest clinical analogy to experimental preparations subjected to warm unprotected arrest. The advantages of this method were perhaps more compelling when cardiopulmonary bypass technology was less highly developed and when materials used for cannulation of the heart and great vessels were not generally available in sizes appropriate for neonates. Although operations under inflow occlusion require a great deal of expertise, they can be performed effectively and safely by experienced surgeons [101].

Profound hypothermia and circulatory arrest

Profound hypothermia and circulatory arrest have permitted early correction in neonates of certain congenital defects that had previously been approached with initial palliation and subsequent repair [102,103]. In animal studies, very low temperatures are associated with greater times to ischemic contracture, less lactate accumulation, and slower losses of ATP stores [104]. Although most surgeons have found profound hypothermia and circulatory arrest to be a useful addition to their therapeutic armamentarium, some investigators have questioned the safety of this technique. In addition to the long-standing reservations that some individuals have regarding the possibility of cerebral injury, concerns have also arisen regarding the possibility of myocardial injury arising directly as a result of the profound hypothermia itself. Rebeyka and associates have described diminished contractile function and loss of compliance in neonatal hearts subjected to profound cooling prior to cardioplegic arrest. Such deterioration did not occur in hearts maintained at normothermia just prior to cold cardioplegic arrest. They have suggested that this increase in myocardial tension is attributable to elevation of intracellular calcium [105]. Profound hypothermia may also cause accumulation of serum catecholamines during circulatory arrest. These catecholamines may then be released into the circulation when flow is reestablished with the possible production of ventricular arrhythmias [106]. It should be noted, however, that the catecholamine levels fell when the patients became normothermic and were separated from bypass.

Despite these concerns, a large number of surgeons have found deep hypothermia not to be associated with increased myocardial injury, and in fact may provide a critical margin of additional protection [107–109]. Profound hypothermia helps to maintain an optimal myocardial temperature and avoids rewarming from the lungs, liver, and other sources of heat in the local environment. These advantages are particularly important in the neonatal heart, because the higher ratio of ventricular surface area to ventricular mass creates a greater susceptibility to rewarming [28]. The combination of chemical cardioplegia and profound hypothermia have demonstrated improved recovery of function in immature hearts in both experimental and clinical studies [28,81].

There are limits, however, to the degree of hypothermia that can be safely employed. Temperatures of 10°C or less may cause accelerated depletion of ATP and CP. It is hypothesized that temperatures this low may cause injury by abolishing energy producing processes while not providing any further reduction in energy losses than is achievable with more moderate degrees of cooling [110].

Warm induction cardioplegia

Warm cardioplegia, used primarily for induction of cardiac arrest prior to systemic cooling, has recently been advocated as an alternative method of protection by those who have reservations about the safety of deep hypothermia and circulatory arrest. Warm induction cardioplegia has been used by Williams and colleagues, who had observed myocardial contracture occurring during induction of hypothermia during cardiopulmonary bypass. These investigators have described a marked reduction in operative mortality in a large group of neonates with a wide variety of congenital heart abnormalities [111]. Additional clinical and experimental studies will be necessary to substantiate the efficacy of this novel and interesting technique.

References

1. Friedman WF. The intrinsic physiologic properties of the developing heart. Prog Cardiovasc Dis 1972;15: 87–111.
2. Parrish MD, Ayres NA, Kendrick BT *et al.* Maturational differences in the isolated isovolumic rabbit heart. Am J Physiol 1986; 251: H1143–8.
3. Jarmakani JM, Nagatomo T, Nakazawa M *et al.* Effect of hypoxia on myocardial high-energy phosphates in the neonatal mammalian heart. Am J Physiol 1978; 235: H475–H481.
4. Klitzner TS. Maturational changes in excitation-contraction coupling in mammalian myocardium. J Am Coll Cardiol 1991; 17:1218–25.
5. Maylie JG. Excitation-contraction coupling in neonatal and adult myocardium of cat. Am J Physiol 1982; 242: H834–H843.
6. Nishioka K, Nakanishi T, George BL *et al.* The effect of calcium on the inotropy of catecholamine and paired electrical stimulation in the newborn and adult myocardium. J Mol Cell Cardiol 1981; 13: 511–20.
7. Riva E, Hearse DJ. Isolated, perfused neonatal rat heart preparation for studies of calcium and functional stability. Ann Thorac Surg 1991; 52: 987–92.
8. Nakanishi T, Okuda H, Nakazawa M *et al.* Effect of acidosis on contractile function in the newborn rabbit heart. Pediatr Res 1985; 19: 482–8.
9. Burrows FA, Williams WG, Teoh KH *et al.* Myocardial performance after repair of congenital cardiac defects in infants and children. Response to volume loading. J Thorac Cardiovasc Surg 1988; 96: 548– 56.
10. Pickoff AS, Singh S, Flinn CJ *et al.* Atrial vulnerability in the immature canine heart. Am J Cardiol 1985; 55: 1402–6.
11. Boudreaux JP, Schieber RA, Cook DR. Hemodynamic effects of halothane in the newborn piglet. Anesth Analg 1984; 63: 731–7.
12. McAuliffe JJ, Hickey PR. The effect of halothane on the steady-state levels of high-energy phosphates in the neonatal heart. Anesthesiology 1987; 67.1231–5.
13. Krane EJ, Su JY. Comparison of the effects of halothane on skinned myocardial fibers from newborn and adult rabbit. I. Effects on contractile proteins. Anesthesiology 1989; 70: 176–81.
14. Caspi J, Coles JG, Benson LN *et al.* Age-related response to epinephrine-induced myocardial stress. A functional and ultrastructural study. Circulation 1991; 84 (Suppl III) III-394–III-399.

15. Konishi T, Apstein CS. Deleterious effects of digitalis on newborn rabbit myocardium after simulated cardiac surgery. J Thorac Cardiovasc Surg 1991;101: 337–41.
16. Harden WR III, Barlow CH, Simson MB *et al.* Temporal relation between onset of cell anoxia and ischemic contractile failure. Myocardial ischemia and left ventricular failure in the isolated, perfused rabbit heart. Am J Cardiol 1979; 44: 741–6.
17. Coles JG, Watanabe T, Wilson GJ *et al.* Age-related differences in the response to myocardial ischemic stress. J Thorac Cardiovasc Surg 1987; 94: 526–34.
18. Hammon JW Jr, Graham TP Jr, Boucek RJ Jr *et al.* Myocardial adenosine triphosphate content as a measure of metabolic and functional myocardial protection in children undergoing cardiac operation. Ann Thorac Surg 1987; 44: 467–70.
19. Yano Y, Braimbridge MV, Hearse DJ. Protection of the pediatric myocardium. Differential susceptibility to ischemic injury of the neonatal rat heart. J Thorac Cardiovasc Surg 1987; 94: 887–96.
20. Grice WN, Konishi T, Apstein CS. Resistance of neonatal myocardium to injury during normothermic and hypothermic ischemic arrest and reperfusion. Circulation 1987; 76 (Suppl V): V-150–V-155.
21. Magovern JA, Pae WE Jr, Miller CA *et al.* The mature and immature heart: Response to normothermic ischemia. J Surg Res 1989; 46: 366–9.
22. Bove EL, Gallagher KP, Drake DH *et al.* The effect of hypothermic ischemia on recovery of left ventricular function and preload reserve in the neonatal heart. J Thorac Cardiovasc Surg 1988; 95: 814–8.
23. Julia PL, Kofsky ER, Buckberg GD *et al.* Studies of myocardial protection in the immature heart. I. Enhanced tolerance of immature versus adult myocardium to global ischemia with reference to metabolic differences. J Thorac Cardiovasc Surg 1990; 100: 879–87.
24. Wittnich C, Peniston C, Ianuzzo D *et al.* Relative vulnerability of neonatal and adult hearts to ischemic injury. Circulation 1987; 76 (Suppl V): V-156–V-160.
25. Chiu RC-J, Bindon W. Why are newborn hearts vulnerable to global ischemia? The lactate hypothesis. Circulation 1987; 76 (Suppl V): V-146–V-149.
26. Bove EL, Stammers AH. Recovery of left ventricular function after hypothermic global ischemia. Age-related differences in the isolated working rabbit heart. J Thorac Cardiovasc Surg 1986; 91: 115–22.
27. Watanabe H, Yokosawa T, Eguchi S *et al.* Functional and metabolic protection of the neonatal myocardium from ischemia. Insufficient protection by cardioplegia. J Thorac Cardiovasc Surg 1989; 97: 50–58.
28. Ganzel BL, Katzmark SL, Mavroudis C. Myocardial preservation in the neonate. Beneficial effects of cardioplegia and systemic hypothermia on piglets undergoing cardiopulmonary bypass and myocardial ischemia. J Thorac Cardiovasc Surg 1988; 96: 414–22.
29. Eton D, Billingsley AM, Laks H *et al.* Effect of P_{CO2}-adjusted pH on the neonatal heart during hypothermic perfusion and ischemia. J Thorac Cardiovasc Surg 1990; 100: 902–9.
30. Lofland GK, Abd-Elfattah AS, Wyse R *et al.* Myocardial adenine nucleotide metabolism in pediatric patients during hypothermic cardioplegic arrest and normothermic ischemia. Ann Thorac Surg 1989; 47: 663–8.
31. Mask WK Abd-Elfattah AS, Jessen M *et al.* Embryonic versus adult myocardium: adenine nucleotide degradation during ischemia. Ann Thorac Surg 1989; 48: 109–12.
32. Grosso MA, Banerjee A, St. Cyr JA *et al.* Cardiac 5'-nucleotidase activity increases with age and inversely relates to recovery from ischemia. J Thorac Cardiovasc Surg 1992;103: 206–9.
33. Mavroudis C, Ebert PA. Hemodilution causes decreased compliance in puppies. Circulation 1978; 58 (Suppl I): I-155–I-159.
34. Schaper J, Schwarz F, Kittstein H *et al.* The effects of global ischemia and reperfusion on human myocardium: quantitative evaluation by electron microscopic morphometry. Ann Thorac Surg 1982; 33: 116–22.
35. Pridjian AK, Levitsky S, Krukenkamp I *et al.* Intracellular sodium and calcium in the postischemic myocardium. Ann Thorac Surg 1987; 43: 416–9.

36. Hamasaki T, Kuroda H, Mori T. Temperature dependency of calcium- induced reperfusion injury in the isolated rat heart. Ann Thorac Surg 1988; 45: 306–10.
37. Kohman LJ, Veit LJ. Neonatal myocardium resists reperfusion injury. J Surg Res 1991; 51: 133–7.
38. del Nido PJ, Nakamura H, Mickle DAG *et al.* Maturational difference in functional/metabolic sequelae of free radical formation on reperfusion. J Surg Res 1989; 46. 532–6.
39. del Nido PJ, Mickle DAG, Wilson GJ *et al.* Evidence of myocardial free radical injury during elective repair of tetralogy of Fallot. Circulation 1987; 76 (Suppl V): V-174–V-179.
40. Breda MA, Drinkwater DC, Laks H *et al.* Prevention of reperfusion injury in the neonatal heart with leukocyte-depleted blood. J Thorac Cardiovasc Surg 1989; 97: 654–65.
41. Bull C, Cooper J, Stark J. Cardioplegic protection of the child's heart. J Thorac Cardiovasc Surg 1984; 88:, 287–93.
42. Boucek RJ Jr, Kasselberg AG, Boerth RC *et al.* Myocardial injury in infants with congenital heart disease. Evaluation by creatine kinase MB isoenzyme analysis. Am J Cardiol 1982; 50: 129–35.
43. Bache RJ, Vrobel TR, Ring WS *et al.* Regional myocardial blood flow during exercise in dogs with chronic left ventricular hypertrophy. Circ Res 1981; 48: 76–87.
44. Bache RJ, Vrobel TR, Arentzen CE *et al.* Effect of maximal coronary vasodilation on transmural myocardial perfusion during tachycardia in dogs with left ventricular hypertrophy. Circ Res 1981; 49: 742–50.
45. Attarian DE, Jones RN, Currie WD *et al.* Characteristics of chronic left ventricular hypertrophy induced by subcoronary valvular aortic stenosis. I. Myocardial blood flow and metabolism. J Thorac Cardiovasc Surg 1981; 81: 382–8.
46. Attarian DE, Jones RN, Currie WD *et al.* Characteristics of chronic left ventricular hypertrophy induced by subcoronary valvular aortic stenosis. II. Response to ischemia. J Thorac Cardiovasc Surg 1981; 81: 389–95.
47. Peyton RB, Jones RN, Attarian D *et al.* Depressed high-energy phosphate content in hypertrophied ventricles of animal and man. Ann Surg 1982; 196: 278–84.
48. Sink JD, Pellom GL, Currie WD *et al.* Response of hypertrophied myocardium to ischemia. Correlation with biochemical and physiological parameters. J Thorac Cardiovasc Surg 1981; 81: 865–72.
49. Swain JL, Sabina RL, Peyton RB *et al.* Derangements in myocardial purine and pyrimidine nucleotide metabolism in patients with coronary artery disease and left ventricular hypertrophy. Proc Natl Acad Sci USA 1982; 79: 655–9.
50. Rabinov M, Chen XZ, Rosenfeldt FL. Comparison of the metabolic response of the hypertrophic and the normal heart to hypothermic cardioplegia. The effect of temperature. J Thorac Cardiovasc Surg 1989; 97: 43–9.
51. Visner MS, Arentzen CE, Crumbley AJ III *et al.* The effects of pressure-induced right ventricular hypertrophy on left ventricular diastolic properties and dynamic geometry in the conscious dog. Circulation 1986; 74: 410–9.
52. Badke FR. Left ventricular dimensions and function during exercise in dogs with chronic right ventricular pressure overload. Am J Cardiol 1984; 53: 1187–93.
53. del Nido PJ, Benson LN, Mickle DAG *et al.* Impaired left ventricular postischemic function and metabolism in chronic right ventricular hypertrophy. Circulation 1987; 76 (Suppl V): V-168–V-173.
54. Merrill WH, Alexander SL, Conkle DM. Coronary blood flow and distribution in right ventricular hypertrophy. J Thorac Cardiovasc Surg 1981; 82: 365–71.
55. Archie JP, Fixler DE, Ullyot DJ *et al.* Regional myocardial blood flow in lambs with concentric right ventricular hypertrophy. Circ Res 1974; 34: 143–54.
56. Manohar M, Thurmon JC, Tranquilli WJ *et al.* Regional myocardial blood flow and coronary vascular reserve in unanesthetized young calves with severe concentric right ventricular hypertrophy. Circ Res 1981; 48: 785–96.
57. Graham TP Jr, Erath HG Jr, Boucek RJ Jr *et al.* Left ventricular function in cyanotic congenital heart disease. Am J Cardiol 1980; 45: 1231–6.

58. Barragry TP, Blatchford JW, Tuna IC *et al.* Left ventricular dysfunction in a canine model of chronic cyanosis. Surgery 1987; 102: 362–70.
59. Visner MS, Arentzen CE, Ring WS *et al.* Left ventricular dynamic geometry and diastolic mechanics in a model of chronic cyanosis and right ventricular pressure overload. J Thorac Cardiovasc Surg 1981; 81: 347–57.
60. Graham TP Jr, Erath HG Jr, Buckspan GS *et al.* Myocardial anaerobic metabolism during isoprenaline infusion in a cyanotic animal model: possible cause of myocardial dysfunction in cyanotic congenital heart disease. Cardiovasc Res 1979;13: 401–6.
61. Bernstein D, Voss E, Huang S *et al.* Differential regulation of right and left ventricular β-adrenergic receptors in newborn lambs with experimental cyanotic heart disease. J Clin Invest 1990; 85: 68–74.
62. Posner P, Prestwich KN, Buss DD. Cardiac maturation in an hypoxic milieu: Implications for arrhythmias in hypoxemic defects. Pediatr Res 1985;19: 64–66.
63. Scheuer J, Shaver JA, Kroetz FW *et al.* Myocardial metabolism in cyanotic congenital heart disease. Cardiology 1970; 55: 193–210.
64. Friedli B, Haenni B, Moret P *et al.* Myocardial metabolism in cyanotic congenital heart disease studied by arteriovenous differences of lactate, phosphate, and potassium at rest and during atrial pacing. Circulation 1977; 55: 647–52.
65. Fujiwara T, Kurtts T, Anderson W *et al.* Myocardial protection in cyanotic neonatal lambs. J Thorac Cardiovasc Surg 1988; 96: 700–10.
66. Silverman NA, Kohler J, Levitsky S *et al.* Chronic hypoxemia depresses global ventricular function and predisposes to the depletion of high-energy phosphates during cardioplegic arrest: Implications for surgical repair of cyanotic congenital heart defects. Ann Thorac Surg 1984; 37: 304–8.
67. Lupinetti FM, Wareing TH, Huddleston CB *et al.* Pathophysiology of chronic cyanosis in a canine model. Functional and metabolic response to global ischemia. J Thorac Cardiovasc Surg 1985; 90: 291–6.
68. Surjadhana A, Rouleau J, Boerboom L *et al.* Myocardial blood flow and its distribution in anesthetized polycythemic dogs. Circ Res 1978; 43: 619–31.
69. Toorop GP, Hardjowijono R, Dalinghaus M *et al.* Effects of nitroprusside on myocardial blood flow and oxygen consumption in conscious lambs with an aortopulmonary left-to-right shunt. Circulation 1990; 81: 319–24.
70. Fixler DE, Saunders KW, Sugg WL. Subendocardial underperfusion during acute aorticopulmonary shunting in anesthetized dogs. Am Heart J 1974; 87: 483–90.
71. Aberdeen E. The total correction of congenital heart disease in infants. Annu Rev Med 1975; 26: 451–64.
72. Corno AF, Bethencourt DM, Laks H *et al.* Myocardial protection in the neonatal heart. A comparison of topical hypothermia and crystalloid and blood cardioplegic solutions. J Thorac Cardiovasc Surg 1987; 93: 163–72.
73. Fujiwara T, Heinle J, Britton L *et al.* Myocardial preservation in neonatal lambs. Comparison of hypothermia with crystalloid and blood cardioplegia. J Thorac Cardiovasc Surg 1991; 101: 703–12.
74. Baker JE, Boerboom LE, Olinger GN. Age-related changes in the ability of hypothermia and cardioplegia to protect ischemic rabbit myocardium. J Thorac Cardiovasc Surg 1988; 96: 717–24.
75. Takach TJ, Glassman LR, Milewicz AL *et al.* Continuous measurement of intramyocardial pH: relative importance of hypothermia and cardioplegic perfusion pressure and temperature. Ann Thorac Surg 1986; 42: 365–71.
76. Balderman SC, Binette JP, Chan AWK *et al.* The optimal temperature for preservation of the myocardium during global ischemia. Ann Thorac Surg 1983; 35: 605–74
77. Hosseinzadeh T, Tchervenkov CI, Quantz M *et al.* Adverse effect of prearrest hypothermia in immature hearts: Rate versus duration of cooling. Ann Thorac Surg 1992; 53: 464–71.
78. Sawa Y, Matsuda H, Shimazaki Y *et al.* Ultrastructural assessment of the infant myocardium receiving crystalloid cardioplegia. Circulation 1987; 76 (Suppl V): V-141–V-145.

79. Singh AK, Corwin RD, Teplitz C *et al.* Consecutive repair of complex congenital heart disease using hypothermic cardioplegic arrest – its results and ultrastructural study of the myocardium. Thorac Cardiovasc Surg 1984; 32: 23–26.
80. Kyosola K, Chambers D, Cankovic-Darracott S *et al.* St. Thomas' Hospital cardioplegia for myocardial preservation during prolonged aortic cross-clamping. Ann Chir Gynaecol 1985; 74: 111–7.
81. Schachner A, Vladutiu A, Montes M *et al.* Myocardial protection in infant open heart surgery. Scand J Thorac Cardiovasc Surg 1983; 17: 101–7.
82. Avkiran M, Hearse DJ. Protection of the myocardium during global ischemia. Is crystalloid cardioplegia effective in the immature myocardium? J Thorac Cardiovasc Surg 1989; 97: 220–8.
83. Diaco M, DiSesa VJ, Sun S-C *et al.* Cardioplegia for the immature myocardium. A comparative study in the neonatal rabbit. J Thorac Cardiovasc Surg 1990; 100:, 910–3.
84. Kempsford RD, Hearse DJ. Protection of the immature myocardium during global ischemia. A comparison of four clinical cardioplegic solutions in the rabbit heart. J Thorac Cardiovasc Surg 1989; 97: 856–63.
85. Baker JE, Boerboom LE, Olinger GN. Cardioplegia-induced damage to ischemic immature myocardium is independent of oxygen availability. Ann Thorac Surg 1990; 50: 934–9.
86. Zweng TN, Iannettoni MD, Bove EL *et al.* The concentration of calcium in neonatal cardioplegia. Ann Thorac Surg 1990; 50: 262–7.
87. Baker EJ IV, Olinger GN, Baker JE. Calcium content of St. Thomas' II cardioplegic solution damages ischemic immature myocardium. Ann Thorac Surg 1991; 52:1993–9.
88. del Nido PJ, Wilson GJ, Mickle DAG *et al.* The role of cardioplegic solution buffering in myocardial protection. A biochemical and histopathological assessment. J Thorac Cardiovasc Surg 1985; 89: 689–99.
89. Lupinetti FM, Hammon JW Jr, Huddleston CB *et al.* Global ischemia in the immature canine ventricle. Enhanced protective effect of verapamil and potassium. J Thorac Cardiovasc Surg 1984; 87: 213–9.
90. Mori F, Miyamoto M, Tsuboi H *et al.* Clinical trial of nicardipme cardioplegia in pediatric cardiac surgery. Ann Thorac Surg 1990; 49: 413–8.
91. Lynch MJ, Bove EL, Zweng TN *et al.* Protection of the neonatal heart following normothermic ischemia: a comparison of oxygenated saline and oxygenated versus nonoxygenated cardioplegia. Ann Thorac Surg 1988; 45: 650–5.
92. DeLeon SY, Idriss FS, Ilbawi MN *et al.* Comparison of single versus multidose blood cardioplegia in arterial switch procedures. Ann Thorac Surg 1988; 45: 548–53.
93. Magovern JA, Pae WE Jr, Waldhausen JA. Protection of the immature myocardium. An experimental evaluation of topical cooling, single-dose, and multiple-dose administration of St. Thomas' Hospital cardioplegic solution. J Thorac Cardiovasc Surg 1988; 96: 408–13.
94. Magovern JA, Pae WE Jr, Waldhausen JA. Age-related changes in the efficacy of crystalloid cardioplegia. J Surg Res 1991; 51: 229–32.
95. Bove EL, Stammers AH, Gallagher KP. Protection of the neonatal myocardium during hypothermic ischemia. Effect of cardioplegia on left ventricular function in the rabbit. J Thorac Cardiovasc Surg 1987; 94: 115–23.
96. Magovern JA, Pae WE Jr, Miller CA *et al.* The immature and the mature myocardium. Responses to multidose crystalloid cardioplegia. J Thorac Cardiovasc Surg 1988; 95: 618–24.
97. Sawa Y, Matsuda H, Shimazaki Y *et al.* Comparison of single dose versus multiple dose crystalloid cardioplegia in neonate. Experimental study with neonatal rabbits from birth to 2 days of age. J Thorac Cardiovasc Surg 1989; 97: 229–34.
98. Kempsford RD, Hearse DJ. Protection of the immature heart. Temperature-dependent beneficial or detrimental effects of multidose crystalloid cardioplegia in the neonatal rabbit heart. J Thorac Cardiovasc Surg 1990; 99: 269–79.

99. Yonenaga K, Yasui H, Kado H *et al.* Myocardial protection by retrograde cardioplegia in arterial switch operation. Ann Thorac Surg 1990;50: 238–42
100. Drinkwater DC, Laks H, Buckberg GD. A new simplified method of optimizing cardioplegic delivery without right heart isolation. Antegrade/retrograde blood cardioplegia. J Thorac Cardiovasc Surg 1990; 100: 56–63.
101. Sade RM, Crawford FA, Hohn AR. Inflow occlusion for semilunar valve stenosis. Ann Thorac Surg 1982; 33: 570–5.
102. Bove EL, Behrendt DM. Open-heart surgery in the first week of life. Ann Thorac Surg 1980; 29: 130–4.
103. Bender HW Jr, Fisher RD, Walker WE *et al.* Reparative cardiac surgery in infants and small children: Five years experience with profound hypothermia and circulatory arrest. Ann Surg 1979;190: 437–43.
104. Wittnich C, Vincenti W, Salerno TA. Comparison of mild and deep hypothermia: do they provide similar protection in all neonatal hearts? Can J Surg 1991; 34: 317–20.
105. Rebeyka IM, Diaz RJ, Augustine JM *et al.* Effect of rapid cooling contracture on ischemic tolerance in immature myocardium. Circulation 1991; 84 (Suppl III): 389–93.
106. Wood M, Shand DG, Wood AJ. The sympathetic response to profound hypothermia and circulatory arrest in infants. Can Anaesth Soc J 1980; 27: 125–31.
107. Barratt-Boyes BG. Corrective surgery for congenital heart disease in infants with the use of profound hypothermia and circulatory arrest techniques. Aust N Z J Surg 1977; 47: 737–44.
108. Yamaguchi M, Imai M, Ohashi H *et al.* Enhanced myocardial protection by systemic deep hypothermia in children undergoing total correction of tetralogy of Fallot. Ann Thorac Surg 1986; 41: 639–46.
109. Di Eusanio G, Ray SC, Donnelly RJ *et al.* Open heart surgery in first year of life using profound hypothermia (core cooling) and circulatory arrest. Experience with 134 consecutive cases. Br Heart J 1979; 41: 294–300.
110. Kaijser L, Jansson E, Schmidt W *et al.* Myocardial energy depletion during profound hypothermic cardioplegia for cardiac operations. J Thorac Cardiovasc Surg 1985; 90: 896–900.
111. Williams WG, Rebeyka IM, Tibshirani RJ *et al.* Warm induction blood cardioplegia in the infant. A technique to avoid rapid cooling myocardial contracture. J Thorac Cardiovasc Surg 1990; 100: 896–901.

PART TWO

Concepts of cardioplegia

5. Cardioplegia with an intracellular formulation

CLAUS J. PREUSSE

Introduction

Cardioplegia, or myocardial protection – the latter expression is the more precisive one – is a very complex procedure. It is not only the aim to arrest the heart by suppression of its electrical and mechanical activities, that means 'cardioplegia', but to protect the heart against ischemia induced injuries.

In the beginning of cardiac surgery when Melrose firstly reported on a reversible intraoperative cardiac arrest [1] after application of a potassium-enriched, citrate containing solution, one was only interested in a complete, but reversible cardiac arrest. Nowadays since we have studied physiological and biochemical basics on myocardial hypoxia, anoxia, and ischemia (either partial or global) we know that myocardial global ischemia – and that is now the topic – may be influenced not only by the conditions during ischemia, e.g. duration and temperature, but also by the pre-ischemic and post-ischemic period. Therefore it is a logical consequence to distinguish between cardioplegia, that special period of ischemic cardiac arrest and myocardial protection, since the degree of myocardial damage during open heart procedure may be influenced by the pre- and post-ischemic periods, as well.

On principle, an optimized myocardial protective method will act on different sites: energetical, metabolic and morphological ones (Table 5.1).

Related to the energetics it must be emphasized that during anaerobic glycolysis, which is the main source for the heart to produce energy during global ischemia, the rate of energy yield is very poor, since instead of 36 moles at aerobiosis only 2 moles adenosine triphosphate (ATP) per mole glucose are produced [2], respectively the ATP gain is slightly higher if glycogen is degraded (1.5 mol ATP per mole lactate) [3]. Therefore an energetical deficit caused by ischemia is developing with increasing ischemic stress. The ischemic stress, however, resulted from both duration of ischemia and organ temperature during ischemia. Since the myocardial energy demand cannot be met with anaerobic glycolysis alone the energy stores of the arrested heart will be depleted during ischemia [4–6]. The efficiency of the anaerobic glycolysis being defined as quotient from energy gain by lactate production to the degraded amount of energy rich phosphates per time unit is no fixed constant, but a variable factor [4,7] This fact implies that the higher the efficiency of the glycolytic production is, the longer the heart will

H.M. Piper and C.J. Preusse (eds): Ischemia-reperfusion in cardiac surgery, 107–134.

Table 5.1. Sites of action of myocardial protection.

I)	Energetics
	a) Phosphocreatine content and its rate of ischemia induced breakdown
	b) ATP content and its rate of ischemia induced breakdown
	c) Glycogen content and the degree of efficiency of anaerobic glycolysis
II)	Metabolism
	a) Rate of developing intra- and extracellular acidosis
	b) Preventing of formation of toxic metabolites (e.g., free radicals)
	c) Lipid metabolism
III)	Morphology
	a) Cellular structures (e.g. nuclei, membranes, mitochondria)
	b) Myocardial tissues (e.g. atria, ventricles, conducting system)
	c) Coronary vessels and endothelial cells

tolerate ischemia provided that the energy demand is not stimulated to an unexpectedly high extent. The metabolic changes during ischemia are partly caused by the above-mentioned production of lactate by the anaerobic glycolysis. The intracellular production of lactate will consequently lead to an increasing intracellular acidosis that finally will inhibit the glycolysis ('self-inhibition of glycolysis') [4]. Therefore all procedures that will help to delay this self-inhibition will prolong the anaerobic glycolytic energy production. On principle such procedures are: continuous or intermittent ante- and/or retrograde cardioplegic delivery respectively buffering of the cardioplegic solution [8–11]. Such different ways of administering cardioplegic solutions or specially composed solutions counteract the proton induced intra- and extracellular acidosis [12].

The production of oxygen free radicals and their deleterious effects have been detected during reperfusion of the ischemic myocardium ('post-ischemic' period) [13]. However it has not yet been proven whether these metabolic products are indeed of critical causal and consequently of critical clinical importance, because of current methodological insufficiencies [14]. Apart from energetical and metabolic alterations caused by ischemia ultrastructural changes also occur, like swelling of mitochondria, cristolysis, loss of matrix granula [15,16]. These morphological changes do not occur *per se* but there is a close correlation between biochemical and morphological changes during global ischemia [7,17,18].

Principle of the Bretschneider method

Contrary to other methods for intraoperative myocardial protection the Bretschneider solution represents a so-called intracellular type of cardioplegic solution. When Bretschneider firstly published this concept for myocardial protection in 1964 it was a procaine containing, sodium poor, and calcium free, still unbuffered solution [6]. The first clinical applications were performed by Søndergaard at Aarhus in Denmark and by Reidemeister in Cologne [19,20]. Shortly after Bretschneider's first report on this new method for myocardial protection Zimmerman and Hülsmann demonstrated deleterious effects during reperfusion, when hearts had been primarily perfused with a calcium free solution; they called it 'calcium paradox' phenomena [21]. These inferior experimental results principally resemble a problem of any kind of cardioplegic solution, since there may be often mutual effects among the various components (ions) of a cardioplegic solution, which may act on sarcolemnal and/or subcellular sites in an unpredictable way. So it is with the mutual effect of sodium and calcium: a reduction of the extracellular sodium content leads via the transsarcolemmal Na^{+}-Ca^{2+} exchange to an overload of intracellular calcium resulting in an activation of the contractile system, respectively, in an increase of the intracellular energy turnover [7]. The Ca^{2+} paradoxical actions of reperfusion may be prevented if the extracellular sodium is lowered to a cyptoplasmic level according the equation $(Ca^{2+}/Na^{+})^2$ (extracellular concentration!) [22–24]. The effect of a low sodium, calcium-free perfusion bases on a delayed depletion of intracellular calcium via the above mentioned exchange mechanism. The calcium-free perfusion may also delay calcium depletion by promoting calcium re-entry. Thus the overload of intracellular space with calcium will be prevented [25,26]. According to these physiological basics the first Bretschneider solution was calcium-free and the sodium concentration was about 10 mM/l [15], according to the experimentally determined intracellular sodium concentration [27]. The potassium concentration of the solution was slightly elevated to ensure a rapid electrical and mechanical inactivation of the heart intraoperatively, while magnesium was kept at a physiological extracellular level. The main osmotic carrier was mannitol. Additionally, procaine was administered to the solution to 'stabilize' the sarcolemmal membranes during ischemia. The influence of this solution from the pre- and intra-ischemic energy demand will be demonstrated in the corresponding chapters of this article. Roughly ten years later the Bretschneider group succeeded in enhancing the efficiency of the anaerobic glycolysis by adding an effective buffer system to the solution [11]. As already mentioned the enhancement of the anaerobic glycolysis may principally be performed by a continuous washout of produced and accumulated protons or by buffering of cardioplegic solution, being conceptually simplier. However, basic physicochemical aspects have to be considered administering a buffer system to a cardioplegic infusate: the buffer must not be toxic, its concentration should be high, it should neither permeate into the intracellular space nor impair the permeation of lactate and hydrogen ions from the intra- to the extracellular space, its pk value should be suitable with regard to the expected buffer range, and its temperature shift should be equivalent to that one of the neutral point of water. Among many buffer substances the only – natural(!) – buffer that fulfilled the requirements was

Table 5.2. Cardioplegic solution Custodiol® (Bretschneider HTK-solution).

NaCl	15 mM
KCl	9 mM
$MgCl_2$	4 mM
K-Ketoglutarate	1 mM
α-Histidine	180 mM
α-Histidine-HCI	18 mM
Tryptophan	2 mM
Mannitol	30 mM
Osmolarity (measured)	290 mosm/kg H_2O
pH (at 25°C)	7.1
pO_2 (at 37°C)	~210 mm Hg
pCO_2 (at 37°C)	~7 mm Hg

histidine. The pk value is 6.1 at 25°C, it is not toxic, the temperature shift is equivalent to neutral point of water, and it does not impair lactate and proton permeation [3,11]. Consequently procaine had to be eliminated from the solution, since the drug was demonstrated to strongly impair the lactate and hydrogen ion permeation into the extracellular space during ischemia; thus the feasible buffer capacity of the dilated extracellular space could not be used [28]. Theoretically carnosine (alanyl-histidine), also a physiological buffer substance is superior to histidine because its pk value is 6.8 at 25°C. The buffer capacity of carnosine is therefore 2.6-fold higher than that of histidine between pH 7.4 and 6.8 [29]. Although the energetical protection during ischemia was nearly the same compared to protection with histidine buffered solution, however, after reperfusion all hearts completely failed to recover functionally and a tremendous enzyme leakage took place [30].

The histidine concentration of the actual Bretschneider solution (Custodiol®, manufactured by Dr. F. Koehler Chemie GmbH, D-6146 Alsbach) was adjusted to 180 mM/I, since at this buffer concentration an optimal protective efficiency could be detected [7]. Besides the hydrophilic amino acid histidine, tryptophane, an amino acid with an aromatic sidebranch being hydrophobic, was added. Finally in the early eighties ketoglutarate, metabolite of the KREBS cycle, was administered to the solution, so that the total composition is now as listed (Table 5.2). For 15 years this solution has been clinically used in Germany and other European countries while the first application in the United States took place in Minneapolis at the end of 1992 [31].

Cardioplegic delivery

Any method of myocardial protection consists of both, the solution and its mode of delivery. The Bretschneider method is well-known to favour high volume application independent whether the solution was unbuffered or not. Related to an optimized energetical protection, it is a necessary prerequisite that the myocardial stores of energy-rich phosphates (CP, ATP) and glycogen are filled up before the onset of global ischemia. For this reason myocardial O_2 consumption has to be lowered to a very low level, since the Bretschneider group has demonstrated the inverse relationship between O_2 consumption and myocardial content of energy-rich phosphates [15,32]. Consequently it should be the aim of any cardioplegic perfusion to lower the energy turnover as much as possible. Besides this temperature-depending process, it is also a time-consuming one [15,33]. After it has been demonstrated in mongrel dogs that a sufficiently long cardioplegic perfusion of about 9 min with the histidine buffered solution resulted in constantly low values of O_2 consumption of 0.14 ml/min/100 g heart weight at about 12°C, corresponding measurements were performed in human hearts during open heart procedures [34]. Figure 5.1 summarizes the measurements in adults (n = 21) and small children (n = 23) at a mean age of 20.8 months and a mean body weight of 9.2 kg. It is evident that even after 7 min of perfusion the difference between the 'arterial' pO_2 and the pO_2 of the coronary venous effluent has not reached a constantly low plateau. This fact implies the necessity of high volume perfusion to achieve an optimized pre-ischemic energy status, independent from the age of the patient. Since it has often been argued that the delayed reduction of O_2 consumption of these perfused hearts is due to the special fomulation of Custodiol®. Therefore we measured myocardial O_2 consumption in patients who had a transaortic subvalvular myectomie because of a hypertrophic obstructive cardiomyopathy (HOCM). Cardiac arrest was induced by St. Thomas' solution or by Custodiol® (Figure 5.2) [35–37]. The upper panel of this figure illustrates myocardial O_2 consumption being calculated by multiplying of arterial-coronary venous pO_2 difference, flow rate of perfusion, and oxygen solubility [34,37]. Independent from the patient population and the cardioplegic solution applied, myocardial energy turnover was lowered to nearly the same degree. The argument that the reduction is mainly temperature dependent can be countered by the time course of myocardial temperature having reached almost constantly low level after about 4 min. Considering weights of these human hearts to be about 500 g the minimally reached O_2 consumption after 7 min of perfusion is 0.2 ml/min/100 g heart weight. So O_2 consumption of completely inactivated, but perfused human hearts is equivalent to the energy turnover of dog hearts under the same conditions [33].

Equilibration of electrolytes happens during cardioplegic perfusion within 3 to 5 min; as well coronary resistance is maximally lowered within the same period. Cardiac lymph flow could be detected, under experimental condition, during the perfusion period even after the hearts were completely inactivated [33,34,36].

Based on experimental and clinical experiences in more than 6000 patients we recommend high volume cardioplegia according to following data: after

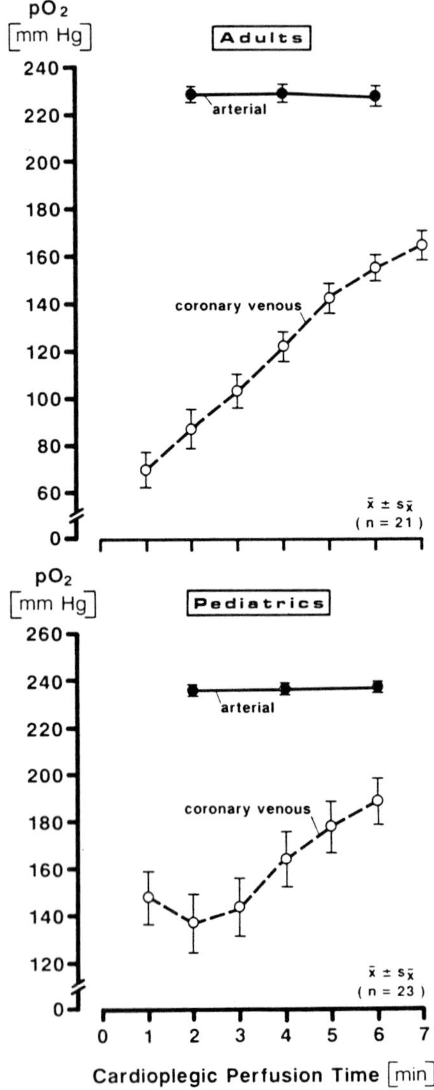

Figure 5.1. Oxygen partial pressure of inflow ('arterial') and of coronary venous effluent ('coronary venous') in adults and children during perfusion with the histidine buffered Bretschneider solution (Custodiol®).

initiation of total cardiac arrest perfusion pressure should be kept at 40–50 mmHg for a period of 7 to 9 min. Hence it follows a perfusion rate of 1 ml/min/g heart weight (estimated) respectively a total amount of 3000 to 4000 ml in adults and 300 to 500 ml in children [38,39]. Such large volumes may keep surgeons using this method, because the large volume cannot be

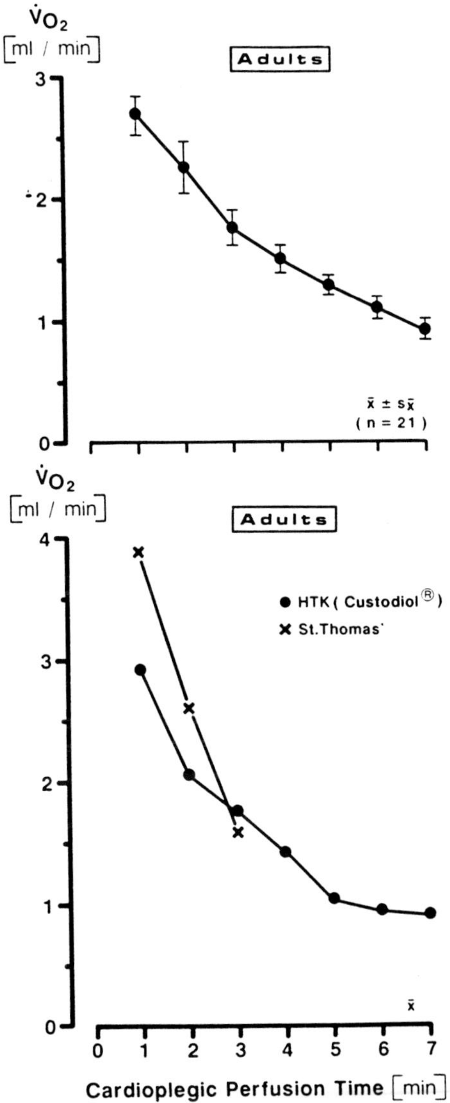

Figure 5.2. Myocardial O_2 consumption of arrested adult human hearts during perfusion with the histidine buffered Bretschneider solution (both panels) and with St. Thomas' solution (lower panel).

used for additional priming of the extracorporeal circulation because of hemodilution, therefore the delivered solution must be rejected after having passed the heart. Consequently this protective method does not allow the use of a double stage venous cannula; therefore we always cannulate the upper and lower caval veins separately [38,39].

It may be criticized that by high volume cardioplegia an unpredictably high blood loss may occur – especially in patients with cyanotic cardiac defects – since the delivered volume must be rejected, otherwise hemodilution by increasing of the prime volume of the heart lung machine is too extreme. We will not neglect that sometimes the autologous blood loss will become a problem, however by using a cell saver system, the problem can be solved. The disadvantage of blood loss during high volume perfusion will be counteracted by the fact that even in patients with long term cardiac arrest of about 180 min, no further cardioplegic perfusion must be performed if no electrical or mechanical ventricular activities are recognized. Using this myocardial protective method, neither additional topical cooling or retrocardial ice jackets, nor intermittent cardioplegic delivery or deeply hypothermic systemic perfusion, is necessary after the single dose high volume application.

The concept of high volume application is not only connected with the Bretschneider method but it has also been proposed by other groups [41,42]. A further argument to deliver large volumes of cardioplegic solution is given by Matsuda and coworkers who have shown, by a clinical study, an inverse relationship between post-ischemic enzyme (CK-MB) loss and delivered solution; the higher the applicated volume per left ventricular mass (LV) the lower the enzyme loss was [43]. However, these interesting results may be misleading with regard to the volume-LV mass relation in pediatrics. In case of very well-vascularized hearts like the neonatal or infant heart, a relatively large volume must be delivered at constant perfusion pressure related to perfusion time and to a standardized unit of heart weight. Since the equilibration procedures are not only volume dependent but also time dependent, small human hearts require higher volumes of solution than relatively less-vascularized adult hearts [33]. This close relationship is experimentally also documented by the Hearse group who demonstrated in rat hearts (small, well-vascularized hearts!) that the entity of both, volume and duration, is necessary to achieve an optimal myocardial protection [44].

Mostly cardioplegic reperfusions are a fixed component of the protective method [for overview see 36]. Contrary to this the histidine buffered Bretschneider solution is only administered initially; a reperfusion with the solution is only necessary if electrical or mechanical (atrial) or ventricular activities are observed even if cardiac arrest exceeds 180 min at moderate systemic temperature, as mentioned above. For cardioplegic reperfusion we recommend a perfusion pressure of about 40 mmHg to deliver about 1 liter of solution, although a higher perfusion pressure for the re-administering of a crystalloid cardioplegic solution has been proposed [45]. Such recommended high perfusion pressures, up to 150 mmHg, bear the risk of evoking an endothelial and/or interstitial edema of the arrested, flaccid heart. Long term perfusion for 60 min, however, with warm Bretschneider solution (25°C) did not injure the myocardium and provided a good functional recovery after delivery was finished [3]. The principle of singledose cardioplegia is of major importance in neonates, because the single dose application provides better myocardial protection in this special patient population [46].

Further details about the specific protocol of the technique of cardioplegic delivery have been published previously by Schulte and Preusse [37–40].

Protection during ischemia

Energetical rationale

It is an objective that myocardium is not able to cover its energy demand during anaerobiosis, so that with progression of ischemia time – to be scientificly exact one should speak of ischemic stress being the entity of both, time of ischemia and temperature during ischemia – an increasing energetical deficit will develop [3–6,12,47,49]. Adenosine triphosphate (ATP) and creatine phosphate (CP) are parameters to evaluate the developing energy deficit. Consequently the efficiency of any method for myocardial protection is in very close relation to its influence on the energy-rich phosphate depletion during ischemia.

The German physiologist Schneider has defined three phases that the ischemic heart muscle passes before it is irreversibly damaged [50]. After cross-clamping of the aorta, the first one is called latency time ('Latenzzeit'), which will last for seconds at normothermia. This period is characterized by the fact that the function is not yet impaired because only the oxygen reserves will be depleted within this period. If intramyocardial O_2 partial pressure (pO_2) is decreased up to 5 mmHg, the next period will start: the period, during which the function will exponentially decrease until it is completely exhausted. Together with the latency time this period is called survival time ('Überlebenszeit'). The period until myocardium is irreversibly damage – including the survival time – is called resuscitation time ('Wiederbelebungszeit') [6,50]. Resuscitation time may be separated into two parts, 'theoretical' and 'practical', as will be shown. Except the latency time, a biochemical rationale may be correlated to all other periods. It could be demonstrated experimentally that survival time is finished if myocardial phosphocreatine content is lowered to 3 μmol/g heart wet weight [6]. However, the mentioned separation of the resuscitation time bases on clinical aspects, because the 'practical' resuscitation time is reached, if it only takes 20 to 30 min after declamping of the aorta to be weaned from extracorporeal bypass. According to Bretschneider such a rapid post-ischemic metabolic, functional and ultrastructural recovery will be achieved if the myocardial ATP content is only depleted up to 4 μmol/g; the limit of the practical resuscitation time is reached [6,15]. The ATP threshold to be equivalent for the 'theoretical' limit of resuscitation (1–2 μmol/g heart wet weight) has been described for ischemic dog myocardium and ischemic rat hearts, among others [4,51,52]. However it is questionable whether an absolute threshold of the reversibility in cellular ATP contents exists [53].

Myocardial survival time varies in dependence of the ionic composition of the cardioplegic solution [3,7,54]. Calcium-poor, magnesium-free solutions cause a significantly higher myocardial phosphate content after 60 min of global ischemia. The phosphate accumulation could be mainly attributed to the decay of CP, since ATP hydrolysis was nearly the same compared to a control group being protected with a calcium-poor, magnesium-rich solution [55]. Survival time was significantly shortened after application of the Kirklin solution, which is a magnesium-free solution compared to other cardioplegic solutions [3,7,54]. The significance of phosphate was pointed out by Kübler and Katz, when they reported on pathophysiological mechanisms of the early myocardial pump failure [49].

It is quite evident that the protection of the heart with Custodiol® leads to a prolongation of both the survival and the resuscitation time compared to a purely ischemic heart (Figure 5.3). The critical level of CP (3 μmol/g) is reached within a few minutes in the ischemia group, while it takes 75 min in the cardioplegically protected group; these data are valid for 25°C. At 15° and 35°C – myocardial temperatures during cardioplegic arrest – the corresponding data are: 170 min and 35 min. Following these data the Q_{10} values for the survival time are 2.3 between 15° and 25°C and 2.1 between 25° and 35°C. Finally, it should be noted that the CP content at the onset of ischemia is much higher in the Custodiol®-group caused by high volume delivery, by which the myocardial energy reserve will be optimized.

It is a striking fact that the rate of ATP decay is much smaller in the Custodiol®-group than in the other group, because the 'critical' ATP content of 4 μmol/g heart wet weight is reached after 280 min compared to about 50 min in the other group.

The reduced anaerobic myocardial energy turnover always leads to a decrease of velocity of the decay of energy-rich phosphates and to a diminished lactate production. Consequently myocardial acidosis will develop slower even if an unbuffered cardioplegic solution is applied (see also Figure 5.4). It is obvious that lactate production starts much later in the Custodiol® group than in the 'ischemia' group. This fact indirectly indicates myocardial energy turnover to be higher in the 'ischemia' group at onset of ischemia. With continuing time of ischemia, lactate is produced at the same rate in both groups. Thus the anaerobic energy production of the electrically and mechanically arrested, nonperfused heart differs from that of the anoxicly perfused heart, since at the onset of ischemia less energy is produced and the rate of energy production is almost independent from myocardial ATP content [4,7,56].

The improvement of the energetical protection after use of the buffered Bretschneider solution is graphically shown in Figure 5.4, in which the time courses of various metabolites (CP, ATP, lactate) during pure ischemia, during cardiac arrest with Custodiol® and – additionally – during cardiac

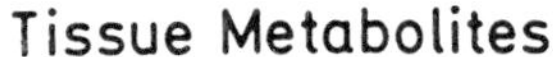

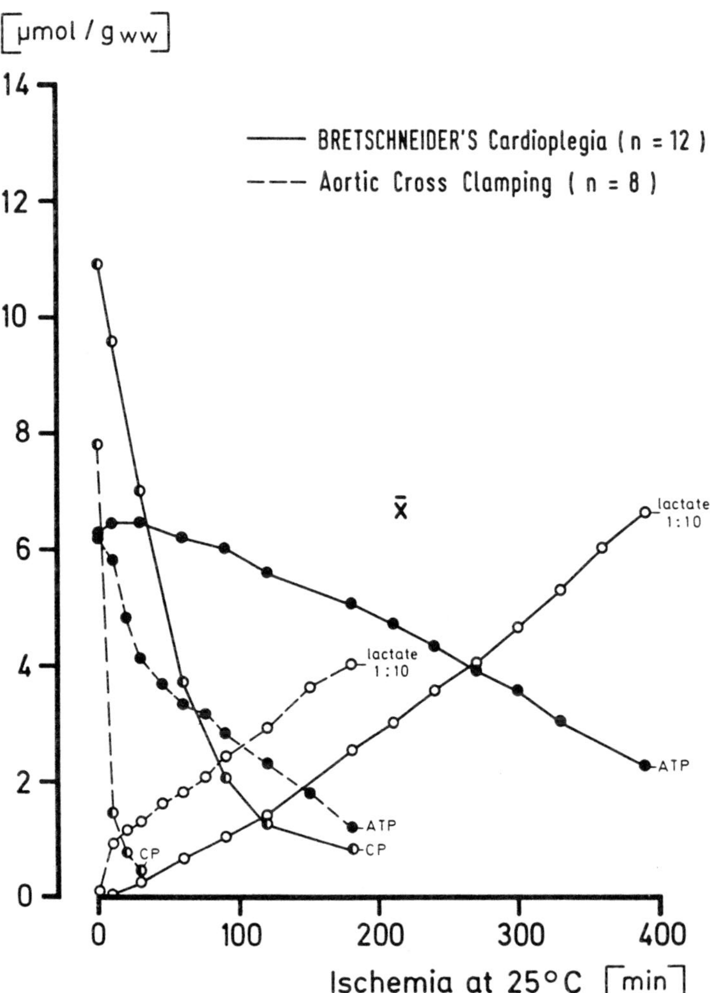

Figure 5.3. Myocardial-CP-, ATP-, and lactate contents during purely ischemic cardiac arrest and during cardiac arrest induced by the histidine buffered Bretschneider solution (Custodiol®). Myocardial temperature was constantly kept at 25°C.

arrest with the unbuffered, procaine-containing Bretschneider solution (middle panel) are listed. The buffer additive has not only lead to prolongation of the survival time but also the resuscitation time was extended, however, to a different degree. This might be a further indirect indication for a myocardial compartmentation of ATP and CP [57].

The application of the amino acid buffered Bretschneider solution leads to a prolongation of the resuscitation time at all temperature ranges. It will

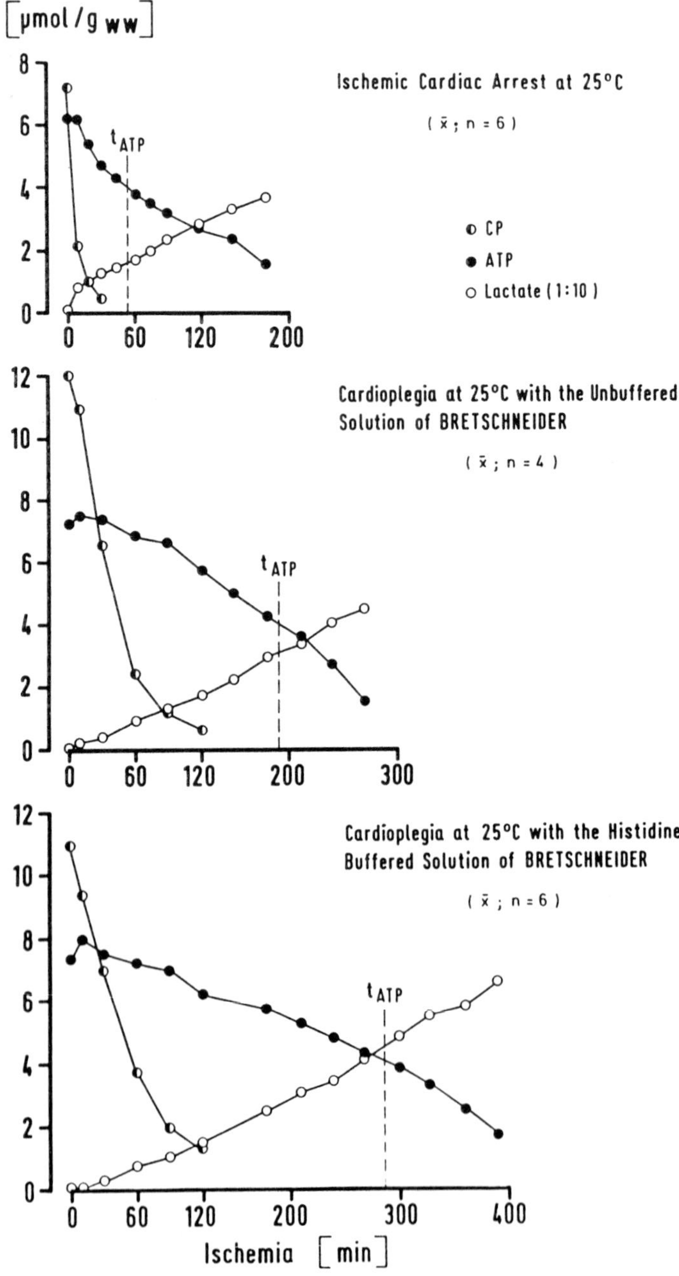

Figure 5.4. Myocardial CP-, ATP-, and lactate contents during purely ischemic cardiac arrest (upper panel), during protection with unbuffered, procaine containing Bretschneider solution (middle panel), and during protection with the histidine buffered Bretschneider solution (Custodiol®) (lower panel). Myocardial temperature was constantly kept at 25°C. Additionally the limit of the 'practical resuscitation time' is listed (for further details see text).

last for about 500 min at 15°C, 280 min at 25°C and 95 min at 35°C. By these data the following Q_{10} values may be calculated: 15° to 25°C 1.8, 25° to 35°C 2.9. So, it should be noted that there is no linear shortening of the resuscitation time with increasing temperature, because the enhancement of myocardial energy turnover gets higher than the anaerobic energy gain by glycolysis. Recent investigations into improvement of myocardial protection have confirmed Bretschneider's concept of a buffered solution, since a formulation with enriched branch chain amino acids as additives to a crystalloid solution leads to a post-ischemic enhancement of ATP and CP in rat hearts [58,59].

The efficiency of the anaerobic glycolysis, being the ratio energy production versus energy turnover during ischemia, was enhanced from 65–70% to about 85% if the histidine was used in the solution [3,4]. As an explanation, two possibilities may exist to improve the energetical status during ischemia: either by reduction of the total energy turnover or by optimization of the efficiency of the anaerobic glycolysis. Up to now it remains unclear which cellular processes may regulate the efficiency of the anaerobic glycolysis and how the histidine buffered solution interferes.

From the cardiac surgeon's point of view intra-ischemic biochemical changes at 25°C are the most important ones, since myocardial temperature during open heart procedure is at least lowered to that range. Therefore, some left ventricular biochemical changes of the nucleotide metabolism and of anaerobic glycolysis at 25°C are graphically presented in Figure 5.5. The products of ATP hydrolysis, ADP and AMP, are transiently enhanced shortly after the onset of ischemia, but during the following anaerobic period they remain at a nearly constant level. These findings are contrary to results published by Spieckermann and Isselhard, who had performed their investigations on purely ischemic canine hearts or on potassium arrested guinea pig hearts [16,60].

Glycogen content is distinctly diminished with increased ischemic stress. However, it must be pointed out that anaerobic glycolysis was never limited by too low a myocardial glycogen concentration. Therefore there is not need to enhance glycogen stores, provided that they are not exhausted by special pathological conditions [60–62]. The addition of ketoglutarate to the histidine buffered solution has not produced significant changes of the anaerobic nucleotide metabolism under experimental conditions.

Buffering rationale

During myocardial ischemia, energy gain is closely linked to lactate production obtained from anaerobic glycolysis. To prevent the inhibition of anaerobic glycolysis by lactate two possibilities principally exist [4,64]: continuous or intermittent coronary perfusion or to use an effective buffer system in the extracellular space. During ischemia, 2 protons will be produced per 2 molecules of lactate; these hydrogen ions originate either from the ATP hydrolysis or from substrate level phosphorylation [63].

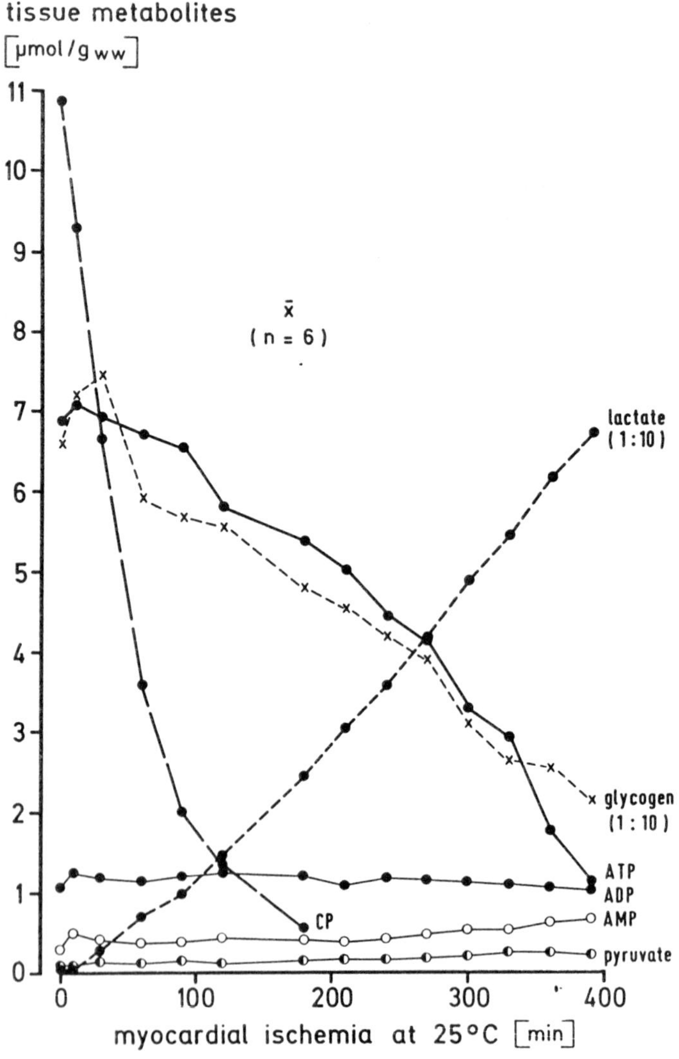

Figure 5.5. Myocardial tissue content of different metabolites of anaerobic glycolysis and of energy rich phosphates during cardiac arrest induced by the histidine buffered Bretschneider solution (Custodiol®) at 25°C.

Continuous washout of accumulated hydrogen ions and an effective buffering will enhance the efficiency of the anaerobic glycolysis to about 85% [3,7,64]. From a practical point of view, the continuous (or intermittent) coronary perfusion during open heart procedures (e.g., valve replacement) is often troublesome, so that the most elegant way to prevent an early intraischemic acidosis is by the enhancement of the myocardial buffer capacity.

The intracellular acidosis caused by ischemic is principally influenced by 'cellular' or 'extracellular' components [65]. The 'cellular' component may be varied by: (a) intensity of proton accumulation; (b) intracellular buffer capacity; (c) K^+ or Na^+/H^+ exchange; (d) membrane permeability for hydrogen ions. The 'extracellular' component depends on: (a) volume of the extracellular space (dilated coronary system!); (b) extracellular buffer capacity. An enhancement of the intracellular buffer capacity might be achieved by an extended perfusion with an almost carbon-dioxide-free cardioplegic solution that will wash out the well-diffusible CO_2 from the extra- and intracellular space [33]. Membrane permeability for hydrogen ions, however, might be inhibited by special anaesthetic drugs with antiarrhythmic properties, like procaine [3,47]. Therefore procaine was eliminated from the histidine buffered solution, because otherwise the adjusted extracellular buffer capacity might not be totally used.

The buffering of myocardial protective solutions and consequently of the ischemic myocardium is conceptually simple, but special aspects of its application make the way of solution difficult. One of the basic assumptions for optimal buffering are the physico-chemical properties (solubility, pK value) and the concentration of the buffer in the solution. It is quite obvious that all cardioplegic solutions with an extracellular formulation – sodium-rich (!) – only have a small osmotic margin to use buffer substances if the solution shall not become hyperosmotic. Contrary to this, all solutions based on an intracellular formulation might be buffered at a high concentration. Consequently the latter ones do have the higher buffer capacity. So, it is with the buffered Bretschneider solution, in which histidine concentration is 180 mM/l. The Bretschneider group could impressively demonstrate an excellent correlation between the buffer capacity of various cardioplegic solutions and the period until an interstitial pH of 6.0 was reached [24]. The pH value of 6.0 was chosen, since phosphofructokinase, the enzyme playing a key role with anaerobic glycolysis, is almost inactivated at that pH value [4]. To avoid an intracellular edema, 'artificial' buffer substances may only be restricted to the extracellular, or vascular, space because the permeation of the buffer into the intracellular space will result in a cellular uptake of water. So the principal restriction of the buffer to the vascular space implies that any enhancement of buffer capacity of the solution by an increase of buffer concentration may only lead to a partial increase of the tissue buffer capacity, since the volume of the myocardial capillary space is 0.5 to 1.0% of total cardiac volume [7,66]. Consequently it is therefore important that the vascular space is completely dilated. Time course of coronary resistance during cardioplegic perfusion indirectly indicates an enlargement of the vascular space with the consequence of an enhanced tissue buffer capacity [34,40]. High volume delivery is again a prerequisite for this enlargement!

The Bretschneider solution (Custodiol®) is adjusted to a pH of 7.1 at 25°C and so fully compensates the 'Rahn effect' [67]. Buckberg's blood cardioplegia is adjusted to pH range from 7.5 to 7.7 depending on warm induction of multidose cardioplegia [9]. It is still a controversial discussion whether to adjust the initial pH of cardioplegic perfusate or to combat the subsequent acidosis. High buffer concentrations and an optimal pK value of the buffer itself are main factors for effectively combating ischemia induced acidosis. Although pK value of carnosine is more ideal (6.8 at 25°C) than histidine (6.1 at 25°C) related to cardiac surgery, it totally failed to improve myocardial protection [24,29,30]. The buffering efficiency of the Bretschneider solution is presented in Figure 5.6. Canine hearts were protected with various myocardial protective methods and the interstitial pH was continuously measured in the ventricular septum by pH glass electrodes [65]. The pH value being reported to be critical limit has been additionally marked (dotted line). If pH values of the myocardial interstice are related to the 'practical' limit of resuscitation time (ATP 4 μmol/g) the corresponding pH values differ depending on the formulation of the cardioplegic solution [65].

Contrary to all other cardioplegic solutions after application of the buffered Bretschneider solution, interstitial pH decreases slowest within the pH range from 7.0 to 6.5, indicating a high buffering efficiency. This pH range is of clinical significance during open heart procedures in hypertrophied human hearts [69]. It may be argued that intra-ischemic lactate, or proton, production is delayed after application of the buffered Bretschneider solution resulting in less acidotic pH values. However, lactate production per time during cardiac arrest was not decreased [7] and secondly the buffering power of the solution was proven if the interstitial pH values of the particular groups (see Figure 5.6) were referred to defined myocardial lactate contents. The differences were striking ($p < 0.001$) indicating the buffering efficiency of the Bretschneider solution [65]. The buffering effect of the Bretschneider solution was confirmed by Tait and coworkers who conducted an experimental study to assess the effect of multidose infusion of various solutions. Only multidose blood cardioplegia and multidose Bretschneider solution prevented a progressive development of myocardial acidosis [70]. In conclusion, it may be confirmed that the buffering power of the histidine buffer is equivalent to that of blood or myocardial tissue [71,72]. However, improvement of myocardial protection and post-ischemic recovery may only be achieved if high potassium concentrations and a high pH level of the solution are avoided [72]. Custodiol® does fulfil all these requirements.

Ultrastructural changes

The close relationship between energy metabolism and ultrastructural changes during ischemia has been demonstrated by various studies [7,15,16,18,73]. After onset of anaerobiosis at first mitochondrial granula disappear; these morphological alterations occur during survival time (CP 3 μmol/g). Afterwards mitochondrial swelling, interstitial and intracellular edema, cristolysis can be analyzed up to the theoretical limit of resuscitation time. Yet these correlations are not valid for each myocardial protective

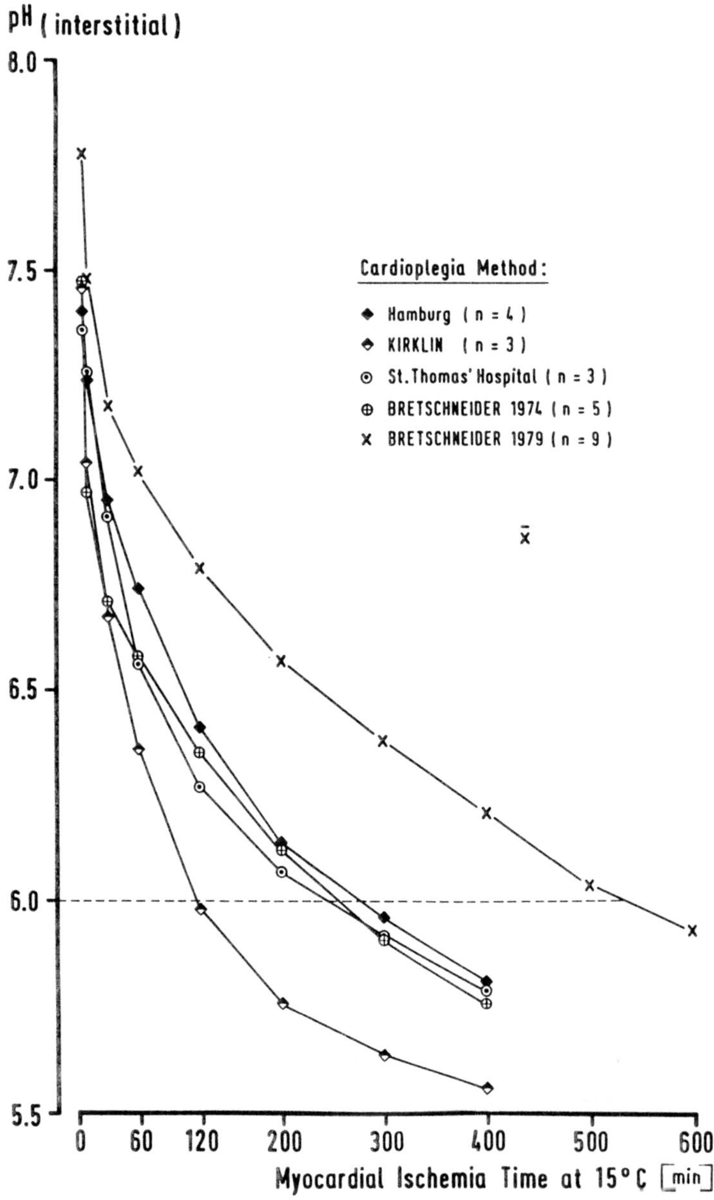

Figure 5.6. Interstitial myocardial pH in canine hearts during cardiac arrest induced by various myocardial protective methods. The Bretschneider solution of 1974 is unbuffered and procaine containing, while that one of 1979 is histidine buffered (Custodiol®). Myocardial temperature was constantly kept at 15C.

method. So every myocardial protective concept may not only be evaluated by its influence on energy preservation but also on ultrastructure, since morphological changes at a defined ATP content (4 μmol/g) differ greatly [7]. Carnosine protected hearts showed an excellent preservation of ATP, but an extremely poor ultrastructural protection [3]. Since post-ischemic recovery completely failed it may be concluded that a poor structural protection coincides with a poor functional recovery under certain circumstances [7]. Schnabel and coworkers could detect that the degree of progression of morphological alterations during ischemia does distinctly vary depending on the myocardial protective method applied [18]. They emphasized that after application of a procaine-containing, magnesium-enriched solution, an intracellular edema develops shortly after the onset of ischemia which progressively increases, while during protection with a magnesium-free, potassium-enriched crystalloid solution an endothelial edema of the capillaries is more pronounced. These alterations were always related to the same – reduced – myocardial ATP content. After application of Custodiol® the ultrastructural alterations also occur, but to a much smaller degree. Contraction bands that occur in the subendocardial layer during pure ischemia – aortic cross clamping at deep hypothermia (25°C) – could be completely prevented by Custodiol® [74]. Cellular and mitochondrial swelling in Purkinje fibres following ischemia (30 min at 25°C) protected by the buffered Bretschneider solution remain moderate [75]. Not only during short-term ischemia but also during long-term cardiac arrest of 240 min at 25°C, the ultrastructure of the myocardium was well protected by the Bretschneider solution. Although mitochondria were swollen and had lost granules some matrix material, the contractile system, and intercalated discs seem to be intact and glycogen granula were still present [76].

The clinical experiences with morphology of ischemic human hearts confirm the experimental ones although the way of cardioplegic delivery of Custodiol® seems to be responsible for different degrees of tissue injury [77]. The morphological alterations in neonatal animal hearts have demonstrated an improved protection if single dose application(!) was used and if an intracellular type solution at pH 7.0 was administered [78,79]. These experimental results confirm Bretschneider's concept and give advice that Custodiol® can be applied in human neonates as well as in adults [80].

Post-ischemic reperfusion

Post-ischemic reperfusion is generally determined by an unmasking of damages developed and caused by ischemia and by specific reperfusion injuries [2,53,81]. The excellent studies by the Buckberg group detected that the post-ischemic damage could be reduced by a specially modified reperfusion before declamping of the aorta [2,82]. Oxygen-free radicals are considered to injure myocardial cells in the early post-ischemic reperfusion period [83].

Although this effect is still controversially discussed, free radical scavengers have been tested to improve myocardial function post-ischemically [53,84]. Blood cardioplegic solutions containing their own endogenous-free radical scavengers were superior to crystalloid cardioplegic solutions. If free radical scavengers were added to the crystalloid cardioplegic reperfusate, cardiac function could be improved [84]. The composition of the Bretschneider solution avoids the risk of injury by oxygen-free radicals since after onset of post-ischemic reperfusion the vascular space is still filled with the histidine solution and histidine is known to be a free radical scavenger. After histidine solution is washed out, blood-own endogenous scavengers will continue protection.

Besides the relationship between post-ischemic myocardial and morphological damages, a close relationship between myocardial energy status and post-ischemic function also exists [3,7,39]. The delayed ATP hydrolysis during ischemia protected by Custodiol® causes higher myocardial ATP contents, after defined ischemic stress, compared to other cardioplegic methods [7,39,54]. After various periods of ischemia up to 300 min with a subsequent post-ischemic reperfusion of 20 min ATP concentrations of canine hearts protected by the Bretschneider solution were distinctly higher – up to 2 μmol/g – compared to other cardioplegic methods [39,54]. However it should be considered that reperfusion was carried out with a modified, crystalloid Tyrode solution. Cardiopulmonary bypass as being practiced routinely in open heart surgery was not used in animal experiments.

The excellent energetical preservation after use of the buffered Bretschneider solution also leads to a faster replenishment of energy stores, although it should be kept in mind that ATP resynthesis is biphasic [85,861]. The fast period which lasts for only minutes is determined by regeneration of ATP from ADP and AMP, while the slow regeneration lasts for hours and days. Herewith, for ATP resynthesis, nucleosides like adenosine, inosine and hypoxanthine are used. During ischemia and during the early post-ischemic reperfusion these nucleosides are washed out since they may permeate cellular membranes. So the less ATP is hydrolysed during ischemia – as it is with Custodiol® protected hearts – the less ATP stores must be replenished post-ischemically. Furthermore it follows that post-ischemic functional recovery is superior if adenine nucleotides are well preserved [87–89].

Myocardial metabolism recovered rapidly after long term cardiac arrest induced by the histidine buffered solution. Re-uptake of lactate could be measured under experimental conditions within 10 min of reperfusion after 210-min-arrest [90]. After cardiac arrest of 300 min (22–24°C storage temperature) protected by the buffered solution, myocardial O_2 consumption was 6.2 ml O_2/min/100 g heart wet weight during the early reperfusion period. To determine the O_2 consumption per beat, basic energy demand of 0.8 ml/min/100 g was subtracted [3]; so after 21 min of reperfusion the actual O_2 consumption per beat of the empty beating hearts was 0.045 ml/100 g/beat [91].

Table 5.3. Reasons of increased post-ischemic coronary resistance.

I)	Vascular component
	a) Endothelial swelling
	b) Vascular tone or spasm
	c) Vasomotorial dysfunction
	d) Beguiling of diastolic period per minute
II)	Myocardial component
	a) Interstitial edema
	b) Intracellular edema
	c) Impaired diastolic relaxation
	d) Regional contractures

Coronary resistance slightly increased during this period of post-ischemic reperfusion [91]. An increased post-ischemic coronary resistance may be induced by several 'vascular' or 'myocardial' reasons (Table 5.3). According to the ultrastructural investigations of Schnabel *et al.*, the slightly elevated coronary resistance may be attributed to a moderate edema of myocytes and capillary endothelia that occurs during cardioplegic arrest with Custodiol®, but that diminishes rapidly during reperfusion [18]. However a marked increase of post-ischemic coronary resistance was never analyzed as reported by Toshima *et al.*, who also had tested the functional recovery of rat hearts being protected by an intracellular-type of cardioplegic solution (Collins solution), in advance [92]. The disadvantageous post-ischemic coronary vasoconstriction in these experiments may be attributed to the extremely high K^+ concentration (117 mM/l) in that solution. The different outcome of post-ischemic myocardial function after protection with 'intracellular' types of cardioplegic solutions demand a specific differentiation to evaluate the protective properties of any cardioplegic solution.

Clinical aspects

The clinical evaluation of the histidine buffered Bretschneider solution (Custodiol®) must consider its pre-ischemic delivery, its intra-ischemic efficiency and the post-ischemic myocardial recovery.

Pre-ischemic delivery is determined by high volume application, characteristic of the Bretschneider method. Although blood loss during cardioplegic perfusion is disadvantageous, the method is favoured by a large number of German cardio-surgical units, since further reperfusions with the solution at certain intervals can be renounced if no atrial or ventricular activities of the heart occur. In our unit such reperfusions must be performed in about 20% of patients [38,39]. Principally, cardioplegic reperfusions bear the risk of washing out traces of bivalent ions, since with progressive ischemia their protein bindings become looser due to myocardial acidosis (see also Figure 5.6). Such loss of bivalent ions will destabilize membranes.

Oxygenation of Custodiol® is unnecessary since myocardial energy demand of the arrested heart is so low that the O_2 content of the solution will cover the oxygen requirements completely. Hence possible deleterious effects of oxygenation will be avoided [93]. Nearly all myocardial protective methods require reperfusion at certain intervals to keep the hearts at a low temperature level. This is not valid for the Bretschneider method since its protective properties will tolerate extended durations of ischemia at moderate hypothermia [38,39,94]. Topical cooling or ice jackets need not be used, except a wet pad placed at the anterior ventricular wall to avoid an exsiccation. Furthermore, temperature measurements, e.g. septal probes, must not be carried out during ischemia.

Although experimental investigations with multidose infusion of the buffered Bretschneider solution have confirmed the excellent preservation of high energy phosphates during long-term storage of donor hearts for transplantation (up to 24 h at 0.5°C),the clinical experiences give evidence not to exceed 4 hours for cold storage [68,95,96]. Recently cardiac re-transplantation of an already transplanted heart has been performed within a very short period using Custodiol® for myocardial protection [97].

To avoid pressure-induced injury of the still-arrested and flaccid heart at the beginning of post-ischemic reperfusion we always perform a way of 'controlled' reperfusion: shortly before declamping of the aorta the systemic perfusion pressure is reduced to 40 mmHg; afterwards the aorta is declamped, while this normothermic low pressure perfusion is kept on for two more minutes before pressure is raised to about 80 mmHg. Metabolic recovery of Custodiol® protected hearts of all age groups happens within 20 min after declamping of the aorta so far that these hearts came off the pump after 20 to 30 min [38]. Figure 5.7 summarizes our metabolic investigations in adults with valve replacements and small children (mean age 20.9 months, mean body weight 9.2 kg). During the first 20 min after declamping of the aorta, simultaneous analyses of arterial and coronary venous lactate concentrations were carried out. With these results we established a re-uptake of lactate in both groups after equivalent ischemic stress [80]. Post-operative inotropic drug support may serve as particular parameter to evaluate the protective efficiency of the Bretschneider method. In a special patient population of 169 patients with acquired heart disease – patients with selective coronary bypass grafting were excluded – who had cardiac arrest either of more than 120 or 150 min, inotropic support (e.g., dobutamine) was given postoperatively in 5.7% (>120 min) or 10.3% (>150 min) (unpublished data).

Post-ischemic or post-operative dysrhythmias may not only be caused by ischemia induced injuries but also by the cardioplegic solution applied. After use of Custodiol® we often observe delayed AV-conduction (atrio ventricular block I°/II°) during the first post-operative hours. However, these

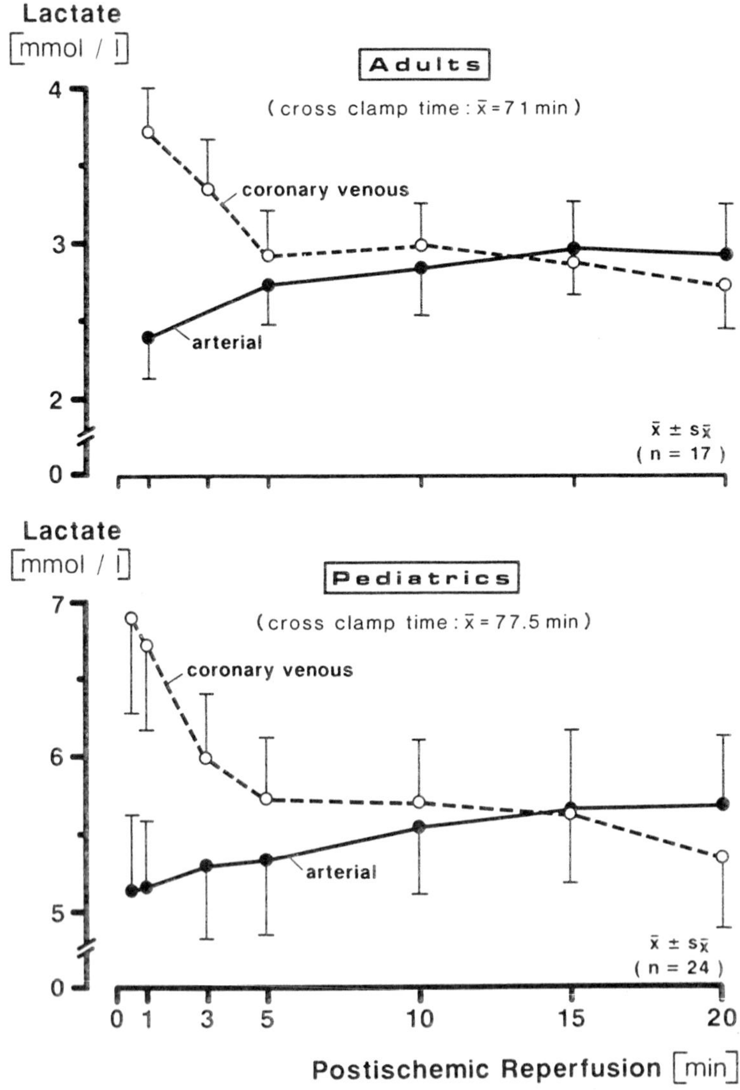

Figure 5.7. Arterial and coronary venous post-ischemic lactate contents in adults and pediatrics after declamping of the aorta. For intraoperative myocardial protection the histidine buffered Bretschneider solution (Custodiol®) was used.

dysrhythmias nearly always disappear within the first post-operative day [39]. Special clinical reports on post-ischemic myocardial rhythm after Bretschneider cardioplegia gave no evidence for long lasting solution induced dysrhythmias [98,99].

Comparative experimental studies with Bretschneider solution and Roe solution detected a better intra-ischemic ATP preservation and a superior functional recovery of canine hearts protected by the Bretschneider method [100]. Clinical studies with different methods for myocardial protection in patients with coronary artery bypass grafting (CABG) have shown no statistically different results between blood cardioplegia and Bretschneider's method [101]. However, unfortunately, the number of patients was too small and the demographic data differed.

In final conclusion, the intracellular approach of the histidine buffered Bretschneider solution causes a good myocardial protection against ischemia – and reperfusion(!) – induced damages in open heart surgery, provided the method is correctly applied. In the meantime the clinical use has been extended to other organs [102].

Within the previous decades, intraoperative myocardial protection in cardiac surgery has been decisively improved, however, it still remains a challenge for experimental and clinical research, since further still unclear metabolic and functional myocardial conditions being previously detected, e.g. stunning, or special cardiac emergency situations, e.g. induced by failed coronary angioplasties, also require optimal intra- and post-ischemic protection [103].

References

1. Melrose DG, Dreyer B, Bentall HH *et al.* Elective cardiac arrest: preliminary communication. Lancet II 1955; 269: 21–2.
2. Buckberg GD. When is cardiac muscle damaged irreversibly? J Thorac Cardiovasc Surg 1986; 92: 483–7.
3. Bretschneider HJ, Gebhard MM, Preusse CJ. Reviewing the pros and cons of myocardial preservation within cardiac surgery. In Longmore DB (ed): Towards safer cardiac surgery. Lancaster: MTP Press Ltd 1981; 21–53.
4. Kübler W, Spieckermann PG. Regulation of glycolysis in the ischemic and anoxic myocardium. J Mol Cell Cardiol 1970; 11: 351–9.
5. Levitsky S, Feinberg H. Biochemical changes of ischemia. Ann Thorac Surg 1975; 20: 21–9.
6. Bretschneider HJ. Überlebenszeit und Wiederbelebungszeit des Herzens bei Normo- und Hypothermie. Verhandl Dtsch Ges Kreislaufforschg 1964; 30: 11–34.
7. Gebhard MM. Pathophysiologie der globalen Ischämie des Herzens. Z Kardiol (Suppl. 4) 1987; 76: 115–29.
8. Menasche P, Subay J, Piwnica A. Retrograde coronary sinus cardioplegia for aortic valve operations: a clinical report on 500 patients. Ann Thorac Surg 1990; 49: 556–64.
9. Buckberg GD. Antegrade/retrograde blood cardioplegia to ensure cardioplegic distribution: operative techniques and objectives. J Card Surg 1989; 4: 216–238.
10. Salerno TA, Christakis GT, Pannos AJ *et al.* Technique and pitfalls of retrograde continuous warm blood cardioplegia. Ann Thorac Surg 1991; 51: 1023–5.
11. Bretschneider HJ, Preusse CJ, Kahles H *et al.* Further improvement in artificial cardiac arrest with subsequent anaerobiosis by combination of various parameters. Pflügers Arch Ges Physiol 1975; 359: R13.
12. Wechsler AS, Abd-Elfattah AS, Murphey CE *et al.* Myocardial protection. J Card Surg 1986; 1: 271–306.

13. Garlick PB, Davies MJ, Slater TS *et al.* Detection of free radical production in the isolated rat heart using a spin trap agent and electron spin resonance. Cir Res 1987; 61: 757–60.
14. Baker JE, Felix CC, Olinger GN *et al.* Myocardial ischemia and reperfusion: Direct evidence for free radical generation by electron spin resonance spectroscopy. Proc Natl Acad Sci USA 1988; 85: 2786–9.
15. Bretschneider HJ, Hübner G, Knoll D *et al.* Myocardial resistance and tolerance to ischemia: Physiological and biochemical basis. J Cardiovasc Surg 1975; 16: 241–60.
16. Spieckermann PG. Überlebens- und Wiederbelebungszeit des Herzens. Berlin-Heidelberg: Springer 1973; 66–72.
17. Schaper J, Mulch J, Bretschneider HJ *et al.* Correlation between morphological and biochemical changes in induced myocardial ischemia for cardiac surgery. In Isselhard W. (ed): Myocardial protection for cardiovascular surgery. Köln: Pharmazeutische Verlagsgesellschaft 1979; 160–9.
18. Schnabel PA, Gebhard MM, Pomykaj T *et al.* Myocardial protection: Left ventricular ultrastructure after different forms of cardiac arrest. Thorac Cardiovasc Surgeon 1987; 35: 148–56.
19. Søndergaard T, Senn A. Klinische Erfahrungen in der Kardioplegie nach Bretschneider. Langenbecks Arch Klin Chir 1967; 3 1 9: 661–5.
20. Reidemeister JC, Heberer G, Gehl H *et al.* Klinische Ergebnisse mit der Kardioplegie durch extrazellulären Natrium- und Calcium-Entzug und Procaingabe. Langenbecks Arch Klin Chir 1967; 319: 701–7.
21. Zimmerman ANE, Hülsmann WC. Paradoxical influence of calcium ions on the permeability of the cell membranes of the isolated rat heart. Nature 1966; 211: 646–7.
22. Noble D. The initiation of the heart beat. Oxford: Clarendon 1979.
23. Langer GA. Sodium: calcium exchange in the heart. Ann Rev Physiol 1982; 44: 431–49.
24. Bretschneider HJ, Gebhard MM, Preusse CJ. Cardioplegia. Principles and problems. In Sperelakis N (ed): Physiology and Pathophysiology of the Heart. Boston: Martinus Nijhoff 1984; 605–16.
25. Dhalla NS, Alto LE, Signal PK. Role of Na^+-Ca^{2+} exchange in the development of cardiac abnormalities due to the calcium paradox. Eur Heart J 1983; 4 (Suppl H): 51–6.
26. Reuter H, Seitz N. The dependence of Ca efflux from cardiac muscle on temperature and external ionic composition. J Physiol 1968; 195: 451–70.
27. Orellano LE, Grebe D, Bretschneider HJ. Fortlaufende Messung der Kalium- und Natriumverluste des Myokards während eines Herzstillstandes durch Koronarperfusion mit natriumarmen, calciumfreien, procainhaltigen, sauerstoffgesättigten kardioplegischen Lösungen. Arch Kreisl Forsch 1967; 53: 264–307.
28. Preusse CJ, Bretschneider HJ, Kahles H *et al.* Use of myocardial extracellular space for prolongation of ischemia tolerance of the heart by variation of myocardial permeability and extracellular buffer capacity. Pflügers Arch Ges Physiol 1976; 365: R3.
29. Gercken G, Bischoff, Trotz M. Effects of carnosine-buffered cardioplegic solutions and different substrates on myocardial metabolism and protection. In Isselhard W (ed): Myocardial protection for Cardiovascular surgery. Koln: Pharmazeutische Verlagsgesellschaft 1979; 170–81.
30. Preusse CJ, Gebhard MM, Bretschneider HJ. Ischemia tolerance and post-ischemic recovery of the heart after use of carnosine and histidine buffered cardioplegic solutions. Pflügers Arch Ges Physiol 1981; 389: R1.
31. Molina E 1992; (personal communication).
32. Kübler W, Grebe D, Orellano LW *et al.* Zur Bewertung des Gewebsgehaltes der energiereichen Phosphate für die Pathogenese der akuten Herzinsuffizienz. In Reindell H, Keul J, Doll E (eds): Herzinsuffizienz: Pathophysiologie und Klinik. Stuttgart: Thieme, 1968: 226–31.
33. Preusse CJ, Gebhard MM, Bretschneider HJ. Myocardial "Equilibration Processes" and myocardial energy turnover during initiation of artificial cardiac arrest with cardioplegic

solution – reasons for a sufficiently long cardioplegic perfusion. Thorac Cardiovasc Surgeon 1981; 29: 71–6.
34. Preusse CJ, Winter J, Schulte HD *et al.* Energy demand of cardioplegically perfused human hearts. J Cardiovasc Surg 1985; 26: 558–63.
35. Braimbridge MV. Equipment for inducing cold cardioplegic arrest. J Thorac Cardiovasc Surg 1979; 77: 323–4.
36. Hearse DJ, Braimbridge MV, Jynge P. Protection of the ischemic myocardium: cardioplegia. New York: Raven Press, 1981: 353–74.
37. Preusse CJ, Schulte HD, Bircks W. High volume cardioplegia. Ann Chir Gynaecol 1987; 76: 39–45.
38. Schulte HD, Preusse CJ, Groschopp C *et al.* Crystalloid cardioplegia – Experience with the Bretschneider solution. In Engelman RM, Levitsky S (eds): A Textbook of Clinical Cardioplegia. New York: Futura Publ Comp, 1982: 199–210.
39. Preusse CJ, Schulte HD. Cardioplegia for Repeat Valve Surgery. In Engelman RM, Levitsky S (eds): A Textbook of Cardioplegia for Difficult Clinical Problems. New York: Futura Publ Comp, 1992: 203–19.
40. Preusse CJ, Winter J, Gebhard MM *et al.* Myocardial equilibration procedures with high-volume cardioplegia. Thai J Surg. 1986; 7: 165–8.
41. Engelman RM, Rousou JH, Lemeshow S. High-volume cardioplegia. J Thorac Cardiovasc Surg 1983; 86: 87–96.
42. Landymore RW, Marble AE, Eng P *et al.* Effect of high-volume cardioplegia on small-amplitude electrical activity during cardioplegic arrest. Eur J Cardiovasc Surg 1991; 5: 395–9.
43. Matsuda H, Maeda S, Hirose HJ *et al.* Optimum dose of cold potassium cardioplegia for patients with chronic aortic valve disease: Determination by left ventricular mass. Ann Thorac Surg 1986; 41: 22–6.
44. Takahashi A, Chambers DJ, Braimbridge MV *et al.* Cardioplegia: relation of myocardial protection to infusion volume and duration. Eur J Cardiovasc Surg 1989; 3: 150–3.
45. Johnson RE, Dorsey LM, Moye SL *et al.* Cardioplegic infusion. J Thorac Cardiovasc Surg 1982; 83: 813–23.
46. Sawa Y, Matsuda H, Shimazaki Y *et al.* Comparison of single dose versus multiple dose crystalloid cardioplegia in neonate. J Thorac Cardiovasc Surg 1989; 97: 229–34.
47. Buckberg GD. A proposed "solution" to the cardioplegic controversy. J Thorac Cardiovasc Surg 1979, 77: 803–15.
48. Feinberg A, Levitsky S. Biochemical rationale of cardioplegia. In Engelman RM, Levitsky S (eds): A textbook of clinical cardioplegia. New York: Futura Publ. Comp 1982: 131–7.
49. Kübler W, Katz A. Mechanism of early "pump" failure of the ischemic heart: Possible role of adenosine triphosphate depletion and inorganic phosphate accumulation. Am J Cardiol 1977; 40: 467–71.
50. Schneider M. Über die Wiederbelebung nach Kreislaufunterbrechung. Thoraxchirurgie 1958; 6: 95–108.
51. Jennings RB, Hawkins HK, Lowe JE *et al.* Relation between high energy phosphate and lethal injury in myocardial ischemia in the dog. Am J Pathol 1978; 92: 187–241.
52. Taegtmeyer H, Roberts AFC, Raine AEG. Energy metabolism in reperfused heart muscle: metabolic correlates to return of function. J Am Coll Cardiol 1985; 6: 864–70.
53. Piper HM. Energy deficiency, calcium overload or oxidative stress: Possible causes of irreversible ischemic myocardial injury. Klin Wochenschr 1989; 67: 465–76.
54. Preusse CJ, Bretschneider HJ, Gebhard MM. Comparison of cardioplegic methods of Kirklin, Bretschneider, and St. Thomas' Hospital by means of biochemical and functional analyses during post-ischemic aerobic recovery period. In Isselhard W (ed): Myocardial protection for Cardiovascular surgery. Köln: Pharmazeutische Verlagsgesellschaft 1979: 184–93.
55. Pernot AC, Ingwall JS, Menasche P *et al.* A P-31 nuclear magnetic resonance evaluation

of various cardioplegic solutions. Langenbecks Arch Klin Chir, Suppl Chir Forum 1981; 364: 51–4.
56. Neely JR, Grotyohann LW. Role of glycolytic products in damage to ischemic myocardium: dissociation of adenosine triphosphate levels and recovery of function of reperfused ischemic hearts. Circ Res 1984; 55: 816–24.
57. Gudbjarnason S, Mathes P, Ravens KG. Functional compartmentation of ATP and CP in heart muscle. J Mol Cell Cardiol 1970;1: 325–30.
58. Schwalb H, Izhar U, Yaroslavsky E *et al.* The effect of amino acids on the ischemic hearts. J Thorac Cardiovasc Surg 1989; 98: 551–6.
59. Schwalb H, Kushnir T, Navon G *et al.* The protective effect of enriched branch chain amino acids formulation in the ischemic heart: A phosphorous – 31 nuclear magnetic resonance study. J Mol Cell Cardiol 1987; 19: 991–8.
60. Isselhard W. Maßnahmen zur Verbesserung der Erholung des Herzens nach Anaerobiose. Langenbecks Arch Klin Chir 1967; 319: 665–75.
61. Conn HL, Wood JC, Morales GS. Rate of change in myocardial glycogen and lactic acid following arrest of coronary circulation. Circ Res 1959; 7: 721–7.
62. Hearse DJ, Stewart DA, Braimbridge MV. Myocardial protection during bypass and arrest. J Thorac Cardiovasc Surg 1976; 72: 880–4.
63. Hochachka PW, Guppy M. Metabolic arrest and control of biological time. Cambridge, Massachusetts, London: Haward University Press, 1987.
64. Kübler W, Spieckermann PG. Changes in myocardial glycolysis and in high energy phosphates during ischemia with intermittent coronary perfusion. Cardiologie 1971; 100–7.
65. Preusse CJ, Gebhard MM, Bretschneider HJ. Interstitial pH value in the myocardium as indicator of ischemic stress of cardioplegically arrested hearts. Basic Res Cardiol 1982; 77: 372–87.
66. Bretschneider HJ. Myocardial protection. Thorac Cardiovasc Surgeon 1980; 28: 295–302.
67. Rahn H, Reeves RB, Howell BJ. Hydrogen ion regulation, temperature and evolution. Am Rev Resp Dis 1975; 112: 165–72.
68. Krug A. Alteration in myocardial hydrogen ion concentration after temporary occlusion: A sign of irreversible damage. Am J Cardiol 1975; 36: 214–7.
69. Khuri SF, Warner KG, Josa M *et al.* The superiority of continuous cold blood cardioplegia in the metabolic protection of the hypertrophied human heart. J Thorac Cardiovasc Surg 1988; 95: 442–54.
70. Tait GA, Booker PD, Wilson GJ *et al.* Effect of multidose cardioplegia and cardioplegic solution buffering on myocardial tissue acidosis. J Thorac Cardiovasc Surg 1982; 83: 824–9.
71. Kresh YJ, Natala C, Bianchi PC *et al.* The relative buffering power of cardioplegic solutions. J Thorac Cardiovasc Surg 1987; 93: 309–11.
72. del Nido PJ, Wilson GJ, Mickle DA *et al.* The role of cardioplegic buffering in myocardial protection. J Thorac Cardiovasc Surg 1985; 89: 689–99.
73. Schaper J, Mulch J, Winkler B *et al.* Ultrastructural, functional, and biochemical criteria for estimation of reversibility of ischemic injury. A study on the effects of global ischemia on the isolated dog heart. J Mol Cell Cardiol 1979; 11: 521–41.
74. Schnabel PA, Schmiedl A, Ramsauer B *et al.* Occurrence and prevention of contraction bands in Purkinje fibres, transitional cells and working myocardium during global ischemia. Virchows Archiv A Pathol Anat 1990; 417: 463–71.
75. Schnabel PA, Richter J, Schmiedl A *et al.* The ultrastructural effects of global ischemia on Purkinje fibres compared with working myocardium: a qualitative and morphometric investigation on the canine heart. Virchows Archiv A Pathol Anat 1991; 418: 17–25.
76. Gebhard MM, Bretschneider HJ, Gersing E *et al.* Bretschneider's histidine-buffered cardioplegic solution: Concept, application, and efficiency. In Roberts AJ (ed): Myocardial protection in cardiac surgery. New York-Basel: Marcel Dekker, 1987: 95–119.
77. Schaper J, Walter P, Scheld H *et al.* The effects of retrograde perfusion of cardioplegic solution in cardiac operations. J Thorac Cardiovasc Surg 1985; 90: 882–7.

78. Breda MA, Drinkwater DC, Laks H *et al.* Improved neonatal heart preservation with an intracellular cardioplegia and storage solution. J Surg Res 1989; 47: 212–9.
79. Sawa Y, Matsuda H, Shimazaki Y *et al.* Comparison of single dose versus multiple dose crystalloid cardioplegia in neonate. J Thorac Cardiovasc Surg 1989; 97: 229–34.
80. Preusse CJ, Kocherscheidt K, Krian A *et al.* Post-ischemic metabolism of infant hearts following either ischemic or cardioplegic arrest. In Crupi G, Parenzan L, Anderson RH (eds): Perspectives in Pediatric Cardiology Vol 2. Mount Kisco: Futura 1990: 223–6.
81. Hearse DJ, Braimbridge MV, Jynge P. Protection of the ischemic myocardium: cardioplegia. New York: Raven Press, 1981: 329–38.
82. Follette DM, Fey K, Buckberg GD *et al.* Reducing post-ischemic damage by temporary modification of reperfusate calcium potassium, pH, and osmolarity. J Thorac Cardiovasc Surg 1981; 82: 221–38.
83. Ferrari R, Ceconi C, Cureelo S *et al.* Oxygen free radicals and reperfusion injury: the effect of ischemia and reperfusion on the cellular ability to neutralise oxygen toxicity. J Mol Cell Cardiol 1986; 18: 67–9.
84. Julia PL, Buckberg GD, Acar C *et al.* Studies of controlled reperfusion after ischemia. J Thorac Cardiovasc Surg 1991; 101: 303–13.
85. Isselhard W, Mäurer W, Stremmel WJ *et al.* Stoffwechsel des Kaninchenherzens in situ während Asphyxie und in der post-asphyktischen Erholung. Pflügers Arch Ges Physiol 1970; 316: 164–93.
86. Isselhard W, Schorn B, Hügel W *et al.* Comparison of three methods of myocardial protection. Thorac Cardiovasc Surgeon 1980; 28: 329–36.
87. Mankad P, Lachno R, Yacoub M. Preservation of adenine nucleotides following ischemia and reperfusion: correlation with functional recovery. Adv Exp Med Biol 1991; 309 A: 279–84.
88. Hearse DJ, Stewart DA, Braimbridge MV. Cellular protection during myocardial ischemia. Circulation 1976; 54: 193–202.
89. Warnecke H, Hetzer R, Franz P *et al.* Standardized comparison of cardioplegic methods in the isolated paracorporal dog heart. Thorac Cardiovasc Surgeon 1980; 28: 322–8.
90. Preusse CJ, Gebhard MM, Bretschneider HJ. Recovery of myocardial metabolism after a 210 minute cardiac arrest induced by Bretschneider cardioplegia. J Mol Cell Cardiol (Suppl 2) 1979; 11: 46.
91. Preusse CJ, Gebhard MM, Schnabel PA *et al.* Post-ischemic myocardial function after pre-ischemic application of propanolol or verapamil. J Cardiovasc Surg 1984; 25: 158–64.
92. Toshima Y, Kohno H, Matsuzaki K *et al.* Collins' solution for cold storage of the heart for transplantation must be reversed with cardioplegic solution before reperfusion. J Thorac Cardiovasc Surg 1992; 104: 1572–81.
93. Lochner A, Lloyd L, Brits W *et al.* Oxygenation of cardioplegic solutions: A note of caution. Ann Thorac Surg 1991; 51: 777–87.
94. Stapenhorst K. Prolonged safe ischemic cardiac arrest using hypothermic Bretschneider Cardioplegia combined with topical cardiac cooling. Thorac Cardiovasc Surgeon 1981; 29: 272–4.
95. Dyszkiewicz W, Minten J, Flameng W. Long-term preservation of donor hearts: the effect of intra- and extracellular-type of cardioplegic solutions on myocardial high energy phosphate content. Mater Med Pol 1990; 22: 147–52.
96. Reichenspurner H, Russ C, Überfuhr P *et al.* Myocardial preservation using HTK-solution for heart transplantation – A multicenter study. Eurotransplant Newsletter 1992; 100: 8–10.
97. Meiser BM, Überfuhr P, Stang A *et al.* Retransplantation of an already transplanted heart. Transplant Proc 1992; 24: 2663–4
98. Panzner R, Wollert HG, Hermann M *et al.* Reperfusion arrhythmias after cardioplegia using Bretschneider-HTK solution. Thorac Cardiovasc Surgeon 1990; 38: 370.
99. Gorlach G, Podzuweit T, Borsutzky B *et al.* Factors determining ventricular fibrillation after induced cardiac arrest. Thorac Cardiovasc Surgeon 1991; 39: 140–2.

100. Wilson GJ, Axford-Gatley RA, Bush BG *et al.* European versus North America cardioplegia: Comparison of Bretschneider's and Roe's cardioplegic solutions in a canine model of cardiopulmonary bypass. Thorac Cardiovasc Surgeon 1990; 38: 10–4.
101. Beyersdorf F, Krause E, Sarai K *et al.* Clinical evaluation of hypothermic ventricular fibrillation, multi-dose blood cardioplegia, and single-dose Bretschneider cardioplegia in coronary surgery. Thorac Cardiovasc Surgeon 1990; 38: 20–9.
102. Kallerhoff M, Blech M, Götz L *et al.* A new method for conservative renal surgery – Experimental and first clinical results. Langenbecks Arch Chir 1990; 375: 340–6.
103. Heusch G. Hibernation, Stunning, Ischemic Preconditioning – neue Paradigmen der koronaren Herzkrankheit? Z Kardiol 1992; 81: 596–609.

6. Cardioplegia with an extracellular formulation

DAVID JOHN CHAMBERS and MARK VINEY BRAIMBRIDGE

Introduction

The clinical use of cardioplegia is now accepted world-wide for all aspects of cardiac surgery. Myocardial protection can be achieved with a number of cardioplegic solutions but, essentially, there are only two types of solution – the 'extracellular-type' and the 'intracellular-type'. The latter has been covered in the preceding chapter.

'Extracellular-type' solutions can be divided into purely crystalloid solutions or those having blood as the vehicle for the cardioplegic component. The next chapter will discuss the concepts underlying the use of blood cardioplegia.

'Extracellular' solutions are based on an ionic formulation similar to that of extracellular body fluids. Thus, they have a relatively normal concentration of sodium (around 100–120 mmol/l) and calcium (around 1.0 mmol/l or slightly lower) but the concentration of potassium ions is elevated. This elevation is usually to around 15–40 mmol/l, which is considerably lower than the normal potassium concentration of an intracellular solution of around 140 mmol/l. The elevated potassium concentration is sufficient to induce rapid diastolic arrest by cellular depolarisation but is not sufficiently high to be classed as an 'intracellular' solution.

The underlying concepts associated with an extracellular crystalloid cardioplegic solution have been designated by Hearse and colleagues [1,2]. These concepts are chemical arrest, hypothermia and the additional protection of individual components. Briefly, the first concept involves the use of agents to induce rapid diastolic arrest. The usual agent to achieve this is an elevated potassium concentration; other agents (such as low (or zero) calcium, elevated magnesium, tetrodotoxin, procaine, calcium antagonists) have also been used. Secondly, hypothermia has been generally recognised as additive to myocardial protection. Some workers, however, have challenged this concept, suggesting that hypothermia is unnecessary. The third component of cardioplegia is the choice of other agents to enhance the protection required to prevent ischemia-induced events. Such components are designed to prevent ionic imbalance, cell swelling, ischemia-induced acidosis and metabolite leakage due to increased membrane permeability.

For the purposes of this chapter, the components of extracellular-type

H.M. Piper and C.J. Preusse (eds): Ischemia-reperfusion in cardiac surgery, 135–179.

crystalloid cardioplegic solutions which may play a role in the protective process are characterised, illustrated by studies from our own laboratory and others, in which each component has been shown to improve (or reduce) myocardial protection in both experimental and clinical studies.

Greater consideration has been given in this chapter to the more controversial aspects of extracellular solutions rather than to those that are more generally accepted.

Types of extracellular crystaloid solutions

Ionic components of extracellular cardioplegic solution

For a cardioplegic solution to be classified as an extracellular-type solution, it has to have a high sodium and a normal calcium concentration (corresponding approximately to those found in the extracellular bathing solutions). Thus, sodium concentrations are normally 100 mmol/l or above and the ionised calcium concentration is normally above 0.5 mmol/l. Potassium remains the most popular ion for arresting the heart in an extracellular solution. Another common ion is magnesium, used either alone (as the cardioplegic component) or in conjunction with potassium. Thus, extracellular solutions are designed to avoid extremes of ionic concentration and to approximate to normal extracellular body fluid composition.

Sodium

Extracellular sodium concentrations have been shown [3] to influence protection of the myocardium. Reducing the sodium level from normal to 120 mmol/l reduces enzyme leakage by some 25%; any further reduction in sodium increases enzyme leakage, which becomes significant below 70 mmol/l. The sodium concentration is inextricably linked to the calcium concentration and the correct stoichiometric relationships have to be maintained. Thus, reducing the sodium concentration requires that the calcium concentration be similarly reduced. These relationships can be extremely complex and highly volume-dependent [4].

Calcium

Extracellular cardioplegic solutions generally contain a 'normal' level of calcium – thus the Tyers' solution contains a calcium concentration of 0.9 mmol/l [5,6]. The clinically introduced St Thomas' Hospital cardioplegic solution No. 1 (STH1) contained a calcium concentration of 2.2 mmol/l [7], based on the formulation of Ringers' solution, whereas, in the original experimental studies in the characterisation of this solution [8], based on Krebs Henseleit bicarbonate buffer [9], a calcium concentration of 2.4 mmol/l was used. In the St Thomas' Hospital cardioplegic solution No. 2 (STH2), the calcium concentration was reduced to 1.2 mmol/l [10]. Previous studies by

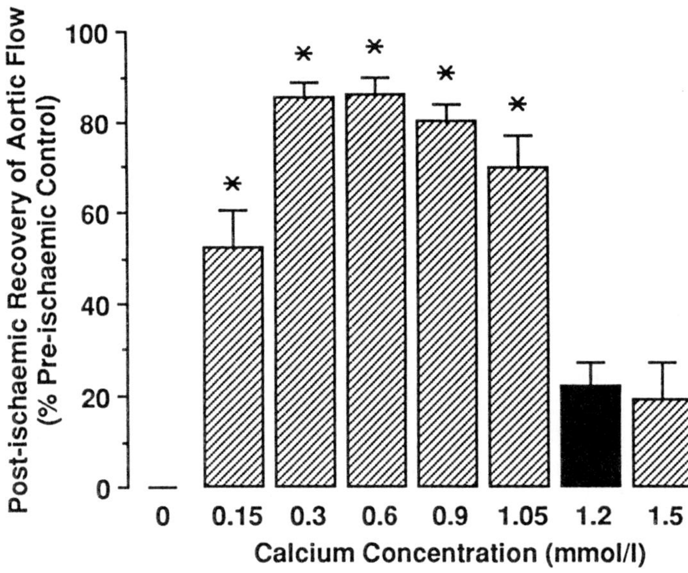

Figure 6.1. Dose-response curve for calcium concentration of St Thomas' Hospital cardioplegic solution No. 2 (STH2) and post-ischemic recovery of aortic flow (expressed as a percent of pre-ischemic control value) in rat hearts subjected to 300 min of hypothermic (20°C) global ischemia. The dark column represents the standard calcium concentration in STH2. Each value is the mean of 6 hearts; bars represent standard error of the mean (SEM). $*p < 0.05$ when compared with standard (1.2 mmol/l) calcium concentration. (Redrawn from: Robinson and Harwood, J Thorac Cardiovasc Surg 1991; 101: 314–25.)

Jynge and colleagues [4,11] had demonstrated the importance of maintaining cellular calcium control and its relationship with the extracellular sodium concentration but it was not until a study by Yamamoto and colleagues [12] that it was shown that 1.2 mmol/l in STH2 was the optimal calcium concentration. This study was carried out in hearts subjected to normothermic global ischemia; a more recent study, using 300 min of hypothermic (20°C) ischemia, demonstrated that the optimal calcium concentration (Figure 6.1) for STH2 at this temperature was 0.6 mmol/l [13]. This was recently confirmed for lower temperatures (7.5°C) and longer (360 min) ischemic durations [14]. Interestingly, a study by Boggs and colleagues [15] had shown that, in a cardioplegic solution based on Krebs Henseleit buffer, either zero calcium or 0.25 mmol/l calcium gave better protection during hypothermic ischemia than did cardioplegia containing 0.75 or 1.25 mmol/l calcium. Thus, the optimal calcium concentration for an extracellular cardioplegic solution remains controversial; however, the danger of instituting a calcium paradox when calcium is completely absent from the cardioplegic solution with sodium remaining high is considerable.

Potassium

Elevation of the potassium concentration (ranging from 15 to 40 mmol/l) is the most commonly used principle for achieving rapid diastolic arrest but it is also a myocardial protective agent in its own right [8]. Elevated potassium activates the potassium channel and repolarises the cardiac cell; hence the sodium channel is inactivated by a reduction of the resting membrane potential to approximately −50 mV, preventing sodium influx during the upstroke of the action potential [16].

The effect of potassium loading on cellular calcium is complex. Mild hyperkalemia inactivates the calcium channel and reduces calcium influx; however, higher potassium concentrations (30–40 mmol/l) activate the calcium channel, increasing calcium influx and promoting calcium overload. Thus, the beneficial effects of a raised potassium have a relatively narrow window, which stresses the importance of dose-response studies for potassium in relation to the other ionic constituents of the cardioplegic solution. These have been well documented by Hearse and colleagues [1] in studies which demonstrated that optimal potassium concentration for myocardial protection varies between 15 and 20 mmol/l. However, on its own, potassium is a relatively inefficient protective agent.

Magnesium

Magnesium can be considered as a cardioplegic agent in its own right, but it is less effective at arresting the heart than is potassium. As an example of this, the Kirsch solution [17] used a high concentration of magnesium aspartate (160 mmol/l), together with procaine (11 mmol/l), given as a bolus injection to induce myocardial arrest.

The inclusion of magnesium in cardioplegic solutions lies in its ability to provide additional myocardial protection. Dose-response studies were originally undertaken by Hearse and colleagues [18] who showed that the optimal concentration was 16 mmol/l. These studies were carried out in hearts subjected to normothermic (37°C) or hypothermic (28°C) ischemia for 30 or 60 min, respectively; more recent studies have demonstrated similar results in hearts subjected to 2 hours of hypothermic (8°C) ischemia [19].

In addition, the relationship between magnesium and calcium has been examined [20]. The addition of 16 mmol/l magnesium to cardioplegic solutions containing either 0, 0.1 or 1.2 mmol/l calcium was beneficial at all concentrations. In contrast, a recent study by Kinoshita [21] demonstrated that a cardioplegic solution containing low calcium (0.1 mmol/l) and zero magnesium provided better myocardial protection in patients than did the standard St Thomas' Hospital solution. Once again, the importance of establishing dose response curves of any ion in relation to other cardioplegic components is emphasised.

Types of solution

High potassium only

A number of extracellular-type solutions have been developed and used clinically throughout the world. The most widely used type is that of elevated potassium only. Gay and Ebert [22] were the first to report on the efficacy of high potassium-containing solutions for protecting the ischemic myocardium. Their solution contained 25 mmol/l potassium and 200 mmol/l sodium but no calcium. Modifications to this solution were made by Roe and colleagues [23], who reduced the sodium concentration to 27 mmol/l and added glucose (278 mmol/l) and Tris buffer (1 mmol/l). Tyers and coworkers [5] introduced a solution based on Normosol® with added potassium (25 mmol/l) and calcium (0.5 mmol/l), together with other components such as acetate and gluconate. This solution was shown clinically to provide good results with an operative mortality of 4.6%.

A number of other extracellular-type solutions were also developed, primarily in the United States, which were all variations on the theme of arrest with high potassium. The Birmingham solution, developed by Conti and colleagues [24], contained 30 mmol/l potassium, 100 mmol/l sodium, 0.7 mmol/l calcium, together with glucose, albumin and mannitol. Many centres developed their own particular solution, the vast majority of which were not tested in experimental studies to anything like the degree of the St Thomas' solution before clinical use. Robinson and colleagues [25] compared several with the St Thomas' Hospital solution and found them to be less than optimally formulated.

Potassium and magnesium (St Thomas' Hospital cardioplegic solution)

The St Thomas' Hospital cardioplegic solution No. 1 was developed and used clinically in 1975 in the UK. This solution, based on high potassium together with high magnesium, is probably the most widely used and is certainly the most intensively researched solution in the world today. The rationale for the development of the St Thomas' solution has been that each component should be present in its optimal concentration, that is, optimal in terms of its synergistic or inter-ionic effects with the other components [8,10].

There are 2 formulations for the St Thomas' Hospital cardioplegic solution. The original solution (St Thomas' No. 1 solution; STH1), which contains 20 mmol/l potassium, 144 mmol/l sodium, 16 mmol/l magnesium, 2.2 mmol/l calcium and 1 mmol/l procaine, was first used clinically in 1975 [7] and continues to be used in the UK. For ease of clinical use it was not buffered and was made by adding a 20 ml ampoule containing 16 mmol/l potassium chloride, 16 mmol/l magnesium chloride and 1 mmol/l procaine to a litre bag of Ringers' solution.

The St Thomas' Hospital cardioplegic solution No. 2 (STH2) differs from the No. 1 solution, with lower potassium (16 mmol/l), sodium (120 mmol/l) and calcium (1.2 mmol/l); the procaine is absent and it contains a small buffering capacity (10 mmol/l bicarbonate). It is the only cardioplegic solution that has been awarded FDA approval for administration in the USA, and is widely available (under the tradename, Plegisol®, manufactured by Abbott Pharmaceuticals) throughout the world. Experimental studies have shown that STH2 provides superior protection to STH1 [26]; this has been validated clinically [27].

Additional components

Many supplements to cardioplegic solutions that were theoretically desirable were introduced following the establishment of cardioplegia as the major method for myocardial protection in the later 1970s.

Glucose/Mannitol/Insulin. Glucose, insulin and potassium (GIK) solutions have been used since 1978 for protection of the ischemic myocardium. Krause and colleagues [28] studied normothermic ischemia in dogs and, using a solution containing 125 g glucose, 10 mmol/l potassium and 12.5 U insulin, showed that pretreatment before 120 min of normothermic ischemia improved post-ischemic function. Lolley and colleagues [29] showed, in a series of patients, that continuous infusion of a solution containing 278 mmol/l glucose, 20 mmol/l potassium, 20 units insulin and 69 mmol/l mannitol improved myocardial protection. It was suggested that the GIK solution improved anaerobic glycolysis together with toxic washout.

A recent study has also suggested that glucose is beneficial when added to the St Thomas' Hospital cardioplegic solution. Von Oppell and coworkers [30] showed, in the isolated rat heart, that addition of an optimal dose of glucose (7–11 mmol/l), coupled with multidose infusions of cardioplegia (every 30 min) throughout a hypothermic ischemic period, was beneficial to the adult myocardium. This was in contrast to earlier studies by Hearse and colleagues [31], again in the isolated rat heart, showing that addition of glucose (11 mmol/l) to the St Thomas' Hospital cardioplegic solution, when used as a single infusion during moderate hypothermia (28°C) together with relatively prolonged ischemia (70 min), was detrimental to post-ischemic recovery.

It is likely that these differences were associated with the intermittent washout of toxic metabolites during multidose infusions of cardioplegia; however, the role of glucose as a beneficial metabolic enhancer during global ischemia remains controversial. It is probable that very specific conditions need to be adhered to for glucose to be beneficial in the clinical setting.

Calcium channel blockers. Calcium channel blockers (calcium antagonists) cause a depression of cardiac function and induce heart block by preventing calcium influx through the myocardial calcium channels. As such, they can be used as cardioplegic agents *per se*. Since a major component of ischemic and reperfusion injury is thought to occur due to calcium overload, calcium channel blockers have been used as adjuncts to extracellular cardioplegic solutions in an effort to reduce myocardial injury.

In a series of studies, Yamamoto and colleagues [32], using rat hearts subjected to normothermic ischemia, demonstrated that diltiazem, nifedipine and verapamil could all exert myocardial protective effects when added to the St Thomas' Hospital cardioplegic solution, with each agent having a characteristic bell-shaped dose-response curve. These effects, however, were temperature dependent, such that, at myocardial temperatures used clinically (20°C), the beneficial effects of these agents was lost. In contrast, a recent study by Murashita and coworkers [33], using adult and neonatal rabbit hearts, showed that diltiazem had no protective effect, even during normothermic ischemia, in either adult or neonates. This suggests species differences in response to calcium antagonists during ischemia and reperfusion.

Delivery of a cardioplegic solution in the clinical setting is often heterogeneous due to coronary artery disease or hypertrophy, with certain areas of the myocardium receiving low volumes of cardioplegia and consequent poor cooling. Calcium antagonists have been suggested as improving delivery of crystalloid cardioplegic solutions to ischemic areas and enhancing myocardial protection in areas of the myocardium that have been inadequately cooled. Experimentally this has been shown to occur by Guyton and colleagues [34] using PlasmaLyte 148®, (Travenol) as an extracellular-type cardioplegic solution (containing an extra 25 mmol/l potassium); nifedipine, but not lidoflazine, was beneficial in terms of post-ischemic recovery in a dog model of heterogeneous cardioplegic delivery. This work was supported by a study by Chiavarelli and coworkers [35] who showed that nifedipine was beneficial as an additive to the University of Alabama Hospitals' cardioplegic solution (an extracellular-type crystalloid solution containing glucose and mannitol) under normothermic ischemic conditions in guinea pig hearts, but that it had no effect in hypothermic ischemia, confirming the conclusions drawn by Yamamoto [32] with the St Thomas' Hospital cardioplegic solution.

In a clinical study, using the St Thomas' solution, Flameng and coworkers [36] demonstrated that, although nifedipine was useful in reducing ATP catabolism in patients undergoing valve operations in which the myocardial temperature rose from 14°C to 25°C, there was no detectable benefit in terms of improved clinical outcome. Other clinical studies, in which verapamil was added to an extracellular-type solution [37], or diltiazem added to an intracellular-type solution [38], showed little, if any, benefit arising from the use of the calcium channel blockers, both studies emphasising the possibility of deleterious side effects such as atrioventricular block and depressed systolic function post-ischemically. Christakis and colleagues [38] have again emphasised the concept that a dose-response study is necessary for each component of cardioplegic solutions used at individual institutions, which has been the St Thomas' style of investigation from the beginning. Overall, the advantages of using calcium channel blockers as additives to cardioplegic solutions are outweighed by their disadvantages.

Procaine/lignocaine. Procaine and lignocaine (lidocaine) are local anaesthetic agents. They have been used in cardioplegic solutions because, at sufficiently high concentrations, they have sodium channel blocking activity [39] which rapidly arrests the heart and provides myocardial protection. These compounds are also thought to have antidysrhythmic properties.

They have been used in a number of 'intracellular' cardioplegic solutions (such as the Bretschneider and Kirsch solutions) at concentrations of 7.4–11.0 mmol/l, at which they have a cardioplegic effect. They have also been used to demonstrate protective effects in extracellular solutions. Harlan and colleagues [40] demonstrated that addition of either 30 mmol/l potassium or 7.4 mmol/l procaine to Krebs Henseleit buffer used as cardioplegic solutions in the isolated rat heart enhanced myocardial protection when compared to Krebs Henseleit alone at either 15°C or 5°C. Procaine was also used as an additive to the St Thomas' Hospital cardioplegic solution No. 1 at a concentration of 1.0 mmol/l [7]; at this concentration it did not have cardioplegic properties *per se* but was added for its potential antidysrhythmic and membrane stabilising effects. Subsequent studies [41] demonstrated that the optimal dose, for both procaine and lignocaine when added to STH2, was 0.05 mmol/l; higher doses had a potentially detrimental effect. Procaine was subsequently excluded from the formulation of the St Thomas' No. 2 solution [10] as the beneficial effects observed were not great and as it had not been passed by the Federal Drugs Administration in the USA.

Antioxidants. After the identification of superoxide dismutase and the linkage of this scavenging system to the xanthine oxidase hypothesis [42,43], oxygen-derived free radical-mediated myocardial injury was suggested as having a possible role during cardiac surgery involving elective cardiac ischemia and reperfusion. The protective effects of superoxide dismutase and catalase, which together prevent the formation of the damaging hydroxyl radical, when added to a modified St Thomas' Hospital cardioplegic solution were first shown by Shlafer and colleagues [44,45]. Enhanced myocardial protection was obtained in either buffer-perfused rabbit hearts or in blood-perfused cat hearts subjected to 2 hours of global ischemia at 27°C before reperfusion. These results were confirmed by Stewart and colleagues [46] in the dog, in which a hyperkalemic saline cardioplegic solution was used. The addition of superoxide dismutase and mannitol to this solution significantly improved post-ischemic function and sarcoplasmic reticulum calcium transport.

Subsequent studies have suggested that hydrogen peroxide is an important component of this ischemia-induced myocardial injury [47]; use of catalase alone (to remove hydrogen peroxide), or the addition of allopurinol (to prevent superoxide radical and hydrogen peroxide formation by inhibiting the generating enzyme, xanthine oxidase), has been shown to be beneficial. These results were supported by studies from our laboratory in which a combination of superoxide dismutase and catalase provided enhanced protec-

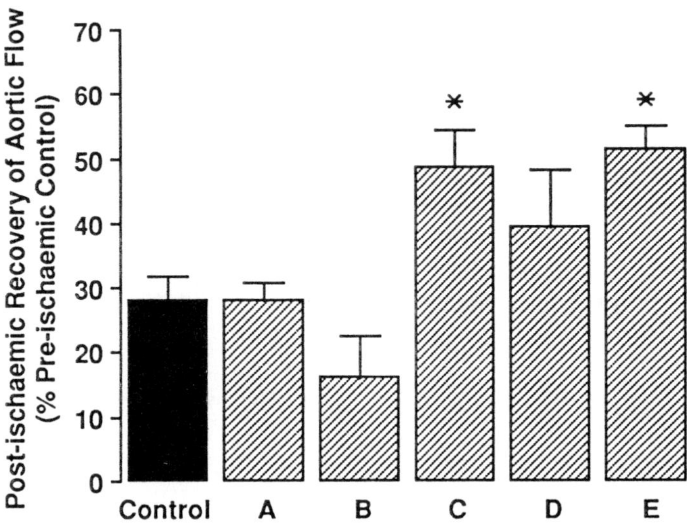

Figure 6.2. Post-ischemic recovery of aortic flow (expressed as a percent of pre-ischemic control value) in rat hearts subjected to 30 min of normothermic (37°C) global ischemia. Each column represents the mean of 6 hearts; bars represent SEM. *$p < 0.05$ compared with control. The solid column represents the control group (no additives), the hatched columns represent the experimental groups. A = superoxide dismutase (SOD) added to STH2 and the reperfusion solution [RS]); B = catalase (CAT) added to STH2 and RS; C = SOD plus CAT added to STH2 and RS; D = SOD plus CAT added to STH2 alone; E = SOD plus CAT added to RS alone. (Redrawn from: Chambers *et al.*, Eur J Cardio-thorac Surg 1987; 1: 37–45.)

tion to the isolated rat heart (Figure 6.2) when included in the cardioplegic or the reperfusion solution [48]. Allopurinol was also shown to be protective when used either as a pretreatment or as an additive to the cardioplegic or reperfusion solution [49].

Metal ions (such as iron) have been implicated as catalysts in the Haber-Weiss reaction for the generation of hydroxyl radicals. Compounds such as deferoxamine (which chelate free metal ions) may be important in preventing post-ischemic free radical-induced myocardial injury during cardiopulmonary bypass when iron may be released from haemolysed red cells. Myers and colleagues [47] showed that the addition of deferoxamine to a modified St Thomas' Hospital cardioplegic solution did not significantly enhance post-ischemic recovery of function in isolated buffer perfused rabbit hearts. In contrast, the addition of deferoxamine to the Hôpital Laribosiere cardioplegic solution (an extracellular-type solution with low (0.25 mmol/l) calcium supplemented with glutamate and mannitol) has been shown both experimentally and clinically to enhance myocardial protection significantly, presumably by preventing the formation of the hydroxyl radical. Deferoxamine was significantly better than using peroxidase to remove hydrogen peroxide [50, 51].

One mechanism whereby deferoxamine may reduce free radical generation is in the activation of neutrophils to produce free radicals after ischemia [52]. The enthusiasm for the xanthine oxidase hypothesis of oxygen-derived free radical generation, whilst being an attractive explanation for ischemia and reperfusion-induced injury after cardioplegia, has been dampened by the recent findings that xanthine oxidase is either absent, or very low in activity, in the human myocardium [53]. There is no doubt, however, that oxygen-derived free radicals play a role in myocardial ischemia and reperfusion-induced injury, but this role has not yet been accurately identified.

Substrate enhancement – high energy phosphates. One of the first and major effects of ischemia is the catabolism of adenosine triphosphate (ATP). It has been suggested from a number of studies that the post-ischemic ATP content of the myocardium correlates with the ultimate recovery of function of the heart, and it is possible that a threshold level of ATP is required below which the heart fails to recover any mechanical function. Consequently, considerable work has been done on methods to maintain or enhance myocardial ATP content during ischemia and reperfusion.

The use of cardioplegia and hypothermia, by inducing rapid arrest and slowing metabolism, reduce high energy phosphate metabolism considerably. During relatively prolonged ischemia, however, these high energy phosphates are slowly metabolised. Various metabolic additives to the cardioplegic solution have been used either to prevent high energy phosphate catabolism or to enhance anaerobic metabolism in an attempt to maintain high energy phosphate content of the myocardium.

Early studies by Hearse and colleagues [8], using the isolated working rat heart, had shown that addition of ATP (10 mmol/l) to a K^+-enhanced bicarbonate buffer improved post-ischemic recovery of aortic flow from 31% to 76%. Subsequent studies by Robinson and colleagues [54] had shown that creatine phosphate (CP), used as an additive to the St Thomas' Hospital cardioplegic solution (STH2), was beneficial to post-ischemic recovery of function at an optimal concentration of 10 mmol/l (Figure 6.3) under conditions of both normothermic and hypothermic ischemia. Further studies [55] showed that ATP added to St Thomas' Hospital cardioplegic solution (STH2) was also effective as an additive protective agent (but at an optimal concentration of 0.1 mmol/l). Furthermore, when used in combination with the optimal concentration of CP (10 mmol/l), there was an even greater protection than with either component alone.

These experimental studies were taken to the clinical field by Chambers and colleagues [56], who showed that, although the addition of 10 mmol/l creatine phosphate to STH2 had no effect on clinical outcome, birefringence

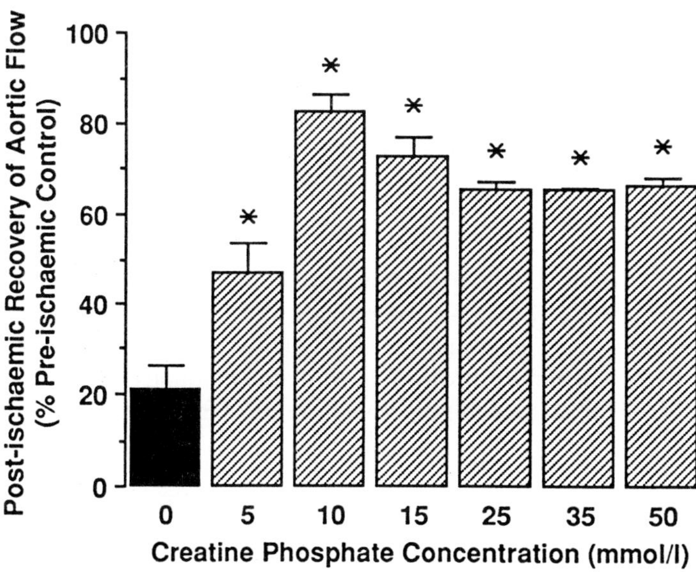

Figure 6.3. Dose-response curve for creatine phosphate concentration added to STH2 and post-ischemic recovery of aortic flow (expressed as a percent of pre-ischemic control value) in rat hearts subjected to 40 min of normothermic (37°C) global ischemia. Each column represents the mean of 6 hearts; bars represent SEM. $^*p < 0.05$ compared with creatine phosphate-free control group (solid column). (Redrawn from: Robinson *et al.*, J Thorac Cardiovasc Surg 1984; 87: 190–200.)

assessment (see later chapter) of myocardial function demonstrated improved myocardial protection at the cellular level.

Recent studies have suggested some mechanisms by which these compounds may be acting. Robinson and Harwood [57] suggested that CP acts by chelating calcium in the cardioplegic solution and showed (in further studies [13]) that reducing the calcium concentration in the St Thomas' Hospital cardioplegic solution (STH2), from 1.2 mmol/l to 0.6 mmol/l during hypothermic ischemia, had a beneficial effect. Similar calcium chelating properties were demonstrated for ATP by Hohl and Hearse [58]. This mechanism has, however, been challenged by Conorev and coworkers [59], who showed that, by titrating the calcium concentration of the cardioplegic solution to compensate for the calcium chelating effect of creatine phosphate, there was no effect on myocardial protection. Instead, Conorev and colleagues suggested that creatine phosphate acts to reduce the effect of oxidative stress, a concept originally proposed by Zucchi and colleagues [60] when they showed that creatine phosphate reduced the detrimental effects induced by perfusing rat hearts with hydrogen peroxide.

Similar studies have been carried out by other groups. Thelin and coworkers [61] investigated the effects of ATP (0.067 mmol/l) or phosphoenolpyruvate (14.4 mmol/l) when added to a modified St Thomas' Hospital cardioplegic solution. They used blood-perfused isolated rat hearts and showed that hearts arrested with ATP-supplemented cardioplegia had significantly improved post-ischemic function and adenylate charge potential when compared with control (non-supplemented) hearts; phosphoenolpyruvate also improved post-ischemic function but to a lesser extent than ATP and a combination of the two compounds had the same effect as ATP alone.

Overall, these results suggest that the use of high energy phosphate compounds as additives to extracellular-type cardioplegic solutions are beneficial. The mechanism by which these compounds are acting is unclear, but it is unlikely that they are increasing the high energy phosphate content of the myocardium. It is generally acknowledged that compounds such as ATP and CP do not cross the cell membrane but, in spite of this, several studies have shown them to be beneficial.

Substrate enhancement – adenine nucleosides. Breakdown products of ATP have also been used in an attempt to prevent the catabolism of ATP or to maintain the adenylate pool and improve nucleotide resynthesis. DeWitt and colleagues [62] showed that addition of 200 μmol/l inosine, added to a bicarbonate buffer modified to resemble St Thomas' cardioplegic solution, was able to reduce the degradation of ATP and total adenine nucleotides and improve post-ischemic functional recovery in isolated crystalloid perfused rat hearts. Inosine (100 μmol/l) has also been shown to be effective as a protective agent when given as a pretreatment to rabbit hearts subjected to global ischemia without cardioplegic arrest, by preserving ATP levels and improving post-ischemic function [63].

Recently, adenosine has enjoyed a renewed interest as a compound which may be of significant benefit to the ischemic myocardium. Adenosine, at a concentration of 10 mmol/l, is an effective cardioplegic agent [64] and was shown to provide additional myocardial protection when compared with potassium-based cardioplegia (20 mmol/l K^+) in isolated crystalloid perfused rat hearts. Other workers have shown similar beneficial effects of adenosine when used as an adjunct to crystalloid (extracellular-type) cardioplegic solutions, although usually at a lower concentration than that used above. Thus, De Jong and colleagues [65] showed that adenosine (1 mmol/l) added to Krebs Henseleit bicarbonate buffer containing 26 mmol/l K^+ induced a significantly shorter time to arrest and improved post-ischemic functional recovery.

Similar studies were carried out by Bolling *et al.* [66] and by Ledingham *et al.* [67] who added adenosine to St Thomas' Hospital cardioplegic solution at concentrations of 200 μmol/l and 3.75 μmol/l, respectively. Both studies showed improved recovery of function in hearts; suggested mechanisms of action were, however, different. At the higher adenosine levels, adenine nucleotides were preserved and it was suggested that the improved function

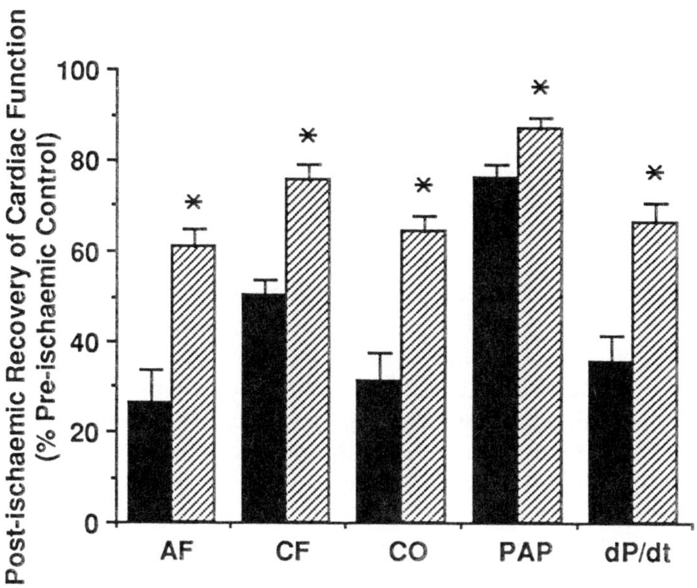

Figure 6.4. Post-ischemic recovery of cardiac function (expressed as percent pre-ischemic control value) in rat hearts reperfused with ordinary reperfusate (solid columns) or reperfusate containing 3.75 μmol/l adenosine (hatched columns). Each column represents the mean of 10 hearts; bars represent SEM. $^*p < 0.05$ compared with control. AF = aortic flow, CF = coronary flow, CO = cardiac output, PAP = peak aortic pressure. (Redrawn from: Ledingham *et al.*, Cardiovasc Res 1990; 24: 247–53.)

was due to accelerated repletion of adenine nucleotide stores [66]. In contrast, the low levels of adenosine used in Ledingham's study [67] did not influence myocardial content of ATP and the improved recovery (Figure 6.4) was suggested to be a consequence of the significantly increased microvasculature coronary flow during reperfusion.

Adenine nucleosides, particularly adenosine, would appear to have a role to play as an additive to cardioplegic solutions. Although there are a number of problems associated with its clinical use (such as a short half-life (1.5 seconds), rhythm and conduction disturbances and induction of physical discomfort), the coronary vasodilator effects of adenosine, particularly during reperfusion may be of significant benefit when reflow complications occur.

Substrate enhancement – amino acids. Amino acid enhancement of cardioplegic solutions has also been advocated as an effective means of improving post-ischemic function. The most commonly used amino acids are glutamate and aspartate, and most studies using these compounds have been done in blood-based cardioplegic solutions (see next chapter; Buckberg). An early study by Rau and coworkers [68] demonstrated the potential benefit of amino acids added to a crystalloid perfusate to which red cells had been added (for a final haematocrit of 20%) in ischemic rabbit septa. Ornithine, glutamate and aspartate at concentrations of 1 mmol/l induced significant improvement in recovery of developed tension compared with controls and it was suggested that the transamination processes involved in the malate-aspartate shuttle were involved in stimulating anaerobic mitochondrial metabolism and producing high-energy phosphates from succinate and succinyl-CoA (substrate level phosphorylation). Pisarenko and colleagues [169] added glutamic acid at a concentration of 1% (equivalent to 67 mmol/l) to oxygenated bicarbonate buffer containing 20 mmol/l K^+ in isolated perfused rat hearts subjected to 30 min global ischemia. Recovery of function in treated hearts was 75% compared to 39% in untreated controls.

More recent studies have concentrated on the effect of amino acids added to cardioplegic solutions used for long-term preservation of hearts prior to transplantation. Gharagozloo *et al.* [70] added glutamate (24 mmol/l) to an extracellular-type crystalloid cardioplegic solution and stored hearts for 8 hours in saline. Following reperfusion with blood, hearts treated with glutamate recovered to almost 100% whereas control hearts deteriorated by approximately 60% in both left and right ventricular function. Aspartate (20 mmol/l) was also shown to have a beneficial effect when added to the St Thomas' Hospital cardioplegic solution [71], in hearts stored for 10 hours at 4°C. Recovery of function was 99% in treated hearts compared to 0% in control, untreated hearts; myocardial ATP content was also significantly greater in the former. All studies using these amino acids suggest that they are involved in transamination reactions associated with the malate-aspartate shuttle which allows substrate level phosphorylation and regenerates NAD which may allow glycolysis to proceed and generate additional ATP.

It would seem that amino acids as additives to extracellular cardioplegic solutions may have a role in the context of long-term preservation, rather than in conventional open heart surgery. Alternatively, they may be of benefit when added to a modified reperfusion solution, enhancing recovery of mitochondrial function.

Alternative techniques

Recent studies have highlighted alternative methods for inducing cardiac arrest. Schubert and colleagues [64] demonstrated the cardioplegic affect of adenosine by inhibition of nodal tissue. In a study designed to compare the effects of adenosine-arrest with that of potassium-arrest, they showed that 10 mmol/l adenosine improved tissue phosphocreatine levels after ischemia; post-ischemic hemodynamic function was significantly improved in comparison to 20 mmol/l potassium. It was speculated that adenosine caused membrane hyperpolarisation in atrial and sinus node tissue, causing inhibition of atrial action potential and atrioventricular block.

The use of the sodium channel blocker, tetrodotoxin (TTX), has also been advocated as a potential mediator in inducing rapid cardiac arrest. An original study by Tyers and colleagues [72] showed that a dose of 14 μg of tetrodotoxin infused into the rat heart induced immediate cardiac arrest. These hearts, subjected to 60 min reperfusion, recovered to 82% of their pre-ischemic function compared with a recovery of only 22% in hearts that had not been so arrested. A more recent study by Sternberg and coworkers [73] used 25 μmol/l TTX to demonstrate that induction of myocardial arrest by maintenance of polarisation gave protection to the ischemic myocardium similar to that of 20 mmol/l potassium-induced arrest. They suggested that TTX maintains the membrane potential at the resting potential, a mechanism of action similar to that advanced for adenosine. In both these studies, arrest was induced significantly more rapidly than with potassium and ventricular pressure during arrest was maintained at a lower level. This suggests that calcium influx during ischemia was lower in adenosine or TTX-induced arrest, which would support theoretical considerations relating to maintenance of diastolic membrane potential rather than slight depolarisation induced by potassium.

Another interesting concept relating to cardioplegic arrest was reported in a study by Wikman-Coffelt and colleagues [74], who used a physiological saline solution containing 10 mmol/l pyruvate and 4% alcohol as a cardioplegic solution and compared this to Roe's solution in isolated rat hearts. They showed that the combination of alcohol as an arresting solution and pyruvate as a substrate provided significantly improved functional and metabolic recovery following 24 hours of storage in the respective solution. Alcohol has been shown to influence transmembrane fluxes of Na^+, K^+ and Ca^{2+} and Cl^-; inhibition of Na^+/Ca^{2+} exchange and Na^+/K^+ ATPase would reduce basal energy-dependent processes. Alcohol also prevents oedema by decreasing intracellular Na^+ concentration. Alcohol caused immediate arrest of the heart, a mechanism that may be similar to that described above for adenosine and TTX.

Although interesting, methods of arrest using compounds other than potassium are unlikely to be taken up clinically for conventional open heart surgery. Where these alternative compounds may have a significant role to play in the future, however, is as an alternative means of protecting the heart for long term preservation prior to transplantation.

Modifications to extracellular crystalloid solutions

Oxygenation

Blood was used as the vehicle for cardioplegic solutions on the hypothesis that oxygen played a role in the beneficial effects. Most crystalloid extracellular-type solutions used experimentally and clinically in the late 1970s were not oxygenated.

Engelman and colleagues [75], however in 1980, reported a comparative study of blood and crystalloid cardioplegia in pigs subjected to 3 hours of global hypothermic ischemia with multidose cardioplegic infusions. Measurement of oxygen availability was greatest with blood cardioplegia with myocardial ATP content maintained. Creatine phosphate decreased to a lesser extent with blood cardioplegia with rebound occurring only with blood and oxygenated-crystalloid solutions. The two solutions, however, were used at different temperatures, so that this study was not well-controlled.

The effect of temperature and oxygen release was investigated by Digerness and colleagues [76]. They showed, using dogs, that crystalloid solutions released all the available oxygen at 10°C or 20°C whereas blood solutions released approximately 40% and 50% at 10°C and 20°C, respectively. Thus, crystalloid solutions saturated with oxygen contain a relatively large amount of oxygen, all of which is potentially available for release. In another study, using dog hearts subjected to 4 hours of cold (4°C) ischemia, oxygenated crystalloid cardioplegia infused every 20 mins was shown to improve post-ischemic cardiac function significantly, maintain significantly higher myocardial ATP levels, reduce oedema formation and reduce ultrastructural injury when compared with aerated crystalloid cardioplegia [77].

Bing and colleagues [78] showed that the addition of washed red cells to a simple extracellular-type cardioplegic solution infused into dog hearts subjected to 120 min of hypothermic (27°C) ischemia resulted in a significant improvement of post-ischemic function when compared with the oxygenated crystalloid solution alone. This solution was, however, devoid of calcium and, in a similar study by Heitmiller *et al.* [79], it was shown that the reduction in post-ischemic function with an oxygenated crystalloid solution could be accounted for by the absence of calcium. Addition of calcium (0.2 mmol/l) was sufficient to improve post-ischemic function from 42% to 79%, compared with blood cardioplegia (containing 0.26 mmol/l calcium) which recovered to 71%. In the study by Bing and colleagues [78] the ischemic temperature and the infusate temperature was 27°C; in contrast, the study by Heitmiller *et al.* [79] used an infusion temperature of 4°C and an ischemic temperature of 10°C. This study emphasises the common deficit of comparing blood cardioplegia with an inadequate crystalloid cardioplegic solution.

Earlier, Magovern and colleagues [80] had demonstrated the importance of temperature on the protective properties of oxygenated crystalloid and blood cardioplegia. Dog hearts were subjected to 90 min of global ischemia at 4°, 10° or 20°C and either oxygenated crystalloid or blood cardioplegia were administered every 30 min. Hearts subjected to 4°C ischemia with crystalloid cardioplegia recovered significantly better than hearts subjected to blood cardioplegia; in contrast, however, this relationship was reversed at 20°C. At 10°C there was no difference between the two groups (Figure 6.5).

In contrast, a study by Rousou and coworkers [81] compared an oxygen-

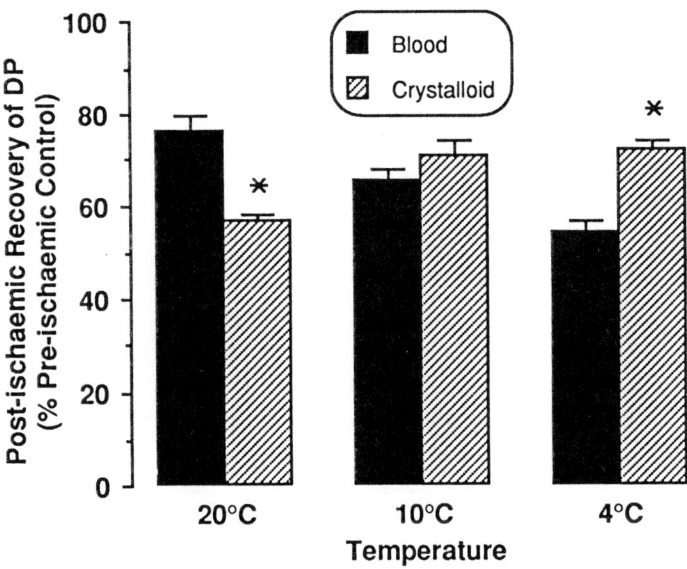

Figure 6.5. Post-ischemic recovery of developed pressure (DP) (expressed as a percent of pre-ischemic control value) in dog hearts subjected to an infusion of blood or crystalloid cardioplegia at 20°C, 10°C or 4°C and maintained at the same temperature for 90 min global ischemia. Each column represents the mean of 7 hearts; bars represent SEM. $*p < 0.05$ compared with blood cardioplegia. (Redrawn from: Magovern *et al.* , Circulation 1982; 66 (Suppl I): I-60–I-67.)

ated crystalloid cardioplegic solution (at 10°C) to blood cardioplegic solutions at various temperatures (10° or 20°C) and haematocrit (10%, 20% or 30%) and concluded that, although temperature was an important factor for protection with blood cardioplegia, haematocrit was unimportant. In addition, they also showed that cold oxygenated crystalloid cardioplegia was as effective as cold blood cardioplegia.

Oxygenation of St Thomas' Hospital cardioplegic solution carried out in experimental studies in rat hearts by Ledingham, Braimbridge and Hearse [82] have demonstrated beneficial effects. Both STH1 and STH2 (Plegisol®) were shown to improve post-ischemic recovery of function after long ischemic periods of 3 and 4 hours at 20°C (Figure 6.6). In addition, there was a significant reduction in post-ischemic arrhythmias and enzyme leakage.

Further studies using the isolated rat heart and the effects of oxygenation of the St Thomas' Hospital cardioplegic solution have been conducted by von Oppell and colleagues [83]. They investigated the effect of different pH changes to the cardioplegic solution resulting from different oxygenation techniques. Use of 100% oxygen gave a pH of approximately 9.1 and this

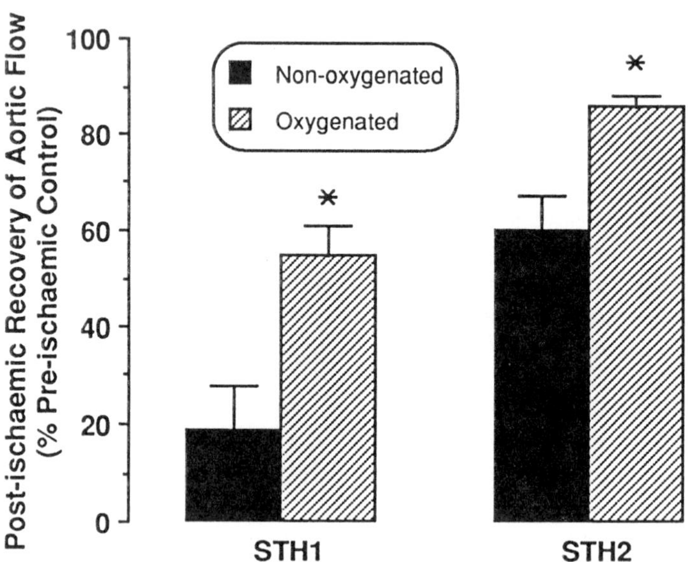

Figure 6.6. Post-ischemic recovery of aortic flow (expressed as a percent of pre-ischemic control value) in rat hearts arrested with either non-oxygenated (solid columns) or oxygenated (hatched columns) STH1 or STH2 and subjected to either 180 min (STH1) or 240 min (STH2) hypothermic (20°C) global ischemia with multidose infusions of cardioplegic solution every 30 min. Each value represents the mean of 10 hearts; bars represent SEM. $^*p < 0.05$ compared with non-oxygenated group. (Redrawn from: Ledingham *et al.*, J Thorac Cardiovasc Surg 1988; 95: 103–11.).

was associated with a reduced recovery of function compared to oxygenation with 95% O_2:5% CO_2 which gave a solution pH of approximately 7.0 and a significantly increased recovery of post-ischemic function. These studies suggest that relative acidity of the solution was beneficial – a somewhat surprising result in view of Ledingham's study with STH1 (which has a pH of between 5.5–7.0) and STH2 (with a pH of 7.8) in which STH2 solution gave significantly better protection to rat hearts than STH1 solution. The study by von Oppell had also demonstrated that addition of perfluorocarbons to the St Thomas' Hospital solution (in which additional oxygen was provided to the myocardium) had conferred no additional protection.

This confirmed a previous study, using dogs, by Tabayashi *et al.* [84] in which a non-oxygenated, an oxygenated and an oxygenated perfluorocarbon cardioplegic solution had been compared. Dogs were subjected to 120 min of global ischemia; recovery was significantly improved in the 2 oxygenated cardioplegia groups and, despite the fluorocarbon providing twice the oxygen content of the oxygenated crystalloid solution, there was no difference in myocardial protection.

Clinical studies were able to demonstrate that oxygenation of extracellular-type cardioplegic solutions was beneficial. Guyton and coworkers [85], in a small subgroup of 12 patients, was unable to show any differences in creatine kinase, myoglobin and lactate release or in oxygen consumption or cardiac work measured 1 hour after reperfusion in oxygenated or control cardioplegic solutions (based on PlasmaLyte®) containing a number of additives (acetate, gluconate, dextrose) but with zero calcium. The same group conducted a larger clinical study, in which 57 coronary bypass patients received non-oxygenated cardioplegic solution and 94 patients received an identical, but oxygenated cardioplegic solution. Analysis showed that, in those patients who had cross-clamp durations in excess of 28 min, a significantly greater release in creatine kinase-MB occurred in those patients receiving non-oxygenated cardioplegia.

In a larger clinical study by Daggett and colleagues [86], in which 400 patients were involved, the addition of red cells (to a haematocrit of 5%) in an extracellular-type solution infused at 4°C significantly improved post-operative outcome in terms of 30 day mortality (6% vs 3%), the incidence of post-operative intra-aortic balloon pump requirement (11.5% vs 4.5%) and the incidence of atrioventricular pacing (13.5% vs 4.0%). Of interest, however, is the fact that the crystalloid solution contained no calcium whereas the addition of 5% red blood cells increased the calcium concentration to 0.20 mmol/l – exactly the calcium concentration in Heitmiller's study [79] which, if added to the crystalloid solution, improved post-ischemic recovery above that of blood cardioplegia at the temperature used in Daggett's study (4°C). It is tempting to speculate, therefore, that a small addition of calcium added to the crystalloid solution advocated by Daggett [86] might have prevented any differences between these 2 groups of patients, again emphasising the pitfalls in blood/crystalloid studies.

A recent study by the authors [87] confirmed clinically the beneficial effect of oxygenation of St Thomas' Hospital cardioplegic solution (STH2) that had been shown in earlier experimental studies [82]. Patients (50) were randomly assigned to STH2 (Plegisol®) with or without oxygenation. Although it was not possible to observe differences in clinical outcome, CK-MB release or ECG changes, measurements of birefringence, a sensitive assessment of the ability of the myofibril to respond to ATP and calcium using polarised microscopy at the cellular level (see details in a later chapter: Darracott-Cankovic), were able to demonstrate significant differences in left ventricular epimyocardium and right ventricular samples obtained at the end of ischemia and after 15 min of reperfusion.

The evidence from both experimental and clinical studies suggests that oxygenation of extracellular crystalloid cardioplegic solutions provides some additional benefit in terms of myocardial protection. Care should, however, be taken in the composition of the gas for oxygenation; as was shown above, the pH of the resultant cardioplegic solution may influence the degree of protection.

Hypothermia

Hypothermia, systemic and topical, has been used successfully in cardiac surgery for over 4 decades as a means of protecting the heart [88,89,90]. From the introduction of extracellular cardioplegic solutions in the 1970s, hypothermia has been a consistent adjunct. Studies from our laboratory [91] in 1975 in the rat heart showed the additive protective effect of potassium arrest to hypothermia. Gillette and coworkers [92] showed that, whereas moderate hypothermia (26°C) failed to protect the dog heart subjected to 60 min of ischemic arrest, more profound hypothermia (18°C) resulted in almost complete recovery of function; elevation of the potassium concentration (to 15 mmol/l) only slightly improved recovery of function further.

In contrast, studies by Rosenfeldt and colleagues [93] using the dog heart subjected to 120 min of ischemia at 20°C, showed a significant improvement in recovery of function (cardiac output, minute work and dP/dt) in the cold cardioplegia group compared to hearts protected with hypothermia alone. These results were confirmed in isolated working rat hearts subjected to 120 min of hypothermic (20°C) ischemic arrest [94].

In a clinical study of 35 patients with coronary and valvular heart disease, Borst and Iversen [95] demonstrated the inhomogeneity of myocardial cooling and concluded that it was essential to minimise intra- and extracavity heat sources, keep systemic temperatures low, drain collateral blood flow, maintain topical cooling and shield the heart from the pericardium.

More recent studies from Rosenfeldt's group [96] have highlighted the importance of temperature combined with cardioplegic infusion volume in hypertrophied hearts. They showed that the induction of arrest was slower in hypertrophied dog hearts, leading to a greater decrease in high-energy phosphate compounds and a larger increase in lactate production than in normal hearts; during arrest, however, no further metabolic differences were observed. Further cooling of the myocardium (from 20°C to 12°C) improved myocardial protection in both groups. Thus, they concluded that, for optimum myocardial preservation during ischemia in hypertrophied hearts, it was critical to induce rapid arrest with an adequate volume of cold cardioplegic solution to lower the myocardial temperature to 12–15°C.

Recently, warm continuous blood cardioplegia has been suggested as an alternative to cold heart protection [97]. However, a recent study by Landymore and colleagues [98] has highlighted the potential for detrimental periods of ischemia occurring during this procedure. The requirement of a bloodless field to carry out coronary anastomoses means that the myocardium will be normothermically ischemic, during which time myocardial oxygen consumption will exceed supply and lactate production will be high.

Hypothermia is an important component of cardioplegic protection, since it contributes to rapid arrest and reduces the rate of myocardial metabolism. Hypothermia can, however, be too severe, resulting in hypothermic injury. Thus, the use of iced-saline slush as a topical coolant should be avoided.

Buffering and pH

This is a difficult field of study. When assessing the buffering requirements of cardioplegic solutions, basic concepts of pH and temperature have necessarily to be considered. The rate of dissociation of water into hydrogen $[H^+]$ and hydroxyl $[OH^-]$ ions becomes reduced as the temperature decreases and the point of neutrality of water shifts in an alkaline direction by approximately 0.015 of a pH unit per °C fall in temperature. This has been reviewed by Rahn and colleagues [99]; intracellular pH remains constant with respect to the neutrality of water due to intracellular protein buffering, predominantly by the alpha imidazole group of histidine residues. Extracellular pH needs to change in line with the intracellular pH changes to maintain acid-base balance; consequently, a relative alkalinity of the extracellular medium is required during hypothermia.

Early studies on the development of the St Thomas' Hospital solution [100] demonstrated the advantages of certain buffers over others, with phosphate and bicarbonate buffers being more effective than lactate when post-ischemic recovery of function was measured. It has been assumed that, when hearts are arrested with a cold cardioplegic solution, an alkaline pH should be used with the increasing alkalinity corresponding to decreasing temperature [101]. This concept was challenged by Nugent and colleagues [102] who reported that, using a crystalloid extracellular cardioplegic solution that was buffered with bicarbonate and titrated to pH levels of 7.1, 7.4 or 7.7, post-ischemic recovery of LV function in dog hearts subjected to 2 hours of 22°C ischemia was better in the acidic group than in the alkaline group. They suggested that acidic cardioplegia may inhibit metabolism and thus increase myocardial protection.

This concept was supported in a study by Bernard and coworkers [103] who looked at similar extracellular crystalloid cardioplegic solutions titrated to pH 7.0, 7.4 and 7.7. The most acidotic solution gave the best preservation of high-energy phosphate compounds and of post-ischemic functional recovery. In addition, these authors determined that, when comparing 20 mM bicarbonate, 20 mM glutamate, 47.5 mM Tris or 64.4 mM histidine buffers, bicarbonate gave the best buffering capacity but glutamate buffer maintained high energy phosphate compounds at the highest level with the most rapid return of aortic flow although ultimate recovery of function was the same with all buffers.

In contrast, Tait and colleagues [104] showed that the buffering capacity of 1.2 mM bicarbonate buffer was 60 times less than that obtained with 195 mM histidine and that even multidose infusions of bicarbonate buffered cardioplegic solution were unable to prevent the development of intramyocardial acidosis during 3 hours of ischemia at 20°C.

The importance of the pH of the cardioplegic solution has also been questioned. Lange and colleagues [105] investigated the mechanism by which intra-myocardial pH decreased. They concluded that the most important component was hypothermia and that the high alkalinity of the cardioplegic solution or the washout of acidic metabolites were of lesser importance. In an interesting study which investigated the role of intramyocardial pH and post-ischemic recovery of function following a period of hypothermic (28°C) ischemia alone, Takach and coworkers [106] demonstrated that, when intramyocardial pH fell below pH 7.0 (pH 6.8 or pH 6.6), post-ischemic recovery was significantly lower than if the intramyocardial pH was pH 7.0 or above, the intramyocardial pH being shown to correlate with the ultimate degree of recovery. Confirmation of this concept was demonstrated in a study by Vander Woude *et al.* [107], using isolated rabbit hearts, in which a bicarbonate-buffered crystalloid cardioplegic solution was compared to an imidazole-buffered solution. Imidazole is the buffering component of histidine and is present in blood in sufficient concentration to be its most important buffer. The use of imidazole was shown to prevent the pH of the coronary sinus effluent falling below pH 7.0 which was consistent with improved recovery of function.

The St Thomas' Hospital cardioplegic solution No. 2 is a bicarbonate-buffered solution which has a pH of 7.8 when exposed to air. It has been demonstrated that oxygenation of this solution improves myocardial protection [82,83]. Depending on the gassing mixture, the pH of the cardioplegic solution is altered; 100% O_2 increases the alkalinity of the solution giving a pH of 9.0, whereas 95% O_2 and 5% CO_2 increases the acidity of the solution to pH 7.0 [108]. A significant improvement in post-ischemic recovery of function was obtained following the use of the St Thomas' solution gassed with 95% O_2 and 5% CO_2 (pH 7.0), together with improved recovery of the sarcolemma. This study confirms those described earlier [102,103] in which acidotic solutions improved preservation.

The optimal pH and the optimal buffering component of extracellular crystalloid cardioplegic solutions remain to be established. Current opinion suggests that an acidic solution provides better protection than an alkalotic solution, in contrast to received opinion that decreased temperature favours alkalosis for the cardioplegic solution.

Methods of infusion

Antegrade versus retrograde

The first component of cardioplegia – rapid diastolic arrest – is dependent on delivering the arresting agent to all areas of the myocardium as rapidly as possible. When cardioplegic solutions were first introduced into clinical practice, they were administered by antegrade infusion via the aortic root or directly by infusion into the coronary ostia [7,109]. It was soon realised, however, that delivery via the antegrade route could be limiting if complete coronary occlusion was present, particularly at low infusion pressures.

One of the first studies to explore an alternative technique, that of infusing the cardioplegic solution retrogradely via the coronary sinus, was reported by Solorzano and colleagues in 1978 [110]. This technique had the advantage of protecting the myocardial mass distal to a coronary occlusion and was not influenced by opening the aorta or by severe aortic insufficiency. Menasché and colleagues [111] confirmed that the technique of coronary sinus cardioplegia was safe and efficacious in patients undergoing aortic valve surgery. In several experimental studies [112,113], using dogs with occluded coronary arteries, a significant improvement in delivery of cardioplegia to the occluded zone was obtained by retrograde coronary sinus infusion in comparison with antegrade cardioplegic delivery. This was associated with improved regional function and regional high-energy phosphate content.

An alternative retrograde infusion technique was advocated by Fabiani and colleagues [114]. Clinical studies by Fabiani and colleagues [114], in a large number of patients, had shown that the technique of retrograde coronary sinus infusion could be associated with damage to the coronary sinus. Consequently, they developed the technique of right atrial delivery with pulmonary artery occlusion with improved left ventricular function and no injury to the coronary sinus.

However, injury to the right ventricle, generated by pressures up to 60 mmHg, was not specifically measured. In a study designed to evaluate whether right ventricular function was compromised by right atrial cardioplegic solution in comparison to continuous retrograde coronary sinus cardioplegic perfusion, Salter and colleagues [115] demonstrated that right ventricular function was severely depressed. Left ventricular function was the same in both groups.

Studies from Buckberg's group [116] have demonstrated that using both antegrade and retrograde cardioplegic infusion adequately protects both the right and left ventricular myocardial mass distal to coronary artery occlusions. These studies, however, were conducted with blood cardioplegia and definitive studies using extracellular-type crystalloid cardioplegia have yet to be undertaken. Controversy remains as to whether right ventricular function is compromised using retrograde cardioplegic infusion.

Multidose versus single dose

Crystalloid cardioplegic solutions, such as the St Thomas' solution, were originally administered as a single infusion regardless of the duration of ischemia [109,117,118]. It was soon realised, from clinical observation and from birefringence assessment [117], that improved myocardial protection could be achieved with multiple infusions of cardioplegia when the ischemic duration was greater that 60 min [119]. It was also shown that extending the ischemic duration to 180 min or longer was detrimental to the myocardium, even with multidose cardioplegic infusions [120], which was subsequently confirmed by Chambers and colleagues [118].

The volume of cardioplegic infusion, together with the duration of infusion, promoted controversy between the proponents of 'extracellular-type' solutions and those of 'intracellular-type' solutions. Jynge and colleagues [4] demonstrated that, using extracellular-type solutions, infusion volume and duration were irrelevant to consistent myocardial protection, whereas intracellular-type solutions (such as that proposed by Bretschneider) were extremely volume and duration dependent. Subsequent studies have confirmed those findings, demonstrating that, for maximal myocardial protection with the St Thomas' Hospital No. 2 solution, the rate of infusion should be not less than 2.0 ml/gm wet wt for a duration of no less than 30 seconds [121]; infusion volumes/durations greater than this did not affect the recovery (Figure 6.7). These results suggest that the commonly used infusion volume of 1000 ml administered clinically is probably the minimum volume necessary for adequate myocardial protection.

Large volumes of cardioplegic infusion can be a problem if they are returned to the circulation on partial bypass. A solution to this problem is to discard these from the right atrium on total bypass, a technique used by the authors at St Thomas' Hospital, though dialysis on bypass is an alternative. An earlier study by Engelman and colleagues [122] had shown that infusing up to 5 litres of an extracellular-type crystalloid cardioplegic solution contributed to increased oxygen utilisation and did not cause any problems, provided the coronary sinus effluent was discarded and absorption was avoided. Similar results, using a modified Tyers' solution (extracellular type), was reported by Saydjari and colleagues [123], who could detect no significant difference between single dose or multiple dose infusion in terms of adenine nucleotide loss or reduction in myocardial function.

In contrast, Preusse *et al.* [124] demonstrated that the Bretschneider solution (intracellular-type) required infusion durations of 7–9 min of cardioplegic solution to reduce the myocardial O_2 consumption to a level consistent with energy demand at the hypothermic temperatures achieved in the myocardium.

Whereas multidose cardioplegic infusions appear to be beneficial in adult hearts, a number of recent studies suggest that they have a detrimental effect in immature/neonatal hearts. The first indication that multidose infusion of extracellular-type cardioplegic solutions might be detrimental was given by Magovern *et al.* [125] who studied the effects of multidose St Thomas' solution in immature (3–4 weeks) rabbit hearts subjected to 60, 90 or 120 min of 4°C global ischemia. When compared with mature hearts, functional recovery was decreased in a time (dose)-dependent manner, suggesting inadequacy

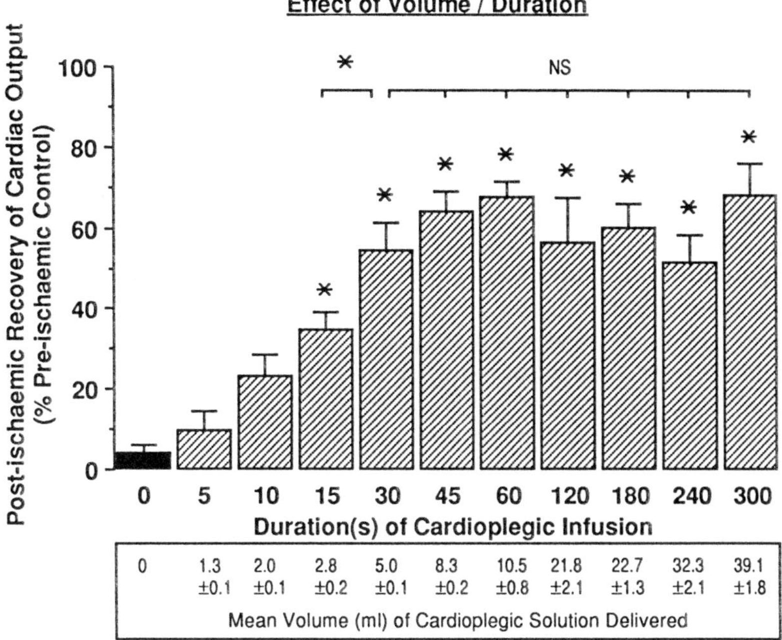

Figure 6.7. Post-ischemic recovery of cardiac output (expressed as a percent of pre-ischemic control value) in rat hearts subjected to various durations of cardioplegic infusion followed by 30 min normothermic (37°C) global ischemia. The solid column represents ischemia alone, cross-hatched column represents hearts protected by a cardioplegic infusion. Each column represents the mean of 6 hearts; bars represent SEM. $*p < 0.05$ compared with control (0) group. (Redrawn from: Takahashi *et al.*, J Thorac Cardiovasc Surg 1988; 95: 730–40.)

of myocardial preservation in the immature myocardium. This study was extended by Magovern and colleagues [126] to show that multidose cardioplegic infusions over ischemic durations of 90 or 120 min at 4°C resulted in significantly reduced post-ischemic recovery when compared with either topical cooling or single dose cardioplegic infusion.

This phenomenon has been studied in more detail by Kempsford and Hearse [127]. They demonstrated that the deleterious effects of multidose administration of St Thomas' Hospital cardioplegic solution No. 2 in neonatal (7–10 day) rabbit hearts was temperature-dependent; at moderate hypothermia (20°C), multidose cardioplegic infusions gave improved protection over single dose infusions. With deeper hypothermic (10°C), however, multidose infusion of St Thomas' cardioplegia was deleterious when compared with single dose or even with hypothermic ischemia alone.

Perfusion pressure

Perfusion pressure is an important component of the delivery and distribution of cardioplegic solutions. Increasing perfusion pressure would be expected to deliver an extracellular cardioplegic solution to more regions of the heart, particularly when coronary stenoses were present. A comparison between the delivery of blood versus crystalloid cardioplegia was carried out by Buckberg's group [128]. They demonstrated that, in dog hearts in which cardioplegia was infused at a constant flow of 250 ml/min, blood cardioplegia produced a significantly greater pressure; in addition, post-stenotic flow was higher with blood cardioplegia resulting in more rapid arrest and lower myocardial temperatures. They suggested that the lower viscosity of crystalloid cardioplegia resulted in a diversion of the solution from the obstructed vessels to the unobstructed vessels, with a reduced coronary vascular resistance and reduced infusion pressure.

In contrast, a more recent study by Eugene and colleagues [129], measuring regional flow by Xenon-133 washout in dogs subjected to moderate, severe and critical LAD stenosis, demonstrated that, although blood cardioplegia generated a higher perfusion pressure, regional perfusion was better with crystalloid cardioplegia under all conditions. Thus, the controversy regarding the efficacy of blood versus crystalloid cardioplegia remains open, even with regard to regional perfusion.

Special applications

Long-term preservation

With the advent of cardiac transplantation, the long-term preservation of donor hearts during transportation has become a priority. A number of studies carried out in the late 1960s and early 1970s had demonstrated that hearts could be preserved for periods of 24 to 72 hours [130–134] with hypothermia, either stored in hyperbaric oxygen [130] or continuously perfused with an extracellular-type solution (but not a cardioplegic solution) throughout the storage duration [131–134]. Most early studies relied on hypothermia alone to achieve this.

The advent of cardioplegia produced an increased interest in studies aimed at achieving long-term preservation, with solutions of both the 'extracellular-type' and the 'intracellular-type' being investigated. Intracellular-type solutions under investigation were predominantly those which had been used with success in long-term preservation of other organs, such as kidney, pancreas and liver. These solutions were the Collins [135] and Sacks [136] solutions and the University of Wisconsin (UW) solution [137]. The predominant extracellular-type solution used for long-term preservation has been the St Thomas' solution or a simple saline-based solution such as Krebs Henseleit bicarbonate buffer with elevated potassium. Preservation of donor hearts can be achieved by arrest (with an appropriate cardioplegic solution) and then storage by immersion in either the same or a different solution.

Although simple storage is the least complicated method for preserving and transporting donor hearts and is the technique used by most cardiac transplantation centres [138], it can lead to inadequate protection and result in poor recovery of function [139]. Despite arrest and profound hypothermia in stored hearts, metabolism will continue, leading to a build-up of toxic metabolites, changes in myocardial pH, increase in oedema and other sequelae. A number of studies have demonstrated the benefits of continuous, low flow perfusion throughout the storage period. Wicomb and colleagues [140] preserved baboon hearts for 20–24 hours, using a hyperosmolar crystalloid cardioplegic solution containing a number of additives (such as procaine, insulin, dextrose and verapamil) together with a hyperosmolar perfusate solution maintained between 4°C and 10°C and infused at a pressure of 8–10 cm H_2O. They used a modified nonpulsatile perfusion apparatus originally described by Proctor and Parker [131] and achieved survival of up to 33 days following orthotopic transplantation before rejection.

Subsequent studies in humans [141] with preservation times up to 17 hours, showed that this technique could be used with success in the human heart. These studies were extended by autotransplanting baboon hearts preserved for 24–48 hours using this technique, with survival of up to 27 months before sacrifice for ultrastructural analysis [142]. Similar studies have been carried out by Burt and colleagues [143,144] using rabbit hearts. They showed that preservation for 24 hours was possible using a Langendorff perfused preparation at either 5°C or 25°C perfused continuously at a pressure of 13 mmHg, and that it was the storage period of 24 hours that caused most damage to the heart, rather than the ischemia and reperfusion associated with removal of the heart and replacement in the recipient.

Studies carried out in the authors' laboratory, investigating the effects of using the St Thomas' Hospital cardioplegic solution for long-term preservation, have shown that rat hearts can be stored for up to 12 hours with good recovery of function, that immersion throughout this period does not influence the post-ischemic recovery (suggesting oedema may not be a critical component of injury) and that 7.5°C was the optimal temperature for long-term storage [145]. We [146] have also demonstrated that, when harvesting hearts for transplantation, an initial warm, rather than cold, infusion of cardioplegic solution to induce arrest, followed by a cold infusion, improves long-term preservation. We have also carried out studies using continuous low flow perfusion with the St Thomas' Hospital solution (Figure 6.8), which has shown that any benefit over simple storage is only obtained over a relatively narrow pressure range (10–30 cm H_2O) and that infusion at lower or higher pressures either leads to deterioration or to similar degrees of recovery, respectively [147].

Recently, there have been a number of long-term comparative studies

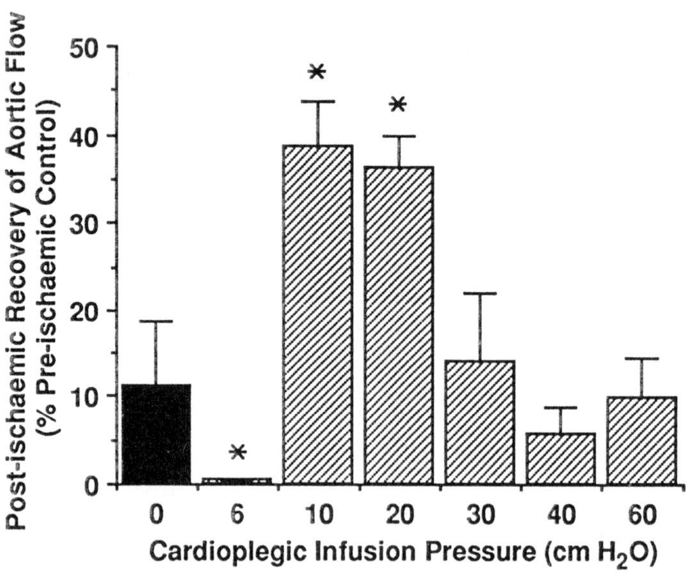

Figure 6.8. Post-ischemic recovery of aortic flow (expressed as a percent of pre-ischemic control value) in rat hearts subjected to 3 min STH2 infusion at 60 cm H_2O and either stored in STH2 (solid column) or continuously infused with STH2 at various infusion pressures (hatched columns) for 480 min at 7.5°C. $^*p < 0.05$ when compared with control (0) group. Each column represents the mean of 6 hearts; bars represent SEM. (Redrawn from: Chambers *et al.*, J Heart Lung Transplant 1992; 11: 665–75.)

between the St Thomas' solution and other crystalloid solutions, most notably the UW solution. St Thomas' solution was shown to provide the best preservation of human right atrial trabeculae following storage for 24 hours when compared to other extracellular-type solutions (modified Krebs Henseleit (K^+ = 15 mmol/l), Krebs Henseleit (K^+ = 4.5 mmol/l) and saline) or an intracellular solution (Euro-Collins solution) in terms of recovery of resting force [148]. Similar results were obtained in a study carried out by Choong and Gavin [149] comparing St Thomas' solution to the UW solution. Whereas hearts stored in UW solution for 5 hours resulted in poor recovery of function (but good recovery of myocardial adenine nucleotide content), preservation with STH produced normal function together with good recovery of myocardial adenine nucleotide content. Surprisingly, in this study the water content of hearts stored with UW solution was significantly greater than that of hearts stored in STH, even though the UW solution contains components (lactobionate and raffinose) specifically included to avoid the formation of oedema during the preservation period.

In contrast, Ledingham and colleagues [150] demonstrated superior preservation with UW solution compared with that of either St Thomas' No. 1 or

No. 2 solutions. Similar results were reported by Yeh *et al.* [151] in terms of post-ischemic ventricular function, water content and myocardial metabolite content; in this study, however, rat hearts were only arrested with the St Thomas' solution and were then stored for 6 hours in saline only.

It would not be surprising if extracellular-type cardioplegic solutions, which were developed for relatively short-term preservation of the myocardium during cardiac surgery, proved to be less than optimal for long-term preservation of donor hearts, but many experimental studies have shown that extracellular-type solutions have proved to be remarkably good at preserving the myocardium, even for relatively long periods.

The immature myocardium

In 1984, Bull, Cooper and Stark [152] published a study which concluded that, in consecutive series of 200 pediatric cardiac surgical patients, there was no difference in mortality between hearts protected by intermittent crossclamping and reperfusion and those protected by cardioplegia. In addition, analysis of the causes of mortality suggested that half could be accounted for by inadequate myocardial preservation. This study led to a renewed interest in the possibility that cardioplegic solutions, developed for adult hearts and used almost universally for both adult and pediatric surgery, are not ideal for preserving the immature myocardium.

Subsequently, however, studies by a number of groups have generated controversy. Isolated neonatal rabbit hearts were shown to have a greater tolerance to ischemia than mature hearts [153] and St Thomas' Hospital cardioplegia (either single or multidose) was shown to be significantly better than hypothermia alone or intermittent infusion with an oxygenated non-cardioplegic solution [154].

In contrast, Corno and colleagues [155] showed that topical hypothermia was better than crystalloid (St Thomas') cardioplegia and was as effective as blood cardioplegia in neonatal (1–5 day) pigs. The presence of normal calcium levels in the St Thomas' solution and the blood cardioplegia was shown to be important for good recovery, since similar solutions with low calcium levels (0.5–0.6 mmol/l) caused poor recovery of function.

These results suggested that neonatal hearts may be more sensitive to calcium. However, an ultrastructural study by Sawa *et al.* [156] in humans, showed that myocardial injury was greater in infants less than 3 months in terms of mitochondrial structure when protected with cold crystalloid GIK cardioplegia (but containing no calcium). In a further study, Sawa *et al.* [157] showed that addition of calcium (1.2 mmol/l) failed to reduce the mitochondrial injury observed previously, whereas addition of prostacyclin analogue together with calcium improved myocardial protection.

Studies from our laboratory showed that, despite the demonstrated increased tolerance to ischemia of the immature myocardium, the St Thomas' Hospital solution was protective [158]. Extracellular-type solutions (St Thomas' and Tyers) appeared to be more protective than intracellular-type solutions (Bretschneider and Roe's); this difference was suggested to be related to their lack of calcium [6]. However Riva and Hearse [159] demonstrated that, in neonatal rat hearts, calcium concentration of the cardioplegic solution appeared to have little influence on post-ischemic recovery. In contrast to these studies where cardioplegia was shown to be beneficial in neonatal hearts, Baker and colleagues [160] reported that hypothermia alone gave better protection to the immature myocardium of rabbits than St Thomas' Hospital cardioplegic solution, which appeared to have a significant detrimental effect when compared to the adult myocardium where it was protective. Further studies from this group [161,162] have suggested that oxygen availability during the pre-ischemic infusion was not a factor in this detrimental effect, whereas the calcium content may be involved. This latter point is in conflict with the study reported by Riva and Hearse [159] but may be associated with the different species used (rabbit and rat, respectively).

As has been discussed earlier, multidose infusions of crystalloid cardioplegic solutions appeared to be detrimental to myocardial recovery after ischemia in the immature myocardium. Using the St Thomas' Hospital cardioplegic solution, Magovern *et al.* [125,126] demonstrated that immature hearts were not protected as well as were adult hearts and that multidose administration was detrimental when compared with single dose cardioplegia or topical cooling alone (Figure 6.9). These studies were confirmed by Kempsford and Hearse [127], who also demonstrated that the detrimental effect of multidose administration was temperature-dependent. Further studies on the temperature-dependent detrimental effect of multidose cardioplegic administration in immature rabbit hearts have suggested that multidose cardioplegia is less effective than hypothermia alone at temperatures below 20°C and that the frequency of administration is also an important factor, although this did not appear to be related to the overall volume of cardioplegia infused [163].

In discussion of the 'immature' myocardium, it is essential to distinguish between neonatal, immature and 'adult' myocardium in both animals and humans, as was clearly shown by Riva and Hearse [159]. It is possible that many of the discrepancies that have arisen revolves around this point. The use of specific cardioplegic solutions for the particular type of myocardium (neonatal, infant or adult) remains a possibility.

Reperfusion

The majority of studies involving reperfusion have used blood cardioplegic solutions, studies which will be detailed in the following chapter. There have, however, been a few studies investigating extracellular solutions.

Good myocardial protection may be negated by poor or inappropriate reperfusion, resulting in so-called 'reperfusion injury'; the use of a modified reperfusion solution to attempt to prevent such injury may be a component

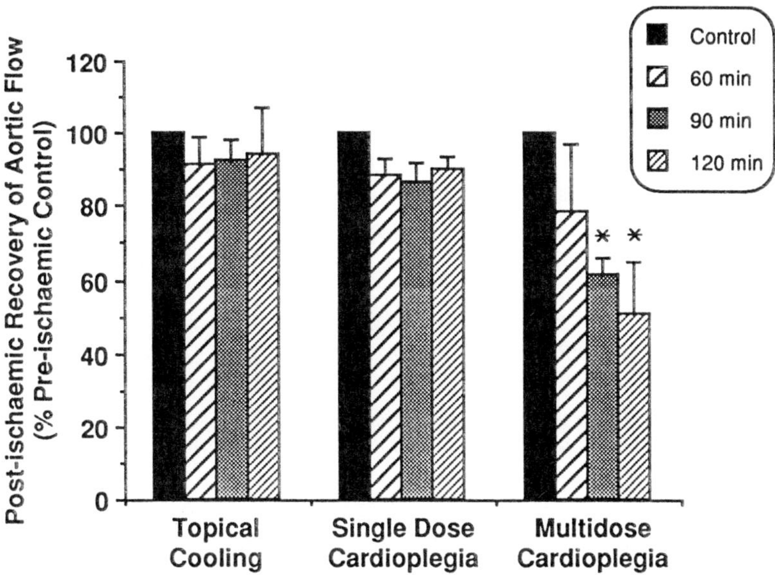

Figure 6.9. Post-ischemic recovery of aortic flow (expressed as a percent of pre-ischemic control value) in immature rabbit hearts subjected to no ischemia (control), 60, 90 or 120 min of global (10°C) ischemia. Hearts were protected either by topical cooling (immersion in saline), a single infusion (at 4°C) of STH2 at the start of ischemia with topical cooling, or multidose infusions (every 30 min) of STH2 with topical cooling. $^*p < 0.05$ when compared with control. Each column represents the mean of 6 hearts; bars represent SEM. (Redrawn from: Magovern *et al.*, J Thorac Cardiovasc Surg 1988; 96: 408–13.)

of good overall myocardial protection. In experimental studies using rat hearts, Menasché and colleagues [164] demonstrated that reperfusion with their cardioplegic solution containing low calcium and high magnesium was significantly less effective than using Krebs Henseleit buffer as the reperfusion solution. If, however, they increased the calcium concentration from 0.25 to 1.0 mmol/l, recovery of post-ischemic function was slightly greater than that achieved with cardioplegia alone. This contrasts with the studies from Buckberg's group using blood-based cardioplegic reperfusion solutions [165], who have shown that reduction of calcium is an important component of preventing reperfusion-induced injury under these conditions.

Menasché and coworkers [164] were also able to demonstrate that addition of glutamate improved post-ischemic recovery of function, even in hearts reperfused with the cardioplegic solution containing the low calcium concentration. Subsequent studies by the same group [166] in patients subjected to open heart surgery for aortic valve disease, showed that use of an extracellular cardioplegic reperfusion solution in high risk patients afforded significant benefit in terms of post-ischemic stroke work index together with a lower incidence of inotropic support.

More recent studies from our laboratory have investigated the effects of using oxygenated St Thomas' No. 1 and No. 2 solutions as reperfusion solutions. We [167] showed that reperfusion with these solutions failed to demonstrate any beneficial effect and, in the case of St Thomas' No. 1 solution, was actually detrimental. Addition of pyruvate to these solutions was beneficial when added to the St Thomas' No. 2 solution but had no effect on the St Thomas' No. 1 solution [168]. Thus, the benefit of crystalloid extracellular cardioplegic solutions as reperfusion solutions remains controversial.

Complications of extracellular solutions

Conduction system

There have been relatively few studies undertaken to determine the effects of crystalloid cardioplegic solutions on the myocardial conduction system. Together with the increasing use of hyperkalemic cardioplegic solutions has been an increase in the incidence of conduction abnormalities following reperfusion; thus, for example, prolonged heart block and supraventricular tachyarrhythmias not infrequently occur after open-heart surgery. These problems have been shown to result mainly from inadequate preservation leading to ischemic injury of the supraventricular conduction system during cardioplegic arrest. The major site of conduction delay was determined to be the AV-node [169].

Subsequent studies have demonstrated the occurrence of low-amplitude electrical activity (LEA), detected in the lower atrial septum, the atrioventricular node-His bundle complex and in the ventricular myocardium. This LEA occurs even at myocardial temperatures below 15°C, when conditions were thought to be adequate for myocardial protection [170]. Re-infusion of hyperkalemic cardioplegia, together with the application of topical hypothermia, decreased the likelihood of LEA during cardioplegic arrest. The site of origin of this LEA has been localised to the region of the atrial septum containing the atrioventricular nodal conduction tissue [171], and it has been shown that the addition of a calcium channel blocker (nifedipine) to the cardioplegic solution prevents LEA, suggesting the involvement of calcium-mediated activation of specialised conduction tissue.

An interesting study by Gundry and colleagues [172] showed that, when comparing blood and crystalloid cardioplegic solutions, there was a significantly greater incidence of perioperative and postoperative conduction disturbances with blood cardioplegia than with crystalloid cardioplegia. This study suggested that blood cardioplegia should be avoided in patients with pre-existing conduction problems; however, it is possible that the problems arise from using topical iced saline slush.

It has been shown clinically at St Thomas' Hospital that an important factor associated with post-occlusion heart block is the temperature of the 'reperfusing' solution. Removing the aortic clamp with the systemic temperature of the patient having been raised to 37°C virtually abolished a previously troublesome incidence of heart block after cold STH cardioplegia.

Preservation of the conduction system remains a little studied area. Postoperative dysrhythmias can be lethal; a specific component of this dysrhythmogenesis in cardioplegic solutions has yet to be identified.

Oedema

Myocardial cell swelling caused by increased water content is a consequence of ischemic injury; although crystalloid extracellular-type cardioplegic solutions are used to reduce ischemic injury, it is theoretically possible that they induce intracellular oedema. Thus, Kay and colleagues [173] found that water content increased by as much as 10% with hypothermic cardioplegia. Although cellular oedema has been shown to be associated with myocardial injury [174], what remains unclear is the extent of injury caused by infusing the extracellular-type cardioplegic solutions themselves. The addition of colloid or mannitol to an extracellular-type solution was shown [175] to prevent myocardial oedema which, in turn, was associated with improved function after infusion.

A recent study by Drewnowska and colleagues [176] showed that St Thomas' Hospital cardioplegic solution (used at 9°C) was hypotonic and induced cell swelling that was not due to hypothermia in the absence of ischemia. This study showed that influx of potassium chloride caused the cell swelling and that it could be partially prevented by replacing the chloride ion with an impermeant anion. They also demonstrated a transient shrinking of the myocardial cells when they were rewarmed using a normothermic Tyrode's solution; this shrinking could be prevented by ouabain, suggesting the involvement of sodium loading via the sodium-potassium pump. In contrast, Darracott-Cankovic and colleagues [177], using microscopic interferometry, showed that oedema was related to the degree of myocardial damage caused during ischemia; well preserved hearts showed no oedema.

The value of the inclusion of hypertonic components to combat the theoretical risk of oedema from extracellular cardioplegic solutions is clearly not proven. For instance, mannitol was shown to be potentially deleterious by Hearse *et al.* [31].

Endothelial damage

Little attention has been focused on the effects of extracellular-type crystalloid cardioplegic solutions on vascular tissue. A comparative study conducted by Carpentier and colleagues [178], in which the toxicity of 11 different cardioplegic solutions were compared to Eagle's culture medium on cultured endothelial cells, demonstrated that extracellular-type solutions (St Thomas' Hospital No. 1, Fabiani No. 1 and Robb-Nicholson solutions, in particular) were damaging, as was the Kirsch solution (intracellular solution); interestingly, Lolley's solution (and the Robb-Nicholson solution) had a considerable delayed cytotoxic effect. Intracellular-type solutions were less toxic and the addition of blood reduced the toxicity of all solutions but did not eliminate the delayed toxicity of Robb-Nicholson's or Lolley's solutions. Similar conclusions were reached by Mattila and coworkers [179] who studied the ultrastructure of coronary arteries infused with a crystalloid cardioplegic solution (similar to St Thomas' No. 1 solution but containing glucose). After 10 min of infusion, severe coronary endothelial damage occurred which could be prevented by the inclusion of blood or albumin.

A recent report from our laboratories has confirmed that infusion of hyperkalemic crystalloid solutions cause vascular damage involving the endothelium or its function [180]. Endothelium derived relaxant factor (EDRF)-induced vasodilation has been shown to be mediated by 5–HT whereas papaverine induces vasodilation via an action on the smooth muscle. Using these compounds, Saldanha and colleagues demonstrated that, after a 30 minute infusion of a modified St Thomas' Hospital cardioplegic solution containing 25 mmol/l potassium, the papaverine response was maintained whereas the 5-HT effect was abolished (Figure 6.10), suggesting cardioplegia-induced damage to the endothelium. Confirmation of these findings were reported by Chiavarelli and colleagues [181] in an ultrastructural study comparing the effects of infusing St Thomas' Hospital or the Alabama cardioplegic solutions with Krebs Henseleit bicarbonate buffer solution after subjecting the hearts to various periods of ischemia and reperfusion. Whilst the myocardium was well preserved with both cardioplegic solutions, the endothelium was damaged by the St Thomas' Hospital solution, together with a tendency towards removal of the endothelial lining. Similar findings have been obtained by von Oppell and colleagues [182] using endothelial cell culture and comparing the St Thomas' solution with the Bretschneider cardioplegic solution and to the Collins and UW preservation solutions. They again found that the St Thomas' solution was the most damaging during hypothermic infusion; however, at normothermic infusion the St Thomas' solution was the least cytotoxic.

Infusion flow rate and pressure are important determinants of both endothelial and myocardial injury; higher flows and pressures cause endothelial damage whereas low flow and pressure increases myocardial ischemic injury [183]. The addition of adenosine to the St Thomas' solution, followed by blood reperfusion with added adenosine has been suggested as a means by which endothelial damage mediated by cardioplegia may be ameliorated, presumably by the increased vasodilation, reducing physical damage and preventing vasoconstrictive effects [184].

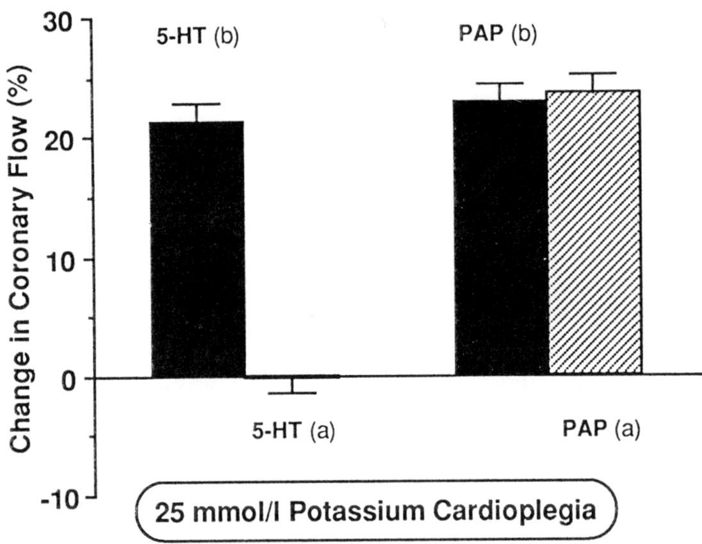

Figure 6.10. Changes in coronary flow (expressed as a percent of drug-free control) in rat hearts in response to 5–hydroxtryptamine (5–HT) at a dose of 1×10^{-7} mol/l and to papaverine (PAP) at a dose of 5×10^{-6} mol/l before (b) and after (a) 30 min continuous infusion of a modified STH2 (containing 25 mmol/l potassium). Each column represents the mean of 8 hearts; bars represent SEM. (Redrawn from: Saldanha and Hearse, J Thorac Cardiovasc Surg 1989; 98: 783–7.)

Extracellular solutions do damage the endothelium in experimental studies. The importance of such damage in the clinical situation, where there is consistent washout by non-coronary collateral flow, is not yet clear.

Particulate contamination

A potential hazard with crystalloid cardioplegic solutions (particularly those based on commercially available intravenous solutions) was demonstrated by Robinson *et al.* [185]. Rat hearts exposed to various solutions which conformed to standard limits established for intravenous solutions caused a progressive reduction in coronary flow which could be partially relieved by nifedipine and almost completely relieved by filtration, suggesting that particle-induced coronary vasoconstriction was the likely mechanism. Further studies into this mechanism demonstrated that focal endothelial injury associated with the 5–HT receptor was probably responsible for transient vasospasm [186]. Following these studies, 8 μm filters were routinely included in the cardioplegic infusion apparatus at St Thomas' Hospital.

Vasoconstriction affects distribution of the cardioplegic solution and is therefore undesirable. Measures to eliminate it can only be beneficial.

Conclusion

Extracellular-type crystalloid solutions have proved the most universally used cardioplegic solutions since their introduction in the 1970s; at one point the St Thomas' solution was used by 40% of the cardiac units of the world. Their advantages have been simplicity and speed of infusion, requiring no pumps nor elaborate equipment, and their consequent cheapness, both combined with overall efficacy of myocardial protection.

Subsequent experience has shown that they still supply the gold standard that has to be surpassed by other solutions. They do have an incidence of dysrhythmias, potential endothelial damage and difficulty with administration of modified reperfusion techniques, but their advantages have outweighed their disadvantages, particularly in units where simplicity of administration and cheapness are important.

Only time will tell whether the current diversity of solutions for myocardial protection for adult and pediatric surgery, for routine cardiac and transplantation surgery, will settle into a well-characterised, clinically proven mode. Till then, extracellular-type solutions will maintain their popularity.

References

1. Hearse DJ, Braimbridge MV, Jynge P. Protection of the ischemic myocardium: cardioplegia. New York: Raven Press, 1981.
2. Hearse DJ. Cardioplegia. Postgrad Med J 1983; 59 (Suppl 2): 11–24.
3. Jynge P. Cardioplegic solutions and sodium-calcium relationships. In Calderera CM, Harris P (eds): Advances in Studies on Heart Metabolism. Bologna: CLUEB 1982; 369–74.
4. Jynge P, Hearse DJ, Braimbridge MV. Protection of the ischemic myocardium. Volume-duration relationships and the efficacy of myocardial infusates. J Thorac Cardiovasc Surg 1978; 76: 698–705.
5. Tyers GFO, Manley NJ, Williams EH *et al.* Preliminary clinical experience with isotonic potassium-induced arrest. J Thorac Cardiovasc Surg 1977; 74: 674–81.
6. Kempsford RD, Hearse DJ. Protection of the immature myocardium during global ischemia. A comparison of four clinical cardioplegic solutions in the rabbit heart. J Thorac Cardiovasc Surg 1989; 97: 856–63.
7. Braimbridge MV, Chayen J, Bitensky L *et al.* Cold cardioplegia or continuous coronary perfusion? J Thorac Cardiovasc Surg 1977; 74: 900–6.
8. Hearse DJ, Stewart DA, Braimbridge MV. Cellular protection during myocardial ischemia. The development and characterisation of a procedure for the induction of reversible ischemic arrest. Circulation 1976; 54: 193–202.
9. Krebs HA, Henseleit K. Untersuchungen uber die Harnstoffbildung im Tierkorper. Hoppe Seylers Z Physiol Chem 1932; 210: 33–66.

10. Jynge P, Hearse DJ, Feuvray D *et al.* The St Thomas' Hospital cardioplegic solution: A characterisation in two species. Scand J Thorac Cardiovasc Surg 1981; (Suppl 30): 1–28.
11. Jynge P. Protection of the ischemic myocardium: cold chemical cardioplegia, coronary infusates and the importance of cellular calcium control. Thorac Cardiovasc Surgeon 1980; 28: 310–21.
12. Yamamoto F, Braimbridge MV, Hearse DJ. Calcium and cardioplegia. J Thorac Cardiovasc Surg 1984; 87: 902–12.
13. Robinson LA, Harwood DL. Lowering the calcium concentration in St Thomas' Hospital cardioplegic solution improves protection during hypothermic ischemia. J Thorac Cardiovasc Surg 1991; 101: 314–25.
14. Takahashi A, Chambers DJ, Braimbridge MV *et al.* Long term hypothermic preservation of the heart: the optimal concentration of calcium in the St Thomas' Hospital cardioplegic solution. J Mol Cell Cardiol 1989; 21 (Suppl II): S.121.
15. Boggs BR, Torchiana DF, Geffin GA *et al.* Optimal myocardial preservation with an acalcemic crystalloid cardioplegic solution. J Thorac Cardiovasc Surg 1987; 93: 838–46.
16. Ettinger PO, Regan TJ, Oldewurtel HA. Hyperkalemia, cardiac conduction and the electrocardiogram: a review. Am Heart J 1974; 88: 360–71.
17. Kirsch U, Rodewald G, Kalmar P. Induced ischemic arrest: clinical experience with cardioplegia in open-heart surgery. J Thorac Cardiovasc Surg 1972; 63: 121–30.
18. Hearse DJ, Stewart DA, Braimbridge MV. Myocardial protection during ischemic cardiac arrest. The importance of magnesium in cardioplegic infusates. J Thorac Cardiovasc Surg 1978; 75: 877–85.
19. Reynolds TR, Geffin GA, Titus JS *et al.* Myocardial preservation related to magnesium content of hyperkalemic cardioplegic solutions at 8°C. Ann Thorac Surg 1989; 47: 907–13.
20. Geffin GA, Love TR, Hendren WG *et al.* The effects of calcium and magnesium in hyperkalemic cardioplegic solutions on myocardial preservation. J Thorac Cardiovasc Surg 1989; 98: 239–50.
21. Kinoshita K, Oe M, Tokunaga K. Superior protective effect of low-calcium, magnesium-free potassium cardioplegic solution on ischemic myocardium. Clinical study in comparison with St Thomas' Hospital solution. J Thorac Cardiovasc Surg 1991; 101: 695–702.
22. Gay WA, Ebert PA. Functional, metabolic and morphological effects of potassium-induced cardioplegia. Surgery 1973; 74: 284–90.
23. Roe BB, Hutchinson JC, Fishman NH *et al.* Myocardial protection with cold, ischemic, potassium-induced cardioplegia. J Thorac Cardiovasc Surg 1977; 73: 366–70.
24. Conti VR, Bertranou EG, Blackstone EH *et al.* Cold cardioplegia versus hypothermia for myocardial protection. Randomized clinical study. J Thorac Cardiovasc Surg 1978; 76: 577–86.
25. Robinson LA, Braimbridge MV, Hearse DJ. Comparison of the protective properties of four clinical crystalloid cardioplegic solutions in the rat heart. Ann Thorac Surg 1984; 38: 268–74.
26. Ledingham SJM, Braimbridge MV, Hearse DJ. The St Thomas' Hospital cardioplegic solution. A comparison of the efficacy of two formulations. J Thorac Cardiovasc Surg 1987; 93: 240–6.
27. Chambers DJ, Sakai A, Braimbridge MV *et al.* Clinical validation of St Thomas' Hospital cardioplegic solution No 2 (Plegisol). Eur J Cardio-thorac Surg 1989; 3: 346–52.
28. Krause BL, Wakefield JSJ, McMillan AB *et al.* Protection of the ischaemic myocardium by glucose-insulin-potassium infusion assessed by ventricular function and electron microscopy. J Cardiovasc Surg 1978; 19: 421–32.
29. Lolley DM, Ray JF, Myers WO *et al.* Reduction of intraoperative myocardial infarction by means of exogenous anaerobic substrate enhancement: prospective randomized study. Ann Thorac Surg 1978; 26: 515–23.
30. von Oppell UO, Du Toit EF, King LM *et al.* St Thomas' Hospital cardioplegic solution.

Beneficial effect of glucose and multidose reinfusions of cardioplegic solution. J Thorac Cardiovasc Surg 1991; 102: 405–12.

31. Hearse DJ, Stewart DA, Braimbridge MV. Myocardial protection during ischemic cardiac arrest. Possible deleterious effects of glucose and mannitol in coronary infusates. J Thorac Cardiovasc Surg 1978; 76: 16–23.
32. Yamamoto F, Manning AS, Braimbridge MV *et al.* Calcium antagonists and myocardial protection during cardioplegic arrest. In Dhalla NS, Hearse DJ (eds): Advances in myocardiology. New York: Plenum Press 1985; 545–62.
33. Murashita T, Hearse DJ, Avkiran M. Effects of diltiazem as an additive to St Thomas' Hospital cardioplegic solution in isolated neonatal and adult rabbit hearts. Cardiovasc Res 1991; 25: 496–502.
34. Guyton RA, Dorsey LM, Colgan TK *et al.* Calcium-channel blockade as an adjunct to heterogeneous delivery of cardioplegia. Ann Thorac Surg 1983; 35: 626–31.
35. Chiavarelli M, Chiavarelli R, Macchiarelli A *et al.* Calcium entry blockers and cardioplegia: interaction between nifedipine, potassium, and hypothermia. Ann Thorac Surg 1986; 41: 535–41.
36. Flameng W, De Meyere R, Daenen W *et al.* Nifedipine as an adjunct to St Thomas' Hospital cardioplegia. A double-blind, placebo-controlled, randomized clinical trial. J Thorac Cardiovasc Surg 1986; 91: 723–31.
37. Guffin AV, Kates RA, Holbrook GW *et al.* Verapamil and myocardial preservation in patients undergoing coronary artery bypass surgery. Ann Thorac Surg 1986; 41: 587–91.
38. Christakis GT, Fremes SE, Weisel RD *et al.* Diltiazem cardioplegia. A balance of risk and benefit. J Thorac Cardiovasc Surg 1986; 91: 647–61.
39. McCall DM. Responses of cultured heart cells to procainamide and lignocaine. Cardiovasc Surg 1978; 12: 529–36.
40. Harlan BJ, Ross D, MacManus Q *et al.* Cardioplegic solutions for myocardial preservation. Analysis of hypothermic arrest, potassium arrest, and procaine arrest. Circulation 1978; 58 (Suppl I): I-114–I-118.
41. Hearse DJ, O'Brien K, Braimbridge MV. Protection of the myocardium during ischemic arrest. Dose-response curves for procaine and lignocaine in cardioplegic solutions. J Thorac Cardiovasc Surg 1981; 81: 873–9.
42. McCord JM, Fridovich I. Superoxide dismutase. An enzymic function for erythrocuprein (hemocuprein). J Biol Chem 1969; 244: 6049–55.
43. Parks DA, Bulkley GB, Granger DM *et al.* Ischemic injury in the cat small intestine: role of superoxide radicals. Gastroenterology 1982; 82: 9–15.
44. Shlafer M, Kane PF, Wiggins VY *et al.* Possible role for cytotoxic oxygen metabolites in the pathogenesis of cardiac ischemic injury. Circulation 1982; 66 (Suppl I): I-85–I-92.
45. Shlafer M, Kane PF, Kirsh MM. Superoxide dismutase plus catalase enhances the efficacy of hypothermic cardioplegia to protect the globally ischemic, reperfused heart. J Thorac Cardiovasc Surg 1982; 83: 830–9.
46. Stewart JR, Blackwell WH, Crute SL *et al.* Inhibition of surgically induced ischemia/reperfusion injury by oxygen free radical scavengers. J Thorac Cardiovasc Surg 1983; 86: 262–72.
47. Myers CL, Weiss SJ, Kirsh MM *et al.* Effects of supplementing hypothermic crystalloid cardioplegic solution with catalase, superoxide dismutase, allopurinol, or deferoxamine on functional recovery of globally ischemic and reperfused isolated hearts. J Thorac Cardiovasc Surg 1986; 91: 281–9.
48. Chambers DJ, Braimbridge MV, Hearse DJ. Free radicals and cardioplegia. Free radical scavengers improve post-ischemic function of rat myocardium. Eur J Cardio-thorac Surg 1987; 1: 37–45.
49. Chambers DJ, Braimbridge MV, Hearse DJ. Free radicals and cardioplegia: allopurinol and oxypurinol reduce myocardial injury following ischemic arrest. Ann Thorac Surg 1987; 44: 291–7.
50. Menasché P, Grousset C, Gaudel Y *et al.* Prevention of hydroxyl radical formation: a

critical concept for improving cardioplegia. Protective effects of deferoxamine. Circulation 1987; 76 (Suppl V): V-180–V-185.
51. Bernard M, Menasché P, Piétri S *et al.* Cardioplegic arrest superimposed on evolving myocardial ischemia. Improved recovery after inhibition of hydroxyl radical generation by peroxidase or deferoxamine. A ^{31}P nuclear resonance study. Circulation 1988; 78 (Suppl III): III-164–III-172.
52. Menasché P, Pasquier C, Bellucci S *et al.* Deferoxamine reduces neutrophil-mediated free radical production during cardiopulmonary bypass. J Thorac Cardiovasc Surg 1988; 96: 582–9.
53. Eddy LJ, Stewart JR, Jones HP *et al.* Free radical-producing enzyme, xanthine oxidase, is undetectable in human hearts. Am J Physiol 1987; 253: H709–H711.
54. Robinson LA, Braimbridge MV, Hearse DJ. Creatine phosphate: an additive myocardial protective and antiarrhythmic agent in cardioplegia. J Thorac Cardiovasc Surg 1984; 87: 190–200.
55. Robinson LA, Braimbridge MV, Hearse DJ. Enhanced myocardial protection with high-energy phosphates in St Thomas' Hospital cardioplegic solution. Synergism of adenosine triphosphate and creatine phosphate. J Thorac Cardiovasc Surg 1987; 93: 415–27.
56. Chambers DJ, Braimbridge MV, Kosker S *et al.* Creatine phosphate (Neoton) as an additive to St Thomas' Hospital cardioplegic solution (Plegisol). Results of a clinical study. Eur J Cardio-thorac Surg 1991; 5: 74–81.
57. Robinson LA, Harwood DL. Exogenous creatine phosphate: favorable calcium-altering effects in St Thomas' Hospital cardioplegic solution. J Am Coll Cardiol 1988; 11: 170A.
58. Hohl CM, Hearse DJ. Vascular and contractile responses to extracellular ATP: studies in the isolated rat heart. Can J Cardiol 1985; 1: 207–16.
59. Conorev EA, Sharov VG, Saks VA. Improvement in contractile recovery of isolated rat heart after cardioplegic ischaemic arrest with endogenous phosphocreatine: involvement of antiperoxidative effect? Cardiovasc Res 1991; 25: 164–71.
60. Zucchi R, Poddighe R, Limbruno U *et al.* Protection of isolated rat heart from oxidative stress by exogenous creatine phosphate. J Mol Cell Cardiol 1989; 21: 67–73.
61. Thelin S, Hultman J, Ronquist G *et al.* Enhanced protection of rat hearts during ischemia by phosphoenolpyruvate and ATP in cardioplegia. Thorac Cardiovasc Surgeon 1986; 34: 104–9.
62. DeWitt DF, Jochim KE, Behrendt DM. Nucleotide degradation and functional impairment during cardioplegia: amelioration by inosine. Circulation 1983; 67: 171–8.
63. Devous MD, Lewandowski ED. Inosine preserves ATP during ischemia and enhances recovery during reperfusion. Am J Physiol 1987; 253: H1224–H1233.
64. Schubert T, Vetter H, Owen P *et al.* Adenosine cardioplegia. Adenosine versus potassium cardioplegia: Effects on cardiac arrest and post-ischemic recovery in the isolated rat heart. J Thorac Cardiovasc Surg 1989; 98: 1057–65.
65. De Jong JW, van der Meer P, van Loon HA *et al.* Adenosine as adjunct to potassium cardioplegia: effect on function, energy metabolism, and electrophysiology. J Thorac Cardiovasc Surg 1990; 100: 445–54.
66. Bolling SF, Bies LE, Bove EL *et al.* Augmenting intracellular adenosine improves myocardial recovery. J Thorac Cardiovasc Surg 1990; 99: 469–74.
67. Ledingham S, Katayama O, Lachno D *et al.* Beneficial effect of adenosine during reperfusion following prolonged cardioplegic arrest. Cardiovasc Res 1990; 24: 247–53.
68. Rau EE, Shine KI, Gervais A *et al.* Enhanced mechanical recovery of anoxic and ischemic myocardium by amino acid perfusion. Am J Physiol 1979; 236: H873–H879.
69. Pisarenko OI, Solomatina ES, Studneva IM *et al.* Protective effect of glutamic acid on cardiac function and metabolism during cardioplegia and reperfusion. Basic Res Cardiol 1983; 78: 534–43.
70. Gharagozloo F, Melendez FJ, Hein RA *et al.* The effect of amino acid L-glutamate on the extended preservation ex vivo of the heart for transplanation. Circulation 1987; 76 (Suppl V): V-65–V-70.

71. Choong YS, Gavin JB. L-aspartate improves the functional recovery of explanted hearts stored in St Thomas' Hospital cardioplegic solution at 4°C. J Thorac Cardiovasc Surg 1990; 99: 510–7.
72. Tyers GFO, Todd GJ, Niebauer IM *et al.* Effect of intracoronary tetrodotoxin on recovery of the isolated working rat heart from sixty minutes of ischemia. Circulation 1974; 49/50 (Suppl II): II-175–II-179.
73. Sternbergh WC, Brunsting LA, Abd-Elfattah AS *et al.* Basal metabolic energy requirements of polarized and depolarized arrest in rat heart. Am J Physiol 1989; 256: H846–H851.
74. Wikman-Coffelt J, Wagner S, Wu S *et al.* Alcohol and pyruvate cardioplegia. Twenty-four-hour in situ preservation of hamster hearts. J Thorac Cardiovasc Surg 1991; 101: 509–16.
75. Engelman RM, Rousou JH, Dobbs W *et al.* The superiority of blood cardioplegia in myocardial preservation. Circulation 1980; 62 (Suppl I): I-62–I-66.
76. Digerness SB, Vanini V, Wideman FE. In vitro comparison of oxygen availability from asanguinous and sanguinous cardioplegic media. Circulation 1981; 64 (Suppl II): II-80–II-83.
77. Bodenhamer RM, DeBoer LWV, Geffin GA *et al.* Enhanced myocardial protection during ischemic arrest. Oxygenation of a crystalloid cardioplegic solution. J Thorac Cardiovasc Surg 1983; 85: 769–80.
78. Bing OHL, LaRaia PJ, Stoughton FJ *et al.* Mechanism of myocardial protection during blood-potassium cardioplegia: a comparison of crystalloid red cell and methemoglobin solutions. Circulation 1984 70 (Suppl I): I-84–I-90.
79. Heitmiller RF, BeBoer LWV, Geffin GA *et al.* Myocardial recovery after hypothermic arrest: a comparison of oxygenated crystalloid to blood cardioplegia. A role of calcium. Circulation 1985; 72 (Suppl II): II-241–II-253.
80. Magovern GJ Jr., Flaherty JT, Gott VL *et al.* Failure of blood cardioplegia to protect myocardium at lower temperatures. Circulation 1982; 66 (Suppl I): I-60–I-67.
81. Rousou JA, Engelman RM, Breyer RH *et al.* The effect of temperature and hematocrit level of oxygenated cardioplegic solutions on myocardial preservation. J Thorac Cardiovasc Surg 1988; 95: 625–30.
82. Ledingham SJM, Braimbridge MV, Hearse DJ. Improved myocardial protection by oxygenation of the St Thomas' Hospital cardioplegic solution. J Thorac Cardiovasc Surg 1988; 95: 103–11.
83. von Oppell UO, King LM, Du Toit EF *et al.* Effect of oxygenation and consequent pH changes on the efficacy of St Thomas' Hospital cardioplegic solution. J Thorac Cardiovasc Surg 1991; 102: 396–404.
84. Tabayashi K, McKeown PP, Miyamoto M *et al.* Ischemic myocardial protection. Comparison of nonoxygenated crystalloid, oxygenated crystalloid, and oxygenated fluorocarbon cardioplegic solutions. J Thorac Cardiovasc Surg 1988; 95: 239–46.
85. Guyton RA, Dorsey LMA, Craver JM *et al.* Improved myocardial recovery after cardioplegic arrest with an oxygenated crystalloid solution. J Thorac Cardiovasc Surg 1985; 89: 877–87.
86. Daggett WM Jr., Randolph JD, Jacobs M *et al.* The superiority of cold oxygenated dilute blood cardioplegia. Ann Thorac Surg 1987; 43: 397–402.
87. Chambers DJ, Kosker S, Takahashi A *et al.* Comparison of standard (non-oxygenated) vs. oxygenated St Thomas' Hospital cardioplegic solution No 2 (Plegisol). Eur J Cardiothorac Surg 1990; 4: 549–55.
88. Bernhard WF, Schwartz HF, Mallick NP. Profound hypothermia as an adjunct to cardiovascular surgery. J Thorac Cardiovasc Surg 1961; 42: 263–74.
89. Greenberg JJ, Edmunds LH. Effect of myocardial ischemia at varying temperatures on left ventricular function and tissue tension. J Thorac Cardiovasc Surg 1961; 42: 84–91.
90. Griepp RB, Stinson EB, Shumway NE. Profound local hypothermia for myocardial protection during open-heart surgery. J Thorac Cardiovasc Surg 1973; 66: 731–41.

91. Hearse DJ, Stewart DA, Braimbridge MV. Hypothermic arrest and potassium arrest: metabolic and myocardial protection during elective cardiac arrest. Circ Res 1975; 36: 481–9.
92. Gillette PC, Pinsky WW, Lewis RM *et al.* Myocardial depression after elective ischemic arrest: subcellular biochemistry and prevention. J Thorac Cardiovasc Surg 1979; 77: 608–18.
93. Rosenfeldt FL, Hearse DJ, Cankovic-Darracott S *et al.* The additive protective effects of hypothermia and chemical cardioplegia during ischemic cardiac arrest in the dog. J Thorac Cardiovasc Surg 1980; 79: 29–38.
94. Hearse DJ, Stewart DA, Braimbridge MV. The additive protective effects of hypothermia and chemical cardioplegia during ischemic cardiac arrest in the rat. J Thorac Cardiovasc Surg 1980; 79: 39–43.
95. Borst HG, Iversen ST. Myocardial temperatures in clinical cardioplegia. Thorac Cardiovasc Surgeon 1980; 28: 29–33.
96. Rabinov M, Chen XZ, Rosenfeldt FL. Comparison of the metabolic response of the hypertrophic and the normal heart to hypothermic cardioplegia. The effect of temperature. J Thorac Cardiovasc Surg 1989; 97: 43–9.
97. Lichtenstein SV, Abel JG, Panos A *et al.* Warm heart surgery: experience with long cross-clamp times. Ann Thorac Surg 1991; 52: 1009–13.
98. Landymore RW, Marble AE, Eng P *et al.* Myocardial oxygen consumption and lactate production during antegrade warm blood cardioplegia. Eur J Cardio-thorac Surg 1992; 6: 372–6.
99. Rahn H, Reeves RB, Howell BJ. Hydrogen ion regulation, temperature, and evolution. Am Rev Resp Dis 1975; 112: 165–72.
100. Hearse DJ, Stewart DA, Braimbridge MV. Myocardial protection during bypass and arrest. A possible hazard with lactate-containing infusates. J Thorac Cardiovasc Surg 1976; 72: 880–4.
101. Buckberg GD. A proposed "solution" to the cardioplegic controversy. J Thorac Cardiovasc Surg 1979; 77: 803–15.
102. Nugent WC, Levine FH, Liapis CD *et al.* Effect of the pH of cardioplegic solution on postarrest myocardial preservation. Circulation 1982; 66 (Suppl I): I-68–I-72.
103. Bernard M, Menasché P, Canioni PJ *et al.* Influence of the pH of cardioplegic solutions on intracellular pH, high-energy phosphates, and postarrest performance. Protective effects of acidotic, glutamate-containing cardioplegic perfusates. J Thorac Cardiovasc Surg 1985; 90: 235–42.
104. Tait GA, Booker PD, Wilson GJ *et al.* Effect of multidose cardioplegia and cardioplegic solution buffering on myocardial tissue acidosis. J Thorac Cardiovasc Surg 1982; 83: 824–9.
105. Lange R, Cavanaugh AC, Zierler M *et al.* The relative importance of alkalinity, temperature, and the washout effect of bicarbonate-buffered, multidose cardioplegic solution. Circulation 1984; 70 (Suppl I): I-75–I-83.
106. Takach TJ, Glassman LR, Ribakove GH *et al.* Continuous measurement of intramyocardial pH: correlation to functional recovery following normothermic and hypothermic global ischemia. Ann Thorac Surg 1986; 42: 31–6.
107. Vander Woude JC, Christlieb IY, Sicard GA *et al.* Imidazole-buffered cardioplegic solution. Improved myocardial preservation during global ischemia. J Thorac Cardiovasc Surg 1985; 90: 225–34.
108. von Oppell UO, King LM, Du Toit EF *et al.* Effect of pH shifts induced by oxygenating crystalloid cardioplegic solutions. Ann Thorac Surg 1991; 52: 903–7.
109. Braimbridge MV, Hearse DJ, Chayen J *et al.* Cold cardioplegia versus continuous coronary perfusion: clinical and cytochemical assessment. In. Longmore DB (ed): Modern Cardiac Surgery. London: MTP Press 1978; 285–98.
110. Solorzano J, Taitelbaum G, Chiu R C-J. Retrograde coronary sinus perfusion for myocardial protection during cardiopulmonary bypass. Ann Thorac Surg 1978; 25: 201–8.

111. Menasché P, Kural S, Fauchet M *et al.* Retrograde coronary sinus perfusion: a safe alternative for ensuring cardioplegic delivery in aortic valve surgery. Ann Thorac Surg 1982; 34: 647–58.
112. Mori F, Ivey TD, Tabayashi K *et al.* Regional myocardial protection by retrograde coronary sinus infusion of cardioplegic solution. Circulation 1986; 74 (Suppl III): III-116–III-124.
113. Masuda M, Yonenaga K, Shiki K *et al.* Myocardial protection in coronary occlusion by retrograde cardioplegic perfusion via the coronary sinus in dogs. Preservation of high-energy phosphates and regional function. J Thorac Cardiovasc Surg 1986; 92: 255–63.
114. Fabiani J-N, Relland J, Carpentier A. Myocardial protection via the coronary sinus in cardiac surgery: comparative evaluation of two techniques. In Mohl W, Wolner E, Glogar D (eds): The Coronary Sinus. Darmstadt: Steinkopff Vertag, 1984: 305–11.
115. Salter DR, Goldstein JP, Abd-Elfattah A *et al.* Ventricular function after atrial cardioplegia. Circulation 1987; 76 (Suppl V): V-129–V-140.
116. Partington MT, Acar C, Buckberg GD *et al.* Studies of retrograde cardioplegia II Advantages of antegrade/retrograde cardioplegia to optimize distribution in jeopardized myocardium. J Thorac Cardiovasc Surg 1989; 97: 613–22.
117. Cankovic-Darracott S, Braimbridge MV, Chayen J. Biopsy assessment of preservation during open-heart surgery with cold cardioplegic arrest. In Chazov E, Saks V, Rona G (eds): Advances in Myocardiology. Plenum Publishing Corporation, 1983; 497–504.
118. Chambers DJ, Darracott-Cankovic S, Braimbridge MV. Clinical and quantitative birefringence assessment of 100 patients with aortic clamping periods in excess of 120 minutes after hypothermic cardioplegic arrest. Thorac Cardiovasc Surgeon 1983; 31: 266–72.
119. Engelman RM, Levitsky S, O'Donoghue MJ *et al.* Cardioplegia and myocardial preservation during cardiopulmonary bypass. Circulation 1978; 58: 107–13.
120. Engelman RM, Rousou JH, Vertrees RA *et al.* Safety of prolonged ischemic arrest using hypothermic cardioplegia. J Thorac Cardiovasc Surg 1980; 79: 705–12.
121. Takahashi A, Chambers DJ, Braimbridge MV *et al.* Optimal myocardial protection during crystalloid cardioplegia. Interrelationship between volume and duration of infusion. J Thorac Cardiovasc Surg 1988; 96: 730–40.
122. Engelman RM, Rousou JH, Lemeshow S. High-volume crystalloid cardioplegia. An improved method of myocardial preservation. J Thorac Cardiovasc Surg 1983; 86: 87–96.
123. Saydjari R, Asimakis G, Conti VR. Effect of increasing volume of cardioplegic solution on post-ischemic myocardial recovery. J Thorac Cardiovasc Surg 1987; 94: 234–40.
124. Preusse CJ, Schulte HD, Bircks W. High volume cardioplegia. Ann Chirurg Gynaecol 1987; 76: 39–45.
125. Magovern JA, Pae WE, Miller CA *et al.* The immature and the mature myocardium. Responses to multidose crystalloid cardioplegia. J Thorac Cardiovasc Surg 1988; 95: 618–24.
126. Magovern JA, Pae WE, Waldhausen JA. Protection of the immature myocardium. An experimental evaluation of topical cooling, single-dose, and multiple-dose administration of St Thomas' Hospital cardioplegic solution. J Thorac Cardiovasc Surg 1988; 96: 408–13.
127. Kempsford RD, Hearse DJ. Protection of the immature heart. Temperature dependent beneficial or detrimental effects of multidose crystalloid cardioplegia in the neonatal rabbit heart. J Thorac Cardiovasc Surg 1990; 99: 269–79.
128. Robertson JM, Buckberg GD, Vinten-Johansen JJ *et al.* Comparison of distribution beyond coronary stenoses of blood and asanguineous cardioplegic solutions. J Thorac Cardiovasc Surg 1983; 86: 80–6.
129. Eugene J, Lyons KP, Ott RA *et al.* Regional myocardial perfusion of cardioplegic solutions. Ann Thorac Surg 1987; 43: 522–26.
130. Kondo Y, Gradel FO, Chaptal P-A *et al.* Immediate and delayed orthotopic homotransplantation of the heart. J Thorac Cardiovasc Surg 1965; 50: 781–9.
131. Proctor E, Parker R. Preservation of isolated hearts for 72 hours. Brit Med J 1968; 296–8.

132. Levitsky S, Williams WH, Detmer DE *et al.* A functional evaluation of the preserved heart. J Thorac Cardiovasc Surg 1970; 60: 625–34.
133. Proctor E, Matthews G, Archibald J. Acute orthotopic transplantation of hearts stored for 72 hours. Thorax 1971; 26: 99–102.
134. Copeland JG, Jones M, Spragg R *et al.* In vitro preservation of canine hearts for 24 to 48 hours followed by successful orthotopic transplantation. Ann Surg 1973; 178: 687–92.
135. Collins GM, Bravo-Shugarman M, Terasaki PI. Kidney preservation for transplantation. Initial perfusion and 30 hours' ice storage. Lancet 1969; ii: 1219.
136. Sacks SA, Petritsch PH, Kaufman JJ. Canine kidney preservation using a new perfusate. Lancet 1973; ii: 1024–8.
137. Swanson DK, Pasaoglu I, Berkoff HA *et al.* Improved heart preservation with UW preservation solution. J Heart Transplant 1988; 7: 456–67.
138. English TA, Foreman J, Gadian DG *et al.* Three solutions for preservation of the rabbit heart at 0°C. A comparison with phosphorus-31 nuclear magnetic resonance spectroscopy. J Thorac Cardiovasc Surg 1988; 96: 54–61.
139. Darracott-Cankovic S, Wheeldon D, Cory-Pearce R *et al.* Biopsy assessment of fifty hearts during transplantation. J Thorac Cardiovasc Surg 1987; 93: 95–102.
140. Wicomb W, Cooper DKC, Hassoulas J *et al.* Orthotopic transplantation of the baboon heart after 20 to 24 hours' preservation by continuous hypothermic perfusion with an oxygenated hyperosmolar solution. J Thorac Cardiovasc Surg 1982; 83: 133–40.
141. Wicomb WN, Cooper DKC, Novitzky D *et al.* Cardiac transplantation following storage of the donor heart by a portable hypothermic perfusion system. Ann Thorac Surg 1984; 37: 243–48.
142. Wicomb WN, Rose AG, Cooper DK *et al.* Hemodynamic and myocardial histologic and ultrastructural studies on baboons from 3 to 27 months following autotransplantation of hearts stored by hypothermic perfusion for 24 or 48 hours. J Heart Transplant 1986; 5: 122–9.
143. Burt JM, Larson DF, Copeland JG. Recovery of heart function following 24 hours preservation and ectopic transplantation. J Heart Transplant 1986; 5: 298–303.
144. Burt JM, Copeland JG. Myocardial function after preservation for 2 hours. J Thorac Cardiovasc Surg 1986; 92: 238–46.
145. Takahashi A, Braimbridge MV, Hearse DJ *et al.* Long-term preservation of the mammalian myocardium. Effect of storage medium and temperature on the vulnerability to tissue injury. J Thorac Cardiovasc Surg 1991; 102: 235–45.
146. Takahashi A, Hearse DJ, Braimbridge MV *et al.* Harvesting hearts for long-term preservation. Detrimental effects of initial hypothermic infusion of cardioplegic solutions. J Thorac Cardiovasc Surg 1990; 100: 371–8.
147. Chambers DJ, Takahashi A, Hearse DJ. Long-term preservation of the heart: The effect of infusion pressure during continuous hypothermic cardioplegia. J Heart Lung Transplant 1992; 11: 665–75.
148. Hendry PJ, Anstadt MP, Plunkett MD *et al.* Optimal temperature for preservation of donor myocardium. Circulation 1990; 82 (Suppl IV): IV-306–IV-312.
149. Choong YS, Gavin JB. Functional recovery of hearts after cardioplegia and storage in University of Wisconsin and in St Thomas' Hospital solutions. J Heart Lung Transplant 1991; 10: 537–46.
150. Ledingham SJM, Katayama O, Lachno DR *et al.* Prolonged cardiac preservation. Evaluation of the University of Wisconsin preservation solution by comparison with the St Thomas' Hospital cardioplegic solutions in the rat. Circulation 1990; 82 (Suppl IV): IV-351–IV-358.
151. Yeh T, Hanan SA, Johnson DE *et al.* Superior myocardial preservation with modified UW solution after prolonged ischemia in the rat heart. Ann Thorac Surg 1990; 49: 932–9.
152. Bull C, Cooper J, Stark J. Cardioplegic protection of the child's heart. J Thorac Cardiovasc Surg 1984; 88: 287–93.
153. Bove EL, Stammers AH. Recovery of left ventricular function after hypothermic global

ischemia. Age-related differences in the isolated working rabbit heart. J Thorac Cardiovasc Surg 1986; 91: 115–22.

154. Bove EL, Stammers AH, Gallagher KP. Protection of the neonatal myocardium during hypothermic ischemia. Effect of cardioplegia on left ventricular function in the rabbit. J Thorac Cardiovasc Surg 1987; 94: 115–23.
155. Corno AF, Bethencourt DM, Laks H *et al.* Myocardial protection in the neonatal heart. A comparison of topical hypothermia and crystalloid and blood cardioplegic solutions. J Thorac Cardiovasc Surg 1987; 93: 163–72.
156. Sawa Y, Matsuda H, Shimazaki Y *et al.* Ultrastructural assessment of the infant myocardium receiving crystalloid cardioplegia. Circulation 1987; 76 (Suppl V): V-141–V-145.
157. Sawa Y, Matsuda H, Shimazaki Y *et al.* Experimental and clinical study of crystalloid cardioplegic solution in neonatal period and early infancy. Effects of calcium and prostacyclin analogue. Circulation 1988; 78 (Suppl III): III-191–III-197.
158. Avkiran M, Hearse DJ. Protection of the myocardium during global ischemia. Is crystalloid cardioplegia effective in the immature myocardium? J Thorac Cardiovasc Surg 1989; 97: 220–8.
159. Riva E, Hearse DJ. Calcium and cardioplegia in neonates: dose-response and time-response studies in rats. Am J Physiol 1991; 261: H1609–H1616.
160. Baker JE, Boerboom LE, Olinger GN. Age-related changes in the ability of hypothermia and cardioplegia to protect ischemic rabbit myocardium. J Thorac Cardiovasc Surg 1988; 96: 717–724.
161. Baker JE, Boerboom LE, Olinger GN. Cardioplegia-induced damage to ischemic immature myocardium is independent of oxygen availability. Ann Thorac Surg 1990; 50: 934–9.
162. Baker EJ, Olinger GN, Baker JE. Calcium content of St Thomas' II cardioplegic solution damages ischemic immature myocardium. Ann Thorac Surg 1991; 52: 993–9.
163. Murashita T, Hearse DJ. Temperature-response studies of the detrimental effects of multidose versus single-dose cardioplegic solution in the rabbit heart. J Thorac Cardiovasc Surg 1991; 102: 673–83.
164. Menasché P, Grousset C, de Boccard G *et al.* Protective effect of an asanguineous reperfusion solution on myocardial performance following cardioplegic arrest. Ann Thorac Surg 1984; 37: 222–8.
165. Allen BS, Okamoto F, Buckberg GD *et al.* Studies of controlled reperfusion after ischemia. IX. Reperfusate composition: benefits of marked hypocalcemia and diltiazem on regional recovery. J Thorac Cardiovasc Surg 1986; 92: 564–72.
166. Menasché P, Dunica S, Kural S *et al.* An asanguineous reperfusion solution. An effective adjunct to cardioplegic protection in high risk valve operations. J Thorac Cardiovasc Surg 1984; 88: 278–86.
167. Chambers DJ, Harvey DM, Venn DJ *et al.* Transient initial reperfusion with oxygenated cardioplegia; contrasting effects of St Thomas' Hospital solutions 1 and 2. Eur Heart J 1992; 13 (Abstract Suppl): P783.
168. Harvey DM, Venn GE, Chambers DJ. Transient initial reperfusion with oxygenated cardioplegia: contrasting effects of substrate addition to St Thomas' solutions 1 and 2. J Mol Cell Cardiol 1992; 24 (Suppl V): 516.
169. Smith PK, Buhrman WC, Levett JM *et al.* Supraventricular conduction abnormalities following cardiac operations. A complication of inadequate atrial preservation. J Thorac Cardiovasc Surg 1983; 85: 105–15.
170. Ferguson TBJ, Smith PK, Lofland GK *et al.* The effects of cardioplegic potassium concentration and myocardial temperature on electrical activity in the heart during elective cardioplegic arrest. J Thorac Cardiovasc Surg 1986; 92: 755–65.
171. Ferguson TBJ, Smith LS, Smith PK *et al.* Electrical activity in the heart during hyperkalemic hypothermic cardioplegic arrest: site of origin and relationship to specialized conduction tissue. Ann Thorac Surg 1987; 43: 373–9.
172. Gundry SR, Sequiera A, Coughlin TR *et al.* Postoperative conduction disturbances: a comparison of blood and crystalloid cardioplegia. Ann Thorac Surg 1989; 47: 384–90.

173. Kay HR, Levine FH, Fallon JT *et al.* Effect of cross-clamp time, temperature, and cardioplegic agents on myocardial function after induced arrest. J Thorac Cardiovasc Surg 1978; 76: 590–603.
174. Ganote CE, Worstell J, Iannotti JP *et al.* Cellular swelling and irreversible myocardial injury: effects of polyethylene glycol and mannitol in perfused rat heart. Am J Pathol 1977; 88: 95–118.
175. Foglia RP, Steed DL, Follette DM *et al.* Iatrogenic myocardial edema with potassium cardioplegia. J Thorac Cardiovasc Surg 1977; 78: 217–22.
176. Drewnowska K, Clemo HF, Baumgarten CM. Prevention of myocardial intracellular edema induced by St Thomas' Hospital cardioplegic solution. J Mol Cell Cardiol 1991; 23: 1215–21.
177. Darracott-Cankovic S, Braimbridge MV, Kyosola K *et al.* Use of microscopic interferometry for measuring changes in water content of small samples of tissue. Cell Biochem Funct 1984; 2: 57–61.
178. Carpentier S, Murawsky M, Carpentier A. Cytotoxicity of cardioplegic solutions: evaluation by tissue culture. Circulation 1981; 64 (Suppl II): II-90–II-95.
179. Mattila S, Harjula A, Mattila I *et al.* Coronary endothelium and cardioplegic solutions. Ann Chirurg Gynaecol 1987; 76: 46–50.
180. Saldanha C, Hearse DJ. Coronary vascular responsiveness to 5–hydroxytryptamine before and after infusion of hyperkalemic crystalloid cardioplegic solution in the rat heart. Possible evidence of endothelial damage. J Thorac Cardiovasc Surg 1989; 98: 783–7.
181. Chiavarelli R, Macchiarelli G, Familiari G *et al.* Ultrastructural changes of coronary artery endothelium induced by cardioplegic solutions. Thorac Cardiovasc Surgeon 1989; 37: 151–7.
182. von Oppell UO, Pfeiffer S, Preiss P *et al.* Endothelial cell toxicity of solid-organ preservation solutions. Ann Thorac Surg 1990; 50: 902–10.
183. Molina JE, Galliani CA, Einzig S *et al.* Physical and mechanical effects of cardioplegic injection on flow distribution and myocardial damage in hearts with normal coronary arteries. J Thorac Cardiovasc Surg 1989; 97: 870–7.
184. Keller MW, Geddes L, Spotnitz W *et al.* Microcirculatory dysfunction following perfusion with hyperkalemic, hypothermic, cardioplegic solutions and blood reperfusion. Effects of adenosine. Circulation 1991; 84: 2485–94.
185. Robinson LA, Braimbridge MV, Hearse DJ. The potential hazard of particulate contamination of cardioplegic solutions. J Thorac Cardiovasc Surg 1984; 87: 48–58.
186. Hearse DJ, Sonmez B, Saldanha C *et al.* Particle-induced coronary vasoconstriction in the rat heart: pharmacological investigation of underlying mechanisms. Thorac Cardiovasc Surgeon 1986; 34: 316–25.

7. Blood cardioplegic strategies during adult cardiac operations

GERALD D. BUCKBERG, BRADLEY S. ALLEN, and
FRIEDHELM BEYERSDORF

Introduction

Pharmacologic cardioplegia was not used widely in the United States until the past fifteen years because of previous reports of left ventricular damage following cold hypertonic potassium citrate blood as introduced by Melrose *et al.* in 1955 [1,2]. Studies by Bretschneider [3], Kirsch [4], and Hearse [5] and their co-workers in Europe and by Gay and Ebert [6] provide a solid framework for the renewed interest in cardioplegia which has resulted in the intraoperative use of pharmacologic cardioplegia by most surgeons throughout the world. Tyers *et al.* [7] showed that the problem with Melrose solution was inappropriate concentration of its constituents, rather than an inappropriate composition. Our studies fully support the original cardioplegic constituents of Melrose solution and we now use safe concentrations of alkaline, hypertonic, potassium citrate, and cold blood to stop the heart whenever we clamp the aorta during clinical surgery [8], the safety of this approach has been confirmed by others [9–12]. Cold cardioplegic solutions are used almost universally to prevent intraoperative myocardial ischemic damage during aortic clamping. This review shows that the inclusion of oxygen in the cardioplegic solution expands the therapeutic scope for clinical cardioplegia. It describes how these same solutions can be delivered warm to allow their use for active resuscitation before ischemia is imposed, and how to avoid and reverse ischemic and reperfusion damage before and after aortic unclamping. It reiterates briefly the principles that must underlie the composition of cardioplegic solutions and puts into perspective the commonality of apparently different pharmacologic approaches to myocardial protection [13]. It focuses primarily on the principles that form the basis for clinical strategies for cardioplegic delivery that can ensure that the selected cardioplegic solution can exert its desired effect and it describes how these can be implemented. Each proposed strategy can be used with oxygenated cardioplegic solutions (regardless of precise composition) and several are applicable to asanguineous cardioplegic solutions devoid of oxygen.

Table 7.1 lists the factors affecting the myocardial energy supply/demand balance during aortic clamping. The two factors affecting supply include oxygenated blood coming from noncoronary collateral blood flow, and intrinsic or extrinsic substrate stores. All surgeons have noted noncoronary col-

H.M. Piper and C.J. Preusse (eds): Ischemia-reperfusion in cardiac surgery, 181–227.

Table 7.1. Myocardial supply/demand balance during aortic cross-clamping.

Supply	Demand
Non-coronary collaterals	Electromechanical activity
Intrinsic substrate stores (glycogen)	Wall tension
	Temperature (metabolic rate)

lateral flow during aortic clamping, as blood appears in the coronary ostia during aortic valve replacement or in the coronary arteriotomy site during coronary revascularization despite a flaccid aorta. The second determinant of supply is myocardial glycogen or exogenous glucose. Oxygenated hearts undergo aerobic metabolism, but the heart receiving little or no oxygen supply must undergo anaerobic metabolism to generate some energy to maintain cell membrane viability. Anaerobic glycolysis requires the presence of substrate (i.e., glucose or glycogen), and a metabolic environment (i.e., buffering) to allow anaerobic energy production. Myocardial oxygen demands are determined principally by electromechanical activity. The heart that is fibrillating or beating while ischemic has a much higher energy requirement than the heart that is arrested. The second determinant of demand is the wall tension within the myocardium, and the third is the myocardial temperature that governs metabolic rate directly.

Cardioplegic prerequisites

Essential prerequisites for clinical use of cardioplegia include (1) use of solution that has been shown to be safe through testing under experimental conditions, especially in models that simulate clinical circumstances; (2) assurance of distribution to all areas of the heart; (3) periodic replenishment to counteract noncoronary collateral washout; (4) strategies for delivering and maintaining cardioplegia that can be adapted to various clinical conditions.

Cardioplegic composition

The objectives of chemical cardioplegia are to stop the heart safely, create an environment for continued energy production, and counteract deleterious effects of ischemia. The principles which underlie the composition of any cardioplegic solution are enumerated in Table 7.2. Most clinically used solutions that embrace these principles likely confer comparably good myocardial protection during ischemia. First, immediate arrest should be produced to lower energy demands and avoid depletion by ischemic electromechanical work. This is especially true with nonoxygenated cardioplegic solutions.

Table 7.2. Pharmacologic Cardioplegia.

Principal	Method
Immediate arrest	K^+, Mg^{++}, Procaine
Hypothermia	10°–20°C
Substrate	Oxygen, glucose, glutamate, aspartate
Appropriate pH (buffer)	THAM, bicarb, phosphate
Membrane stabilization	Ca^{++}, ?Steroids, ?Procaine, Ca^{++} antagonist, O_2 radical scavenger

Conversely, high-energy stores may be enhanced when cardioplegia is induced with oxygenated solution [14] and delay in asystole is less problematic. Studies [15] show substantial adenosine triphosphate (ATP) store reduction during the brief period of electromechanical activity preceeding normal pharmacologic cardioplegia with asanguineous solutions. Arrest can be achieved either by use of potassium, magnesium, procaine, or perhaps some hypocalcemic solution. Second, myocardial temperature should be lowered to reduce metabolic rate. This can be achieved usually with perfusion hypothermia with a cold cardioplegic solution. Lowering cardiac temperature to 8–10°C does not reduce energy requirements much below those achieved at 15–20°C myocardial temperature (0.3 vs. 0.15 ml/100 g per min). Recurrence of electromechanical activity may, however, occur when the cardioplegic solution is washed out so that cardioplegic infusions at 4–8°C are used and have been shown recently to be safe with blood [16]. Third, substrate (i.e., glucose or glycogen) should be provided for continued anaerobic or aerobic energy production (or both) during aortic clamping. The energy available during both induction of cardioplegia and with replenishments is far greater if oxygen (i.e., blood) is used in the cardioplegic vehicle, especially if the cardioplegic solution is enriched with precursors of Krebs cycle intermediates (i.e., glutamate or aspartate) [17]. Fourth, there must be an appropriate pH to achieve a reasonable state of metabolism during hypothermia. Consequently, a buffer is necessary in all cardioplegic solutions. Tris(hydroxymethyl) aminoethane (THAM), bicarbonate, phosphate, or perhaps some other buffer may be used and reports confirm the benefits of optimizing the small energy output of anaerobic glycolysis during ischemia by buffering the cardioplegic solution [18]. Fifth, there must be some degree of membrane stabilization in the form of exogenous additives or avoidance of intentional hypocalcemia; calcium-free cardioplegic solutions can damage the vital sarco lemmal membrane [19]. Calcium antagonists (i.e., verapamil, nifedipine, diltiazem, etc.) that block calcium cellular entry may be important future cardioplegic additives [20–22]. Their routine incorporation in cardioplegic solutions must be delayed until more information is available about how to counteract their continuing action after extracorporeal circulation is discontinued and normal calcium homeostasis is needed. The role of steroids and procaine and how they affect membrane stabilization is uncertain although many studies of these agents have been reported and will continue. Oxygen radical scavengers (i.e., superoxide dismutase [23], catalase, allopurinol, coenzyme Q_{10}[CoQ_{10}] [24]) may be useful potential cardioplegic additives to counteract the cytotoxic oxygen metabolites that can produce profound changes in membrane phospholipids during ischemia and reperfusion [25]. Sixth, myocardial edema always accompanies ischemic damage so that some attention must be directed to both the osmolarity and colloid osmotic pressure of the cardioplegic solution to avoid producing edema iatrogenically during cardioplegic infusions [26].

Blood versus asanguineous cardioplegia

The need to provide oxygen in the cardioplegic solution continues to be questioned despite experimental and clinical studies establishing the superiority of oxygenated cardioplegic solutions [8–12]. The vehicle for providing oxygen may be blood [8], fluorocarbons [27], stroma-free hemoglobin [27], oxygen dissolved in crystalloid [28]. We have selected blood as the cardioplegic vehicle, since this physiologic source of oxygen is available readily in the extracorporeal circuit, and its use limits hemodilution when large volumes of cardioplegia are needed.

An additional advantage of a blood cardioplegic vehicle is ensurance of the buffering capacity of blood proteins, especially histidine imidazole groups [29]. Furthermore, the rheologic benefits on the microvasculature afforded by erythrocytes enhance papillary muscle perfusion compared with oxygenated crystalloid cardioplegia and reduce coronary vascular resistance and edema formation [28]. The erythrocytes of blood cardioplegia also contain abundant endogenous oxygen free radical scavengers (i.e., superoxide dismutase, catalase, and glutathione) [30], which may reduce oxygen-mediated injury during reperfusion. Our experimental studies show that the salutary effects of controlled blood cardioplegic reperfusion are impaired markedly when endogenous red blood cell glutathione and catalase are blocked pharmacologically [31].

Concerns over use of cold blood cardioplegia stem from: (1) producing possible unfavorable shifts in the oxyhemoglobin dissociation curve with resultant impairment of oxygen unloading at the cellular level; (2) the theoretic potential of blood sludging if $<15°C$ temperatures are used; (3) potentially better distribution of asanguineous solutions beyond coronary stenoses; (4) heretofore complex delivery systems with blood cardioplegia (the oxygen source).

We have addressed these concerns and found the following: First, O_2 uptake exceeds basal demands by as much as 10-fold during 4°C blood cardioplegic reinfusions during the period of prolonged aortic clamping [16]

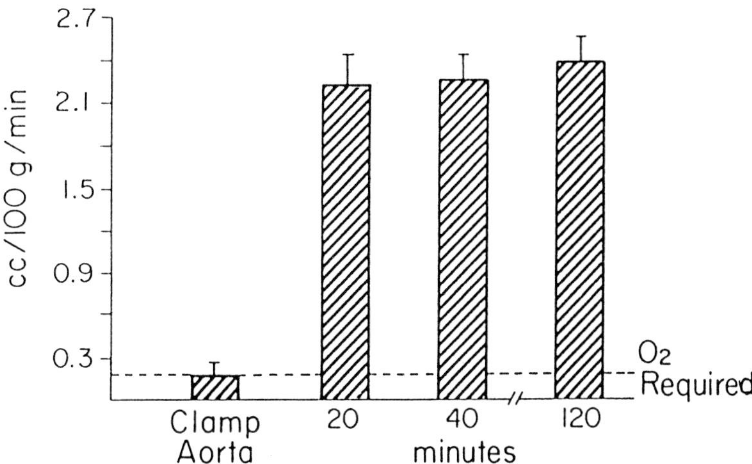

Figure 7.1. Myocardial oxygen uptake during 4°C blood cardioplegic infusions. Note: 1) very low myocardial oxygen demands (O_2 requirement), indicating by hatched line during cardioplegic induction (clamped aorta); 2); O_2 uptake 10 X in excess of basal demands with cardioplegic replenishmen at 20 min intervals.

(Figure 7.1). Second, 4°C cardioplegia can be delivered safely for a period of up to 4 hours of aortic clamping so that colder temperatures of blood cardioplegic perfusate can be used clinically without concern (Figure 7.2) [32]. Third, comparison of 250 mL/min infusions of asanguineous and blood 4°C cardioplegic solutions show that the reduced viscosity of asanguineous cardioplegia results in a lower aortic pressure. The consequent higher aortic pressure with blood cardioplegia allows superior cardioplegic delivery beyond obstructed coronaries and better myocardial cooling (5°C) (Figure 7.3). These findings suggest that the decreased viscosity of asanguineous cardioplegia causes diversion of cardioplegic solutions away from the obstructed vessels to the normal coronary bed [33]. Fourth, as shown in Figure 7.4, a disposable blood cardioplegic delivery system has been developed and used over the past several years to avoid the need for reservoirs, hand-mixing of solutions and delay [16]. This system uses differential volumes of two tubing diameters to mix pump blood with cardioplegic solutions appropriately and instantaneously.

The advantages of oxygenated cardioplegic solutions over oxygen-free solutions are obvious when attention is directed to the energy availability with these two vehicles. With asanguineous cardioplegia, myocardial viability

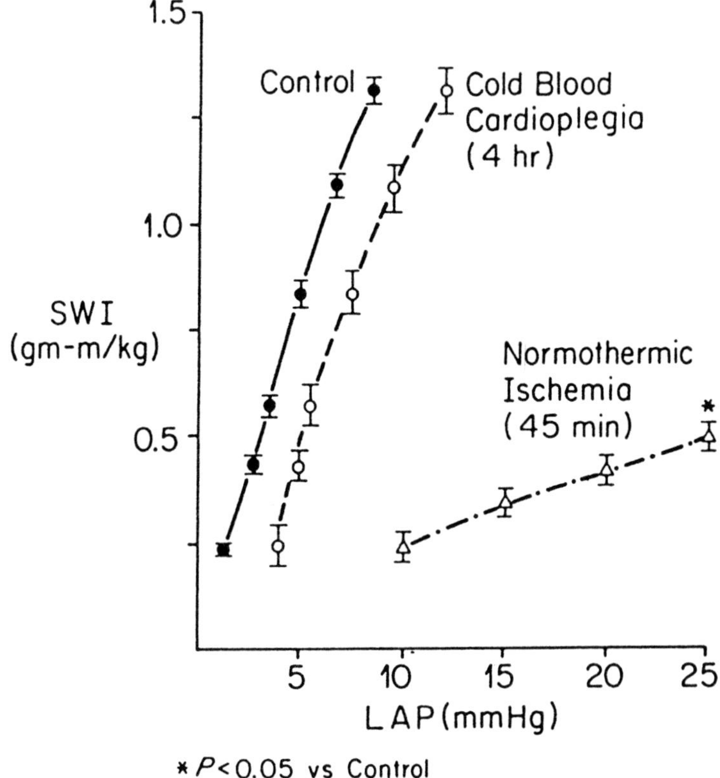

Figure 7.2. Postischemic myocardial performance during inscription of left ventricular function curves 30 minutes after unclamping the aorta. Note: (1) marked depression in function following 45 minutes of normothermic ischemia and (2) normal function after 4 hrs of multidose cold blood cardioplegia. LAP = left atrial pressure; SWI, stroke work index.

must depend on the small amount of energy (2 mol of ATP per mol of glucose metabolized) produced by anaerobic metabolism. Bretschneider *et al.* have emphasized the importance of maintaining aerobic metabolism (36 moles of ATP per mole of glucose metabolized) while the heart is stopped pharmacologically in order to avoid wasting energy stores uselessly by allowing the heart to do electromechanical work during asanguineous cardioplegic perfusion [3]. The use of blood as the vehicle for cardioplegic delivery (Table 7.3) has the obvious advantages of: (1) keeping the heart oxygenated while it is being arrested; (2) allowing reoxygenation when the cardioplegic solution is replenished; (3) avoiding reperfusion damage (to be discussed below); (4) minimizing hemodilution; (5) having endogenous oxygen radical scavengers, buffers, and onconicity.

The critical importance of using an oxygenated cardioplegic solution was

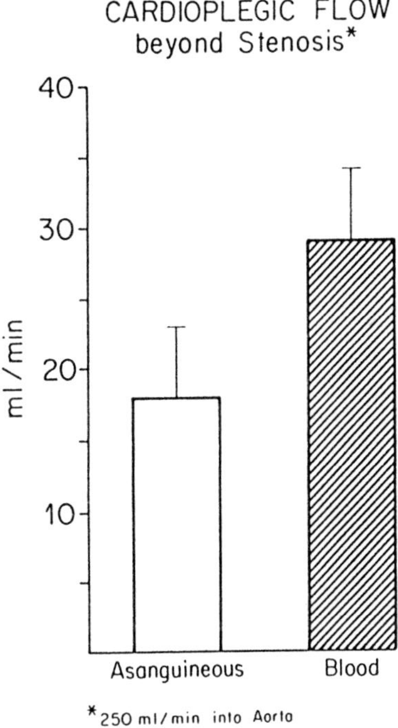

Figure 7.3. Cardioplegic flow beyond coronary stenosis when cardioplegic solution is given at 250 mL/min into aorta. Note the better flow beyond stenosis with blood than asanguineous cardioplegia.

emphasized in a report [34] comparing asanguineous to oxygenated cardioplegia (blood and fluorocarbons) in hypertrophied hearts, whereby the experimental model simulates more closely the clinical conditions confronted when operations are performed in patients with advanced cardiac disease. Table 7.4 enumerates the principles that underlie a clinically tested blood cardioplegic solution that contains the blood constituents shown to provide for ideal reperfusion of ischemic myocardium [35]. The standard cardioplegic solution contains 500–600 uM/L, calcium without glutamate or aspartate, but the cardioplegic solution used for warm cardioplegic induction and warm reperfusion contains glutamate and aspartate and a lower ionic calcium (150–250 μmol/L) achieved by adding more citrate phosphate dextrose (CPD) (discussed later in this chapter). Diltiazem is not available currently for routine use in the United States. Figure 7.5 shows the protective effect of multidose blood vs. asanguineous cardioplegia using two solutions of comparable composition during 2 hours of aortic clamping in the experimental setting. The recovery of contractility is greater than normal with blood cardioplegia, reflecting, perhaps the cardiac effects of the catecholamine release occurring with extracorporeal circulation. Good recovery also

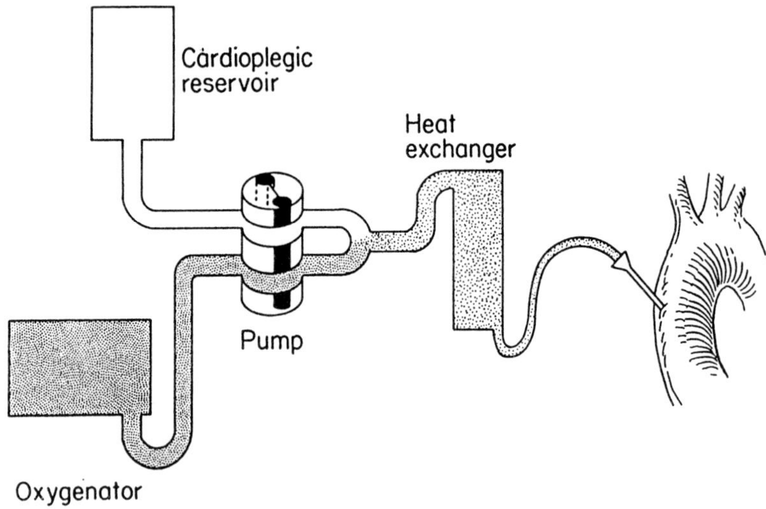

Figure 7.4. Cardioplegic delivery system in current clinical use.

Table 7.3. Blood cardioplegia.

Oxygenation during arrest
Reoxygenation during replenishment
Avoids reperfusion injury
Avoids Hemodilution
Endogenous
Oxygen radical scavengers
Buffers
Onconicity

occurs with asanguineous cardioplegia, but it is slightly less than complete. Figure 7.6 shows a similar early salutary effect in matched groups of 16 high-risk patients (i.e., extending MI, ejection fraction <0.30) where we compared the effects of blood cardioplegia to asanguineous cardioplegia with the same ingredients. Table 7.5 shows the pooled results and indicates that blood cardioplegia resulted in a lower incidence of postoperative ECG abnormalities and inotropic needs but did not avoid completely enzymatic evidence of myocardial damage (Table 7.6).

No attempt was made to distribute either cardioplegia solution beyond stenoses in these patients. We continue to see the highest level of enzymes in patients who have coronary disease, hypertrophied left ventricles, or when these two lesions are combined. These data have led to the development of

Table 7.4. Cardioplegic solution.

Principal	Constituent	Final concentration
Provide oxygen	Blood	Hct 20–30%
Maintain arrest	KCl	12–16 mg/L
Buffer acidosis	Tham	pH 7.5–7.6
Avoid edema	Glucose	>400 mOsm
Restore substrate	Glucose	>400 mg%
	Aspartate	13 mM
	Glutamate	13 mM
Limit calcium entry	CPD	500–600 μM Ca^{++}
	Diltiazem	300 μgm/kg body weight

CPD, citrate phosphate dextrose; HCT, hematocrit.

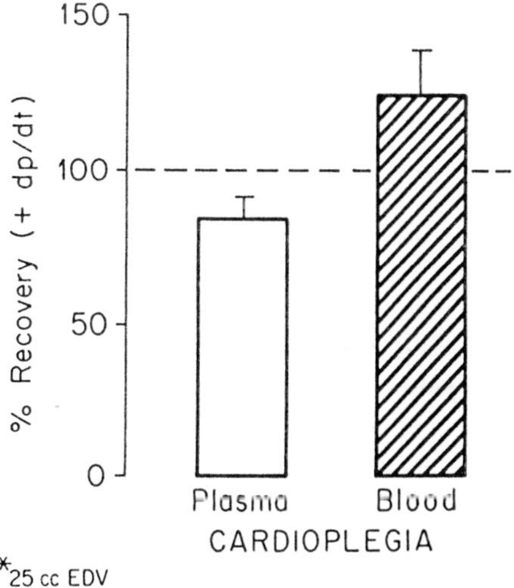

Figure 7.5. Myocardial performance (25 cc end/diastolic volume) after 2 hrs of aortic clamping with either multidose asanguineous (plasma) or blood cardioplegia with comparable constituents. Note the slight depression in postischemic performance with asanguineous cardioplegia, and the better postischemic performance with blood cardioplegia. (The above normal contractility probably reflects the effects of catecholamines normally released during extracorporeal circulation on the well-protected myocardium).

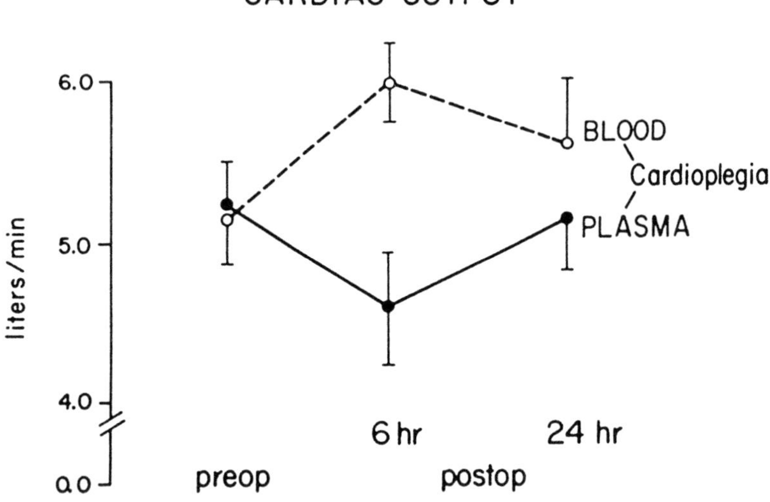

Figure 7.6. Postoperative cardiac output in patients undergoing comparable operations and receiving either blood or asanguineous (plasma) cardioplegia. Note the similarity in transitory increase in cardiac performance following blood cardioplegia and slight depression following asanguineous cardioplegia at 6 hours (see Figure 7.14).

Table 7.5. Pharmacologic cardioplegia.

	Asanguineous %	Blood %
Infarcts	6	0
Abnormal ECG	44	13
Circulatory support	12	0
Death	6	6

ECG: electrocardiogram.

Table 7.6. Postoperative enzymes.

Enzyme (@ 18 hr)	Beating Empty or Intermittent ischemia	Blood Cardioplegia
CPK	1251 ± 127	796 ± 43*
CPK-MB	20 ± 3	13 ± 1
SGOT	99 ± 18	59 ± 4

$p < 0.05$.
CPK, creatine phosphokinase; CPK-MB, CPK-myocardial band; SGOT, serum glutamic-oxaloacetic transaminase.

Table 7.7. Blood cardioplegic induction.

Cold
Global Hypothermia
Prompt Asystole
Warm
"Active resuscitation"

additional strategies to induce, distribute and maintain, and reperfuse with cardioplegic solutions that have increased the safety of cardiac operation and expanded the uses of oxygenated cardioplegic solutions.

Operative strategy

The strategies for clinical cardioplegia may be separated into the phases of (1) induction, (2) maintenance and distribution, and (3) reperfusion.

Cardioplegic induction

Cardioplegia may be given immediately after extracorporeal circulation has begun, provided that the pulmonary artery is collapsed to attest to the adequacy of venous return. This avoids admixture of the cardioplegic solution with systemic blood which traverses the lung because it is not captured by the venous cannula. Starting the infusion shortly before aortic clamping ensures aortic valve competence. The volume, rate, and temperature of cardioplegic administration are determined by the mass and pathophysiologic status of the heart before arrest is initiated.

Cold induction

Cardioplegic induction in operations on hearts with reasonably normal energy reserves is intended to (1) stop the heart promptly to lower oxygen demands, (2) produce hypothermia to reduce O_2 demands further, and (3) create an environment which allows continuous anaerobic energy production during intervals between cardioplegic replenishments in order to *prevent* ischemic damage (Table 7.7). An initial cold (4–8°C) cardioplegic solution contains a high concentration of the arresting agent (i.e., 20–25 mEq/L, KCl). It will produce asystole promptly. Global arrest occurs usually within 30 seconds but may he delayed for 1–2 minutes in patients with coronary disease due to maldistribution of cardioplegia beyond stenotic or occluded arteries. Palpation of the aorta or measurement of infusion pressure will allow detection of aortic incompetence if it is caused inadvertently. Cardioplegic solutions stop the heart by depolarizing the cell membrane. The optimal concentration of cardioplegic agent (i.e., KCL) is that amount required to produce and maintain arrest. Higher cardioplegic potassium concentrations (i.e., 15–30 mEq/L) are necessary to produce and to maintain asystole, but raising $K^+ > 30$ mEq/L is unnecessary during cardioplegic induction, and only increases the potential for systemic hyperkalemia. Arrest occurs more quickly with asanguineous than with blood cardioplegia, since depolarization combines with anoxia and perfusion hypothermia to halt electromechanical activity. Cardioplegic K^+ can be reduced to 8–10 mEq/L during subsequent cold cardioplegic infusions (i.e., multidose cardioplegia; see Cardioplegic Maintenance below) since perfusion or topical hypothermia potentiate the effectiveness of any cardioplegic potassium concentration. The initial cardioplegic flow rate differs with oxygenated and nonoxygenated cardioplegic solutions. Maintenance of the selected flow rate after arrest produces transmural cooling by delivering the total volume of cardioplegic solution. We induce global cardioplegia with a 4–8°C blood cardioplegic flow rate of 250–350 mL/min. depending on cardiac size, and continue the infusion for 3 min (i.e., 750–1000 total dose in nonhypertrophied hearts). Greater volumes of cardioplegia (i.e., 1000–1500 mL) are required when there is increased left ventricular mass [36]. There should be minimal concern over the duration of cardioplegic induction or rapidity of arrest with oxygenated cardioplegic solutions since the heart receives oxygen continually during the cardioplegic infusion. Conversely, delivery of asanguineous cardioplegic solutions at higher flow rates (i.e., 400–500 mL/min) shortens the time to arrest and minimizes the duration of anoxic aortic clamping.

Failure to produce arrest within 1–2 minutes may be due to: (1) incomplete aortic clamping; (2) aortic insufficiency produced by distortion of the noncoronary cusp by a large right atrial cannula; (3) incomplete decompression by the venous cannula resulting in admixture of venous blood returning to the left heart and diluting of the cardioplegic solution; (4) inadvertent failure to add sufficient potassium to the cardioplegic solution. Palpation of the left ventricle during cardioplegic induction allows detection of left ventricular distention which occurs if venous drainage is inadequate or aortic insufficiency has been produced. Corrective measures include readjusting the position of the venous cannula within the right atrium and/or moving it away from the coronary cusp. Discontinuation of the cardioplegic infusion and immediate ventricular venting are necessary if these maneuvers fail to produce decompression. Undue concern should not be directed toward reducing the temperature of the cardioplegic solution much below 10°C since minor differences in solution temperature (i.e., between 5° and 10°C) will not produce major differences in myocardial temperature or oxygen demands during the brief interval of cardioplegic infusion, especially after the heart is arrested. The oxygen requirements of the arrested heart at 20°C are extremely low at 0.3 ml/100 gm/min and are reduced only to 0.15 mL/100 gm/min at 10°C [3,37]. Conversely, the oxygen requirements of the beating or fibrillating heart are 2–3 mL/100 gm/min at comparable temperatures [9,37]. Consequently, preoccupation with obtaining a predetermined level of myocardial cooling after arrest in areas supplied by occluded arteries or stenotic vessels will delay the operation unnecessarily. Deeper regional hypothermia can be achieved readily by distribution of cardioplegic solution through the grafts after they are constructed (see Cardioplegic Distribution, below).

Cardioplegic infusions may cause myocardial edema (especially if the myocardial cells are ischemia), if perfusion pressure is allowed to become excessive (i.e., >80 mmHg) since the myocardial contractile force and muscle tone which limit fluid flux mechanically are overcome by pharmacologic asystole, and hypothermia interferes with normal cell volume regulation by decreasing the effectiveness of the Na^{+}/K^{+} pump. The extent of edema which can be produced during cardioplegic infusion is determined by the interaction of the Starling forces which govern fluid flux. These include the perfusion pressure as well as the oncotic and osmotic pressures of the solution, the electromechanical status of the myocardium and the integrity of the capillary bed. We have, for example, caused temporary myocardial edema iatrogenically in a normal heart by inducing cold cardioplegia with a hypo-oncotic, hypo-osmotic crystalloid cardioplegic solution under experimental conditions [26]. Clinical cardioplegic perfusion pressures of 80–100 mmHg are probably safe during cardioplegic induction since myocardial electromechanical activity persists during part of the infusion, the full extent of perfusion hypothermia is not instantaneous, and the integrity of the capillary bed has not yet been altered by ischemic damage. Conversely, keeping perfusion pressure at or below 50 mmHg during reinfusions and reperfusion will limit edema when cardioplegic replenishments are delivered to myocardial regions containing capillary endothelial cells that may have been damaged because they did not receive adequate cardioplegic protection during previous infusions.

Delivery of cardioplegia at predetermined pressure in coronary patients does not assure even distribution beyond stenoses. Simultaneously, myocardium in regions supplied by unobstructed arteries may become edematous if the arrested heart is perfused at high perfusion pressures. The surgeon and perfusionist should be aware of the actual or estimated perfusion pressure to avoid producing edema.

Warm induction

Cardiac operations upon ischemic hearts (i.e., cardiogenic shock. extending myocardial infarction, hemodynamic instability before bypass) or in patients with advanced left or right ventricular hypertrophy or dysfunction pose more difficult problems in myocardial protection. Depletion of energy reserves and glycogen stores are common in such hearts; they (1) are less tolerant to ischemia during aortic clamping, (2) cannot sustain cell metabolism when blood supply is interrupted, and (3) use oxygen inefficiently during reperfusion [38,39]. Oxygenated cardioplegic solutions are particularly well suited

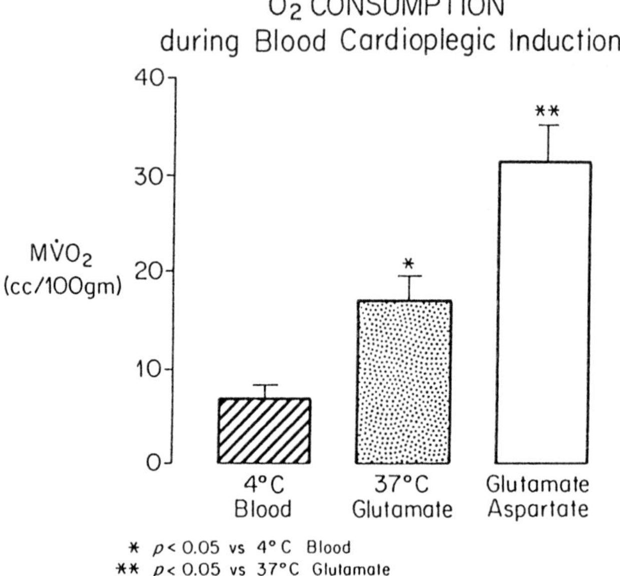

Figure 7.7. Oxygen consumption during induction of blood cardioplegia. Note: (1) twice as much oxygen consumed by hearts given warm (37°C) glutamate blood cardioplegia compared to cold (4°C) blood cardioplegia, (2) >3-fold increase in oxygen consumption by aspartate enrichment of warm glutamate blood cardioplegia. MVO_2, myocardial oxygen consumption.

for use in patients with energy-depleted hearts since they prevent further energy loss during induction, avoid reperfusion damage [40] and improve metabolic recovery when administered warm [41]. The induction of blood cardioplegia in the energy depleted heart is, in a sense, the first phase of reperfusion.

A brief (i.e., 5 min) infusion of warm oxygenated cardioplegic solution can be used as a form of *active resuscitation* in energy-depleted hearts [38] which must undergo prolonged (i.e., 2 hrs) subsequent aortic clamping. Normothermia optimizes the rate of cellular repair, and enrichment of the oxygenated cardioplegic solution with amino acid precursors of Krebs cycle intermediates (aspartate and glutamate) improves oxygen utilization capacity. Substrate enriched warm (37°C) blood cardioplegic induction results in myocardial oxygen uptake in energy depleted hearts (subjected to 45 min of normothermic global ischemia) which exceeds basal requirements markedly (Figure 7.7) and results in improved recovery despite two additional hours of aortic clamping with multidose blood cardioplegia (to simulate the time needed for operative repair) [42,43] (Figure 7.8). The extra oxygen may be used to repair cell damage and to replace the energy stores (creatine phosphate) which can be used to sustain anaerobic metabolism during the ischemic

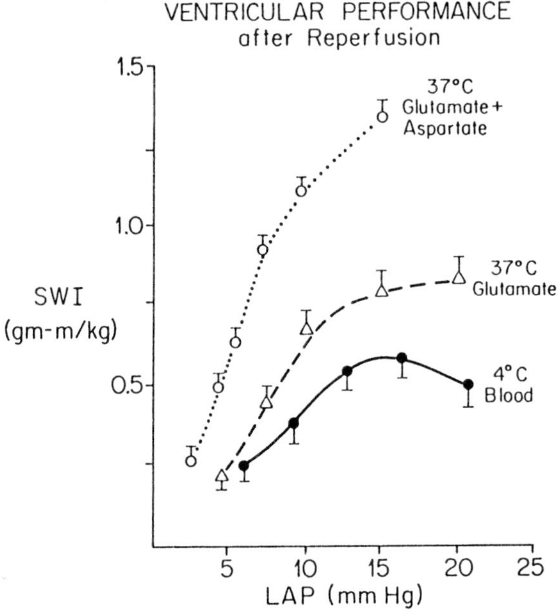

Figure 7.8. Left ventricular performance 30 minutes after blood reperfusion. Note: (1) normal ventricular performance after warm (37°C) induction of aspartate enriched glutamate blood cardioplegia; (2) moderate depression in ventricular performance after warm induction with glutamate blood cardioplegia; (3) severe depression in ventricular function after cold (4°C) blood cardioplegia. LAP, left atrial pressure; SWI, stroke work index.

intervals until the next cardioplegic replenishment. Left ventricular venting during warm induction lowers wall tension maximally [44].

In contrast to cold cardioplegic induction, the duration of cardioplegic delivery during normothermic induction is more important than the volume of cardioplegia given because the heart takes up oxygen over time and not by dose. Whereas the basal myocardial oxygen requirements of the healthy heart subjected to normothermic arrest are only 1 mL/100 g per min or 5 mL/100 g during 5 min, the energy-depleted heart consumes approximately 25–30 mL O_2 over a 5-min induction interval under experimental conditions [17,45]. Administration of this same cardioplegic volume for 1 min would allow only 20% of the oxygen to be used compared to the fivefold greater O_2 uptake which can occur when the same volume of cardioplegia is given over 5 minutes.

The operation does not need to be prolonged during warm induction of oxygenated cardioplegia. Distal anastomoses into occluded left anterior descending or right coronary arteries can be constructed in coronary operations provided aortic insufficiency is not produced by distorting the heart. More immediate arrest during warm induction of blood cardioplegia occurs

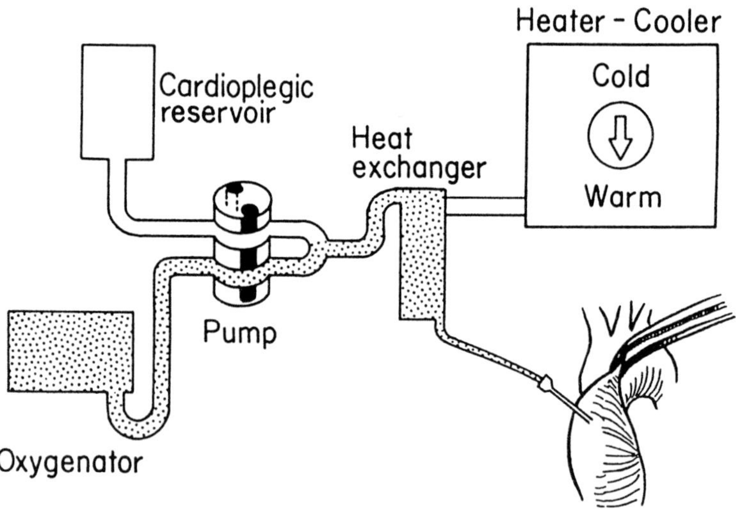

Figure 7.9. Method of warm cardioplegic induction (see text for description).

when the concentration of the cardioplegic agent is increased (i.e., to 25 mEq/L K^+). Normothermia is assured by circulating warm water through the heat-exchanger used for cardioplegic mixing and delivery (Figure 7.9). Warm cardioplegic induction *must* be followed by the administration of cold cardioplegia to provide perfusion hypothermia to *prevent* ischemic damage during the subsequent period of aortic clamping. The prolonged aortic clamping during cardioplegic induction (5 min of warm and 3–5 min of cold blood cardioplegia) does not add ischemia when the cardioplegic ingredients are mixed with blood or some other form of oxygen (i.e., fluorocarbons, bubbled oxygen, or stroma-free hemoglobin). The technique of warm cardioplegia is particularly useful in patients with cardiogenic shock [46], especially when adding it to the other principles of myocardial protection (Table 7.8, Figure 10), see later discussion.

Maintenance and distribution of cardioplegla

Cardioplegic maintenance

All hearts receive some noncoronary collateral blood flow via pericardial connections. The volume of this flow is variable [47], but is sufficient to wash away all cardioplegic solutions with the exception of those given to donor

Table 7.8. Complications.

	Blood cardioplegia	
	Cold blood (11 pts)	Warm glutamate (12 pts)
New arrhythmias	1	0
New St-T change	1	1
New MI	0	1
Deaths (30 days)	2	0

MI: myocardial infarction.

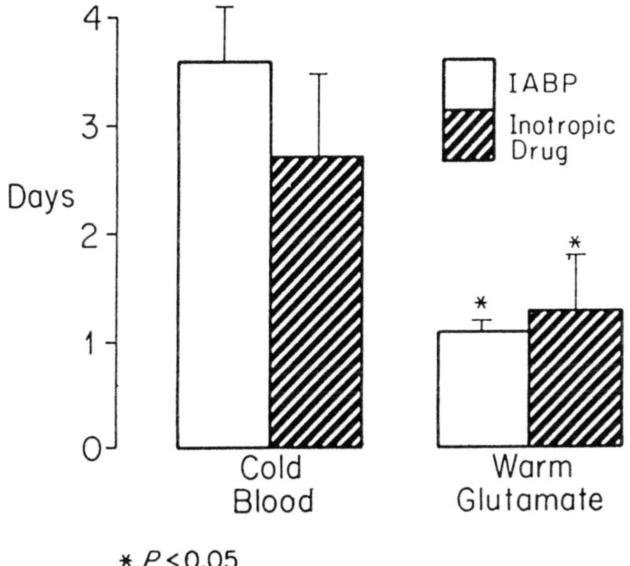

Figure 7.10. Days of postoperative hemodynamic support. Note the earlier discontinuation of intraortic balloon counterpulsation (IABP) and inotropic support in patients receiving warm glutamate cardioplegic induction (warm glutamate).

hearts excised for subsequent transplantation. Myocardial temperature increases after the cardioplegic solution is discontinued, as the heart is rewarmed by the noncoronary collateral blood flow which has the same temperature as the systemic perfusate. Efforts at controlling noncoronary collateral flow by reducing either systemic flow rate or systemic perfusion pressure, or by using profound levels of systemic hypothermia (<25°C) must be tempered by the recognition of the possible hematologic consequences of deep hypothermia, and the potential deleterious effects of hypoperfusion of other vital organs (brain and kidney) at low systemic flow rates. Recurrent ventricular activity is uncommon if systemic temperature is kept between 25° and 30°C despite cardioplegic washout.

The clinical presence of noncoronary collateral flow is evident by (1) refilling of blood in the coronary arteries during revascularization procedures, (2) back-bleeding from the coronary ostia during aortic valve replacement, and (3) recurrence of electromechanical activity after cardioplegic administration, especially during the systemic rewarming phase. Periodic replenishment of the cardioplegic solution at approximately 20-min intervals counteracts noncoronary collateral washout. Multidose cardioplegia is necessary even if electromechanical activity does not return since low-level electrical activity may precede recurrence of visible mechanical activity, and can lead to delayed recovery if cardioplegic replenishment is not provided [48]. Periodic replenishment (1) maintains arrest, (2) restores desired levels of hypothermia, (3) buffers acidosis, (4) washes acid metabolites away which inhibit continued anaerobiosis, (5) replenishes high-energy phosphates if the cardioplegic solution is oxygenated, (6) restores substrates depleted during ischemia [49] and (7) counteracts edema with hyperosmolarity.

Cardioplegic replenishment with low-potassium (8–10 mg/L) solutions limits systemic hyperkalemia. Replenishment of oxygenated cardioplegic solutions at 200–250 mL/min over 2 min ensures a gentle perfusion pressure to avoid edema, and allows enough time for the heart to use the delivered oxygen. Myocardial oxygen uptake may exceed basal demands by as much as 10-fold during each 2 min replenishment [16]. Asanguineous cardioplegic solutions without oxygen should be reinfused after similar intervals, but anoxic solutions should be given as a fixed volume and as rapidly as possible to limit the duration of anoxia, provided perfusion pressure does not exceed 50 mmHg. Limiting perfusion pressure to reduce potential edema formation in newly revascularized myocardium also minimizes mechanical damage to the vein graft. High pressure in the delivery system during cardioplegic reinfusions should direct suspicion toward the possibility of (1) obstruction of the infusion cannula or (2) kinking or twisting of one of the grafts.

Inspection and/or palpation of the aorta during reinfusions allows detection of aortic insufficiency which will interfere with cardioplegic delivery. The most frequent causes of aortic incompetence in the absence of aortic valvular disease are distortion of the aortic valve by (1) a large right atrial cannula against the noncoronary sinus, (2) the retractor or sutures during mitral valve replacement, or (3) failure to remove retrocardiac pads used to improve exposure during valve replacement and/or coronary revascularization.

Cardioplegic distribution

Coronary operations

The ensurance of adequate cardioplegic solution distribution is especially important in coronary patients where maldistribution of flow is the reason for operation. Our studies show that it is safer to clamp the aorta for 2 to 4

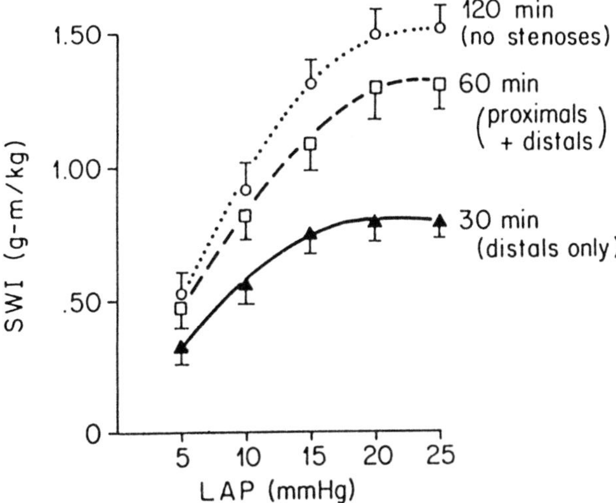

Figure 7.11. Left ventricular performance after blood cardioplegic infusion in dogs with no stenosis, and those where attempts were made to distribute the cardioplegic solution beyond stenosis. Note the partial recovery following 30 minutes of aortic clamping when no attempt was made to distribute the cardioplegic solution, and the normal performance following 120 minutes of aortic clamping when cardioplegic distribution was unimpeded.

hours with good cardioplegic distribution than for as little as 30 min when the same cold cardioplegic solution is given without attempts to deliver it beyond coronary stenoses [50–52] (Figure 7.11). Homogeneous hypothermia is not a necessary immediate goal provided the heart remains arrested. The myocardial oxygen requirements of asystole are so low at 22°C (0.3 mL/100 g per min) that they cannot be reduced substantially by reducing temperature further. Prompt fall in myocardial temperature will be achieved by perfusion of cardioplegia through the grafts after distal anastomoses are constructed. Determination of the order of grafts by review of the preoperative arteriogram allows planning for cardioplegic delivery regionally beyond stenoses. Landymore *et al.* report that myocardium supplied by totally occluded vessels is cooled more slowly than muscle supplied by stenotic or open arteries when cardioplegia is given only through the proximal aorta [53]. Optimal distribution may be achieved if totally occluded vessels with large coronary flow distribution are grafted first, followed by grafting of vessels with significant stenoses, and finally by grafting into areas with the least stenoses or regions receiving the smallest coronary flow distribution. The only exception to this suggested order of grafting is in patients with cardiogenic shock secondary to extending myocardial infarction (>24 hours after coronary occlusion) and this will be discussed separately.

Possible strategies to ensure cardioplegic distribution include (1) constructing proximal grafts before aortic clamping, (2) constructing all anastomoses during a single period of aortic clamping, (3) perfusing cardioplegic solution through the grafts after each distal anastomosis is completed, and (4) delivering retrograde cardioplegia through either the right atrium or coronary sinus. Special techniques for graft perfusion into areas of recent myocardial infarction (i.e., naturally occurring occlusion or angioplasty occlusion) will be discussed in Reperfusion, below.

Proximal grafts first. This method ensures that distribution of cardioplegia is determined by the resistance of the coronary vascular bed of the grafted vessel. The construction of proximal anastomoses on cardiopulmonary bypass avoids increasing left ventricular afterload unnecessarily and unknowingly. Precise estimation of graft length is essential as there is less margin for error than when distal anastomoses are made first.

All anastomoses during aortic clamping. This method prolongs the duration of aortic clamping but ensures cardioplegic delivery provided each proximal anastomosis is accomplished immediately after each distal anastomosis. The obligatory prolongation of aortic clamping is counterbalanced by the improved cardioplegic distribution as shown in a recent report by Weisel *et al.* [54]. Prolongation of aortic clamping may be problematic if complete revascularization is not possible, as no protection can be offered to areas of contracting muscle that cannot be revascularized due to unsuitable distal vessels. Retrograde cardioplegic administration circumvents this problem by ensuring distribution to areas supplied by obstructed vessels [55,57], and can be delivered during construction of proximal anastomoses to further limit the ischemic duration while the aorta is clamped. The construction of all anastomoses during a single period of aortic clamping also circumvents possible dislodgement of atheromatous intraaortic debris during application of a tangential aortic clamp.

Perfusion through grafts. This method does not prolong aortic clamping and allows somewhat easier estimation of graft length, especially with sequential grafts. Care must be taken to avoid kinking during reinfusions. Each cardioplegic reinfusion should be delivered through all completed grafts. This can be accomplished with a cardioplegic delivery system that ensures equal resistance through the cannulae delivering cardioplegic solution to the aorta and grafted arteries. Use of a manifold with multiple sidearms allows the same system to deliver warm noncardioplegic blood to the distal myocardium while proximal anastomoses are constructed after aortic unclamping (see Reperfusion below).

Retrograde Cardioplegia. This method has several theoretical advantages which include (1) distribution of cardioplegia in diffuse coronary disease, especially when all areas cannot be revascularized, (2) avoidance of the need for direct coronary cannulation and possible late ostial stenoses in patients undergoing aortic valve replacement, (3) exclusion of the need for aortotomy and cannulation of the coronary ostia in patients with minimal aortic regurgitation who do not require aortic valve replacement, (4) ability to give cardioplegia during mitral valve operations without removing the valve retractor [56].

The need for both routes of cardioplegic delivery in coronary operations is emphasized by experimental and clinical data [55–58]. We have shown poor cardioplegic distribution to jeopardized myocardium with antegrade infusions under conditions of experimentally simulated coronary stenosis [55,57], redistribution of cardioplegic flow away from vulnerable subendocardial muscle. In addition, the inability of cold antegrade cardioplegia to protect ischemic myocardium has been confirmed by others [59,60]. Conversely, retrograde cardioplegia is directed preferentially toward subendocardial muscle despite occlusion of the arterial vessel supplying the jeopardized region. The right ventricle is not protected consistently by retrograde cardioplegia, as right ventricular cooling and post-bypass functional recovery are somewhat variable in experimental studies of isolated cold retrograde cardioplegia. Recent preliminary clinical observations suggest that antegrade and retrograde cardioplegia supply different vascular beds, as glucose and O_2 uptake increase, and lactate washout occurs when switching from antegrade to retrograde cardioplegia, or from retrograde to antegrade cardioplegia (Figure 7.12) [61].

Retrograde cardioplegia may become particularly useful in coronary patients who receive internal mammary artery grafts since antegrade cardioplegia cannot presently be delivered through the proximally intact mammary artery. Current retrograde methods are somewhat cumbersome because they may require double venous cannulation with tourniquets on the cavae, control of the pulmonary artery, and decompression of the aorta. They also require a greater volume of cardioplegia and longer interval before arrest is produced, and may be less consistent than antegrade techniques.

Infusion of the cardioplegic solution through the right atrium with isolation of the right heart as described by Fabiani and Carpentier [62] cools the right ventricle directly by intracardiac hypothermia as well as by retrograde perfusion through thebesian veins. Failure to maintain right ventricular distention occurs when the cavae or pulmonary artery are not occluded completely, or if there is an atrial septal defect. Direct coronary sinus cannulation as described by Menache requires right atriotomy and direct coronary sinus cannulation [63]. Coronary sinus cardioplegia alone is effective during aortic replacement but may not protect the right ventricle because of problems of distribution [62]. Additional efforts at right ventricular protection by topical hypothermia may be needed when this technique is used in patients with right

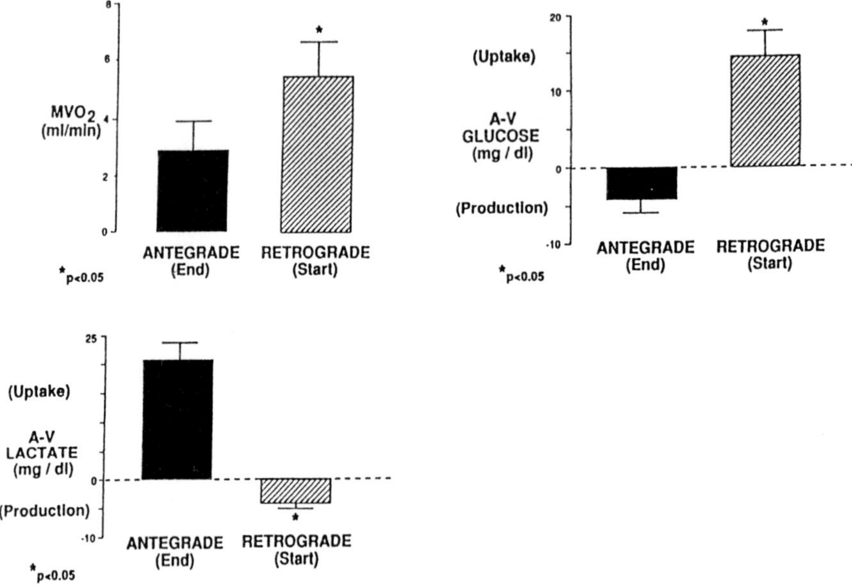

Figure 7.12. Metabolic measurements during warm cardioplegic induction at the end of antegrade (solid bar) and at beginning of retrograde (hatched bar) administration in 26 patients. Note: a) Myocardial O_2 uptake increase when switching from antegrade to retrograde delivery, b) glucose consumption increases and c) lactate consumption switches to production when changing from antegrade to retrograde delivery. A similar pattern was observed when switching from retrograde to antegrade delivery in separate studies.

ventricular hypertrophy or failure. Further experience with both retrograde methods is needed before they can be evaluated fully.

The delay in arrest with retrograde cardioplegia can be offset by combining an initial antegrade cardioplegic infusion to provide for rapid asystole with subsequent retrograde cardioplegia to ensure cardioplegic distribution. Excellent heart protection can be achieved by combining the antegrade and retrograde techniques in coronary patients as reported recently [64]. These results strongly support the conclusion that cardiac surgeons must eventually add retrograde cardioplegic techniques to their armamentarium of ways to ensure cardioplegic distribution. The clinical adoption of retrograde techniques has been slow, despite abundant experimental and clinical data attesting to their usefulness. The principal reason for the delay in clinical acceptance seems to stem from the more cumbersome operative techniques needed for retrograde cardioplegia. Most cardiac surgery in adult patients is performed with a single venous cannula. The need for double cannulation of the venae cavae and isolation of these vessels, right atriotomy and handholding of cannulas (coronary sinus retrograde cardioplegia), or isolation of the pulmonary artery (right atrial retrograde cardioplegia), and large volumes

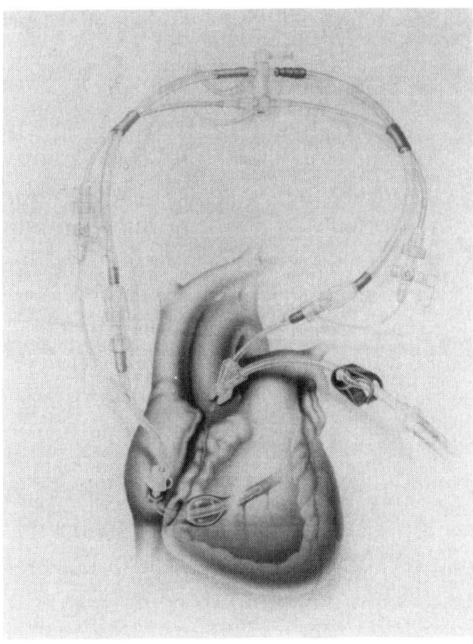

Figure 7.13. Method of delivering antegrade/retrograde cardioplegia to ensure protection to jeopardized myocardium (shaded area and distribution of occluded left anterior descending coronary artery), and areas with open coronary vessels. The aortic vent flow clamp is open during delivery of retrograde dose, which drains primarily through the thesbian and is captured by the 2-stage venous cannula. Note that coronary sinus cannulation can be accomplished transatrially, using a self-inflating balloon catheter with a contained pressure port and thereby avoid SVC and IVC isolation and cannulation and right atriotomy.

of cardioplegic solution needed to fill the right heart to produce arrest has generated limited enthusiasm for and acceptance of retrograde techniques.

Antegrade/retrograde cardioplegia

We have recently developed a simplified clinical technique of retrograde cardioplegia delivery, employing a self-inflating/deflating low pressure balloon on a retrograde cannula, which avoids the need for right heart isolation by allowing coronary sinus cannulation without opening the right atrium (Figure 7.13). This method has allowed retrograde cardioplegia to be used without making cumbersome changes in the conduct of the operation. The superior distribution of cardioplegic delivery afforded by combining the antegrade with retrograde cardioplegia has added substantially to our cardioplegic techniques. We *now routinely use both antegrade and retrograde cardioplegia in all patients undergoing aortic coronary bypass grafting, and valve replacement or repair*. This technique has increased further the safety of the blood cardioplegic technique that we have used in all of our adult and pediatric

Table 7.9. Antegrade/retrograde blood cardioplegia.

CABG	77
Shock or EF < 0.2 or AMI	33
Re-ops	14
AVR and/or MVR	33
Dissecting aortic aneurysm	3
Pediatric CHD	3
Mortality	116 pts (1.7%)

Types of operation where combined antegrade/retrograde blood cardioplegia was used: CABG, coronary artery bypass grafting; AVR, aortic valve replacement; MVR, mitral valve replacement, CHD, congenital heart disease.

patients over the past 10 years. Normally we divide the blood cardioplegic volume delivered equally between antegrade and retrograde cardioplegia during all phases of cardioplegic administration (i.e., warm induction, multi-dose cold blood cardioplegic replenishments, and warm reperfusion).

Initial experience with antegrade/retrograde cardioplegia

The types of operations where combined antegrade/retrograde cardioplegia has been used is summarized in Table 7.9. Transatrial insertion of the Retroplegia@ cannula into the coronary sinus has been successful in all patients, and we could position the retrograde catheter before starting bypass in more than 90% of instances. Partial bypass to expose the coronary sinus surface has been needed in the others to facilitate cannula placement, and right atriotomy never has been necessary. No coronary sinus injury has occurred and we have never had to reposition the cannulae. Compression of the IVC-RA junction to raise coronary sinus pressure (>25 mmHg) has been needed in approximately half the cases in our earlier experience. This has led to our placing the mattress suture lower in the RA wall to minimize intra-atrial redundancy, advancing the cannula to the coronary sinus left atrial junction to limit dislodgement during cardiac retraction, and stopping the cardioplegic infusion between the antegrade and retrograde dose. We raise flow to 200–250 mL/min over 10–15 seconds to limit recoil of the cannula from the coronary sinus to ensure good retrograde distribution. These maneuvers have ensured adequate coronary sinus pressure during infusion, and avoided the need for this minor maneuver in most instances.

Overall mortality was 1.7%, and both deaths occurred in high risk patients with extending myocardial infarctions. This combined antegrade/retrograde approach has expanded our use of IMA grafts in high risk patients who otherwise would have received vein grafts because of previous inability to provide reliable cardioplegic distribution to the jeopardized muscle supplied

Table 7.10. Advantages of combined antegrade/retrograde cardioplegic techniques.

Advantages
Prompt arrest
Ensure distribution (IMA, AI)
Limit CP volume
Uninterrupted valve procedures
Avoid ostial cannulation
Flush coronary debris/air

IMA, Internal mammary artery; AI, aortic insufficiency; CP, cardioplegia.

by the left anterior descending coronary artery. Preliminary data in a subset of coronary operations shows that deeper hypothermia of the anterolateral ventricle and septum (11°C vs. 15°C, $p < 0.05$ range 9–13°C vs. 12–22°C) when the 4–8°C blood cardioplegic infusions are given both antegrade and retrograde, versus only antegrade. The amount of debris that is flushed retrograde from the distal cut orifices of previously placed vein grafts has been surprising. We hope that the availability of retrograde perfusion will reduce the damage produced by atheromatous embolization during dissection in coronary reoperations and will also provide a treatment option in the event of inadvertent coronary air embolism. The other advantages of this combined technique are enumerated in Table 7.10 and were discussed previously.

Proponents of different techniques of intraoperative myocardial protection have traditionally, and for uncertain reasons, taken adversarial positions (i.e., ischemic arrest versus ventricular fibrillation, blood versus crystalloid cardioplegia, antegrade versus retrograde cardioplegia). The fundamental issue is the development of a thoughtful strategy for cardioplegic distribution, and this can be achieved by combining the benefits of both antegrade and retrograde cardioplegic techniques. We suspect that application of this combined strategy will allow more critically ill patients to undergo safe internal mammary artery grafting and to experience the same complete immediate recovery of regional and global function shown in patients who receive vein grafts.

Myocardial protection during coronary reoperations

The increasing frequency of coronary reoperations require special attention toward developing operative strategies that are flexible and provide protection against potential intraoperative damage that would not occur during the primary coronary revascularization. Intraoperative myocardial injury can occur sometimes before aortic clamping if vein grafts are compressed during dissection of the heart in preparation for cannulation or exposure of arteries for subsequent grafting. Functioning grafts sometimes contain atheromatous debris that can undergo inadvertent distal embolization when they are compressed. This problem can be circumvented in several ways. First, the prebypass dissection can be confined to exposing the aorta and right atrium to minimize graft compression, and the remainder of the dissection carried out after extracorporeal circulation is begun and the heart is decompressed and arrested with cardioplegic solution. Second, some surgeons prefer to transect the functioning grafts and perform new anastomoses to avoid graft embolization and to increase graft longevity. Third, the technique of retrograde cardioplegia is particularly well suited for flushing out atheromatous debris that might have embolized during cardiac mobilization. We have been surprised and delighted with the capacity of retrograde administration to remove particulate matter from grafts (and presumably from coronary arteries and capillaries) when doses are given and the effluent of the transected graft is inspected.

In some instances, the predominance of coronary blood flow is provided by functioning grafts. The presence of these conduits ensures cardioplegic distribution during antegrade induction and multidose maintenance, but the heart is particularly vulnerable to damage if they are occluded by the tangential clamp while proximal anastomoses are constructed during rewarming. In these instances, it is preferable to do all proximal and distal anastomoses during a single interval of aortic clamping as described in Cardioplegic Distribution, above. The induction and maintenance of cardioplegic arrest is particularly problematic in patients with functioning mammary grafts (or prior Vineburg operations), since these conduits carry noncardioplegic blood and delay arrest and/or cause early return of electromechanical activity. This potential problem can be circumvented by dissection of the mammary pedicle and temporary occlusion of the graft during aortic clamping. Retrograde cardioplegia is particularly useful when a functioning mammary graft supplies a substantial muscle mass. An alternate strategy in patients with functioning internal mammary artery (IMA) grafts is that of intermittent aortic clamping for each distal anastomosis with use of either ischemic arrest or, preferentially, a dose of antegrade cold cardioplegia to protect areas supplied by patent coronary arteries. The proximal anastomoses are constructed while the aorta is clamped tangentially and the temporary occluder is removed from the IMA pedicle to provide intermittent reperfusion after each interval of aortic clamping.

Aortic valve replacement

Preoperative coronary angiography is helpful to determine (1) if there are coronary arterial stenoses that require bypass grafting, (2) the length of the left main coronary artery (i.e., separate cannulation of the left anterior descending and left circumflex may be necessary if the left main coronary artery is short or if branching occurs at the ostia), and (3) the distribution of the right coronary artery (i.e., if it is dominant and supplies the inferior left ventricular wall). Performance of distal grafts first and distribution of cardioplegia through both the newly constructed grafts and the coronary ostia will optimize the strategy for myocardial protection during combined aortic valve replacement in coronary revascularization.

The underlying valvular lesion (i.e., stenosis or insufficiency) is the principle determinant of how cardioplegia is induced. The total volume of cardioplegia used during induction must be increased (i.e., to 1000–1500 mL) to provide satisfactory cooling of the increased left ventricular muscle mass caused by hypertrophy. Arrest can be achieved without opening the aorta in patients with aortic stenosis, but aortotomy and direct cannulation of the coronary ostia is required in patients with aortic insufficiency unless retrograde cardioplegia is used. Alternation of infusions through the left and right coronary cannula ensures distribution into the vascular bed supplied by each vessel. Intermittent reinfusions are given every 20–30 min unless a very brief procedure is anticipated. Direct infusion into the right coronary artery is important if (1) there is right ventricular hypertrophy or pulmonary hypertension or (2) the right coronary artery supplies substantial branches to the diaphragmatic surface of the left ventricle. Exposure of the right coronary ostium is facilitated by eversion of the aortic lip and counterpressure on the right ventricular outflow tract as described recently [65]. To avoid prolonging the operation unnecessarily, attempts to cannulate the right coronary artery should be abandoned if there is failure after a reasonable effort. This limitation of right coronary cardioplegic delivery can be counterbalanced by provision delivery of retrograde cardioplegia, maintenance of topical hypothermia and by administering a more prolonged warm cardioplegic reperfusate after aortic unclamping (to be discussed later in this chapter).

Reperfusion

Reperfusion injury is defined as the functional, metabolic, and structural alterations caused by reperfusion after a period of temporary ischemia (i.e., aortic clamping) [43]. The potential for this damage exists during all cardiac operations because the aorta must be clamped to produce a quiet bloodless field. Reperfusion damage is characterized by (1) intracellular calcium accumulation [66], (2) explosive cell swelling with reduction of postischemic blood flow and reduced ventricular compliance [66,67], and (3) inability to utilize delivered oxygen, even when coronary flow and oxygen content are ample [35,68]. Our studies show that the fate of myocardium jeopardized by global and regional ischemia is determined more by the careful control of the conditions of reperfusion and composition of the reperfusate than by the duration of ischemia itself [69]. *The cardiac surgeon is in the unique position to counteract the potential of reperfusion damage since the conditions of reperfusion and the composition of the reperfusate are under the surgeon's immediate control.*

Post-ischemic reperfusion damage after global ischemia can be avoided or

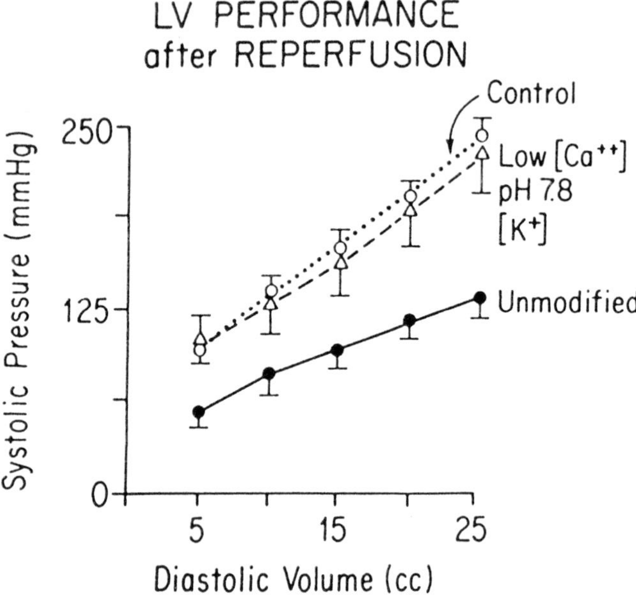

Figure 7.14. Left ventricular performance 30 minutes after one hour of topical hypothermic ischemic arrest. Note the normal postischemic performance when a blood cardioplegic reperfusate containing low calcium, high pH, was given just prior to removal of the aortic clamp, and the depressed myocardiai performance when the reperfusate was unmodified.

minimized by substituting a brief (i.e., 3- to 5-min) warm (37°C) blood cardioplegic infusion during the initial phase of reoxygenation for the normal blood reperfusion which would be provided by aortic unclamping [35] (Figure 7.14). The principles (Table 7.11) that are addressed during controlled reperfusion include (1) reoxygenation with blood to start aerobic metabolism for energy production to repair cellular injury, (2) delivery of the reperfusion over *time* rather than by *dose* to maximize O_2 utilization [70], (3) lowering energy demands by maintaining temporary cardioplegia to allow the limited O_2 ability to be channeled toward reparative processes [71], (4) replenishing substrate (i.e., glutamate) which allows optimal aerobic energy production to occur [42], (5) making the reperfusate pH alkalotic to counteract tissue acidosis and optimize enzymatic and metabolic function during recovery [72], (6) temporarily reducing ionic calcium available to enter the cell (i.e., chelation with citrate phosphate dextrose) [73], (7) inducing hyperosmolarity and decreasing perfusion pressure (i.e., 50 mmHg to reduce and minimize reperfusion edema) [74,75], and (8) warming the reperfusate to 37°C to optimize the rate of metabolic recovery [43,76]. Hypothermic reperfusion is not used because it retards metabolic rate and slows repair [77,78].

Clinical studies by Teoh *et al.* document the metabolic and functional value

Table 7.11. Warm cardioplegic reperfusion.

Principle	Method
Provide O_2	Blood
Optimize metabolism	Normothermia
Duration	5–10 mm
Maintain asystole	KCI
Replenish substrate	Glutamate/aspartate
Reverse acidosis	Buffer
Limit Ca^{++}	CPD
Counteract edema	Hyperosmolarity
	Gentle pressure

CPD, citrate phosphate dextrose.

of using a warm blood cardioplegic reperfusate strategy in elective coronary operations, and we use a warm blood reperfusate before aortic unclamping in *all* operations. Reports by Menasche *et al.* support the benefits of reperfusion cardioplegia even when oxygen is not added [76]. The capacity to avoid or minimize reperfusion damage by reperfusion cardioplegia makes this technique a valuable adjunct to the cardiac surgeon's armamentarium, especially if cardioplegic distribution has been problematic, or if aortic clamping has been prolonged. We have used reperfusion cardioplegia as the primary form of cardiac protection (to avoid reperfusion injury) when homogeneous cardioplegic delivery was questionable through a large right coronary artery or if early branching of left main artery required selective cannulation of anterior descending and circumflex branches during aortic valve replacement. Starting systemic and cardioplegic rewarming about 5 min before unclamping the aorta ensures normothermia in the 8–10 mEq/L K + oxygenated blood cardioplegic reperfusate which is the same solution used during multidose cold cardioplegia. Delivery of this reperfusate at 150 mL/min for 3–5 minutes avoids high reperfusion pressure (i.e., 50 mmHg). Longer infusions (i.e., 5–10 min) may be useful if there has been poor cardioplegic distribution during the preceding aortic clamping interval (i.e., through large right coronary artery which was not perfused during aortic valve replacement or if the last distal coronary anastomoses was made into a vessel with a large myocardial flow distribution). Reperfusion cardioplegia must be delivered into *all* grafts *and* into the aorta in coronary patients to ensure its distribution. The warm cardioplegic reperfusate may be used also to evacuate air from the aorta through the suture line during aortic valve replacement. Recurrence of cardiac electromechanical activity during reperfusion cardioplegia is rare despite the low potassium concentration. The warm reperfusate should be discontinued and the aortic clamp removed if electromechanical activity recurs (i.e., beating or fibrillating) while it is being infused. Electromechanical activity resumes usually 1–2 min after aortic unclamping unless there is systemic hyperkalemia. Failure to recover contractility requires temporary ventricular pacing to avoid the myocardial edema that may follow prolonged perfusion of the flaccid heart. Palpation of the left ventricle detects distention so that a vent can be inserted if necessary. Recurrent asystole after placing the tangential clamp in coronary operations suggests that coronary flow has been interrupted by the clamp. Routine palpation of the proximal aorta allows estimation of the adequacy of coronary perfusion pressure and provides grounds for reapplication of the tangential clamp if the proximal aorta is flaccid.

Reperfusion after acute myocardial infarction

Precise control of the conditions of reperfusion and composition of the reperfusate is especially important in patients undergoing revascularization for acute evolving myocardial infarction [69]. The principles of reperfusate composition discussed previously for use after global ischemia are applicable directly to reperfusion after regional ischemia and the same reperfusate may be used. Delivery of the warm reperfusate selectively into the ischernic region after removing the aortic clamp following completion of all distal anastomoses concentrates the reperfusate in the area most vulnerable to reperfusion damage. We prolong the duration of regional 37°C cardioplegic reperfusion (i.e., through the graft) to 20 min because experimental studies show that postischemic O_2 uptake does not return to baseline levels until this interval has elapsed [70]. 0ther proximal anastomoses can be accomplished during this prolonged segmental cardioplegic reperfusion. Keeping reperfusion pressure gentle (i.e., below 50 mmHg) limits edema and avoids disruption of microvasculature [80,81], and venting ensures low energy demands in the reperfused segment [44]. Restriction of flow to a maximum of 50 mL/min simplifies the procedure. Lower reperfusion pressure (i.e., <50 mmHg) may not revascularize subendocardial muscle optimally, but salvage of overlying midmyocardium and epicardial muscle may convert the potential transmural necrosis to a subendocardial infarction. Application of the aforementioned technique has resulted in early recovery of regional contractility in a preliminary series of 16 patients revascularized after an average of 10 hours of acute coronary occlusion [69]. Subsequently, a multicenter analysis [82] of the treatment of acute coronary occlusion documented the superiority of surgically controlled reperfusion over medically uncontrolled reperfusion using PTCA by showing that it accomplishes more completely the primary goals of revascularization; restoring segmental contractility and lowering mortality (Table 7.12, Figure 7.15). This surgical experience [82] in 156 patients from six centers confirmed our preliminary findings of the benefits of the controlled reperfusion strategy [69,83] and is contrasted to the results in five major series of 1203 patients treated medically by PTCA [84–88]. The improved outcome, including substantial recovery of regional contractile function in 87% of patients, occurred despite longer ischemic time (6.3 vs. 3.9 hrs) and where a larger proportion of surgical

Table 7.12. Results of medically uncontrolled reperfusion by PTCA vs. controlled surgical reperfusion by CABG after acute coronary occlusion.

Reperfusion	PTCA (uncontrolled) (n = 1203)			CABG (controlled) (n = 156)		p value
Ischemic time[a]	3.9 hrs			6.3 hrs		<0.05
Mortality	Pts	Range	%	Pts	%	
Overall	105/1203	(7.2–11%)	(8.7%)	6/156	(3.9%)	<0.05
High Risk Subgroups[b]						
LAD occlusion	39/331	(10–12%)	(11%)	9/95	(5%)	NS
3 vessel disease	27/158	(15–20%)	(17%)	0/66	(0%)	<0.05
Age >70 years	21/109	(17–25%)	(19%)	1/22	(5%)	NS
Failure to reperfuse	26/82	(15–50%)	(32%)	0/0	(0%)	<0.05
Pre op shock	49/114	(41–57%)	(43%)	6/66	(9%)	<0.05

[a]Time from chest pain to reperfusion (PTCA) or bypass (CABG).
[b]Each of the 5 reports did not include *all* subgroups.
n = number of patients.
PTCA, percutaneous transluminal coronary angioplasty; CABG, coronary artery bypass grafting.

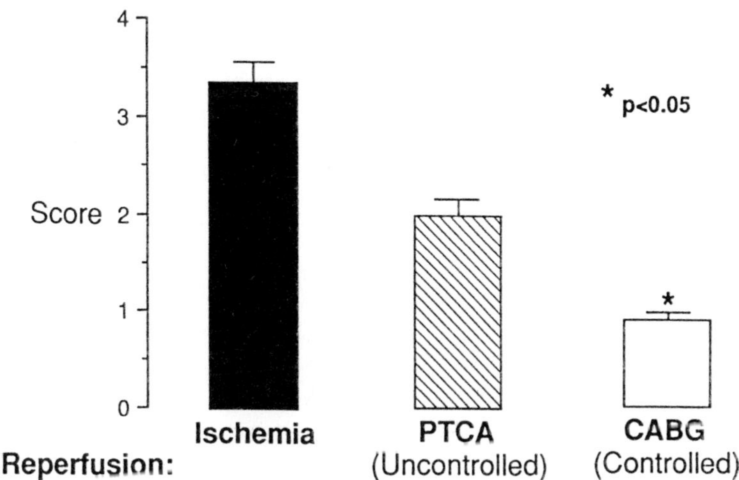

Figure 7.15. Regional myocardial wall motion during acute coronary occlusion (ischemia) and following medically uncontrolled reperfusion (PTCA) or surgically controlled reperfusion (CABG). Note the improved return of regional wall motion in the surgical group despite longer ischemic times (see Table XIII). Regional myocardial wall motion score: 0 = normal motion, 1 = mild to moderate hypokinesis, 2 = severe hypokinesis, 3 = akinesis, 4 = dyskinesis. PTCA, percutaneous transluminal coronary angioplasty; CABG, coronary artery bypass grafting.

patients fell into the high-risk categories of LAD occlusion, 3-vessel disease, age >70 yrs, and cardiogenic shock, as defined in reports of medical revascularization with uncontrolled reperfusion [84–97]. The absence of a prospective randomized trial and failure to include the results of uncontrolled reperfusion from the participation centers are obvious limitations of this study design, but we do not believe that failure to provide this information nullifies the implications of this data.

Warm non-cardioplegic flow through distal grafts

Adequate reperfusion beyond coronary stenoses cannot occur when proximal anastomoses are constructed after aortic unclamping. We have shown experimentally [52] and Weisel has shown clinically [54] that lactate washout persists until the coronary obstruction is bypassed by connecting the graft to the aorta. Warm noncardioplegic blood reperfusion through the grafts can be used to circumvent this problem if proximal grafting is carried out after aortic unclamping whether blood or asanguineous cardioplegia has been employed. Distal graft reperfusion with normal blood hastens cardiac rewarming, (2) washes out residual cardioplegic solution, (3) ensures adequate reperfusion pressure beyond residual stenoses, and (4) facilitates estimation of graft length.

Reversal of the order of proximal grafting from that used for cardioplegic delivery (i.e., connecting the most important graft to the aorta last) optimizes normal blood reperfusion to the largest revascularized region for as long as possible before the tangential clamp is removed. Unobstructed normal blood reperfusion can be provided readily by either removing the cardioplegic tube from the roller head used to deliver blood cardioplegia, or via a side branch from the arterial line. The same vein introducer cannulae placed into the proximal ends of the vein grafts for multidose cardioplegia can be used to deliver *both* the warm cardioplegic reperfusate and warm noncardioplegic blood.

Cardiogenic shock secondary to extending infarction

All of these aforementioned principles of myocardial protection were applied to a recent series of patients with cardiogenic shock secondary to left ventricular power failure, where medical mortality exceeds 75% [98,99] and surgical mortality is 30%–60% [99,100]. Surgical mortality was reduced to approximately 7% [101] (Figure 7.16, Table 7.13) by (1) warm induction of blood cardioplegia to repair cellular processes and replenish energy stores before clamping [46], (2) multidose cardioplegia to minimize energy loss during aortic clamping [102], (3) glutamate and aspartate enrichment of blood cardioplegic solutions to replenish substrate utilized during ischemia [17], (4) ensuring adequate distribution of cardioplegic solutions through the bypassed grafts to protect regions beyond stenoses [52] (5) grafting viable areas first

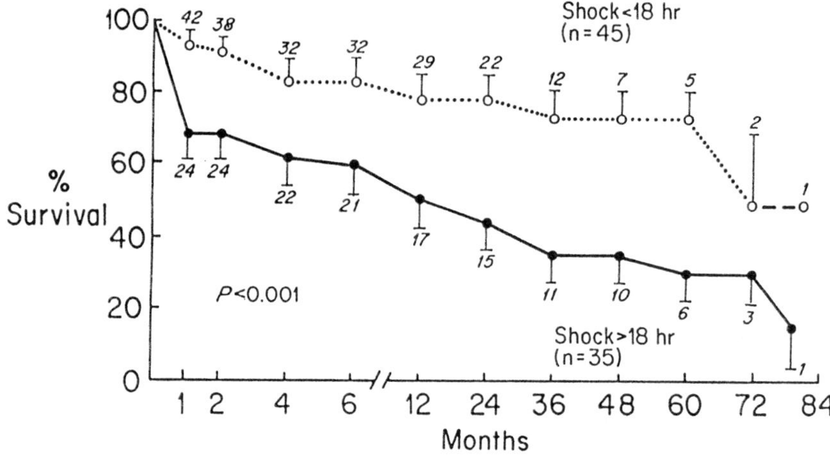

Figure 7.16. Coronary artery bypass grafting after cardiogenic shock: influence of time of operation after cardiogenic shock (n = 80, deaths = 35). p. Wilcoxin, mean ± standard error; italics indicate patients alive and well.

Table 7.13. Influence of time of CABG (n = 80, deaths = 35) after cardiogenic shock.

Time (mo)	Shock <18 hr (n = 45)	Shock >18 hr (n = 35)
1	0.93 ± 0.04	0.69 ± 0.08
12	0.78 ± 0.06	0.51 ± 0.08
24	0.78 ± 0.06	0.45 ± 0.08
36	0.74 ± 0.08	0.36 ± 0.08
48	0.74 ± 0.08	0.36 ± 0.08
60	0.74 ± 0.08	0.31 ± 0.08
72	0.49 ± 0.21	0.31 ± 0.08

CABG, coronary artery bypass graftlng.

to offer maximum protection of the portions of myocardium responsible for supporting the circulation, (6) warm reperfusion of blood cardioplegia to lessen reperfusion damage [35], (7) ensuring adequate blood perfusion of grafted regions while proximal anastomoses are being constructed (Figure 7.17), and (8) early operation to prevent development of preoperative organ failure or progressive loss of ischemic remote myocardium. The gratifying clinical results are due to careful application of *all* aspects of operative strategy (Table 7.14). Our surgical approach is based on our interpretation of the pathophysiology of cardiogenic shock with special reference to the remote myocardium. Cardiogenic shock after acute myocardial infarction usually develops 24–72 hr after acute coronary occlusion even though acutely ischemic muscle stops contracting immediately, is maximally dysfunctional initially, and never contributes to cardiac output before operation [103–108].

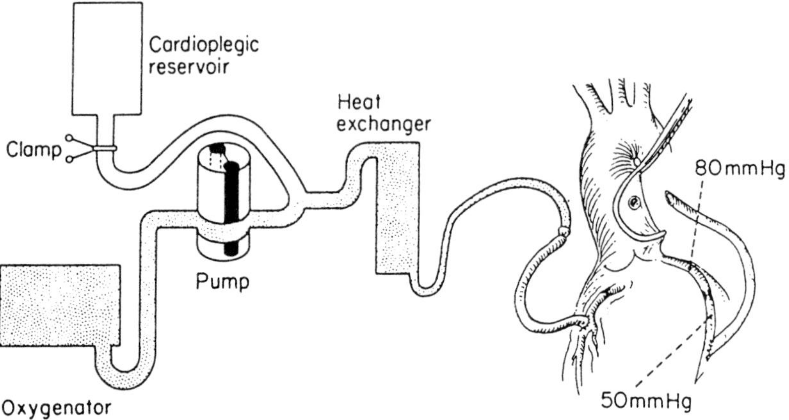

Figure 7.17. Method of graft perfusion during proximal anastomosis (see text for description).

Table 7.14. Operative strategy – cardiogenic shock.

Warm blood cardioplegic induction
Substrate enrichment (glutamate, aspartate)
Graft viable areas first
Multidose cold blood cardioplegia
Ensure distribution through grafts
Warm blood cardioplegic reperfusate
Distal graft perfusion during proximals

Ischemic muscle remains viable for a variable period of time [103] and is a source of chest pain, but there is no evidence that infarct extension worsens infarcting muscle function. Maintenance of systemic output is dependent, therefore, on the ability of adjacent remote myocardium to develop and sustain compensatory hypercontractility. We observed experimentally that LV power failure after an otherwise non-lethal anterior (LAD) infarction (i.e., $<30\%$ LV muscle mass) is caused principally by a progressive decline in remote muscle function when there is associated circumflex stenosis [104,109,110]. Remote muscle contractility becomes impaired if its volume is diminished by previous infarction or if it is ischemic. Consequently, delayed cardiogenic shock (24–72 hours after acute myocardial infarction) occurs because viable muscle in the distribution of stenotic arteries fails to maintain the compensatory hypercontractility which is responsible for ensuring adequate cardiac output [111].

Our operative strategy is designed to ensure maximum myocardial protection and immediate optimal function to this viable functioning muscle. Therefore, grafts are placed first into contracting muscle, especially into arteries with large flow distributions [46]. Vessels supplying regions with smaller functioning muscle mass are grafted next. The last graft(s) are placed into the infarcted region. For example, if cardiogenic shock evolves gradually after a large anterolateral infarction, the right coronary artery and circumflex arteries should be grafted before the left anterior descending and diagonal vessels. Distribution of cold cardioplegia through all grafts into newly revascularized segments should be accomplished after each anastomosis is completed to maximize protection of these regions. We do not believe that there is one isolated aspect of our approach that ensures success, just as there is no single component of the blood cardioplegic solution (i.e., temperature, hypocalcemia, buffering, substrate, hyperosmolarity, etc.) that guarantees perfect protection.

Conventional treatment of cardiogenic shock includes maximum pharmacologic and mechanical support with coronary artery bypass grafting only in balloon dependent patients or in those whose condition improves sufficiently to allow semi-elective revascularization. This concept of "stabilization to buy time" is not borne out by the results. Early operation (<18 hrs) allowed a 93% early survival (Figure 7.16, Table 7.13) and avoided preoperative organ failure. Conversely, delay of operation (>18 hrs) prolonged the need for inotropic support, caused more leg complications from the intraaortic balloon, allowed organ failure to develop, prolonged hospitalization, and increased early and late mortality rates. We suspect that progressive remote muscle necrosis occurred while circulatory support was prolonged and impaired subsequent functional recovery.

Topical hypothermia

Topical cooling is a useful adjunct when problems in cardioplegic distribution are anticipated (i.e., during aortic valve replacement when the right coronary artery cannot be perfused, especially if there is right ventricular hypertrophy, or in coronary patients with diffuse coronary disease or occluded right coronary arteries where right ventricular protection is not possible). Topical hypothermia is most helpful during valve replacement where there is ventricular hypertrophy, as cold solution can be introduced also directly into the ventricular cavity to achieve the endocardial cooling which is more difficult from the myocardial surface.

Topical cooling retards the recurrence of electromechanical activity by keeping myocardial temperature low and counteracts the effects of coronary collateral washout of the cardioplegic solution. Surface cooling may not be essential with multidose cardioplegia since the oxygen requirements of the arrested heart below 20°C are extremely low. The value of topical hypothermia is limited most in coronary patients because (1) the heart must be removed from the pericardial well for all but very proximal left anterior descending and right coronary anastomoses, and (2) injury to the phrenic nerve (especially with ice slush) may cause unavoidable respiratory complications [112,113] which may be problematic in elderly patients.

We recently reviewed 150 consecutive coronary patients undergoing coronary artery bypass grafting (50 with topical ice slush, 50 with 4°C saline, and 50 without topical cooling) [114]. Patients that received ice slush topical hypothermia had a higher incidence of phrenic nerve palsy (9/50 vs. 3/50 vs. 0/50, $p < 0.05$), pleural effusion (25/50 vs. 7/50 vs. 9/50, $p < 0.05$), and atelectasis (33/50 vs. 34/50 vs. 18/50, $p < 0.05$). Conversely, there was no improved protection afforded by the use of topical cooling as measured by postoperative cardiac outputs, EKG changes, postoperative enzymes, inotropic requirements or deaths. We therefore do not use topical hypothermia during coronary operations if complete revascularization is possible, even if there is cardiogenic shock.

Secondary cardioplegia

Inadequate myocardial protection becomes apparent only when extracorporeal circulation is discontinued and cardiac performance is depressed. Most surgeons have observed that temporary resumption of extracorporeal circulation results in some hemodynamic improvement but does not always allow complete recovery. Oxygen demands are reduced by "resting the heart" and simultaneous oxygen delivery to postischemic cells is ensured by maintaining a reasonable perfusion pressure. Delivery of abundant oxygen does not, however, assure that the cell can use its oxygen [39–41] to repair ischemic or reperfusion damage or reconstitute a depressed energy store. We have found that further recovery and *reversal of damage* is possible if the heart is rearrested by providing a brief (5-min) continuous 37°C blood cardioplegic solution during the time-frame allocated for prolonging extracorporeal circulation, especially when the cardioplegic solution is enriched with the precursors of Krebs cycle intermediates (i.e., glutamate and aspartate).

These studies have lead the present authors to conclude that some of the limitation of the postischemic heart's capacity to utilize oxygen is related to myocardial loss of these key Krebs cycle intermediates during ischemia; glutamate and aspartate are now included in all cardioplegic infusions given at our institution. The normothermic (37°C) blood cardioplegic solution used to rearrest the heart restores oxidative metabolism toward normal and results in near complete functional recovery (Figure 7.18). We have termed this intervention *secondary cardioplegia* and we believe that by lowering oxygen demands with secondary cardioplegia, one allows oxygen uptake to be channeled toward reparative processes rather than wasting it on needless electromechanical work. Secondary cardioplegia has also been found useful in 29 treating troublesome ventricular arrhythmias which may be refractory to conventional countershock and pharmacologic agents [115].

As more is learned about the characteristics of reperfusion injury, it should be possible to develop cardioplegic solutions and reperfusates with the ions, substrates, and possible cofactors that will avoid or reverse completely ischemic and reperfusion damage. This extended use of blood cardioplegia

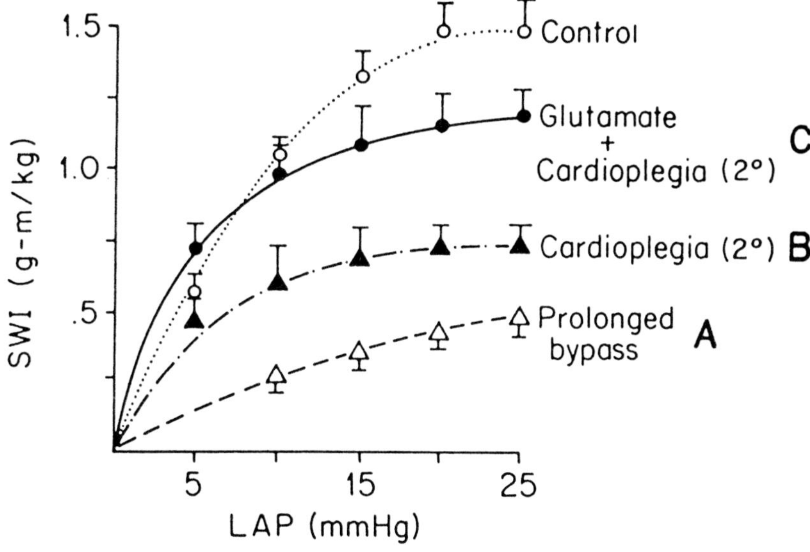

Figure 7.18. Left ventricular performance following 45 minutes of normothermic ischemic arrest when (a) bypass was prolonged without producing secondary cardioplegia, (b) secondary cardioplegia was administered for 5 minutes and (c) glutamate was added to secondary cardioplegic solution. Note the near normal recovery with substrate enhancement of secondary cardioplegic solution with glutamate.

indicates that the surgeon may now play an active role in reversing myocardial injury due to the present limitations of cardioplegic techniques.

Occasionally, intractable ventricular fibrillation (sometimes progressing to asystole) develops after an otherwise successful cardiac operation. The heart becomes severely energy depleted if fibrillation continues, since the diastolic pressure generated during CPR will not adequately perfuse the subendocardium [116,117]. Temporary cardiopulmonary bypass ensures more adequate peripheral perfusion, facilitates defibrillation, but the beating heart requires substantial amounts of oxygen [37,118,119] and the damaged myocardial cells have a reduced capacity to take up oxygen [40,41]. Under these circumstances, a prolonged infusion of amino acid enriched cardioplegic solution on total vented bypass may aid in repair of ischemically damaged cardiac muscle. This concept is based on our experience with prolonged regional ischemia, where we could restore contractility and mitochondrial energy generating capacity after 6 hrs of LAD occlusion [83], and could resuscitate hearts with 2 hrs of intractable ventricular fibrillation under conditions of simulated multi-vessel disease [109]. The heart must be kept arrested on total vented bypass to reduce oxygen demands maximally (to 1 cc/100 gm/min) to achieve optimal benefit. The cardioplegic dose is given over 20 min as oxygen is consumed over time rather than by dose.

We have applied this concept clinically in patients who developed intractable ventricular fibrillation perioperatively who underwent an otherwise successful operation. Careful attention is directed toward maintaining adequate cerebral perfusion pressure during CPR, especially during transit to the operating room for placement on total vented bypass and prolonged secondary cardioplegic infusion for myocardial resuscitation. Total vented bypass is begun as quickly as possible, and aspartate/glutamate blood cardioplegia (37°C at 150 cc/min) is delivered antegrade for 20 minutes immediately after aortic clamping. The heart is kept in the beating empty state for 30 minutes after removing the aortic clamp and extracorporeal is then discontinued gradually. We reported recently survival of 11 of 14 patients who underwent secondary cardioplegia to treat intractable perioperative ventricular fibrillation [120]. 0ur data, both experimental and clinical, suggests that complete revascularization is a prerequisite for success of this salvage approach [121]. The clinical availability of percutaneous technology may allow prompt initiation of cardiopulmonary bypass to support the systemic circulation and facilitate defibrillation during transfer to the operating room for secondary cardioplegic administration. This aggressive approach may offer a more optimistic outcome for patients who would otherwise succumb after an seemingly successful operation.

Warm blood cardioplegia without hypothermia

Bigelow, in 1950 at the University of Toronto, introduced hypothermia as an important component of myocardial protection that slows cardiac metabolism while limiting ischemic injury during the periods of aortic cross-clamping needed to optimize operative conditions to provide a quiet bloodless field. The studies of Shumway and Lower in 1959 reinforced this cardioprotective strategy [122]. These observations led to the surgical axiom that "all is well if the heart is made as cold as possible" and that there is a "battle against the clock" when the aorta is clamped. Recent data on the cardioprotective benefits of warm blood cardioplegia suggests that these axioms are outdated, and that intraoperative damage is related more to "how the heart is protected" rather then "how long the aorta is clamped".

Hypothermia may also impose certain adverse consequences, including shifting the oxygen-hemoglobin dissociation curve leftward, retarding sodium potassium ATPase to promote edema, reducing membrane stability, increasing blood viscosity, and activating platelets, leukocytes and complement [123,124]. These concerns led the surgical team at the University of Toronto (where hypothermia was introduced) to suggest warm blood cardioplegia without hypothermia as a cardioprotective strategy, where the patient and the heart are maintained at 37°C and the cardioplegic flow is delivered continually when feasible. This concept is based on the fact that electromechanical arrest substantially decreases myocardial oxygen requirements to low levels (from 10 mL/100 gm/min to 1 mL/100 gm/min) with little further reduction in O_2 demands accomplished by adding profound hypothermia. Therefore, they propose that myocardial oxygen demands can be met with continuous warm cardioplegia as long as the heart is kept arrested [123,125]. This occurs only if there is *homogenous and adequate* distribution of cardioplegic solutions and this has yet to be proven. Unfortunately, there is no current experimental infrastructure for the clinical application of this attractive hypothesis, although preliminary results in patients are encouraging [123,124,126]. The continuous warm cardioplegic approach is in contrast to early attempts of 37°C continuous coronary perfusion with normal blood where the energy requirements remain high when the heart was either kept beating or fibrillated. An added potential advantage of this method is that ischemia is avoided if 37°C blood cardioplegic flow is continuous and post-ischemic reperfusion injury cannot occur by maintaining the heart in a constant aerobic state. Additionally, the resumption of cardioplegic flow if it must be interrupted intermittently for technical reasons (i.e., blood obscuring the operative field) may limit reperfusion damage by delivering a warm reperfusate. The composition of the cardioplegic solution will assume increased importance if it is used as a reperfusate, in addition to a solution to prevent ischemic injury. Finally, systemic normothermia may limit the possible detrimental effects of hypothermic cardiopulmonary bypass on coagulation and other organ systems.

Lichtenstein reported superior clinical results (compared retrospectively to continuous cold blood cardioplegia) using continuous warm antegrade blood cardioplegia, and Salerno reported gratifying results with the continuous warm retrograde blood cardioplegic infusions. The retrograde technique was adopted because of the possible advantages in (1) patients with coronary disease where coronary stenosis might limit antegrade distribution and (2) valve operations where mitral valve retractors can make the aortic valve incompetent and to exclude the need for direct coronary perfusion catheters in aortic operations, since these may lead to late ostial injury. Despite these encouraging early clinical findings, subsequent experimental data shows some limitations of the warm continuous cardioplegic technique and several questions remain unanswered (see below). Several studies show the superiority of intermittent cold antegrade and antegrade/retrograde blood cardioplegic techniques over continuous warm antegrade or retrograde cardioplegia, especially in protecting areas of jeopardized myocardium [59,60]. Furthermore, when continuous warm antegrade or retrograde cardioplegia was interrupted intermittently, as must be done clinically to optimize visualization during construction of distal anastomoses, intermittent cold antegrade/retrograde cardioplegia provided superior results [127]. These observations emphasize that both warm and cold cardioplegic techniques, as well as antegrade and retrograde methods of delivering may be useful and complementary rather than adversarial techniques in the cardiac surgeons armamentarium, especially when cardioprotective strategies are formulated to reduce and avoid damage to myocardial beds that are in jeopardy of injury.

Additional missing data on the role of warm heart surgical techniques includes (1) what flow rates are needed to adequately supply the arrested heart, and will continuous infusion ensure all areas receive sufficient flow to meet metabolic needs, (2) how long can the blood flow be interrupted safely before ischemic changes take place if perfusion must be stopped because blood obscures the operation field, and how can these changes be overcome with resumption of cardioplegic flow, (3) what is the ideal cardioplegic composition (i.e., is it different from the composition used for intermittent cold blood cardioplegia), (4) does warm heart surgery (with the patient at 37°C) lead to increased bleeding due to the inherently higher flow rates that must maintained, (5) will cerebral complications increase if non-pulsatile flows with inherently lower perfusion pressure are used? and (6) will more fatal "perfusion accidents" occur due to the limited time (3–4 minutes) available to the perfusionists to stop extracorporeal circulation and correct the problem before cerebral damage occurs. Finally, experimental and clinical studies have demonstrated that the normal and ischemically damaged heart can be protected safely for 2–4 hrs of aortic clamping with intermittent cold blood cardioplegia especially if bracketed with an interval of warm induction and reperfusion to "resuscitate" the heart and "limited reperfusion injury" (see earlier sections on Blood Cardioplegia and Warm Induction). These intermittent cardioplegic techniques provide the ideal technical conditions of a bloodless field needed for surgical precision, while simultaneously ensuring metabolic correction of the consequences of ischemia, which are minimized by hypothermic protection. Consequently, abandonment of cold cardioplegic techniques in favor of the warm approach is not recommended until a sufficient infrastructure of data is accumulated to answer the aforementioned questions. We suspect that warm blood cardioplegic techniques will become adjunctive to hypothermic techniques, rather than a replacement for them.

Conclusions

The versatility of blood cardioplegia provides the cardiac surgeon with an extremely powerful tool to actively treat the jeopardized myocardium as well as to prevent ischemic damage, provided attention is directed toward ensuring adequate delivering of the cardioplegic solutions. No exogenous blood is needed to deliver blood cardioplegia, as a readily available blood source exists within the extracorporeal circuit during all cardiac operations when the patient's blood volume mixes with the clear priming fluid. The expense of depriving the patient of the potential benefits of blood cardioplegia includes increased perioperative mortality, prolonged intensive care unit stays, and development of late cardiac fibrosis owing to necrosis caused by less adequate protection, and far outweighs the monetary cost of its use.

The aforementioned benefits of enhanced oxygen carrying capacity, active resuscitation, avoidance of reperfusion damage, limitation of hemodilution, provision of onconicity, buffering, rheologic effects, and endogenous oxygen free radical scavengers enumerate only the known benefits of using blood as the vehicle for delivering oxygenated cardioplegia. We are confident that further studies will reveal other naturally occurring blood components (i.e., enzymes, cofactors, substrates, electrolytes) that are important and would otherwise need to be added to any artificially constructed solution.

References

1. Melrose DG, Dreyer B, Bentall HH. Elective cardiac arrest. Lancet 1955; 2: 21.
2. Waldhausen JA, Braunwald NS, Bloodwell RD. Left ventricular function following elective cardiac arrest. J Thorac Cardiovasc Surg 1960; 39: 813.
3. Bretschneider HJ, Hubner G, Knoll D *et al.* Myocardial resistance and tolerance to ischemia: Physiological and biochemical basis. J Cardiovasc Surg 1975; 16: 241.
4. Kirsch U, Rodewald G, Kalmar P. Induced ischemic arrest. J Thorac Cardiovasc Surg 1972; 63: 121.
5. Hearse DJ, Stewart DA, Braimbridge MV. Cellular protection during myocardial ischemia. Circulation 1976; 54: 193.
6. Gay WA Jr, Ebert PA. Functional, metabolic, and morphologic effects of potassium-induced cardioplegia. Surgery 1973; 74: 284.
7. Tyers GFO, Todd GJ, Niebauer IM. The mechanism of myocardial damage following potassium citrate (Melrose) cardioplegia. Surgery 1975; 78: 45.
8. Follette DM, Mulder DG, Maloney JV Jr *et al.* Advantages of blood cardioplegia over continuous coronary perfusion and intermittent ischemia. J Thorac Cardiovasc Surg 1978; 76: 604–19.
9. Roberts AJ, Moran JM, Sanders JH. Clinical evaluation of the relative effectiveness of multidose crystalloid and cold blood potassium cardioplegia in coronary artery bypass graft surgery. Ann Thorac Surg 1982; 33: 421–33.
10. Cunningham JN, Catinella FP, Spencer FC. Blood cardioplegia – experience with prolonged cross-clamping. In Engelman RM, Levitsky S (eds.): A Textbook of Clinical Cardioplegia. Mt. Kisco, New York: Futura Publishing Co 1982; 242–64.
11. Fabiani JN, Perier P, Chelly J. Blood versus crystalloid cardioplegia. In Engelman RM, Levitsky S (eds.): A Textbook of Clinical Cardioplegia. Mt. Kisco, New York: Futura Publishing Co 1982; 285–95.
12. Catinella FP, Cunningham JN, Adams PX. Myocardial protection with cold blood potassium cardioplegia during prolonged aortic cross-clamping. Ann Thorac Surg 1 982; 33: 228–33.
13. Buckberg GD. A proposed "solution" to the cardioplegic controversy. J Thorac Cardiovasc Surg 1979; 77: 803–15.
14. Catinella FP, Cunningham JN Jr, Spencer FC. Myocardial protecion during prolonged aortic cross-clamping. J Thorac Cardiovasc Surg 1984; 88: 422–43.
15. Peyton RB, Van Tright P, Pellam GL. Improved tolerance to ischemia in hypertrophied myocardium by preischemic enhancement of adenosine triphosphate. J Thorac Cardiovasc Surg 1982; 84: 11–15.
16. Buckberg GD, Dyson CW, Emerson RC. Techniques for administering clinical cardioplegia: Blood cardioplegia. In: Levitsky S, Engelman RM (eds): A Textbook of Clinical Cardioplegia. Mt. Kisco, New York: Futura Publishing Co 1982.
17. Rosenkranz ER, Okamoto F, Buckberg GD *et al.* Aspartate enrichment of glutamate blood cardioplegia in energy-depleted hearts after ischemic and reperfusion injury. Safety of prolonged aortic clamping with blood cardioplegia. J Thorac Cardiovasc Surg 1986; 91: 428–35.

18. Vander Woude JC, Christlieb IY, Sicard GA. Imidazole-buffered cardioplegic solution: Improved myocardial preservation during global ischemia. J Thorac Cardiovasc Surg 1985; 90: 225–34.
19. Langer GA. Control of calcium movement in the myocardium. Eur Thorac J 1983; 4: 5–11.
20. Yamamoto F, Manning AS, Braimbridge MV. Cardioplegia and slow calcium channel blockers. Studies with verapamil. J Thorac Cardiovasc Surg 1983; 86: 252–61.
21. Clark RE, Christlieb IY, Henry PD *et al.* Nifedipine. A myocardial protective agent. Am J Cardiol 1979; 44: 825–31.
22. Standeven JW, Jellinek M, Menz LJ *et al.* Cold blood potassium diltiazem cardioplegia. J Thorac Cardiovasc Surg 1984; 87: 201–12.
23. Steward JR, Blackwell WH, Crute SL. Inhibition of surgically induced ischemia/reperfusion injury by oxygen free radical scavengers. J Thorac Cardiovasc Surg 1983; 86: 262–72.
24. Okamoto F, Allen BS, Buckberg GD *et al.* Supplemental role of intravenous and intracoronary CoQ_{10} in avoiding reperfusion damage. Studies of controlled reperfusion after ischemia: Reperfusate composition. J Thorac Cardiovasc Surg 1986; 92: 573–82.
25. McCord JM. Oxygen-derived free radicals in postischemic tissue injury. N Eng J Med 1985; 312: 159–63.
26. Foglia RP, Steed DL, Follette DM *et al.* Iatrogenic myocardial edema with potassium cardioplegia. J Thorac Cardiovasc Surg 1979; 78: 217–22.
27. Elert O, Ottermann U. Cardioplegic hemoglobin perfusion for human myocardium. In Myocardial Protection for Cardiovascular Surgery. Pharmazeutische Verlagsgesellschaft, 1979: 134–43.
28. Bodenhamer RM, DeBoer LWV, Geffin GA. Enhanced myocardial protection during ischemic arrest. Oxygenation of a crystalloid cardioplegic solution. J Thorac Cardiovasc Surg 1983; 85: 769–80.
29. Reeves RB. What are normal acid-base conditions in man when body temperature changes? , In Rahn H, Prakash O (eds): Acid-base regulation and body temperature. Boston: Martinus Nijhoff, 1985; 13–32.
30. Van Asbeck B, Hoidal J, Vercellotti GM *et al.* Protection against lethal hyperoxia by tracheal insufflation of erythrocytes: role of red cell glutathione. Science 1985; 227: 756–8.
31. Julia PL, Buckberg GD, Acar C *et al.* XXI. Superiority of blood cardioplegia over crystalloid cardioplegia in limiting reperfusion damage: Importance of endogenous oxygen free-radical scavengers in red blood cells. Reperfusate composition. J Thorac Cardiovasc Surg 1991; 101: 303–13.
32. Cauvin C, Loutzenhiser R, Hwang O *et al.* Alpha1-adrenoceptors induce Ca influx and intracellular Ca release in isolated rabbit aorta. Eur J Pharmacol 1982; 84: 233–5.
33. Robertson JM, Buckberg GD, Vinten-Johansen J. Comparison of distribution beyond coronary stenoses of blood and asanguineous cardioplegic solutions. J Thorac Cardiovasc Surg 1983; 86: 80–6.
34. Novick RJ, Stefaniszyn HJ, Michel RP. Protection of the hypertrophied pig myocardium. A comparison of crystalloid, blood, and Fluosol-DA cardioplegia during prolonged aortic clamping. J Thorac Cardiovasc Surg 1985; 89: 547–66.
35. Follette DM, Fey K, Buckberg GD *et al.* Reducing postischemic damaqe by temporary modification of reperfusate calcium, potassium; pH, and osmolarity. J Thorac Cardiovasc Surg 1981; 82: 221–38.
36. Matsuuda H, Maeda S, Hirose H. Optimum dose of cold potassium cardioplegia for patients with chronic aortic valve disease: Determination by left ventricular mass. Ann Thorac Surg 1986; 41: 22–6.
37. Buckberg GD, Brazier JR, Nelson R *et al.* Studies of the effects of hypothermia on regional myocardial blood flow and metabolism during cardiopulmonary bypass. I. The adequately

perfused beating, fibrillating and arrested heart. J Thorac Cardiovasc Surg 1977; 78: 87–94.

38. Rosenkranz ER, Vinten-Johansen J, Buckberg GD *et al.* Benefits of normothermic induction of cardioplegia in energy-depleted hearts, with maintenance of arrest by multidose cold blood cardioplegic infusions. J Thorac Cardiovasc Surg 1982; 84: 667–76.
39. Kane JJ, Murphy ML, Bissett JK *et al.* Mitochondria function, oxygen extraction, epicardial S-T segment changes and tritiated digoxin distribution after reperfusion of ischemic myocardium. Am J Cardiol 1975; 36: 218–24.
40. Lazar HL, Buckberg GD, Manganaro AJ. Reversal of ischemic damage with amino acid substrate enhancement during reperfusion. Surgery 1980; 88: 702–9.
41. Lazar HL, Buckberg GD, Manganaro AM. Myocardial energy replenishment and reversal of ischemic damage by substrate enhancement of secondary blood cardioplegia with amino acids during reperfusion. J Thorac Cardiovasc Surg 1980; 80: 350–9.
42. Rosenkranz ER, Okamoto F, Buckberg GD. The safety of prolonged aortic clamping with blood cardioplegia. II. Glutamate enrichment in energy-depleted hearts. J Thorac Cardiovasc Surg 1984; 88: 401–10.
43. Rosenkranz ER, Buckberg GD. Myocardial protection during surgical coronary reperfusion. J Am Coll Cardiol 1983; 1: 1235–46.
44. Allen BS, Okamoto F, Buckberg GD *et al.* XIII. Critical importance of total ventricular decompression during regional reperfusion. Studies of controlled reperfusion after ischemia: Reperfusate conditions. J Thorac Cardiovasc Surg 1986; 92: 605–12.
45. Hoffman JIE, Buckberg GD. Transmural variation in myocardial perfusion. In Yu PN, Goodwin JF (eds). Philadelphia: Lea and Febiger, 1976.
46. Rosenkranz ER, Buckberg GD, Mulder DG *et al.* Warm induction of cardioplegia with glutamate-enriched blood in coronary patients with cardiogenic shock who are dependent on inotropic drugs and intraaortic balloon support: Initial experience and operative strategy. J Thorac Cardiovasc Surg 1983; 86: 507–18.
47. Brazier J, Hottenrott C, Buckberg GD. Noncoronary collateral myocardial blood flow. Ann Thorac Surg 1975; 19: 425–35.
48. Ferguson TB, Smith PK, Buhrman WC. Studies on the physiology of the conduction system during hyperkalemic, hypothermic cardioplegic arrest. Surg Forum 1983; 34: 302–4.
49. Penhkurinen KJ, Takala TES, Nuutinen EM. Tricarboxylic acid cycle metabolites during ischemia in isolated perfused rat heart. Am J Physiol 1983; 244: H281–H8.
50. Robertson JM, Vinten-Johansen J, Buckberg GD *et al.* I. Safety of prolonged aortic clamping with blood cardioplegia. Glutamate enrichment in normal hearts. J Thorac Cardiovasc Surg 1984; 88: 395–401.
51. Hilton CJ, Teubl W, Acker M *et al.* Inadequate cardioplegic protection with obstructed coronary arteries. Ann Thorac Surg 1979; 28: 323.
52. Becker H, Vinten-Johansen J, Buckber GD. Critical importance of ensuring cardioplegic delivery with coronary stenoses. J Thorac Cardiovasc Surg 1981; 81: 407–515.
53. Landymore RW, Tice D, Trehan N. Importance of topical hypothermia to ensure uniform myocardial cooling during coronary artery bypass. J Thorac Cardiovasc Surg 1981; 82: 832–6.
54. Weisel RD, Hoy FDY, Baird RJ. Improved myocardial protection during a prolonged cross-clamp period. Ann Thorac Surg 1983; 36: 664.
55. Partington MT, Acar C, Buckberg GD *et al.* II. Nutritive blood flow distribution in normal and jeopardized myocardium. Studies of retrograde cardioplegia. J Thorac Cardiovasc Surg 1989; 97/4: 613–22.
56. Buckberg GD, Drinkwater DD, Laks H. Antegrade/retrograde blood cardioplegia to ensure cardioplegic distribution: Operative techniques and objectives. J Card Surg 1989; 4: 216–38.
57. Partington MT, Acar C, Buckberg GD *et al.* I. Advantages of antegrade/retrograde

cardioplegia in jeopardized myocardium. Studies of retrograde cardioplegia. J Thorac Cardiovasc Surg 1989; 97/4: 605–12.

58. Buckberg GD. Recent advances in myocardial protection using retrograde blood cardioplegia. Eur Heart J 1989; 10/Supple H: 43–8.
59. Matsuura H, Lazar HL, Yang X *et al.* Warm vs. cold blood cardioplegia: is there a difference? Surg Forum 1991; 42: 231–2.
60. Diehl JT, Pontoriero M, Connolly R *et al.* Alternative Methods of Retrograde cardioplegia delivery: Effects on preservation of the ischemic left ventricle after acute coronary artery occlusion and reperfusion. Aats 1992; 60–1. (Abstract)
61. Beyersdorf F. Personal Communication. J Thorac Cardiovasc Surg 1992; (Submitted).
62. Fabiani JM, Carpentier AF. Comparative evaluation of retrograde cardioplegia through the coronary sinus and the right atrium. Circulation 1983; 68: III-251.
63. Menasche P, Kural S, Fauchet M. Retrograde coronary sinus perfusion: A safe alternative for ensuring cardioplegic delivery in aortic valve surgery. Ann Thorac Surg 1982; 34: 647–58.
64. Diehl JT, Eichhorn EJ, Konstam MA. Efficacy of retrograde coronary sinus cardioplegia in patients undergoing myocardial revascularization: A prospective randomized trial. Ann Thorac Surg 1988; 45: 595–602.
65. Sud A. Identification of right coronary ostium. Correspondence to the Editor. Ann Thorac Surg 1985; 40: 97.
66. Jennings RB, Ganote CE. Structural changes in myocardium during acute ischemia. Circulation Research 1974; 35: III-156–III-172.
67. Kloner RA, Ellis SG, Lange R *et al.* Studies of experimental coronary artery reperfusion. Effects on infarct size, myocardial function, biochemistry, ultrastructure and microvascular damage. Circulation 1983; 68: I-8–I-15.
68. Wood JA, Hanley HG, Entman JL. Biochemical and morphological correlates of acute experimental myocardial ischemia in the dog. IV. Early mechanisms during very early ischemia. Circulation Research 1979; 44: 52–62.
69. Allen BS, Buckberg GD, Schwaiger M *et al.* XVI. Consistent early recovery of regional wall motion following surgical revascularization after eight hours of acute coronary occlusion. Studies of controlled reperfusion after ischemia. J Thorac Cardiovasc Surg 1986; 92: 636–48.
70. Allen BS, Okamoto F, Buckberg GD *et al.* XII. Considerations of reperfusate "duration" vs "dose" on regional functional, biochemical, and histocriemical recovery. Studies of controlled reperfusion after ischemia: Reperfusate conditions. J Thorac Cardiovasc Surg 1986; 92: 594–604.
71. Follette DM, Steed DL, Foglia RP. Reduction on postischemic myocardial damage by maintaining arrest during initial reperfusion. Surg Forum 1977; 28: 281–3.
72. Follette D Fey K, Livesay J *et al.* Studies on myocardial reperfusion injury. I. Favorable modification by adjusting reperfusate pH. Surgery 1977; 82: 149–55
73. Allen BS, Okamoto F, Buckberg GD *et al.* IX. Benefits of marked hypocalcemia and diltiazem on regional recovery. Studies of controlled reperfusion after ischemia: Reperfusate composition. J Thorac Cardiovasc Surg 1986; 92: 564–72.
74. Foglia RP, Buckberg GD, Lazar HL. The effectiveness of mannitol after ischemic myocardial edema. Surg Forum 1980; 30: 320–3.
75. Engelman RM, Spencer FC, Gouge TH. Effect of normothermic anoxic arrest on coronary blood flow distribution of pigs. Surg Forum 1974; 25: 176–9.
76. Menasche P, Grousset C, de Boccard G. Protective effect of an asanguineous reperfusion solution on myocardial performance following cardioplegic arrest. Ann Thorac Surg 1984; 37: 222–8.
77. Lazar HL, Buckberg GD, Manganaro A *et al.* Limitations imposed by hypothermia during recovery from ischemia. Surg Forum 1980; XXXI: 312–5.
78. Metzdorff MT, Grunkemeier GL, Starr A. Effect of initial reperfusion temperature on myocardial preservation. J Thorac Cardiovasc Surg 1986; 91: 545–50.

79. Teoh KH, Christakis GT, Weisel RD *et al.* Accelerated myocardial metabolic recovery with terminal warm blood cardioplegia. J Thorac Cardiovasc Surg 1986; 91: 888–95.
80. Okamoto F, Allen BS, Buckberg GD *et al.* XIV. Importance of ensuring gentle vs sudden reperfusion during relief of coronary occlusion. Studies of controlled reperfusion after ischemia. Reperfusate conditions. J Thorac Cardiovasc Surg 1986; 92: 613–20.
81. Jennings RB, Reimer KA. Factors involved in salvaging ischemic myocardium: effect of reperfusion of arterial blood. Circulation 1983; 68: I-25–I-36.
82. Allen BS. Buckberg GD. Fontan F *et al.* Superiority of controlled surgical reperfusion vs. PTCA in acute coronary occlusion. J Thorac Cardiovasc Surg 1992; (in Press).
83. Allen BS, Okamoto F, Buckberg GD *et al.* XV. Immediate functional recovery after 6 hours of regional ischemia by careful control of conditions of reperfusion and composition of reperfusate. Studies of controlled reperfusion after ischemia. J Thorac Cardiovasc Surg 1986; 92: 621–35.
84. Stack RS, Califf RM, Hinohara T *et al.* Survival and cardiac event rates in the first year after emergency coronary angioplasty for acute myocardial infarction. J Am Coll Cardiol 1988; 11: 1141–9.
85. Miller PF, Brodie BR, Weintraub RA *et al.* Emergency coronary angioplasty for acute myocardial infarction. Arch Intern Med 1987; 147: 1565–70.
86. Rothbaum DA, Linnemeier TJ, Landin RJ *et al.* Emergency percutaneous transluminal coronary angioplasty in acute myocardial infarction. a 3 year experience. J Am Coll Cardiol 1987; 10:264–72.
87. Erbel R, Pop T, Henrichs KJ *et al.* Percutaneous transluminal coronary angioplasty after thrombolytic therapy: A prospective controlled randomized trial. J Am Coll Cardiol 1986; 8: 485–95.
88. O'Keefe JH Jr, Rutherford BD, McConahay DR *et al.* Early and late results of coronary angioplasty without antecdent thrombolytic therapy for acute myocardial infarction. Am J Cardiol 1989; 64: 1221–30.
89. Wilcox RG, Olsson CG, Skene AM *et al.* Trial of tissue plasminogen activator for mortality reduction in acute myocardial infarction. Anglo-Scandinavian Study of Early Thrombolysis (ASSET). Lancet 1988; 11: 525–30.
90. GISSI. Effectiveness of intravenous thrombolytic treatment in acute myocardial infarction. Lancet 1986; 1: 397–402.
91. GISS1-2. A factorial randomised trial of alteplase versus streptokinase and heparin versus no heparin among 12,490 patients with acute myocardial infarction. Lancet 1990; 336: 65–71.
92. ISIS-2. Randomised trial of intravenous streptokinase, oral aspirin, both, or neither among 17,187 cases of suspected acute myocardial infarction: ISIS-2. Lancet 1988; 349–60.
93. Rogers WJ. Update on recent clinical trials of thrombolytic therapy in myocardial infarction. J Invasive Cardiol 1991; 3: 11A–19A.
94. The ISAM Study Group. A prospective trial of intravenous streptokinase in acute myocardial infarction (I.S.A.M.). N Engl J Med 1986; 314: 1465–71.
95. AIMS Trial Study Group. Effect of intravenous apsac on mortality after acute myocardial infarction: preliminary report of a placebo-controlled clinical trial. Lancet 1988; I: 545–9.
96. Qhman EM, Califf RM. Thrombolytic therapy: overview of clinical trials. Coronary Artery Disease 1990; 1: 23–33.
97. Topol EJ, Califf RM, George BS *et al.* A randomized trial of immediate versus delayed elective angioplasty after intravenous tissue plasminogen activator in acute myocardial infarction. N Engl J Med 1987; 317: 581–8.
98. Page DL, Caulfifeld JB, Kastor JA *et al.* Myocardial changes associated with cardiogenic shock. N Engl J Med 1971; 285: 133–7.
99. Johnson SA, Scalon RJ, Loeb HS. Treatment of cardiogenic shock in myocardial infarction by intraaortic balloon counterpulsation and surgery. Am J Med 1977; 62: 687–92.
100. Mundth ED, Buckley JM, Daggett WF. Surgery for complications of acute myocardial infarction. Circulation 1972; 45: 1279–91.

101. Allen BS, Rosenkranz ER, Buckberg GD *et al.* VI. Myocardial infarction with LV power failure: A medical/surgical emergency requiring urgent revascularization with maximal protection of remote muscle. J Thorac Cardiovasc Surg 1989; 98: 691–703.
102. Nelson R, Fey K, Follette DM. The critical importance of intermittent infusion of cardioplegic solution during aortic cross-clamping. Surg Forum 1976; 26: 241–3.
103. Beyersdorf F, Allen BS, Acar C. *et al.* I. Evidence for preserved cellular viability after 6 hours of coronary occlusion. Studies on Prolonged Acute Regional Ischemia. J Thorac Cardiovasc Surg 1989; 98: 112–26.
104. Beyersdorf F, Acar C, Buckberg GD *et al.* III. Early natural history of simulated single and multi-vessel disease with emphasis on remote myocardium. J Thorac Cardiovasc Surg 1989; 98: 368–80.
105. Beyersdorf F, Okamoto F, Buckberg GD *et al.* II. Implications of progression from dyskinesis to akinesis in the ischemic segment. Studies on prolonged Regional Ischemia. J Thorac Cardiovasc Surg 1989; 98: 224–33.
106. Banka VS, Helfant RH. Temporal sequence of dynamic contractile characteristics in ischemic and non-ischemic myocardium after acute coronary ligation. Am J Cardiol 1974; 34: 158–62.
107. Kloner RA, Przyklenk K, Lange R *et al.* Reperfusion pathophysiology. In Roberts AJ (ed.): Myocardial protection in cardiac surgery. New York: Marcel Dekker 1987; 29–52.
108. Kerber RE, Marcus ML, Ehrhardt J *et al.* Correlation between echocardiographically demonstrated segmental dyskinesis and regional myocardial perfusion. Circulation 1992; 520: 1097.109. Beyersdorf F, Acar C, Buckberg GD *et a!.* IV. Aggressive surgical treatment for intractable ventricular fibrillation after acute myocardial infarction. J Thorac Cardiovasc Surg 1989; 98: 557–66.
110. Beyersdorf F, Acar C, Buckberg GD *et al.* V. Metabolic support of remote myocardium during LV power failure. J Thorac Cardiovasc Surg 1989; 98: 567–79.
111. Widimsky P, Gregor P, Cervenka V. Diffuse left ventricular hypokinesis in cardiogenic shock; its cause or consequence? Cor Vasa 1984; 26: 27–31.
112. Benjamin JJ, Cascade PN, Rubenfire M *et al.* Left lower lobe atelectasis and consolidation following cardac surgery: the effect of topical cooling on the phrenic nerve. Radiology 1982; 142: 11–4.
113. Marco JD, Hahn JW, Barner HB. Topical cardiac hypothermia and phrenic nerve injury. Ann Thorac Surg 1977; 23: 235–7.
114. Allen BS, Buckberg GD, Rosenkranz ER *et al.* Topical cardiac hypothermia in coronary patients: An unnecessary adjunct to cardioplegic protection and cause of pulmonary morbidity. J Thorac Cardiovasc 1992; (In Press).
115. Robicsek F. Biochemical termination of sustained fibrillation occurring after artificially induced ischemic arrest. J Thorac Cardiovasc Surg 1984; 87: 143–5.
116. Hottenrott C, Maloney JV Jr, Buckberg GD. Studies of the effects of ventricular fibrillation on the adequacy of regional myocardial flow. III. Mechanism of ischemia. J Thorac Cardiovasc Surg 1974; 68: 634–45.
117. Buckberg GD, Hottenrott CE. Ventricular fibrillation: its effect on myocardial flow, distribution and performance. Ann Thorac Surg 1975; 20: 76–85.
118. Allen BS, Rosenkranz ER, Buckberg GD *et al.* VII. The high oxygen requirements of dyskinetic cardiac muscle. Studies of controlled reperfusion after ischemia. J Thorac Cardiovasc Surg 1986; 92: 543–52.
119. Hottenrott CE, Towers B, Kurkji HJ *et al.* The hazard of ventricular fibrillation in hypertrophied ventricles during cardiopulmonary bypass. J Thorac Cardiovasc Surg 1973; 66: 742–53.
120. Beyersdorf F, Kirsh MM, Buckberg GD *et al.* Warm glutamate/aspartate-enriched blood cardioplegic solution for perioperative sudden death. J Thorac Cardiovasc Surg 1992; 104: 1141–7.
121. Mooney MR, Arom KV, Joyce LD. Emergency cardiopulmonary bypass support in patients with cardiac arrest. J Thorac Cardiovasc Surg 1991; 101: 450–4.

122. Shumway NE, Lower RR. Hypothermia for extended periods of anoxic arrest. Surg Forum 1959; 10: 563–3.
123. Lichtenstein SV, Ashe KA, el Dalati H *et al.* Warm heart surgery. J Thorac Cardiovasc Surg 1991; 101: 269–74.
124. Salerno TA, Houck JP, Barrozo CA *et al.* Retrograde continuous warm blood cardioplegia: a new concept in myocardial protection. Ann Thorac Surg 1991; 51: 245–7.
125. Lichtenstein SV, Salerno TA, Slutsky AS. Warm continuous cardioplegia is preferable to intermittent hypothermic cardioplegia for myocardial protection during cardiopulmonary bypass: pro and con. J Cardiothorac Anesth 1990; 4: 279–81.
126. Lichtenstein SV, Abel JG, Panos A *et al.* Warm heart surgery: Experience with long cross-clamp times. Ann Thorac Surg 1991; 52: 1009–13.
127. Matsuura H, Lazar HL, Yang XM *et al.* Detrimental effects of interrupting warm blood cardioplegia during coronary revascularization. Aats 1992; 62–3. (Abstract)

PART THREE

Clinical application of cardioplegia

8. High volume perfusion

IRVIN B. KRUKENKAMP, CHRISTOPHER A. CALDARONE, PAUL BURNS, and SIDNEY LEVITSKY

Modern operative myocardial management strategies have evolved considerably in the brief 35 year history of cardiac surgery supported by extracorporeal circulation. From the early techniques employing normothermic ischemia ('clamp and run') to a variety of hypothermic cardioplegic ischemic modalities (crystalloid vs. blood, intermittent vs. continuous, antegrade vs. retrograde), to the novel modern approach of nonischemic warm continuous blood cardioplegia, the cardiac surgeon continues to seek an optimal operative environment in which to conduct complicated cardiac and major vascular repairs. The initial and, indeed, ongoing goal of all myoprotective strategies is not only to provide a quiet, bloodless operative field for a prolonged time in which to effect the desired surgical repair, but also to minimize any ischemic damage to the heart, thereby preserving biochemical and mechanical cardiac function postoperatively. Simply stated, the goal is to maintain myocardial energy and substrate supply in excess of electromechanical and biochemical demand during the time of operation. Thus, modern operative myocardial management strategies optimize the relationship of energy supply to consumption by maintaining aerobic (or anaerobic) substrate metabolism. The capacity of the myocardium to provide metabolic activity in excess of demand will be dependent upon not only the temperature and composition of the perfusate administered during the aortic cross-clamp interval, but also on the distribution, duration and volume of the perfusion. Hence, the topic 'High volume perfusion' presented in this chapter.

The term 'High volume perfusion' implies that alternative methods, e.g., 'Low volume perfusion' might optionally be considered. We would suggest that neither case is necessarily key to providing a quiescent surgical field and effective myocellular preservation. As a minimum requirement the perfusion technique must effectively (1) prevent depletion of high energy phosphate stores, (2) maintain aerobic (or anaerobic) metabolism, (3) minimize and/or remove acidic metabolic by-products, (4) provide substrate for cellular and subcellular repair processes, (5) maintain ionic gradients, (6) prevent destructive metabolism such as lipid peroxidation or oxygen tree radical generation and (7) prepare the myocardium energetically and metabolically for the resumption of electromechanical activity upon removal of the aortic cross-clamp. In addition, high (or low) volume perfusate, which is usually collected in the venous reservoir along with systemic venous return, must have minimal

H.M. Piper and C.J. Preusse (eds): Ischemia-reperfusion in cardiac surgery, 231–242.

deleterious effects (e.g., hyperkalemia, hyperglycemia, hemodilution) in the systemic extracorporeal perfusion circuit. Obviously, the extensive variety of techniques cited briefly above indicates the many 'solutions' to these myoprotective goals. The purpose of the present chapter will be to develop both biological and surgical rationales for the modern management of clinical ischemia and reperfusion, with emphasis on the perfusion volume necessary to optimize myoprotective technique.

Biological rationale

Changes in cellular and subcellular structure and function attendant to ischemia induced by aortic cross-clamping are exceedingly complex. Moreover, they are frequently confounded by a variable extent of pre-existing ischemic insults (i.e., by total or subtotal coronary arterial occlusion) and compensatory processes, e.g., chronic coronary arterial collateral channel development. Heretofore, the following basic principles of intraoperative myocardial protection have been considered incontrovertible [1]; (1) immediate induction of complete electromechanical arrest to prevent useless expenditure of energy stores, (2) adequate hypothermia to reduce metabolic requirements, (3) appropriate buffering of ischemically accumulated metabolic acids during aortic cross-clamping and (4) avoidance of intracellular edema related to (high volume) cardioplegic perfusion. These will be discussed subsequently.

Rapid arrest

The initiation of cardiac arrest lowers the metabolic demand by minimizing depletion of high energy phosphate compounds used for electromechanical work. Modern arrest methodologies include elevating extracellular potassium or magnesium, depleting intracellular calcium or sodium and application of local anesthetics or calcium antagonists. The myocardium is thereby rendered unexcitable and remains in diastolic arrest. Since *in vivo*, a significant noncoronary collateral coronary flow not uncommonly washes away the arresting agent, intermittent reinfusions (at 20 to 30 min intervals) or continuous perfusion of cardioplegia are required. Although the optimal dosage of administered potassium ion to maintain electromechanical quiescence and prevent postoperative rhythm disturbances has yet to be defined, practical usage of concentrations between 15 and 30 meq/L have proven efficacious [2].

Intuitively high volume cardioplegia techniques, such as those of Bretschneider, Lichtenstein or Salerno [3–5], should modulate the total amount of potassium administered to obviate postoperative atrioventricular conduction block or supraventricular tachyarrhythmias. This point however, is further obfuscated by the experimental work suggesting that atrioventricular conduction is preserved following potassium cardioplegic arrest and that rhythm disturbances are instead attributable to ischemic injury due to inadequate atrial and atrial septal hypothermia [6] However, Flack and associates have identified a lower incidence of postoperative conduction disturbances when using continuous high volume potassium warm cardioplegia compared to traditional cold techniques [7]. Interestingly the incidence of supraventricular arrhythmias was not affected by the cardioplegic method (warm vs. cold, 35 vs. 34%).

Hypothermia

The heart is an obligate aerobic organ, deriving energy from the mitochondrial oxidation of glucose, free fatty acids, lactate, pyruvate, acetate, ketone bodies and amino acids. Over 75% of the coronary arterial oxygen is extracted during a single passage through the myocardium. Even in the non-working, vented state supported by total extracorporeal circulation, the heart consumes about 3 to 5 ml O_2 per minute/100 gm LV [8]. Initiation of cardiac asystole at normothermia reduces this oxygen demand to about 1 ml O_2 per minute/100 gm LV, or by roughly 80% [9]. Hypothermic perfusion to 15°C or less affords further reduction of the oxygen requirement to less than 0.5 ml O_2 per minute/100 gm LV [10,11]. Indeed, these data are consistent with VanHoff's law for most living systems which suggests that each 10°C decrement in temperature reduces metabolic activity by about 50%. It is this minimal, yet nonzero, metabolic need that must be met during periods of aortic cross-clamping to prevent the deleterious depletion of energy and substrate stores, independently of the cardioplegic vehicle or perfusion rate deemed convenient to the surgeon.

Cardiac cooling may be effected by a number of methods including topically applied iced saline, intracavitary cold saline irrigation, periventricular 'cooling jackets', and by cold intracoronary perfusates. Additionally, systemic perfusion rate may be decreased as well as the perfusate temperature to delay cardiac rewarming. Total extracorporeal circulation effected by snaring caval tapes around the individually cannulated superior and inferior venae cavae limits endocardial rewarming from systemic venous return. Intracoronary cold cardioplegic delivery provides transmural cooling, the efficacy of which is facilitated by continuous infusion as opposed to the intermittent reinfusion technique.

Buffering

Hydrogen ions are produced within the myocyte as breakdown products from metabolic processes such as ATP hydrolysis and reduction of pyruvate to lactate. Metabolic acid accumulation alters coronary vascular resistance and perturbs cationic equilibrium such that potassium is lost from the myocyte and calcium accumulates. Additionally, as hydrogen ion concentration increases, anaerobic energy production via glycogenolysis and anaerobic glycolysis is attenuated. Thus, buffering of intracoronary perfusates is an obvious means of reducing tissue acidosis.

The optimal pH and ideal buffering system remains to be elucidated. It must be understood that pH and buffering capacity, although both representing in some way the quantity of protons in solution, have nevertheless distinctly separate connotations. pH refers mathematically to the *concentration* of hydrogen ions in a particular solution or tissue. Buffering capacity denotes the ability of that particular solution to maintain a neutral pH with the addition of hydrogen ions. The issue is further confounded by the Rosenthal effect, which is the finding that in all physical solutions, pH rises 0.0134 units for each °C of hypothermia [12].

Most clinically used cardioplegic formularies favor alkalinization. Although bicarbonate is a commonly used buffer, it is an extracellular buffer with a low buffering capacity at physiologic pH (7.4). In contrast, the histidine-imidazole buffering system afforded by the proteins in blood cardioplegia provides a large buffering capacity. Supplementation of crystalloid cardioplegia with this protein-based buffer has been shown to be salutary [13].

Tissue edema

The arrested heart accumulates tissue edema during ischemia probably due to impairment of transmyocardial fluid transport either from derangements of cell-volume regulation during ischemia or from altered lymphatic and venous flow patterns. The addition of osmolar agents such as mannitol or glucose, and/or oncotic agents such as albumin, dextran or erythrocytes, to cardioplegic formulae help minimize interstitial edema [14]. Furthermore, cardiac perfusion at excessive pressure during arrest may exacerbate cardiac fluid accumulation from the fragile coronary vasculature [15]. This is particularly true of retrogradely administered cardioplegia where the monitored coronary sinus pressure should remain less than 40 to 45 mmHg to avoid edema [5,16,17]. When the aortic cross-clamp is removed, controlled hypotension during the initial few minutes of reperfusion may prevent edema formation. However, perfusate osmolarities above 400 mOsm should be avoided to obviate cardiac dehydration. The perfusion duration and perfusate volume of osmotically active coronary perfusates remain actively investigated with regards to their effect on myocardial edema.

Surgical rationale

A hallmark of the 35 year evolution of modern cardiothoracic surgical practice is the broad range of operative management problems presently discussed for newborn, neonatal, young adult, adult and senescent myocardium, as differences in ultrastructure, biochemistry and mechanical performance are readily apparent [18,19]. Even a cursory review of modern literature on myocardial perfusion yields controversies regarding antegrade vs. retrograde delivery, ideal perfusate temperature (cold vs. warm) and numerous special issues, e.g., myocardial management in the setting of acute regional ischemia or in dilated or hypertrophied myocardium. While it is beyond the scope of this chapter to resolve any of these issues, it may be useful to examine the surgical rationale for one modern intraoperative myocardial management strategy, with emphasis on the volume of perfusion.

Warm heart surgery

In 1987 Lichtenstein and colleagues at University of Toronto initiated a program of non-ischemic warm cardiac surgery supported on warm extracorporeal circulation. They suggest in their 1991 report of 121 patients undergoing coronary artery bypass grafting using this technique [4], that it provides for an unhurried repair of complex defects with patients weaned from bypass without inotropic or mechanical support in normal sinus rhythm. This novel method is clearly in contradistinction to the heretofore incontrovertible principle of hypothermic myopreservation noted above. As perfusion volume and route play a central role in the development of this technique, let us examine its development as a model to evaluate 'High volume perfusion'.

Central to hypothermic myocardial management is the principle that cardiac metabolism is significantly attenuated by cold temperature during finite periods of aortic cross-clamping and ischemic arrest. Moreover, the heart must be reperfused following the ischemic interval and any ischemia related metabolic derangements or changes in myocellular membrane integrity or osmotic homeostasis become evident as 'reperfusion injury'. Theoretically, a period of warm asystolic quiescence would provide for nonischemic arrest, a limited period of post cross-clamp removal 'reperfusion', and abolition of any potentially deleterious effects of myocardial hypothermia.

In consideration of the differences in myocellular metabolism, one might question the efficacy of a technique that may apparently *not* attenuate biochemical processes during the cross-clamp period. However, the decrease in oxygen demand from the working (off bypass) heart to one supported on total extracorporeal circulation and empty beating amounts to approximately 80% [8]. Simply arresting the electromechanical activity associated with the empty-beating state further reduces the myocardial oxygen consumption to approximately 0.5 ml O_2/min/100 gm LV [9,10]. Cooling the heart from this state also effects a lowering of MVO2, but only to the 0.3 to 0.5 ml O_2/min/100 gm LV, a rather small additional benefit [11]. This is a relatively small difference in myocardial energy requirement, particularly when the ischemic interval is held quite short. Indeed, the advantage of warm continuous blood cardioplegia is that the heart is *not* ischemic. The aortic cross-clamp in effect separates the systemic circulation receiving normal, non-cardioplegic blood perfusion from the aortic root perfusion of potassium-laden arresting solution of blood cardioplegia. The only time that the heart is ischemic is when the aortic root perfusion is turned off, such as when it is necessary to clear the operative field to construct critical portions of an end to side aortocoronary bypass graft. Upon removing the aortic cross-clamp, one only needs to wait for the washout of the arresting solution and resumption of a coordinated rhythm before weaning the patient from extracorporeal circulation.

In consideration of the biological rationale for myocardial management strategies, warm blood cardioplegia fulfills several of the 'incontrovertible' principles. The major benefit of blood as an intracoronary perfusate is its ability to carry and unload oxygen to myocellular tissue. Clearly the oxygen carrying capacity of blood cardioplegia at normothermia, even at modest hematocrits, is superior to that of crystalloid based formularies. Secondly, the serum proteins, red cells and hemoglobin afford a large concentration of histidine-imidazole moieties which act as an ideal buffer system, both in terms of perfusate pH as well as buffering capacity. Thirdly, the formed elements and serum proteins also provide an appropriately physiologic osmotic environment for the myocytes to limit myocardial edema formation and concomitant changes in myocardial compliance.

The major thrust of this modern technique of intraoperative myocardial management is that the constituents and technique of myocellular perfusion during the non-ischemic cross-clamp interval minimize the ischemic insult resulting from the operative procedure. The rationale is to *eliminate* the insult. However, upon further reflection, several potential limitations and advantages become evident. For example, what is the delivery of warm perfusate distal to coronary obstruction? What perfusion rate at what hematocrit is necessary to provide adequate oxygen and substrate at normothermia to maintain the heart nonischemic? Can warm blood cardioplegia be safely delivered retrogradely? At what perfusion pressure and rate? Is there advantage to using this technique in the course of an acute ischemic insult, i.e., acute coronary obstruction, e.g., failed transluminal coronary angioplasty? Can this technique be applied to all ventricles, dilated or hypertrophied? These surgical problems will be discussed subsequently.

Route of administration

In the setting of total or subtotal coronary arterial occlusion, one must be concerned with the distribution of any intracoronary perfusate administered either antegradely or retrogradely. Clinical practice using cold, antegrade cardioplegia has clearly demonstrated, by measurement of myocardial temperature, that collateral channels provide for transmural and ischemic/non-ischemic border zone perfusion (and cooling). However, it is not known what volume of cardioplegia (and therefore oxygen, substrate and buffering capacity) are delivered to jeopardized regional areas. Moreover, with cold techniques, one often depends on alternative methods to effect cardiac cooling, e.g., topical iced saline, a cooling jacket, systemic hypothermia, etc.

With warm myocardial management strategies, the distribution of cardioplegia distal to coronary arterial obstruction is also critical, but more difficult to assess, as the advantage of measuring temperature differentials is lost by maintaining normothermia. Monitoring electrical activity is regionally nonspecific and easily obviated by adjusting either the dose of cations in the cardioplegic regimen or administering a larger volume of arresting solution. To date, a clinically applicable probe to directly assess regional myocellular metabolic activity is not available.

Alternatively, one may administer warm (or cold) blood cardioplegia retrogradely via the coronary sinus. A soft cannula is introduced through the right atrial free wall and by manual palpation is advanced into the coronary sinus as far as it will go. Proper positioning may be confirmed by the return of 'black', markedly desaturated coronary sinus blood and by recording of coronary sinus pressure which approaches venous pressure and varies with the cardiac cycle. Further evidence of proper cannula position is gained inferentially when the aortic crossclamp is applied and retroperfusion started. The coronary sinus pressure should rise with the institution of perfusion. Generally, a pressure of 40 to 45 mmHg is maintained (to avoid transmyocardial edema formation) with a flow rate of 125 cc/min or greater. Abrupt changes in the coronary sinus pressure, e.g., from 40 to 0 mmHg, generally indicate catheter dislodgment into the right atrium.

Since the coronary venous anatomy is that of multiple interconnected transmural venous sinusoids, theoretically, perfusion via these vascular channels 'retrogradely' will provide adequate delivery of cardioplegia distal to total or subtotal coronary arterial obstruction [20,21]. In the case of cold methods, this may be confirmed by a falling intramyocardial temperature. With warm technique, one will observe 'black', desaturated blood emanating from the coronary arterial ostia (and out of the aortic root vent needle) or from the opened coronary artery about to be bypassed. However, laboratory investigation in pigs and dogs has questioned the regional distribution of retrogradely administered coronary sinus perfusates, particularly to the right ventricular free wall, portions of the interventricular septum and left ventricular lateral wall [22,23]. Although clinical evidence of right (or left) ventricular failure attributable to inadequate retrograde cardioplegic delivery is uncommon, the issue of regionally heterogeneous perfusion in man remains unsolved.

Metabolic demand

Optimal delivery of oxygen and substrate for aerobic metabolism is of prime importance in warm cardioplegic myocardial management methods. Maintaining mitochondrial oxidative phosphorylation to regenerate ATP from ADP and AMP theoretically limits myocardial ischemic injury evident during reperfusion and, thus, better prepares the heart for resumption of electromechanical performance to support the systemic circulation upon separation from total cardiopulmonary bypass. However, the precise flow rate and hemoglobin concentration for continuous perfusion of the arrested heart have not been thoroughly investigated.

Recently, Yau and colleagues at the University of Toronto have reported [24] a prospective randomized controlled trial to determine the optimal flow rates and hemoglobin concentrations for continuous normothermic blood cardioplegia compared with standard intermittent cold blood cardioplegia. Thirty-five patients were randomized to receive varying combinations of hemoglobin concentration (50 vs. 80 g/l) and cardioplegia flow rates (<80 vs. >80 ml/min). Standard intermittent cold blood cardioplegia resulted in a significantly greater accumulation of ADP and AMP during the ischemic interval, indicating impairment in mitochondrial function. The low hemoglobin low flow warm blood cardioplegia increased both myocardial oxygen utilization and coronary sinus blood flow after releasing the aortic cross clamp. These data are indicative of a relative ischemic insult with a reperfusion or 'payback' hyperemia. In contrast, continuous normothermic blood cardioplegia at high flow and hemoglobin concentration provided the best metabolic and functional recovery. Theoretically, a higher hemoglobin concentration would deliver a greater percentage of the myocardial oxygen demand during the arrest interval compared to a more dilute solution. This would then afford a margin of safety during periods of decreased or zero flow.

However, higher flow rates of cardioplegia generally result in a larger total volume of administration. When this exceeds 3 liters, one must be cautious of the total amount of potassium ion and glucose infused, as hyperkalemic hyperglycemia may result. Although handled well by the infusion of insulin and/or diuretic, the total duration of cardiopulmonary bypass may be prolonged. Moreover, one must be cautious not to further hemodilute the patient with the crystalloid component of the blood cardioplegia which could dictate a need for administering blood and blood components, the hazards of which are well recognized. Finally, when a higher total volume of cardioplegia is used, one must be concerned about its effects on myocardial edema formation and resultant passive compliance. Indeed, myocardial compliance was affected in both low flow, low hemoglobin and high flow, high hemoglobin groups in the Toronto series.

Unusual circumstances

Operative myocardial management using continuous warm blood cardioplegia frequently requires cessation of cardioplegic flow in order to construct complicated distal aortocoronary anastomoses or to clear the operative field to place valve sutures. However, repeated episodes of normothermic ischemia resulting from the interruption of cardioplegic flow may have detrimental effects on subsequent myocardial mechanical performance. Accordingly, we investigated [25] 24 swine randomized to receive continuous warm

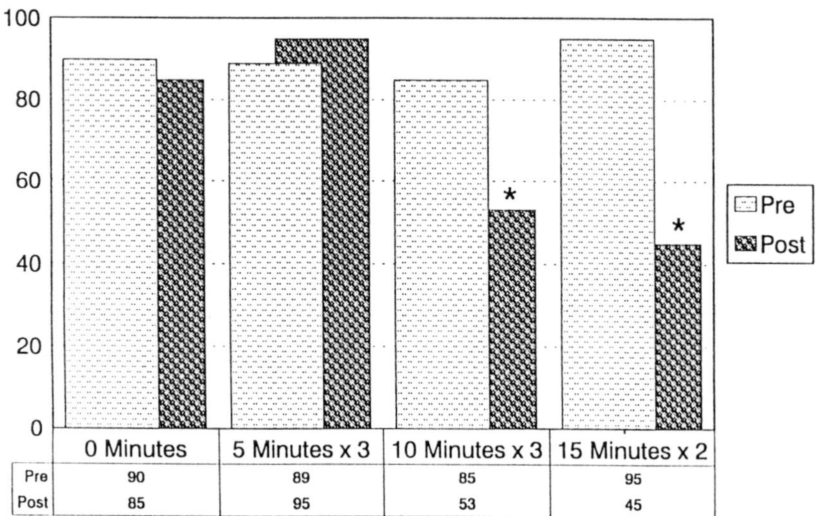

	0 Minutes	5 Minutes x 3	10 Minutes x 3	15 Minutes x 2
Pre	90	89	85	95
Post	85	95	53	45

Figure 8.1. Illustrated are the afterload independent preload recruitable stroke work contractility data for 24 swine (6 each group) undergoing warm cardioplegic arrest. Note that there was good preservation of systolic function when cardioplegia was either not interrupted or interrupted for less than 15 min. When cardioplegia was interrupted for longer than 15 min (the right two groups), functional recovery was significantly reduced (*$P < 0.01$ vs. Preischemia).

blood cardioplegia with either no interruption, three 5 min interruptions, three 10 min interruptions or two 15 min interruptions. A 5 min period of 'payback' reperfusion was allowed between interruptions of cardioplegic flow. Contractility (Figure 8.1) assessed by the slope of the linear preload recruitable stroke work relationship was not significantly changed by uninterrupted or three 5 min interruptions of warm blood cardioplegic perfusion. In contrast, the longer periods of cardioplegic flow cessation (and therefore normothermic ischemia) resulted in significant 38% and 53% depressions of systolic cardiac performance. From these data it was concluded that three successive interruptions longer than 5 min each, or a total normothermic ischemic time longer than 15 min, results in inadequate myocardial protection with depressed left ventricular contractile function.

In another series, we investigated whether continuous retrograde warm blood cardioplegia would be of benefit in the situation of acute regional ischemia where stunned, but still viable myocardium, could potentially be resuscitated during the period of cardiac arrest required for emergent surgical

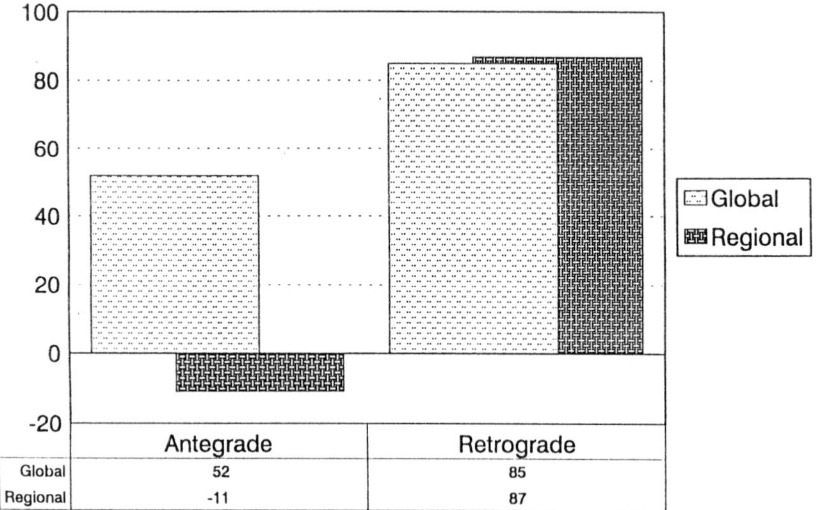

Figure 8.2. This graphic depicts the recovery of systolic function normalized as a percentage of preischemic values for 18 swine undergoing either antegrade or retrograde cardioplegic arrest in the setting of an acute (LAD) coronary arterial occlusion. Note that both regionally and globally, recovery of mechanical function was significantly impaired by the antegrade delivery route (*P < 0.01 each).

revascularization [26]. Eighteen swine were subjected to mid-LAD occlusion followed by one hour of either antegrade or retrograde warm cardioplegic arrest. LAD occlusion was released 20 min after cardiac arrest, mimicking surgical revascularization. Postischemic recovery of global contractile function was 85% following retrograde cardioplegia in contrast to the 52% recovery with antegradely administered cardioplegia (Figure 8.2). Regional stroke work was similarly preserved (87%) with the retrograde but significantly depressed (−11%) with the antegrade perfusion ($P < 0.01$). These data, in contrast to those of Lichtenstein and colleagues [27], suggest that with acute regional ischemia, both global and ischemic zone regional systolic function are depressed by antegrade continuous warm blood cardioplegia. Retrograde normothermic cardioplegia affords adequate protection of contractile performance.

Finally, one might consider the intraoperative myocardial management of critical aortic stenosis with left ventricular hypertrophy. Usually there is concomitant aortic insufficiency, rendering antegrade cardioplegic techniques complicated by left ventricular dilatation during infusion. An ideal methodology would be retrograde perfusion, as this obviates the complication of ventricular distention, as well as the necessity of direct coronary ostial cannulation during subsequent reinfusions (or continuous infusion) when the aortic root is opened. However, due to the large ventricular mass, one must also consider whether delivery of cardioplegia retrogradely adequately perfuses the myocardium transmurally. This issue is not resolved. Additionally, the optimal hematocrit and perfusion rate have *not* been determined for hypertrophied myocardium, particularly with the use of continuous warm cardioplegia. Intuitively, a higher volume (perhaps > 150 cc/min) at a higher hematocrit would supply sufficient oxygen and substrate to support the oxidative metabolism of the thickened myocardium. This, likewise, remains to be elucidated.

Summary

Through this chapter we have attempted to describe both surgical and biological rationale for the development of modern intraoperative myocardial management strategies to provide an optimal environment in which to conduct complicated cardiac and major vascular repairs. Although perfusion volume is but one of the many facets of myoprotective technique, it assumes a more central role in the new era of warm cardioplegic methodologies. We hope that the 'solved' and unresolved questions described herein will motivate further investigations.

References

1. Silverman NA, DelNido PJ, Krukenkamp IB *et al.* Biologic rationale for formulation of antegrade cardioplegic solutions. In Chitwood, WR Jr (ed): Myocardial preservation: clinical application. Cardiac Surgery: State of the Art Review, Vol. 2, No. 2. Philadelphia, 1988.
2. Silverman NA, Wright R, Levitsky S *et al.* Efficacy of crystalloid cardioplegic solutions in patients undergoing myocardial revascularization. J Thorac Cardiovasc Surg 1985; 89: 90.
3. Bretschneider HJ, Hubner G, Knoll D *et al.* Myocardial resistance and tolerance to ischemia. J Cardiovasc Surg 1975; 16: 241.
4. Lichtenstein SV, Ashe KA, Dalati HE *et al.* Warm Heart Surgery. J Thorac Cardiovasc Surg 1991; 101: 269–74.
5. Salerno TA, Houck JP, Barrozo CAM *et al.* Retrograde continuous warm blood cardioplegia: A new concept in myocardial protection. Ann Thorac Surg 1991; 51: 245–7.
6. Hicks GL Jr., Salley RK, DeWeese JA. Calcium channel blockers. An intra-operative and postoperative trial in women. Arm Thorac Surg 1984; 37: 319.
7. Flack JE, Hafer J, Engelman RM *et al.* Effect of normothermic blood cardioplegia on postoperative conduction abnormalities and supraventricular arrhytmias. Circulation (Suppl II) 84: II-687.
8. Krukenkamp IB, Silverman NA, Sorlie D *et al.* Oxygen utilization during isovolumic pres-

sure-volume loading: Effects of prolonged extracorporeal circulation and cardioplegic arrest. Ann Thorac Surg 1986; 41: 407–12.
9. Gibbs CL, Papadoyannis DE, Drake AJ *et al.* Oxygen consumption of the nonworking and potassium chloride-arrested dog heart. Circ Res 1980; 47: 408–17.
10. Chitwood WR, Sink JD, Hill RC *et al.* The effects of hypothermia on myocardial oxygen consumption and transmural coronary blood flow in the potassium-arrested heart. Ann Surg 1979; 190:106–16.
11. Krukenkamp IB, Silverman NA, Sorlie D *et al.* Myocardial energetics after thermally graded hyperkalemic crystalloid cardioplegic arrest. J Thorac Cardiovasc Surg 1986; 92: 56–62.
12. Rahn H, Reeves RB, Howell BJ *et al.* Hydrogen ion regulation, temperature and evolution. Am Rev Respir Dis 1975; 112: 165.
13. Vander Woude JC, Christlieb IY, Sicard GA *et al.* Imidazole-buffered cardioplegic solution: Improved myocardial preservation during global ischemia. J Thorac Cardiovasc Surg 1985; 90: 225.
14. McGoon DC. The ongoing quest for ideal myocardial protection. J Thorac Cardiovasc Surg 1985; 89: 639.
15. Johnson RE, Doresey LM, Moye SJ. Cardioplegic infusion: The sate limits of pressure and temperature. J Thorac Cardiovasc Surg 1982; 83: 813.
16. Menasche P, Subayi JB, Piwnica A. Retrograde coronary sinus cardioplegia tor aortic valve operations: A clinical report on 500 patients. Ann Thorac Surg 1990; 49: 556–64.
17. Salerno TA, Christakis GT, Abel J *et al.* Technique and pitfalls of retrograde continuous warm blood cardioplegia. Ann Thorac Surg 1991; 51: 1023–5.
18. Pridjian AK, Levitsky S, Krukenkamp IB *et al.* Developmental changes in reperfusion injury: Comparison of intracellular ion accumulation in ischemic and cardioplegic arrest. J Thorac Cardiovasc Surg 1988; 96(4): 577–81.
19. Misare BD, Krukenkamp IB, Levitsky S. Age-dependent sensitivity to unprotected cardiac ischemia: The senescent myocardium. J Thorac Cardiovasc Surg 1992; 103: 60–6.
20. Hammond G, Austen G. Drainage patterns of coronary arterial flow as determined from the isolated heart. Am J Physiol 1967; 212: 1435–40.
21. Hutchins G, Moore W, Hatton E. Arterial-venous relationships in the human left myocardium: anatomic basis for countercurrent regulation of blood flow. Circulation 1986; 74: 1195–202.
22. Stirling MC, McClanahan TB, Schott RJ *et al.* Distribution of cardioplegic solution infused antegradely and retrogradely in normal canine hearts. J Thorac Cardiovasc Surg 1989; 98: 1066–76.
23. Caldarone CA, Krukenkamp IB, Misare BD *et al.* Myocardial distribution of retrograde warm blood cardioplegia. Surg Forum 1992; 43: 205.
24. Yau TM, Weisel RD, Micke DAG *et al.* Optimal delivery of blood cardioplegia. Circulation 1991; 84(Supp III): 380–8.
25. Misare BD, Krukenkamp IB, Caldarone *et al.* Can continuous warm blood cardioplegia be safely interrupted? Surg Forum 1992; 43: 208.
26. Misare BD, Krukenkamp IB, Lazer ZP *et al.* Retrograde is superior to antegrade continuous warm blood cardioplegia for acute cardiac ischemia. Circulation 1992; 86 (Suppl II): II-393.
27. Lichtenstein SV, Abel JG, Salerno T. Warm heart surgery and results of operation for recent myocardial infraction. Ann Thorac Surg 1991; 52: 455–60.

9. Intermittent coronary perfusion

HAGEN D. SCHULTE

This contribution is dedicated to

Prof. Dr. Wolfgang Bircks

since 1958 involved in the development and accurate performance of cardiovascular surgery and the establishment of a sufficient and effective care of patients with heart disease of all age groups.

Summary

Intermittent coronary perfusion with the use of global hypothermia is one of the oldest techniques in cardiac surgery to allow the management of congenital defects and acquired coronary, valvular or myocardial diseases. With the introduction and further developments of quite different aspects of cardioplegic myocardial preservation – and this development is not yet finished – the technique of intermittent coronary perfusion was more or less completely replaced by cardioplegic methods.

In our unit, intermittent coronary perfusion was used in combination with total body hypothermia and hemodilution since 1959, and performed especially for coronary revascularisations from 1970 until today. During the past 10 years, more and more cardiac centers reported their results using this simple, effective and safe technique for patients with sole coronary artery disease and coronary revascularisation.

In this chapter we describe the effects of hypothermia, our procedure for hypothermic extracorporeal circulation and the use of intermittent coronary aortic cross-clamping with ischemia and reperfusion, mainly in patients with the need of coronary artery revascularisation.

Whether the newly discussed aspects of warm cardiac surgery will be effective and safe enough need further experimental and clinical investigations for a final judgement.

Introduction

Continuous coronary perfusion under normal pressure and volume conditions during systole (10–30 %) and mainly during diastole (70–90 %) of the cardiac cycle in sinus rhythm is essential for a beating and efficiently working heart. Normal cardiac function can be disturbed by a number of congenital malfor-

H.M. Piper and C.J. Preusse (eds): Ischemia-reperfusion in cardiac surgery, 243–253.

mations and acquired coronary, myocardial, and valvular diseases, each with their particular consequences for the heart and for the patient. Knowledge about these diseases and their side effects is of utmost importance, because today in many cases there is an inclination to influence, to improve or to eliminate the cause of the disease by surgical procedures.

For these types of operations, it is usually necessary that the cardiac surgeon can work on a quiet, non-beating, empty and bloodless, flaccid heart for repair, correction, reconstruction, partial or total replacements or palliative procedures on heart and vessels.

This means that the diseased, predamaged heart must be protected against additional lesions caused by the inevitable ischemic period needed to perform these cardiovascular surgical procedures safely. This protection of the myocardium is mandatory, because afterwards, and after weaning the patient off the supporting cardio-pulmonary bypass, the corrected heart must be able to work properly and maintain an adequate cardiac output for an efficient whole body perfusion.

One of various techniques of myocardial protection is *intermittent coronary perfusion* in combination with perfusion hypothermia for cooling of the whole body, in addition to the myocardium. This technique is in clinical practice since the introduction of cardio-pulmonary bypass, and allows the surgeon to perform the necessary procedure in two or more aortic cross-clamping periods, each followed by a myocardial reperfusion to finish the cardiac procedure under safe conditions.

Hypothermia

Based on the first experimental experiences with hypothermia by Grosse-Brockhoff and Schoedel [1], Bigelow *et al.* [2], Swan [3], Thauer [4], Brendel [5] and others, as well as the first successful clinical experiences, the technique for open heart surgery using surface hypothermia and circulatory arrest was introduced in our hospital in February 1955 [6–8]. Hypothermia continued to be a basic method for myocardial protection, with the introduction of cardio-pulmonary bypass in February 1959 [9,10].

A number of experimental and clinical publications gave credit to the techniques of cardiopulmonary bypass and hypothermia and demonstrated clearly and in detail the effectiveness and safety of moderate hypothermia and intermittent aortic cross-clamping and coronary reperfusion [11–22].

For maintaining myocardial aerobic metabolism and normal function the oxygen requirement is about 8–10 ml O_2 per 100 g heart weight and minute under normothermic conditions. During ischemia the O_2 reserve is small. Thus the metabolic change from aerobic to anaerobic glycolysis after about eight contractions is not sufficient to cover the energy-demand for adequate cardiac contractions and function. It results in an increase of lactate, decrease of pH and loss of phosphocreatine (CP). During the initial 'survival time' in

Table 9.1. Perfusion hypothermia.

Grade of hypothermia (rectal, °C)	O_2–consumption (% of normal)	Perfusion volume (l/min/m^2)	Myocardial ischemic tolerance (min)	Circulatory arrest tolerance (min)
Normothermia				
37–36	100	2.4	5	1–2
Mild hypothermia				
35–32	90–80	2.0–2.4	10	2–4
Moderate hypothermia				
31–25	60–40	1.8–2.0	15–20	5–15
Deep hypothermia				
24–20	35–25	1.5	20–30	20–45
Profound hypothermia				
<20	10	0.5	60	45–60

the period during which some contractile function is still present, energy is provided from the myocardial O_2-reserve, by glycolysis and use of the reserves of energy-rich phosphates. The limit of the 'survival time' is marked by a concentration of CP of about 3 μmol/g. During this time the heart should be resuscitable without longer reperfusion time [12,13].

An increase of the myocardial tolerance to ischemia can be achieved by hypothermia, which results in a considerable retardation of metabolic needs and O_2-demand. The relation between temperature and ischemic tolerance of the myocardium is described by the temperature-coefficient Q-10, i.e., the factor by which ischemic tolerance is prolonged in time when the temperature is reduced by 10°C. Under clinical conditions, taking into consideration a diseased predamaged myocardium, the Q-10 value is about 2.0, which means that the ischemic tolerance time is doubled with a temperature decline of 10°C.

For clinical use, we differentiate five temperature ranges (Table 9.1). For each range the O_2-demand in percentage of normal, the necessary perfusion volume during cardio-pulmonary bypass, the myocardial ischemic tolerance time, and the expected time of safe circulatory arrest can be specified [13,15,16,23]. External cooling of the heart to about 28°C has also been shown to be useful, resulting in a reduction of the oxygen requirement by about 59%. Perfusion cooling leading to an average body temperature of 29°C can reduce the O_2 demand to less than 25%.

In order to reduce possible intramyocardial temperature gradients during cold perfusion, additional topical cooling of the heart can be performed by irrigating the pericardial sac with 6–8°C cold Ringer's lactate or saline solution.

The earlier application of a local saline ice-slush was abandoned after the historical description of localized subepicardial muscle cell necrosis and bleedings [24–26]. However, Barner *et al.* [27] and Robicsek [28], after long-

Table 9.2. Hemodilution for priming of the extracorporeal circuit.

Hemoglobin (g/dl)	Ringer's lactate (ml/kg BW)	Additional (ml/kg BW)
<13	25	(fresh donor blood)
13–17	35	
17–20	25	10 (fresh plasma)
>20	25	20 (fresh plasma)
Neonates, small children	5–30	fresh donor blood

term use of ice-slush, could not confirm any damage of the myocardium or phrenic nerve.

The main protective effects of hypothermia are the reduction of metabolism, O_2-demand, and heart rate [12,15,17]. But there are a number of side effects also worth considering. For instance, hypothermia increases the blood viscosity which is followed by a higher perfusion pressure resulting in vascular (intimal and medial) damage and development of subendocardial edema. Therefore,an adequate blood dilution using Ringer's lactate solution is performed in close relation to the hemoglobin-value of the patient at the time of surgery (Table 9.2). This process can already be initiated by our practice of preoperative donation of own blood by the patient, and fluid compensation by partial replacement of Ringer's lactate solution, three and two days before the scheduled cardiac surgery. The collected blood will be retransfused to the patient during or at the end of surgery. For the time of cardiopulmonary bypass we aim at a reduced hematocrit level of 30–32%.

During perfusion hypothermia and blood dilution the autoregulatory mechanisms of perfusion are not able to act properly. This results usually in a critical drop of the arterial pressure and can be avoided by starting with a warm prime and slow introduction of the extracorporeal circulation until 100% of the calculated cardiac output is taken over by the external circuit. The cooling process is then started by a stepwise reduction of the blood temperature to <27°C. During the hypothermic perfusion phase an arterial pressure of 50–80 mm Hg is acceptable.

Hypothermia has – as already described – a direct negative chronotropic effect, but it may also confer an indirect positive inotropic effect as a result of an intraoperative catecholamine redistribution. The latter may also influence the effect of anesthetic drugs with a possible reduction of their effectiveness.

The influence of hypothermia on muscle and vascular tension is also noteworthy. In our clinical practice the heart usually starts fibrillating after an additional topical cooling. In the fibrillating heart the compliance of the myocardium will increase with a lowering of the temperature. In the empty beating heart the compliance may decrease, resulting in an impediment of coronary blood flow or development of myocardial edema. A reduction of coronary reserve may persist for a longer period even after completion of the surgical intervention. In total, however, hypothermia under optimal conditions and regular control of several parameters during cardio-pulmonary bypass seems to be an effective and safe method of time-limited myocardial protection.

During perfusion hypothermia the cardiac and pulmonary functions can, in general, be adequately replaced. Upcoming problems are mostly related to errors and technical failures or to changes in metabolism, tissue perfusion, and cardiovascular hemodynamics [30]. Rewarming usually causes no problems if done correctly until a rectal temperature of the patient of 34°C is reached. In this period the patient needs some respiratory, perhaps also metabolic and cardiovascular support until he is awake and reacting nearly normally.

The favourable effects of cooling on metabolism and O_2-demand enable the surgeon, anesthesiologist and pump-technician in the clinical practice of extracorporeal perfusion, under adequate control measurements, to reduce considerably the perfusion volume and blood flow (also during ischemia and considerable paracoronary blood flow). Cooling leads to an increased tolerance of the organ to ischemia, and to the possibility to safely prolong the period of circulatory arrest. The overview of important parameters given in Table 9.1 helps to avoid a critical transition of the ischemic tolerance time, which would lead to additional functional and morphological damage of the myocardium.

The recent discussion about warm conditions and ischemia with certain special cardioplegic additives and effective myocardial protection need further investigation before a final judgement can be obtained [29,22].

Clinical application of different techniques for myocardial protection

The technique of intermittent myocardial ischemia by aortic cross-clamping and coronary reperfusion in combination with hypothermia has been in clinical use since the introduction of extracorporeal circulation for cardio-pulmonary bypass including the possibility of temperature exchange. In Düsseldorf, this method has been in use since February 1959 for the surgical correction of congenital malformations, which cannot be performed within one reasonable cross-clamp time of up to 15 min.

Especially with the introduction of open mitral valve reconstruction and replacement in 1962 and myocardial revascularisation techniques by Vineberg [30] in 1970 and coronary artery bypass grafting by Favaloro [31] in 1971, in our unit the technique of intermittent cross-clamping was the method of choice and performed in far more than 10,000 patients.

For patients with aortic lesions the method of elective tube coronary perfusion with 32°C warm blood under pressure, and volume control using coronary perfusion pumps, was successfully performed with a beating heart during the operative procedure.

Since November 1978 cold crystalloid Bretschneider high volume cardioplegia [32] was performed in nearly all clinical cases, except for those who needed only coronary artery revascularisation. In these patients the successful technique of intermittent myocardial ischemia by aortic cross-clamping and coronary reperfusion was continued.

Present technique of intermittent coronary perfusion

After longitudinal midsternal incision, splitting of the sternum and pericardium, inspection of the heart and measurement of the actual LA-pressure, mostly the left internal mammary artery (LIMA), sometimes also the right sided artery (RIMA), is preserved.

Arterial (aortic) cannulation is prepared by two purse-string sutures just below the truncus arteriosus on the convex part of the ascending aorta. Following partial aortic clamping a stitch incision is made within the purse-string sutures and a metallic aortic cannula is inserted into the aorta with release of the aortic clamp.

For venous blood return to the extracorporeal circuit, using bubble or membrane-oxygenators, two separate purse-string sutures are made (around the bases of the right atrial appendage, lower part of the RA-wall) and two venous cannulas are introduced which later on will be positioned into the superior and inferior vena cava, to guarantee unprohibited venous backflow.

The prime of the extracorporeal circuit is bloodless (Ringer's lactate solution + heparine) using 25 ml/kg body weight. Cardiopulmonary bypass with low pulsatile blood flow (2.4 l/min/square under body surface) is started slowly to avoid a drop of arterial pressure under nearly normothermic conditions until the extracorporeal circuit takes over 100% of the calculated heart-time-volume. Stepwise cooling is then introduced until 5 min cold perfusion with a blood-temperature of $<27°C$ is reached. During the early cooling phase a left vent is always placed in the LV via the right upper pulmonary vein and the left atrium (LA).

During the last minute of the cooling period 8°C cold saline or Ringer's solution is poured into the pericardial sac, which usually leads to ventricular fibrillation (VF). Electrical introduction of VF is only necessary in very few patients.

The site of the peripheral first anastomosis will be cleared properly and the exposed part of the coronary artery will be incised.

Usually we start with the RCA, followed by the marginal branches, the diagonal branch and finally with the LAD. The LIMA-LAD anastomosis is the last peripheral anastomosis. In case of acutely necessary revascularisations, for instance after PTCA complication, the first anastomosis is performed to the affected coronary artery.

Before incision of the coronary artery and cross-clamping of the ascending aorta, the saphenous vein or arterial graft are prepared for anastomosis and the first stitch of 5–0 or 6–0 monofil suture material is properly placed to start continuous suturing.

After cross-clamping the ascending aorta the coronary incision is extended and the anastomosis starts and continues for 7–10 min. In more,complicated cases, including endarterectomy, a cross-clamping time of up to 20 min will be tolerated. After aortic cross-clamping the perfusate temperature is elevated to 32°C, and cooling to <27°C starts again about one minute before the expected declamping of the aorta.

The suture of the anastomosis is knotted after outflow of blood for debubbling and control of leaks. The coronary reperfusion period lasts at least 5 min after each performed anastomosis, also in case of institution of sequential anastomoses.

The proximal open end of the vein graft is then connected to the blood perfusion line with a blunt metallic head which, under use of a coronary perfusion pump with pressure and volume control, allows the coronary blood flow to be estimated through the newly constructed bypass via the distal anastomosis to the subsequent coronary artery system and myocardium. Depending on the size of the coronary artery an adequate anastomosis and the vein graft, the usually measured flow rate is between 50 and 150 ml/min. In case of good central flow before cross-clamping the proximal coronary artery should be occluded from outside. Otherwise the obtained flow-rate will not be accurate. But usually we can rely on the measurements, because the coronary flow through the anastomosis is measured at the same pressure as the indicated arterial perfusion pressure.

This easy technique, performed during late reperfusion time, gives rough information about the distal flow capacity of the affected coronary artery and a good control of the distal anastomosis concerning patency and anastomotic leaks.

The preparation of the next anastomosis then starts in an identical procedure until all scheduled peripheral anastomoses are completed.

In situations with no or poor control blood flow after incision of the affected coronary artery, the aorta will not be cross-clamped and remains open, but the perfusion blood temperature is also allowed to increase to 32°C.

The arterio-coronary anastomosis (LIMA-LAD) – as indicated before – will be performed as the last peripheral one. Then the proximal aorto-venous anastomoses are constructed after oblique partial clamping of the anterior part of the ascending aorta, adequate aortic incision and using a 4.0 mm punch. Rewarming of the patient starts after the cross-clamping of the aorta for the last peripheral anastomosis. Electrical defibrillation of the heart is usually possible after finishing the first proximal anastomosis. The total reperfusion time takes at least 20 min until a rectal temperature of the patient of 34°C is reached.

After reducing the left vent and after application of bipolar retractable ventricular and atrial pacemaker leads, and introduction of a pressure line

Table 9.3. Coronary artery revascularisation using intermittent coronary perfusion and hypothermia.

Author	Year	No of patients	✝	%
Reul	1975	200	3	1.5
Akins	1984	500	2	0.4
Bonchek	1992	3000	44	1.5
Antunes	1992	229	2	0.9
Kalmar*	1992	25680	682	2.6
Duesseldorf	1986–1991	3244	78	2.4

* Annual German Cardiac Surgery Registry 1991 (unselected, including CPL).

into the LA, the patient is slowly weaned off cardio-pulmonary bypass under simultaneous arterial and LA-pressure controls.

All blood from the extracorporeal circuit (tubing, oxygenator, venous reservoir) will be retransfused to the patient. He also will get back his own preoperative donated blood. By using this technique coronary revascularisations can be performed in about 68% of our patients without the transfusion of foreign blood or its components.

Discussion

Since the introduction of various cardioplegic methods and techniques, most surgeons completely changed their intraoperative management concerning myocardial protection for all operative procedures. During recent years, publications are increasing in which the authors support, more and more, the technique of intermittent coronary perfusion because of its simple application and its demonstrated effectiveness and safety, also in older and higher risk patients [19–22].

We can also support the favourable reports. We have not yet performed a prospective comparing study between patients operated by intermittent coronary perfusion and those under cardioplegia. But by comparing our results on a yearly basis with the mean results of all German Centers there was, up to now, no reason for changing our technique for coronary revascularisation (Table 9.3). The surgical results seem acceptable even though a very high rate of performed PTCA-procedures results in a surgical patient collective which shows more severe alterations of the coronary artery system, more reduced myocardial function, and contains more older and multimorbid patients than in earlier years. The latter group of patients nowadays are certainly referred to surgery, but were refused several years ago. The surgical results seem acceptable (Table 9.3).

In a multivariate analysis of 3,000 operated patients Bonchek *et al.* [21] found the risk factors which were independent predictors of operative death:

Patients older than 70 years had a higher risk than younger patients as well for elective (1.6%: 0.17%) as for emergency operations (5.8%: 0.82 %). The early mortality rate of women was significantly higher (20/795: 2.5%) than of men (24/2205: 1.1%). Also impaired LV-function is a high risk factor, especially in patients with severe LV-dysfunction (EF $<$ 30%). Other risk factors were the preoperative need of IABP, and the urgency of operation. This group, with a large experience of operated patients using intermittent coronary perfusion mentioned several reasons of preference of intermittent cross-clamping, which we can support in most parts based on our own experiences.

1. Routine coronary artery bypass grafting requires only brief myocardial ischemia times for constructions of the distal anastomosis.The residual time between two ischemic periods can be used for flow measurement, exposure of other effected coronary arteries, preparation of the graft and performance of the proximal anastomosis.
2. The brief ischemic intervals at mild or moderate hypothermia are rapidly reversible using adequate reperfusion in a vented heart and during ventricular fibrillation.
3. The effectiveness of antegrade cardioplegic perfusion is compromised by occluded or stenosed coronary arteries, which makes it mandatory to perfuse the heart also via the coronary venous sinus.

These techniques do not exclude the wash-out effect of the noncoronary collateral blood flow, which in contrary is beneficial during intermittent coronary perfusion, except it may disturb the performance of a distal anastomosis.

4. Continuous warm retrograde cardioplegic perfusion must also be interrupted for performing the distal anastomoses.
5. The avoidance of cardioplegic solutions eliminates the described possibility of injuring the graft endothelium by hyperkalemic solutions.
6. For coronary reoperations cardioplegia is preferred despite the above described advantages.

Antunes *et al.* [22] stress some points which demonstrate the advantage of this type of myocardial protection:

1. Efficient decompression of the heart is necessary.
2. Limitation of the cross-clamp time to 10 min, which is acceptable for an experienced surgeon and under the precondition of only mild general hypothermia.

As our patients are much colder (27°C), they will tolerate clamping times up to 20 min quite safely. And a younger, less experienced cardiac surgeon usually needs more time for completion of a distal anastomosis!

3. During this limited ischemic time of 10 min other procedures, such as

endarterectomies, can be performed including repair of left ventricular aneurysms, which can also be done in our experience without myocardial ischemia. Because of the light rate of intraventricular thrombotic formations we prefer an initial clamping of the aorta until the aneurysm is opened and thrombotic material is identified and removed.
4. The use of only mild hypothermia lower the side effects considerably, especially concerning its influence on the peripheral vascular resistance.

As mentioned before hypothermia was always considered as an important base of myocardial protection, however, the recently introduced techniques of warm or normothermic cardioplegia have to be followed very careful.

5. Another mentioned technical aspect is the secondary hemodiluton by the cardioplegic solution. We always discard the cardioplegic solution, which, however, makes it necessary to close the SVC and IVC around the venous cannulas.

Conclusions

Intermittent coronary perfusion using cross-clamping and mild or moderate hypothermia represents an effective and easy-to-perform technique for myocardial protection, with low costs especially suitable for patients who need primary elective coronary revascularisation. Possible rates of mortality and morbidity of operated patients are mostly dependent on a number of risk factors (age, sex, LV dysfunction, preoperative myocardial insufficiency, urgency of surgical treatment) and not on the technique of myocardial protection (intermittent coronary perfusion, different types of cardioplegia).

Good results for primary, isolated coronary revascularisations are nowadays also highly dependent on the recent medical and technical advances concerning preoperative management, anesthesiology, cardio-pulmonary bypass, surgical skill and experience, avoidance of foreign blood, postoperative monitoring, intensive therapy, and rehabilitation.

References

1. Grosse-Brockhoff F, Schoedel W. Das Bild der akuten Unterkühlung im Tierexperiment. Arch Experim Path und Pharmakol 1943; 241: 417.
2. Bigelow WG, Lindsay WK, Greenwood WF. Hypothermia. Its possible role in cardiac surgery. Ann Surgery 1950; 132: 849.
3. Swan H. The current status of hypothermia. Arch Surg 1954; 69: 597.
4. Thauer R. Ergebnisse experimenteller Kreislaufuntersuchungen bei Hypothermie. Thoraxchir 1956; 4: 522.
5. Brendel W. Kreislauf in Hypothermie. Verh Dtsch Ges Kreislaufforschung 1957: 33
6. Zindler M. Künstliche Hypothermie für Herzoperationen mit Kreislaufunterbrechung. Forschungsbericht des Landes Nordrhein-Westfalen. Westdeutscher Verlag: Köln 1961; 996.
7. Zindler M, Dudziak R, Eunike S *et al.* Surface hypothermia for heart operations with circulatory arrest. Intern Anesthes Clinics 1965; 3: 733–55.

8. Zindler M, Dudziak R, Eunike S *et al.* Erfahrungen bei 1290 künstlichen Hypothermien für Herz- und Gefäßoperationen. Anaesthesist 1966; 15: 69–75.
9. Derra E. Der Vorhofseptumdefekt und sein operativer Verschluß unter Sicht des Auges in Unterkühlungsanästhesie. Dtsch Med Wschr 1955; 80: 1277–80.
10. Derra E. The surgical treatment of congenital valvular pulmonary stenosis under direct vision during hypothermia. German Med Monthly 1957; 2: 129–32.
11. Borst HG. Experimentelle Untersuchungen über die kombinierte Anwendung von extrakorporalem Kreislauf und Hypothermie. II. Zur Frage der adäquaten Perfusion in Hypothermie. Langenbecks Arch Klin Chir 1963; 303: 380–403.
12. Bretschneider HJ. Überlebenszeit und Wiederbelebungszeit des Herzens bei Normo- und Hypothermie. Verh Dtsch Ges Kreislaufforschung 1964; 30: 11–34.
13. Arnold G, Lochner W. Die Temperaturabhängigkeit des Sauerstoffverbrauchs stillgelegter künstlich perfundierter Warmblüterherzen zwischen 34° und 4°C Pflügers Arch Ges Physiol 1965; 284: 169–75.
14. Hoffmeister HE. Stoffwechseluntersuchungen am menschlichen Herzen bei intermittierender Koronarperfusion. Langenbecks Arch Klin Chir 1967; 319: 336–41.
15. Bircks W, Pulver, KG. Erfahrungswerte der Tolerabilität und notwendigen Dauer der Koronarischämie in der Kardiochirurgie. Langenbecks Arch Klin Chir 1967; 319: 697.
16. Schulte HD, Derra E Jr., Herzer JA *et al.* Ischemic tolerance of the human heart during extracorporeal circulation; Clinical experience. J Cardiovasc Surg 1975; 16: 283–7.
17. Buckberg GD, Brazier JR, Nelson RL *et al.* Studies of the effects of hypothermia on regional myocardial blood flow and metabolism during cardio-pulmonary bypass. I. The adequately perfused beating, fibrillation and arrested heart. J Thorac Cardiovasc Surg 1977; 73: 84–7.
18. Laks H, Barner HB, Strandeven JW *et al.* Myocardial protection by intermittent perfusion with cardioplegic solution vs. intermittent coronary perfusion with cold blood. J Thorac Cardiovasc Surg 1978; 78: 158–72.
19. Akins CW. Noncardioplegic myocardial preservation for coronary revascularisation. J Thorac Cardiovasc Surg 1984; 88: 174–81.
20. Bonchek LI, Burlingame MW. Coronary artery bypass surgery. J Thorac Cardiovasc Surgery 1987; 93: 261–7.
21. Bonchek LI, Burlingame MW, Vazales BE *et al.* Applicability of noncardioplegie coronary bypass to high-risk patients. Selection of patients, technique, and clinical experience. J Thorac Cardiovasc Surg 1992; 103: 230–6.
22. Antunes MJ, Bernardo JE, Oliveira JM *et al.* Coronary artery bypass surgery with intermittent aortic cross-clamping. Europ J Cardiothorac Surg 1992; 6: 189–94.
23. Schulte HD, Güttler J. Grundlagen und Durchführung der extrakorporalen Zirkulation beim Erwachsenen – Das Düsseldorfer Verfahren. In Preusse CJ, Schulte HD (eds): Extrakorporale Zirkulation – Heute –. Darmstadt: Steinkopff-Verlag 1991; 37–54.
24. Poche R, Ohm HG. Lichtmikroskopische, histochemische und elektronenmikroskopische Untersuchungen des Herzmuskels vom Menschen nach reduziertem Herzstillstand. Arch Kreislauff 1963; 41: 86.
25. Speicher CE, Ferrigan, Wolfson SK *et al.* Cold injury of the myocardium and pericardium in cardiac hypothermia. Surg Gyn Obst 1962; 114: 659–65.
26. Lynen F. Herzstillstand durch isolierte Organunterkühlung mit Kochsalz-Eisschnee. Med Diss Düsseldorf 1963.
27. Barner HB, Standeven JW Jellinek M *et al.* Topical cardiac hypothermia for myocardial preservation. J Thorac Cardiovasc Surg 1977; 73: 856–67.
28. Robicsek F. Discussions of Griepp RB. J Thorac Cardiovasc Surg 1973; 66: 731–41.
29. Lichtenstein SK, Fremes SE, Abel JG *et al.* Technical aspects of warm heart surgery. J Card Surg 1991; 6: 278–85.
30. Vineberg AN. Development of an anastomosis between the coronary vessels and a transplanted internal mammary artery Canad med Ass J 1946; 55: 117–21.
31. Favaloro RG. Saphenous vein graft in the surgical treatment of coronary artery disease. Operative technique. J Thorac Cardiovasc Surg 1968; 58: 178–82.
32. Bretschneider HJ. Myocardial Protection. Thorac Cardiovasc Surg 1980; 28: 295–302.

10. Retrograde perfusion

PHILIPPE MENASCHE

Over the past years, retrograde coronary sinus perfusion (RCSP) has been increasingly used as a means of delivering cardioplegic solutions during surgically-induced ischemic arrest. More recently, the introduction of normothermic continuous blood cardioplegia has further contributed to expand the indications of the retrograde approach. The purpose of the present review is therefore to provide an update of the indications, techniques and pitfalls of coronary sinus cardioplegia.

1. Anatomical background

The anatomy of the coronary venous system has been the subject of extensive reports [1]. Consequently, only the features that are most relevant to RCSP of cardioplegic solutions will be outlined in this section.

1.1. A solution which is infused into the coronary sinus splits into two fractions. The largest fraction (which accounts for approximately 70% of the retroperfusate) shunts directly into the cardiac cavities, primarily those of the right side, through the thebesian system. This extensive network appears therefore well suited for delivering core cooling and cardioplegic additives throughout the thickness of the myocardium. In addition, this non-nutritive fraction of the retrograde flow is likely to exert topical cooling effects on the endocardium as it egresses into the heart chambers. This can be relevant to protection of the conduction system from ischemic damage and the related occurrence of postoperative rhythm and conduction abnormalities. The remaining fraction of retroperfused solutions (which therefore represents approximately 30% of the coronary sinus infusate) takes the capillary-to-arteriole route and drains into the aortic root through the coronary ostia, predominantly the left one. Although of limited magnitude, this retrograde nutritive flow seems to be still sufficient for matching the reduced energy demands of the arrested, vented heart, whether cold or normothermic, thereby providing a rationale for the delivery of blood cardioplegia in a retrograde fashion.

1.2. Dog studies have consistently demonstrated an extensive permeation

H.M. Piper and C.J. Preusse (eds): Ischemia-reperfusion in cardiac surgery, 255–266.

of the left ventricle by solutions infused into the coronary sinus whereas retroperfusates poorly distribute to the right ventricle, the atria and the basal portion of the interventricular septum. However, for anatomic and pathologic reasons that will be discussed further herein, maldistribution of coronary sinus infusates within the human heart does not seem to be a real issue in clinical practice.

1.3. The coronary venous system is never affected by atherosclerosis. In fact, coronary artery disease stimulates the development of venous channels [2], which should further enhance the efficacy of RCSP in delivering cardioplegia in inflow-restricted myocardial areas.

2. Indications

2.1. *Valve operations*

Procedures on the *aortic valve* probably represent the ideal indication for the implementation of retrograde coronary sinus cardioplegia. This is particularly true if the primary disease is aortic valve regurgitation because of the serious drawbacks inherent to anterograde techniques of cardioplegia delivery both for inducing and for maintaining arrest in this particular condition. Namely, induction of arrest can be achieved either by (1) aortic root infusion with simultaneous manual compression of the left ventricle, but this maneuver can be traumatic and is not consistently successful in forcing cardioplegic solution to flow into the coronary ostia instead of leaking through the incompetent valve, or by (2) selective coronary artery perfusion, but in spite of the recent improvements in catheter design, this technique is not devoid of the risk of traumatic injury that can lead to acute dissection or late stenosis [3]. Obviously, as soon as the aorta has been opened, maintenance of arrest by multidose cardioplegia can only be achieved through selective ostial cannulation which in addition to the previously mentioned risk of intimal injury, has the disadvantage of obscuring the operative field at the time of catheter positioning and perfusion. In the case of pure aortic stenosis, initial asystole can be expeditiously achieved by an aortic root infusion but the administration of supplemental doses of cardioplegia similarly requires direct coronary artery perfusion which can be particularly hazardous when calcified plaques surround the coronary ostia, as commonly occurs in this subset of patients.

All of these shortcomings are eliminated by the use of coronary sinus cardioplegia. This approach has two unquestionable advantages: (1) it avoids the risk of cannulation- and perfusion-related coronary arterial damage, and (2) it allows cardioplegia delivery not to interfere with the surgical procedure because the retroperfusion catheter remains secured within the coronary sinus during the whole period of aortic occlusion, thereby allowing cardioplegic infusions to be repeated whenever necessary without interrupting the operation. At most, cardioplegia can be delivered in a continuous fashion. Even in this case, we have never found the backflow of solution that egresses through the coronary ostia to be a real surgical nuisance. Further, the fact that the coronary sinus catheter is away from the operative field which remains therefore consistently clear from perfusion cannulae is a real advantage, in particular when the aortic root is of small size or, alternatively, when a complex and lengthy procedure has to be performed on the ascending aorta such as repair of aneurysm, dissection or periannular abscesses. It should be stressed that our extensive experience with coronary sinus cardioplegia in aortic valve surgery [3] has clearly demonstrated that these well-documented technical advantages of the retrograde approach were obtained without compromising the quality of intraoperative myocardial protection which is strictly comparable to that achieved with the use of conventional anterograde techniques of cardioplegia delivery. Additional likely advantages of coronary sinus cardioplegia in the setting of aortic valve surgery include (1) a reduced incidence of postoperative supraventricular arrhythmias and conduction defects, presumably because of an improved cooling of the interatrial septum by that large fraction of the retroperfusate which shunts directly into the heart chambers [4], and (2) an effective distribution of cardioplegia beyond coronary artery occlusions (see further), a pattern of atherosclerotic disease which is not uncommon in patients with aortic valve lesions. Finally, some experimental studies [6] have suggested that retrograde cardioplegia would better protect hypertrophied myocardium than anterograde techniques do (probably because of the capacity of the thebesian system to behave as an effective vehicle for delivering core cooling throughout all layers of the heart), and this could be particularly relevant to patients with long-standing aortic valve stenosis.

The indications of retrograde coronary sinus cardioplegia are more limited in *mitral valve* surgery because both initial and subsequent cardioplegia deliveries can be accomplished simply and effectively through the aortic root. It is our opinion that only the following circumstances provide a rationale for the use of RCSP in this subset of patients: (1) the performance of a double valve procedure, because the coronary sinus approach avoids to loose the time required for reestablishing exposure of the coronary ostia if cardioplegic reinfusion has to be given during the mitral valve operation, (2) the performance of a redo valve procedure, because continuously delivered retrograde cold cardioplegia may avoid an extensive dissection of the heart for the sole purpose of implementing topical cooling, and (3) the use of normothermic blood cardioplegia, because distortion of the aortic valve by the left atrial retractor is unlikely to allow for an effective coronary artery perfusion if cardioplegia is given through the aortic root.

2.2. *Coronary bypass operations*

Coronary sinus cardioplegia can also be beneficial to patients that undergo *coronary artery bypass grafting* procedures. The idea of using the retrograde approach in this type of surgery has stemmed from the awareness that anterograde methods of cardioplegia delivery fail to provide homogeneous distribution of cooling and cardioplegic ingredients to inflow-restricted myocardial areas planned for being revascularized by saphenous grafts until distal anastomoses have been constructed (direct graft perfusion then becomes effective), and are still unable to offer adequate protection to inflow-restricted areas than cannot be bypassed or are planned for revascularization by a pedicted arterial conduit (in general, the internal thoracic artery). The recognition that inhomogeneous distribution of cardioplegic solutions correlated with an impaired functional recovery of the most poorly protected regions [7] that could eventually compromise the result of an otherwise technically successful operation, has therefore stimulated the development of alternative strategies of cardioplegia administration. This issue of cardioplegic maldistribution has thus been thought to be most appropriately addressed by RCSP because of both the extensive development of the venous network across the myocardium and its consistent freedom from obstructive lesions, regardless of the extent of disease in the corresponding arterial system. These expectations have actually been met by the results of numerous experimental studies [for a review, see ref. 8]. In brief, these studies have consistently demonstrated that in the presence of a left coronary artery obstruction, RCSP was more effective than anterograde techniques for ensuring adequate distribution of cooling and cardioplegia distal to that obstruction, and that these patterns of improved distribution correlated with a better recovery of function following cross-clamp removal. Recently, contrast echocardiography has provided direct visual evidence that whereas acute simultaneous occlusion of the left anterior descending and left circumflex coronary arteries resulted in 65% reduction in perfusion by aortic root cardioplegia, it had no effects on retrograde cardioplegia distribution [9], thereby supporting the concept that the coronary sinus technique would provide superior protection to left ventricular areas subserved by occluded arteries.

Unfortunately, these experimental findings have not been corroborated by clinical results as all human trials [for a review, see ref. 8] that have compared the two routes for cardioplegia delivery have failed to document any real benefit of RCSP over aortic root perfusion. A likely reason for this discrepancy is that the coronary artery lesions of the patients included in these trials were not the most suitable for the expected benefits of retrograde cardioplegia to be readily apparent. Namely, these patients seem to have been at rather low risk as far as the anatomic patterns of their coronary artery disease are concerned. Given the fact that coronary artery stenoses up to 90% do not necessarily preclude adequate cooling of the corresponding myocardial area by anterogradely delivered cardioplegic solutions [10], in particular if this area is abundantly collateralized, it is not unexpected that the route of cardioplegia infusion has not been a critical determinant of postoperative outcome in these low-risk patient groups. In contrast, our experience suggests that it is only in the presence of *total* (or subtotal) coronary artery occlusion (as opposed to stenosis) that retrograde cardioplegia is likely to offer significantly improved protection [11], not only because this anatomic pattern of coronary artery disease most closely mimicks the type of experimental preparation used for demonstrating the superiority of RCSP, but also because it is only when supplying arteries were *totally* (or subtotally) occluded that RCSP has been thermographically shown to ensure more effective cooling of the ischemic segment than aortic root perfusion did during bypass surgery in man [10].

This has led us to consider that patients with at least complete occlusion of a major coronary vessel, whether chronic or acute (as may occur after a failed angioplasty) were probably the elective candidates for retrograde delivery of cardioplegia, especially if the occlusion is part of a multivessel disease and/or involves an artery that subserves a poorly collateralized area. This line of reasoning leads to extend the indications of RCSP to patients undergoing redo coronary procedures as in this group the risk of inefficacy of anterograde methods due to the usual occlusion of native coronary arteries cumulates with that of distal emboli of atheromatous debris down patent saphenous vein grafts [12]. Patients that require combined procedures on the coronary arteries and the aortic root represent a third subset in which there is a sound justification for using RCSP as the previously mentioned technical advantages of the retrograde approach combine with the potential for an improved myocardial protection.

2.3. *Other indications*

Coronary sinus cardioplegia can also be helpful during repair of *complex congenital heart lesions*, such as transposition of the great arteries [13].

The right atriotomy, which is frequently inherent to these repair procedures, makes coronary sinus cannulation particularly easy whereas avoidance of selective ostial perfusion required for reinfusing cardioplegia if an aortotomy has been performed, appears especially appealing in this pediatric age group.

Finally, RCSP has emerged as an attractive means of delivering cardioplegic solutions during the implantation phase of *heart transplantation*. It is now well admitted that graft preservation must not be limited to the static storage period but has to be pursued until ultimate blood reperfusion. In this setting, additional doses of cardioplegia are increasingly given during donor heart implantation and it is less cumbersome to do so through the coronary sinus than by any of the anterograde methods (selective coronary artery cannulation or direct aortic root perfusion after cross-clamping of the distal aortic stump). In our practice, RCSP of cardioplegic blood (the temperature of which is progressively rewarmed from 30°C to 37°C) is started after completion of the left atrial anastomosis and then proceeds uninterrupted during construction of the three remaining anastomoses until aortic unclamping, which allows a significant shortening of the ischemic interval between the end of cold storage and the onset of reperfusion (in fact, this interval becomes limited to the time required for suturing the donor heart's left atrium to that of the recipient).

3. Techniques of coronary sinus cardioplegia

3.1. *Cannulation*

The coronary sinus can be cannulated under direct vision or blindly, through the right atrial wall. Cannulation of the sinus under direct vision has been our technique of choice since the beginning of our experience with retrograde cardioplegia in the early eighties. It allows to control accurately the location of the catheter, an advantage which is counterbalanced by the need for bicaval cannulation and snares. Details of the 'open' technique have been previously described [4] and only the key procedural steps will be outlined. They include (1) an anteriorly located right atriotomy, parallel to the atrioventricular sulcus, to gain direct access to the coronary sinus ostium, (2) a gentle inflation of the balloon with saline solution until it occludes the lumen of the sinus, (3) maintenance of the inflated balloon at the ostium of the sinus to prevent blockade of proximally draining venous tributaries, and (4) gentle traction of the catheter back toward the right cavity to ensure that it is properly wedged and will therefore remain self-secured into the lumen of the sinus during the ensuing period of aortic cross-clamping. Alternatively, one can place a purse-string suture around the intraatrial rim of the coronary sinus orifice and prevent backflow of cardioplegic solution by tightening it around the catheter, the balloon of which is then only minimally inflated.

Blind cannulation of the coronary sinus by means of a stylet-guided catheter which is introduced through a right atrial stab wound is the second technical option. Its major advantage is to allow concomitant venous return through a single cannula, which has accounted for its rapid gain in popularity. The technical modalities of this blind approach have already been extensively described [14,15] and we shall only comment on some maneuvers that we have found helpful for achieving successful blind coronary sinus catheterization. They include (1) introduction of the catheter through the *lower* part of the right atrium, (2) placement of the catheter *after* that of the venous cannula in order to avoid the former to be dislodged by the latter, (3) placement of the catheter with the patient on *partial* bypass to avoid any hemodynamic compromise during attempts at coronary sinus catheterization, and (4) if necessary, gentle upward retraction of the diaphragmatic aspect of the right ventricle to give a straightforward direction to the coronary sinus and therefore facilitate its intubation.

3.2. *Perfusion*

Coronary sinus cardioplegia should be delivered under pressures in the range of 30–40 mmHg as it is known since a long time that higher perfusion pressures are injurious to the sinus and to the myocardium [8]. In practice, pressure can now be easily monitored owing to the pressure line which is featured by commercially available retroperfusion catheters. Alternatively, one can rely upon flow rate to ensure that retrograde cardioplegia is appropriately delivered. At the time we were using cold crystalloid cardioplegia, we had found flow rates in the range of 100 ml/min to correlate with perfusion pressures that were kept below the safety threshold of 40 mmHg and, in our practice, had discontinued routine pressure monitoring for looking at flow exclusively. Interestingly, higher retrograde flow rates (200 ml/min) have been reported to be safe with the use of *cold* blood cardioplegia [14]. The more recent practice of *warm* blood cardioplegia [16] has led to the recognition that this technique results in a fairly specific pattern of pressure/flow relationship in that its markedly vasodilating effects allow to achieve high retrograde flows (routinely in the range of 150 to 200 ml/min) while maintaining much lower perfusion pressures than would have been expected from the observations made in the ‘cold era’ (these pressures are frequently in the range of 20–30 mmHg in spite of flow rates as high as those mentioned above). Because the rate of cardioplegia delivery is a critical determinant of oxygen delivery under normothermic conditions, one should take advantage of these coronary vasodilating effects and not allow the flow rate to fall below 150 ml/min. This is specially important when a self-inflatable balloon is used for retroperfusion because these balloons do not consistently occlude the lumen of the coronary sinus completely. The subsequent backflow of cardioplegia into the right atrium results in that the amount of nutritive flow which is effectively delivered is lower than that predicted from the preset value, thereby eventually leading to myocardial underperfusion and ischemia.

Further, normothermic blood cardioplegia is a technique which, in our experience, makes pressure monitoring absolutely mandatory, not so much for preventing overpressurization-induced coronary sinus injury than for checking that the catheter has not been inadvertently dislodged. It is clear that any undetected recoil of the catheter into the right atrium is likely to have catastrophic consequences since it would induce a state or normothermic ischemia. The observation that dark blood is coming out of the coronary ostia or the distal coronary arteriotomies provides a fairly reliable indicator that retrograde delivery of blood cardioplegia is effective but this type of information is not available during mitral valve procedures. The continuous recording of a typical coronary sinus pressure tracing is thus probably the safest means of ensuring that the catheter is properly located. Should a pressure drop suddenly occur, the positioning of the retroperfusion cannula should be carefully inspected, which is not always easy, in particular in redo procedures where the undersurface of the heart may have not been freed from pericardial adhesions. It can then be helpful to vary the flow rate of the cardioplegia delivery pump and to assess whether the pressure changes accordingly. If a doubt persists, we would not hesitate to adopt an alternative strategy such as opening of the right atrium for placing the catheter under direct vision (this can be done after temporary cross-clamping of the superior vena cava and snaring of the inferior vena cava around the one-stage venous cannula which, after closure of the atriotomy, is then pulled back into the atrium). Another option is to switch to anterograde cardioplegia delivery.

It should finally be stated that within the aforementioned range of pressures and flows, myocardial edema is not a real concern due to the large runoff of retroperfusates and the additional use of an aortic root sucking vent (except for aortic valve cases where the aortotomy provides a natural drainage pathway).

4. Pitfalls of coronary sinus cardioplegia

4.1. *Delay in cardiac arrest*

It is a fact that retrograde cardioplegia does not arrest the heart as quickly as anterograde methods do. Fortunately, neither our experience [4] nor that of others [17] suggest that this negative feature of the coronary sinus route has detrimental effects upon the postoperative outcome, most likely because the ischemic damage inherent to the brief prearrest period of persisting electromechanical activity is minimized by the protection yet exerted at that stage by hypothermia (topical and systemic) and/or oxygen when blood cardioplegia is used.

Whatsoever, this shortcoming of RCSP can be easily overcome by inducing initial arrest through the aortic root [18], except in patients with significant aortic valve regurgitation. In these patients, it is not necessarily much longer to achieve asystole by cannulating the coronary sinus as soon as the aorta has been cross- clamped (in case of cannulation under direct vision, the right atriotomy can have been done previously to permit immediate catheterization) than by opening the aorta, looking for the coronary ostia and cannulating them prior to the onset of cardioplegic perfusion. Incidentally, since we use normothermic blood cardioplegia, we have found, in a few coronary artery bypass patients, that some degree of electromechanical activity persisted at the completion of the initial aortic root infusion of cardioplegia and only ceased completely when the cardioplegia line was switched to the retrograde coronary sinus catheter.

4.2. *Coronary sinus injury*

Like any invasive procedure, RCSP can create iatrogenic injuries. However, our rate of traumatic complications (0.6%) in aortic valve patients [4] competes well with that of coronary arterial lesions following direct ostial cannulation [6]. Overall, all the clinical studies of retrograde coronary sinus cardioplegia have established that, when properly handled, this technique yields a high safety record.

Coronary sinus injuries occurring during cardioplegia delivery can be due to balloon overinflation or excessively high perfusion pressures ('jet lesions'). The availability of transatrial cannulation techniques has virtually eliminated the risk of balloon-related injury when the balloon is of the auto-inflatable type, but still carries the potential for venous perforation by the stylet. For this reason, inadvertent dislodgement of the catheter during the procedure should *always* be managed by withdrawal of the catheter followed by its repositioning with the help of the stylet and *never* by introduction of the stylet within the catheter while the latter is still inside the heart. On the other hand, safety devices have been incorporated in some retrograde delivery systems [19] that allow to shut off the flow should the pressure exceeds a preset upper limit. However, a sudden increase in recorded pressure can be due only to wedging of the catheter in a branch of the sinus or to its kinking during cardiac manipulations, in particular when the heart is lifted to expose the left obtuse marginal system. This should be promptly recognized and dealt with by withdrawing the catheter 1 or 2 cm until restoration of normal infusion pressures, not by discontinuing perfusion, which could have detrimental effects under normothermic conditions.

Punctual perforations of the coronary sinus or of one its large tributaries are usually easy to repair by fine polypropylene sutures. Conversely, a laceration of the sinus causing an extensive hematoma along the atrioventricular groove can be best treated by a large pericardial patch overlaying the injured area and sutured, far away, to the epicardium. Occasionally, a small hematoma without overt evidence of bleeding can (and probably should) be left untouched. Whenever a venous injury, irrespective of its type, is recognized during the cross-clamping period, it is obviously mandatory to discontinue retrograde perfusion immediately and to switch to an anterograde method of cardioplegia delivery for ensuring uninterrupted myocardial protection during repair (if any) of the injury and completion of the remainder of the cardiac procedure.

The potential severity of coronary sinus lesions leads to emphasize the main safety guidelines that should permit to prevent them. These guidelines include (1) atraumatic manipulations of the catheter, (2) gentle balloon inflation if manually controlled (a small degree of leak around the balloon, which may occur when the diameter of the juxtaatrial portion of the sinus is unusually large, is by far preferable to attempts at obtaining an excessively tight fit between the inflated balloon and the venous wall), (3) positioning of the inflated balloon at the ostium of the sinus to reduce mechanical stress on the underlying wall of the venous conduit (in practice, this can only be achieved with the use of the 'open' technique) and (4) careful monitoring of the parameters of perfusion, whatever pressure or flow.

4.3. *Inadequate preservation of the right ventricle*

Animal studies, whether using dyes, resins or radiolabeled microspheres, have consistently shown that solutions injected into the coronary sinus poorly permeated the right ventricle and the basal portion of the interventricular septum [8,20]. Conversely, right ventricular failure has not been reported to be a *clinically* significant complication following the use of coronary sinus cardioplegia in humans [21]. Whereas this discrepancy can be accounted for by the protective effects of *hypothermia* when topical cooling of the right ventricle is used (which has been the case in all of the clinical studies of retrograde cardioplegia), this explanation is no longer tenable when blood cardioplegia is *normothermically* delivered through the coronary sinus, an approach which, until now, has not been reported to cause clinically detectable right ventricular dysfunction [22].

Given the fact that the backflow of cardioplegic solution through the right coronary ostium is consistently lower than that coming out of the left one, it is assumed that although of small magnitude, the retrograde nutritional pathway of the right ventricle is still sufficient to meet its low residual oxygen requirements when it is arrested. In addition, a potential contribution of the noncapillary retrograde flow to right ventricular preservation cannot be excluded. It is noteworthy that in the human heart, some of the veins that drain the right ventricular blood flow directly into the cardiac cavities are connected with tributaries of the coronary sinus [1]. Owing to these anastomoses, the noncapillary retrograde pathways can vehicle cardioplegic blood infused through the coronary sinus and might therefore provide some degree of oxygenation to the thin-walled right ventricle by a simple diffusion mechanism. Hence, our commitment to keep the balloon catheter seated around the intraatrial rim of the coronary sinus orifice to avoid balloon-related blockade of the ostia of the terminal branches of the sinus that drain right ventricular and septal areas and, more specifically, of the posterior interventricular vein as this branch is a major constituent of the anastomotic network between the coronary sinus system and the venous drainage pathways of the right ventricle. Whatsoever, irrespective of the mechanism of protection, retrograde coronary sinus cardioplegia is likely to be more effective for preserving right ventricular function than anterograde cardioplegia is when a complete occlusion of the right coronary artery is superimposed upon global ischemic arrest [23].

It should be clearly stated that the preceding comments pertain to RCSP – not to the alternative route for cardioplegia delivery, that is, right atrial cardioplegia. Although this technique has been reported to yield satisfactory clinical results [24,25], it has gained only little popularity, most likely because of the repeatedly expressed concerns about right ventricular distension inherent to intraatrial infusion of cardioplegic solution while the pulmonary artery is cross-clamped, and the subsequent potential for impairment of right ventricular function [26]. In an attempt to overcome this problem of right ventricular overdistension, Nakamura and colleagues [27] have recently described a technique, named right atrial perfusion cooling, that basically involves a double-lumen cannula of which one is used for right atrial infusion and the other for right ventricular drainage of cardioplegic solution. The clinical applicability of this variant of the right atrial approach still remains to be determined.

In conclusion, retrograde delivery of cardioplegia through the coronary sinus has now achieved a safety and efficacy record which makes it worth being fully included in our armamentarium of myocardial preservation techniques. It is hoped that future improvements in catheter design will make RCSP still safer and easier to handle while increasing experience with this technique should help in better identifying the patient groups that are most likely to benefit from cardioplegia delivery in a retrograde fashion.

References

1. Lüdighausen MV. Nomenclature and distribution pattern of cardiac veins in man. In Mohl W, Faxon D, Wolner E (eds): Clinics of CSI. Darmstadt: Steinkopff Verlag 1986; 13–32.
2. Ratajczyk-Pakalska E. Thebesian veins in the human hearts with atherosclerotic lesions in the coronary arteries. In Mohl W, Faxon D, Wolner E (eds): Clinics of CSI. Darmstadt: Steinkopff Verlag 1986; 141–5.
3. Pennington DG, Dincer B, Bashiti H *et al.* Coronary artery stenosis following aortic valve replacement and intermittent intracoronary cardioplegia. Ann Thorac Surg 1982; 33: 576–84.
4. Menasche P, Subayi JB, Piwnica A. Retrograde coronary sinus cardioplegia for aortic valve operations: A clinical report on 500 patients. Ann Thorac Surg 1990; 49: 556–64.
5. Menasche P, Maisonblanche P, Bousseau D *et al.* Decreased incidence of supraventricular arrhythmias achieved by selective atrial cooling during aortic valve replacement. Eur J Cardio-Thorac Surg 1987; 1: 33–6.
6. Chitwood WR. Myocardial protection by retrograde cardioplegia: Coronary sinus and right atrial methods. In Cardiac surgery: state of the art reviews. Philadelphia: Hanley and Belfus 1988; 2: 197–218.
7. Dorsey LM, Colgan TK, Silverstein JI *et al.* Alterations in regional myocardial function after heterogeneous cardioplegia. J Thorac Cardiovasc Surg 1983; 86: 70–9.
8. Menasche P, Piwnica A. Cardioplegia by way of the coronary sinus for valvular and coronary surgery. J Am Coll Cardiol 1991; 18: 628–36.
9 Aronson S, Lee BK, Liddicoat JR *et al.* Assessment of retrograde cardioplegia. Distribution using contrast echocardiography. Ann Thorac Surg 1991; 52: 810–4.
10. Shapira N, Lemole GM, Spagna PM *et al.* Antegrade and retrograde infusion of cardioplegia: Assessment by thermovision. Ann Thorac Surg,1987; 43: 92–7.
11. Menasche P, Subayi JB, Veyssie L *et al.* Efficacy of coronary sinus cardioplegia in patients with complete coronary artery occlusions. Ann Thorac Surg 1991; 51: 418–23.
12. Snyder HE, Smithwick W III, Wingard JT *et al.* Retrograde coronary sinus perfusion. Ann Thorac Surg 1988; 46: 389–90.
13. Yonenaga K, Yasui H, Kado HJ *et al.* Myocardial protection by retrograde cardioplegia in arterial switch operation. Ann Thorac Surg 1990; 50: 238–42.
14. Drinkwater DC, Laks H, Buckberg GD. A new simplified method of optimizing cardioplegic delivery without right heart isolation. Antegrade/retrograde blood cardioplegia. J Thorac Cardiovasc Surg 1990; 100: 56–64.

15. Gundry SR, Sequiera A, Razzouk A *et al.* Facile retrograde cardioplegia: Transatrial cannulation of the coronary sinus. Ann Thorac Surg 1990; 50: 882–7.
16. Lichtenstein SV, Ashe KA, El Dalati H *et al.* Warm heart surgery. J Thorac Cardiovasc Surg 1991; 101: 269–74.
17. Fiore AC, Naunheim KS, Kaiser GC *et al.* Coronary sinus versus aortic root perfusion with blood cardioplegia in elective myocardial revascularization. Ann Thorac Surg 1989; 47: 684–8.
18. Kalmbach T, Bhayana JN. Cardioplegia delivery by combined aortic root and coronary sinus perfusion. Ann Thorac Surg 1989; 47: 316–7.
19. Sutter FP, Goldman SM, Clancy M *et al.* Continuous retrograde blood cardioplegia. Ann Thorac Surg 1991; 51: 136–7.
20. Crooke GA, Harris LJ, Grossi EA *et al.* Biventricular distribution of cold blood cardioplegic solution administered by different retrograde techniques. J Thorac Cardiovasc Surg 1991; 102: 631–8.
21. Menasche P, Kucharski K, Mundler O *et al.* Adequate preservation of right ventricular function following coronary sinus cardioplegia. A clinical study. Circulation 1989; 80 (Suppl 3): 19–24.
22. Lichtenstein SV, Fremes SE, Abdel JG *et al.* Technical aspects of warm heart surgery. J Cardiac Surg 1991; 6: 278–85.
23. Diehl JT, Kaplan E, Dresdale AR *et al.* Effects of atrial cardioplegia on the ischemic right ventricle after acute coronary artery occlusion and reperfusion. Ann Thorac Surg 1989; 48: 829–34.
24. Fabiani JN, Deloche A, Swanson J *et al.* Retrograde cardioplegia through the right atrium. Ann Thorac Surg 1986; 41: 101–2.
25. Eichhorn EJ, Diehl JT, Konstam MA *et al.* Protective effects of retrograde compared with antegrade cardioplegia on right ventricular systolic and diastolic function during coronary bypass surgery. Circulation 1989; 79: 1271–81.
26. Salter RD, Goldstein JP, Abd-Elfattah A *et al.* Ventricular function after atrial cardioplegia. Circulation 1987; 76(Suppl 5): 129–40.
27. Nakamura Y, Fukamachi K, Masuda M *et al.* A new method of retrograde cardioplegic administration. J Thorac Cardiovasc Surg 1990; 99: 335–44.

11. Cardiac arrest by ventricular fibrillation

CARY W. AKINS

Hypothermic fibrillatory arrest without aortic occlusion is a technique of myocardial preservation that has been utilized for many years in cardiac surgery. In our institution the basic tenets of this method of myocardial preservation were developed in the late 1960s by Dr. Eldred Mundth and associates during the initiation of coronary artery bypass grafting [1]. During the 1970s several modifications in the technique were made as better understanding of myocardial protection evolved.

Operative principles of hypothermic fibrillatory arrest

The principles of hypothermic fibrillatory arrest without aortic occlusion that are currently followed, particularly during coronary artery bypass grafting, include:

1. Early heparinization and aortic cannulation.
2. Proximal vein-to-aorta anastomoses prior to atrial cannulation and the institution of cardiopulmonary bypass.
3. Administration of beta blocking agents after the induction of anesthesia, as tolerated by the patient, to lower the pulse rate to 50 or less, if the patient is not preoperatively sufficiently beta blocked.
4. Addition of mannitol to the bypass priming solution.
5. Systemic hypothermia to 25°–28°C.
6. Pericardial irrigation with 4°C Ringer's lactate solution.
7. Maintenance of systemic perfusion pressure on cardiopulmonary bypass of 80–100 mmHg.
8. Elective, but not electrically sustained, ventricular fibrillation.
9. Routine left ventricular venting through the right superior pulmonary vein.
10. Avoidance of aortic cross-clamping.
11. Local vessel occlusion with vinyl tapes for distal vein or internal mammary artery to coronary anastomoses.
12. Initial grafting of most ischemic zone first, if possible.
13. Grafting of diseased left lateral (circumflex) coronary arteries before

H.M. Piper and C.J. Preusse (eds): Ischemia-reperfusion in cardiac surgery, 267–278.

internal mammary artery grafting of diseased anterior arteries to avoid traction on the mammary pedicle.
14. Complete revascularization, whenever possible.

Research evidence for the principles of hypothermic fibrillatory arrest

Several research reports were published in the early 1970s which questioned the efficacy of hypothermic fibrillatory arrest for myocardial preservation during coronary grafting. Thus it would be appropriate to review the research literature that supports the principles of hypothermic fibrillatory arrest.

In 1974 Hottenrott and associates [2] reported that electrically sustained ventricular fibrillation in animals, when compared to spontaneous fibrillation, was deleterious to regional myocardial blood flow. In the same report the authors noted that with spontaneous fibrillation at normothermia there was increased oxygen consumption, greater proportional flow to the subendocardium and no detrimental effects on myocardial structure. Thus, in the technique of hypothermic fibrillatory arrest, electrical current may be used very briefly to initiate fibrillation once the heart is cooled, but it is not used to sustain fibrillation.

In a companion article Hottenrot and Buckberg [3] reported that distension of the normothermic, fibrillating heart was deleterious. Routine left ventricular venting through the right superior pulmonary vein is a tenet of the technique. In recent years I have used a personally designed left ventricular vent that allows the continuous, direct measurement of left ventricular pressure to aid the perfusionist in keeping the heart empty while at the same time avoiding excessive suction.

In 1979 Vinas and coworkers [4] documented the benefits of systemic hypothermia on coronary blood flow in fibrillating animal hearts on bypass. At 30°C, as compared to 37°C, fibrillating hearts demonstrated less oxygen consumption, decreased coronary blood flow, and less lactate production. Thus, systemic hypothermia to 28°C was one of the original tenets of hypothermic fibrillatory arrest. With the more recent emphasis on internal mammary artery grafting to the left anterior descending system, which may require somewhat longer periods of time to accomplish a distal anastomosis, we have begun to lower the systemic temperature on cardiopulmonary bypass routinely to 25°C.

During the 1970s the importance of maintaining adequate systemic perfusion pressure with this technique while on cardiopulmonary bypass became obvious. In 1975 Baird and colleagues [5] reported that in fibrillating animals during cardioplumonary bypass perfusion pressures of less than 60 mmHg resulted in decreased subendocardial blood flow. However, in the same study the authors demonstrated that if the perfusion pressure was kept constantly above 80 mmHg, total left ventricular blood flow was greater in the empty-fibrillating heart than in the empty-beating or normal, working heart. Maintenance of the perfusion pressure at 80 mmHg also maintained good subendocardial perfusion. Several years later Cox and associates [6] reported similar findings in nonhypertrophied animal hearts, where at normothermia with perfusion pressures maintained between 70 and 100 mmHg, there were no ischemic changes in empty-fibrillating hearts while on cardiopulmonary bypass. Then in 1982 Spadoro and coworkers [7] demonstrated that there was no lactate production in fibrillating hearts if the perfusion pressure were maintained greater than 65 mmHg. They also noted that coronary vascular resistance was less in fibrillating hearts in comparison to beating hearts, and thus coronary blood flow was greater.

If there is a key principle of the technique of hypothermic fibrillatory arrest, it is the maintenance of an adequate perfusion gradient across the myocardium by keeping the systemic perfusion pressure between 80 and 100 mmHg while at the same time keeping the left ventricular pressure near 0 mmHg with left ventricular venting. The systemic perfusion pressure is maintained first by adjusting flow through the cardiopulmonary bypass pump, usually keeping a flow of greater than 40 to 50 cc per kg while the patient is cool. If much higher flows are required, then the systemic vascular resistance can be increased with the infusion of phenylephrine directly into the pump. If systemic vascular resistance is too high and flows of less than 40 cc per kg per minute still yield systemic hypertension, then systemic vascular resistance is lowered either with additional anesthetic agents or the infusion of nitroprusside. Continuous display of the monitored sytemic blood pressure and left ventricular pressure makes the necessary moment-to-moment adjustments of the cardiopulmonary bypass pumps easier for the perfusionist.

Obviously the maintenance of a perfusion gradient across the myocardium is only useful if one can avoid the imposition of global myocardial ischemia caused by aortic cross-clamping. The deleterious effects of a period of global ischemia that is superimposed upon a heart that is already regionally ischemic was clearly demonstrated by Horneffer and associates [8,9] in 1985. They documented the extension of additional infarction in hearts that had a period of global ischemia imposed during the early phases of regional infarct evolution.

More recently some investigators have evaluated the effects of ventricular fibrillation on myocardial mechanics. In 1990 Krukenkamp and colleagues [10] evaluated the effects of ventricular fibrillation coincident with normothermic ischemia on post-ischemic myocardial energetics when quantitated in the same heart under constant and defined nonworking conditions. Their data demonstrated no detectable differences in post-ischemic energetics in empty-fibrillating and empty-beating hearts, particularly when measured in the vented and adequately perfused state. Additionally the authors noted that their results verified their prior findings of the preservation of mitochondrial respiratory function and high-energy phosphate levels that had previously been demonstrated in porcine tissue bioassays following comparable intervals of ischemic ventricular fibrillation. Similarly in 1992 Yaku and coworkers

[11] reported that ventricular fibrillation for 20 to 40 minutes did not depress postfibrillatory contractility as long as coronary perfusion by blood was maintained at normal levels.

The feasibility of extending the use of hypothermic fibrillatory arrest to procedures other than coronary artery bypass grafting has recently been investigated by Bradley and colleagues [12], who studied the effects of fibrillatory arrest in fetal lambs in utero. They demonstrated that during normothermic bypass with fibrillatory arrest, blood flow to the endocardium and epicardium of both right and left ventricles and the flow ratios were preserved. After bypass, blood flow to all areas was increased, even if the mean arterial pressure was lowered with nitroprusside.

In the 1980s the potential free-radical scavenging effects of mannitol were elucidated by Magovern and coworkers [13] and Scott and associates [14]. Given that information and also because of its relatively benign ability to increase urine output on bypass and thus reduce edema, mannitol was subsequently routinely added to the bypass-priming solutions.

Most recently I have been impressed that patients who are having hypothermic fibrillatory arrest for coronary artery bypass grafting seem to behave better clinically if they are well beta blocked prior to cardiopulmonary bypass. My hypothesis is that adequate beta blockade may reduce myocardial oxygen consumption even during ventricular fibrillation. This supposition is currently being evaluated in the laboratory. Until the results are available, we have begun a policy of instituting beta blockade after anesthesia induction and prior to cardiopulmonary bypass in patients who come to the operating room who are not adequately beta blocked and who will tolerate the administration of beta blocking agents. We have observed that the advent and growth in the use of calcium channel blockers to treat ischemic heart disease has resulted in many patients being sent to operation without adequate concomitant beta blockade.

In one of the few studies that compared hypothermic ventricular fibrillation to hyperkalemic crystalloid cardioplegic methods, Grotte and associates [15] investigated the effects of the two techniques during 90 minutes of bypass in dogs. Hemodynamics were studied with left ventricular function curves, total and regional coronary blood flow with radioactive microspheres, and myocardial morphology with ultrastructural analysis of left ventricular biopsy specimens. Recovery of ventricular function was 97% for fibrillating hearts and 95% for potassium-arrested hearts, a difference that was not statistically significantly different. In fibrillating hearts total coronary blood flow doubled and sustained a three-fold increase during recovery. Also endocardial to epicardial flow ratios increased 21% with a sustained increase of 57% during recovery. Lactate load early after intervention was eight times greater in the potassium-arrested hearts. The authors summarized their results, "Therefore, at hypothermia, the vented fibrillating heart appears to be as well protected as the cross-clamped potassium-arrested heart".

The importance of attempting to achieve complete revascularization in every patient coming to operation with coronary artery disease cannot be overemphasized. In every study where it was carefully evaluated as an incremental risk factor for operative and late deaths and symptom relief, complete revascularization has been demonstrated to be an overwhelmingly important contributor to improved results [16–20].

Reported clinical results with hypothermic fibrillatory arrest

We have published several reports describing the clinical results with hypothermic fibrillatory arrest, especially for coronary artery bypass grafting. Our first report of the technique in 1984 [21] documented the results in 500 consecutive patients having isolated, non-emergency coronary grafting from August, 1979 through June, 1982. Of the 500 patients, 483 had primary revascularization and 17 reoperative grafting. Mean age of the study group was 57.1 years, and women made up only 12.8% of the group. The average number of grafts per patient was 3.8, and no patient had an internal mammary artery graft. Hospital mortality was 0.4% (2/500), and perioperative myocardial infarction, defined as either new Q waves of elevation of the myocardial fraction of creatine kinase above 40 IU, occurred in nine patients (1.8%). Actuarial survival at three years was 95.8%, not statistically significantly different from that for a matched cohort from the general population.

In 1986 we reported the results of left ventricular aneurysm resection with or without coronary bypass grafting during hypothermic fibrillatory arrest in 100 consecutive patients having their operations between December, 1977 and September, 1984 [22]. The mean age of the study group was 57.2 years, and 17% of the group was women. The average number of associated coronary bypass grafts per patient (performed in 97 patients) was 3.2. Postoperative pressor agents were required in 21% of patients, and 2% required postoperative intra-aortic balloon pumping. Hospital mortality was 2% (2/100), and perioperative myocardial infarction was documented in 1%. Actuarial survival at 73 months was 77.0%. Improved survival was noted for patients with anterior left ventricular aneurysms if the left anterior descending or diagonal branches had concomitant bypass grafting.

To assess the efficacy of the technique in patients with acute ischemia, in 1987 we reported the results of isolated myocardial revascularization during hypothermic fibrillatory arrest in 127 patients requiring emergency bypass grafting, of whom 109 patients (85.8%) had a preoperative intra-aortic balloon pump, 97 patients (76.3%) required intravenous nitroglycerin, and 12 (9.4%) had recently received thrombolytic therapy [23]. The bypass grafting was a reoperative revascularization in 4 patients (3.1%). Bypass grafting was performed within one week of an acute myocardial infarction in 47 patients (37%). The mean number of grafts per patient was 4.1. One patient (0.8%) died in hospital, and one patient (0.8%) suffered a perioperative myocardial infarction. Actuarial survival at 45 months was 90.8%.

Our report in 1987 [24] extended the evaluation of the technique in non-emergency, isolated myocardial revascularization to 1000 patients having their procedures between August, 1979 and November, 1984. Mean age for that population was 58.2 years, and women comprised 14.9%. Primary revascularization was performed in 96.2% of the group and reoperative grafting in 3.8%. The mean number of grafts per patient was 4. Hospital mortality occurred in 0.4% (4/1000), and perioperative infarction in 1.8% (18/1000). The study focused on the event-free survival of the patients. Actuarial survival at five years was 91.6%. Actuarial event-free rates at five years were 97.7% for myocardial infarction, 99.4% for percutaneous transluminal coronary angioplasty, 99.5% for reoperative surgical myocardial revascularization, and 88.6% for all combined morbidity and mortality.

Utilizing a similar approach for comparative purposes, in 1989 we reported a group of 1000 consecutive patients having non-emergency, isolated, primary coronary artery bypass grafting from March, 1981 through May, 1986, and compared the results to those of 389 patients having first-time, non-emergency percutaneous transluminal coronary angioplasty during the same time period [25]. The surgical cohort averaged 59.3 years of age, and 15% were women. The average number of grafts per patient was 4.2. Hospital mortality in the surgical cohort was 0.4% (4/1000), and the perioperative infarction rate was 1.7% (17/1000). Actuarial survival at five years was 92.7%. Actuarial event-free rates at five years were 96.4% for myocardial infarction, 99.5% for percutaneous transluminal coronary angioplasty, 98.8% for reoperative bypass grafting, and 88.9% for all combined morbidity and mortality. Only diminished ejection fraction and advanced age predicted late mortality.

Because of the growing application of left internal mammary artery grafting to diseased anterior wall coronary arteries, in 1990 we evaluated the efficacy of hypothermic fibrillatory arrest as a technique of myocardial preservation when arterial grafts were utilized [26]. As a basis for comparison 1000 patients having primary, non-emergency bypass grafting with only saphenous veins from March, 1981 through June, 1989, were compared to 500 patients having at least one internal mammary artery graft during the same time period. Saphenous vein patients had a mean age of 65.5 years, and 84% were male; internal mammary artery patients had a mean age of 60.4 years, and 91% were male. The average number of grafts per patient was 4.3 for the saphenous group and 4.1 for the internal mammary group. Hospital mortality and perioperative infarction for the saphenous vein versus the internal mammary artery groups were 0.6% versus 0.8%, and 1.8% versus 3.6%, respectively.

Finally in 1992 we published a report describing the efficacy of hypothermic fibrillatory arrest during reoperative myocardial revascularization in the presence of patent but atherosclerotically diseased vein bypass grafts, a cohort of patients known for higher operative complication rates because of difficulty with obtaining adequate global cardioplegia and also because of the incidence of atheroembolization [27]. In that study 91 patients having reoperative revascularization in the presence of patent, diseased saphenous vein grafts

Table 11.1. Operative procedures and patient populations during hypothemic fibrillatory arrest: 1980–1991.

Operation	Patients	Mean age (years)	Female
Isolated primary CABG[a]	2512	60.7	15.2%
Non-emergency	2240		
Emergency	272		
Reoperative CABG	198	59.8	10.6%
Non-emergency	164		
Emergency	34		
LVA[b] ± CABG	120	58.9	17.5%
Non-emergency	104		
Emergency	16		
Total	2830	60.6	15.0%

[a] CABG – coronary artery bypass grafting.
[b] LVA – left ventricular aneurysmectomy.

(Group I) were compared to 73 patients having reoperative grafting but who had only totally occluded or undiseased prior grafts (Group II). While operative mortality was 2.2% for Group I and 4.1% for Group II, myocardial infarction rates were 6.5% and 5.5%, respectively.

Summary of clinical results with fibrillatory arrest for coronary grafting

Because all of the above-mentioned reports focused on different subsets of patients with ischemic heart disease, the following will present a summary of our results with hypothermic fibrillatory arrest without aortic occlusion for all patients having operations performed between January, 1980 and December, 1991. During that time-frame 2830 consecutive patients had either isolated, primary or reoperative coronary artery bypass grafting or left ventricular aneurysm resection with or without associated coronary grafting (Table 11.1). Of the total group, 2512 patients had primary, isolated coronary artery bypass grafting (of whom 272 had their grafting performed as an emergency procedure), 198 had reoperative myocardial revascularization, and 120 had resection of a left ventricular aneurysm (of whom 118 had associated coronary bypass grafting). This review will look at the results for the group as a whole and also for each of the three categories described above.

For the patients having isolated coronary artery bypass grafting the average age was 60.7 years, with 15.2% of the population being female (Table 11.1). Over the twelve years of the study the average age of the group rose from 56.8 years in 1980 to 64.8 years in 1991 (Figure 11.1). Another major trend during the study time-frame was the trend of increasing number of bypass grafts per patient, rising from 3.8 grafts per patient in 1980 to a high of 4.9

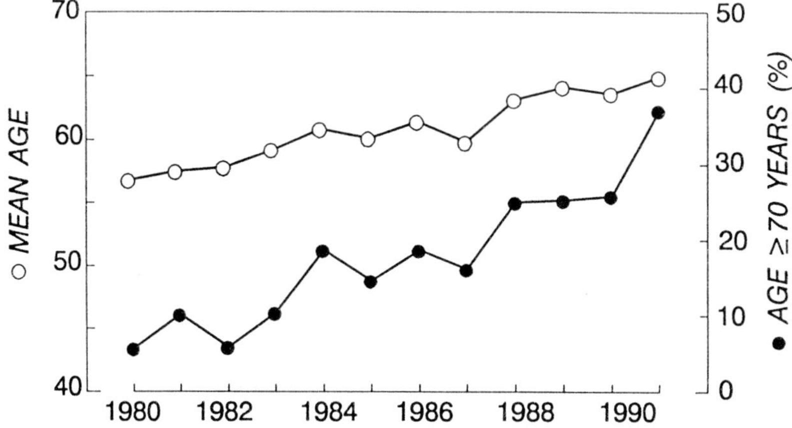

Figure 11.1. Trends in age of isolated coronary artery bypass patients: 1980–1991.

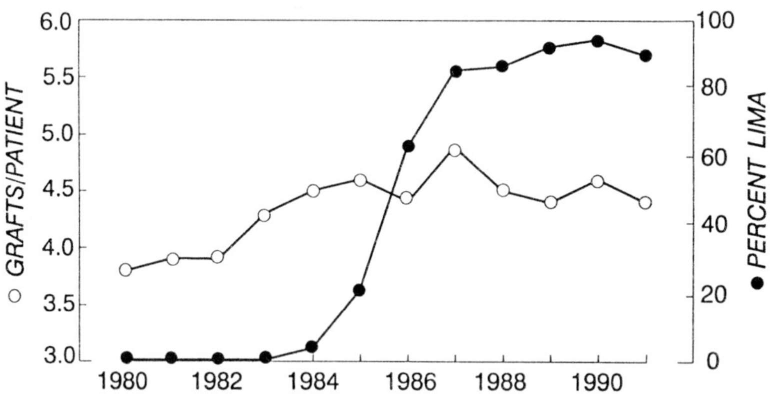

Figure 11.2. Trends in grafts per patient and use of internal mammary artery grafts in isolated coronary artery bypass patients: 1980–1991.

in 1987. The growth of internal mammary artery grafting is illustrated in Figure 11.2, with internal mammary artery grafting beginning in 1984, when 3.4% of patients had mammary grafts and rising to a high of 93.6% in 1990. Of the subset of 272 patients who had emergency, isolated coronary grafting, 204 patients (75.0%) had an intra-aortic balloon in preoperatively. Additionally 54 patients (2.1%) underwent concomitant carotid endarterectomy, and 22 patients (0.9%) required coronary endarterectomy.

The incidence of reoperative revascularization by year also changed gradually during the study interval, rising from 2.3% of all isolated bypass operations in 1980 to 17.0% in 1991. The average age of the reoperative patients was 59.8 years, and 10.6% of the group was female. The reoperative bypass

Table 11.2. Operative results with hypothermic fibrillatory arrest: 1980–1991.

Operation	Hospital mortality	IABP[c]	Myocardial infarction
Isolated primary CABG[a]	40/2512 (1.6%)	50/2512 (2.0%)	51/2512 (2.0%)
Non-emergency	25/2240 (1.1%)		
Emergency	15/272 (5.5%)		
Reoperative CABG	6/198 (3.0%)	19/198 (9.6%)	9/198 (4.5%)
Non-emergency	4/164 (2.4%)		
Emergency	2/34 (5.9%)		
LVA[b] ± CABG	5/120 (4.2%)	4/120 (3.3%)	4/120 (3.3%)
Non-emergency	5/104 (4.8%)		
Emergency	0/16 (0)		
Total	51/2830 (1.8%)	73/2830 (2.6%)	64/2830 (2.3%)

[a] CABG – coronary artery bypass grafting.
[b] LVA – left ventricular aneurysmectomy.
[c] IABP – intraoperative or postoperative intra-aortic balloon pump.

grafting was an emergency operation in 28 patients (14.1%), of whom 19 were on the intra-aortic balloon pump preoperatively. The average number of grafts per patient was 3.6 for the reoperative patients (varying from 1 to 7), of which 60.6% were internal mammary artery grafts.

For the patients having left ventricular aneurysm resection the average age was 58.9 years, and women comprised 17.5% of the group. Of the entire group, 18 (15.0%) were emergency operations, all performed with an intra-aortic balloon pump in place preoperatively, and 3 (2.5%) were reoperations. The average number of grafts per patient for the 118 (98.3%) patients having concomitant bypass grafting was 3.7 (varying from 1 to 7), including 20.0% who received internal mammary artery grafts.

The hospital mortality rates for the various subgroups are listed in Table 11.2. The overall mortality for all 2830 patients in the review was 1.8%, varying from 1.1% for primary, isolated, non-emergency coronary artery bypass graft patients, to 5.5% for primary, isolated emergency coronary grafting, to 3.0% for reoperative revascularization patients, to 4.2% for patients having left ventricular aneurysm resection with or without coronary bypass grafting. For the total population intraoperative or postoperative intra-aortic balloon pumping was required in 2.6%, and 2.3% of all patients suffered a perioperative myocardial infarction.

If one looks at the operative results in terms of operative priority, the 2508 non-emergency procedures had a cumulative hospital mortality of 1.4%; while for the total of 322 patients having emergency operations of all types, the hospital mortality was 5.3%. Examining the operative mortality results in more 11. detail (Table 11.3), one sees that gender and operative priority have a major impact on the hospital mortality for various subgroups. For example, males less than 70 years of age with non-emergency, primary coronary artery bypass grafting have a hospital mortality of 0.6% compared

Table 11.3. Hospital mortality by operative priority and gender.

Operative priority	Deaths/patients (%)	
	Age <70 years	Age ≥70 years
Non-emergency		
Male	9/1629 (0.6%)	4/281 (1.4%)
Female	4/234 (1.7%)	8/91 (8.8%)
Emergency		
Male	6/162 (3.7%)	3/51 (5.9%)
Female	5/40 (12.5%)	1/24 (4.2%)

to 8.8% for females 70 years of age or older who have non-emergency, first-time coronary grafting. The effects of operative priority are also obvious, except for the subgroups with too few patients.

Summary assessment of hypothermic fibrillatory arrest

In light of the foregoing information, the following is a summary of the potential advantages and disadvantages of hypothermic fibrillatory arrest without aortic occlusion. The potential advantages of hypothermic fibrillatory arrest as a technique of myocardial preservation, chiefly for coronary artery bypass grafting include:

1. Aortic cross-clamping and cannulation for cardioplegia delivery are avoided, thus minimizing possibilities for trauma to the aorta.
2. Global myocardial ischemia is avoided, something of particular importance in the presence of acute ischemia.
3. Bypass grafts can be performed in any sequence; specifically internal mammary artery grafting does not have to be delayed until the last anastomosis.
4. Myocardial protection during reoperative myocardial revascularization in the face of patent bypass grafts, particularly internal mammary artery grafts is less complicated.
5. In general the technique is simpler, less cumbersome, quicker and less expensive than techniques employing administration of cardioplegia solutions.
6. Fluid and potassium loads of cardioplegia solutions are avoided.

The potential disadvantages of hypothermic fibrillatory arrest for myocardial preservation include:

1. Retraction of the heart for exposure of lateral and posterior wall coronary arteries may be more difficult because of the constantly perfused state of the heart; although it may not be much different than techniques utilizing continuous cardioplegia delivery.

2. Partial occlusion of the ascending aorta is still necessary for the performance of proximal saphenous vein anastomoses.
3. Distal conduit to coronary artery anastomoses require local occlusion of the coronary arteries to limit blood flow into the operative field which creates the possibility for local arterial damage.
4. Local coronary artery occlusion for distal anastomoses can create local short-term myocardial ischemia in the absence of good collateral circulation to the distal myocardial bed.
5. The operative field is more bloody, but often not much more so than that seen with continuous blood cardioplegia techniques.

Thus, hypothermic fibrillatory arrest without aortic occlusion has been demonstrated both in the laboratory and in extensive clinical utilization to be a safe and effective method of myocardial preservation, particularly for coronary artery bypass grafting and also left ventricular aneurysmectomy.

References

1. Mundth ED, Harthorne JW, Buckley MJ *et al.* Direct coronary arterial revascularization for segmental occlusive disease. Surgery 1970; 61: 168–81.
2. Hottenrot C, Maloney JV, Buckberg G. Studies of the effects of ventricular fibrillation on the adequacy of regional myocardial blood flow. I Electrical vs. spontaneous fibrillation. J Thorac Cardiovasc Surg 1974; 68: 615–25.
3. Hottenrot C, Buckberg G. Studies of the effects of ventricular fibrillation on the adequacy of regional myocardial blood flow. II. Effects of ventricular distension. J Thorac Cardiovasc Surg 1974; 68: 626–33.
4. Vinas JF, Fewel JG, Arom KV *et al.* Effects of systemic hypothermia on myocardial metabolism and coronary blood flow in the fibrillating heart. J Thorac Cardiovasc Surg 1979; 77: 900–7.
5. Baird RJ, Dutka F, Okumori M *et al.* Surgical aspects of regional myocardial blood flow and myocardial pressure. J Thorac Cardiovasc Surg 1975; 69: 17–29.
6. Cox JL, Anderson RW, Pass HI *et al.* The safety of induced ventricular fibrillation during cardiopulmonary bypass in nonhypertrophied hearts. J Thorac Cardiovasc Surg 1977; 74: 423–32.
7. Spadoro J, Bing OHL, Gaasch WH *et al.* Effects of perfusion pressure on myocardial performance, metabolism, wall thickness, and compliance. J Thorac Cardiovasc Surg 1982; 84: 398–405.
8. Horneffer PJ, Gott VL, Gardner TJ. Reperfusion before global ischemic arrest improves the salvage of infarcting myocardium. Ann Thorac Surg 1985; 40: 504–8.
9. Horneffer PJ, Gott VL, Gardner TJ. The deleterious effect of global ischemia on an evolving myocardial infarction. Surg Forum 1984; 35: 308–11.
10. Krukenkamp I, Badellino M, Levitsky S. Effects of ischemic ventricular fibrillation on myocardial mechanics and energetics in the porcine heart. Surg Forum 1990; 41: 239–40.
11. Yaku H, Goto Y, Futaki S *et al.* Ventricular fibrillation does not depress postfibrillatory contractility in blood- perfused dog hearts. J Thorac Cardiovasc Surg 1992; 103: 514–20.
12. Bradley SM, Hanley FL, Duncan BW. Regional myocardial blood flow during cardiopulmonary bypass in the fetal lamb. Surg Forum 1990; 41: 203–5.
13. Magovern GJ, Bolling ST, Casal AS *et al.* The mechanism of mannitol in reducing ischemic injury: hyperosmolarity or hydroxyl scavenger? Circulation 1984; 70(Suppl I): I-91–I-95.

14. Scott JA, Khaw BA, Locke EJ *et al.* The role of free radical-mediated processes in oxygen-related damage in culture murine myocardial cells. Circ Res 1985; 56: 72–7.
15. Grotte GJ, Levine FH, Kay HR *et al.* Effect of ventricular fibrillation and potassium-induced arrest on myocardial recovery in hypothermic hearts. Surg Forum 1980; 31: 296–8.
16. Bartel AG, Behar VS, Peter RH *et al.* Effects of aortocoronary bypass surgery on treadmill exercise. Circulation 1973; 48: 141–48.
17. Cukingnan RA, Carey JS, Wittig JH *et al.* Influence of complete revascularization on relief of angina. J Thorac Cardiovasc Surg 1980; 79: 188–93.
18. Loop FD, Cosgrove DM, Lytle BW *et al.* An 11–year evolution of coronary arterial surgery (1967–1978). Ann Surg 1979; 190: 444–55.
19. Kirklin JW, Naftel DC, Blackstone EH *et al.* Summary of a consensus concerning death and ischemic events after coronary artery bypass grafting. Circulation 1989; 79(Suppl I): I-81–I-91.
20. Sergeant P, Lesaffre E, Flameng W *et al.* Internal mammary artery: Methods of use and their effect on survival. Eur J Cardiothorac Surg 1990; 4: 72–8.
21. Akins CW. Noncardioplegic myocardial preservation for coronary revascularization. J Thorac Cardiovasc Surg 1984; 88: 174–81.
22. Akins CW. Resection of left ventricular aneurysm during hypothermic fibrillatory arrest without aortic occlusion. J Thorac Cardiovasc Surg 1986; 91: 610–8.
23. Akins CW. Early and late results following emergency isolated myocardial revascularization during hypothermic fibrillatory arrest. Ann Thorac Surg 1987; 43: 131–7.
24. Akins CW, Carroll DL. Event-free survival following nonemergency myocardial revascularization during hypothermic fibrillatory arrest. Ann Thorac Surg 1987; 43: 628–33.
25. Akins CW, Block PC, Palacios IF *et al.* Comparison of coronary artery bypass grafting and percutaneous transluminal coronary angioplasty as initial treatment strategies. Ann Thorac Surg 1989; 47: 507–16.
26. Akins CW. Myocardial preservation with hypothermic fibrillatory arrest for coronary grafting. J Mol Cell Cardiol 1990; 22: S44.
27. Akins CW. Repeat coronary operation in the presence of patent but atherosclerotically diseased vein bypass grafts. In Engelman RM, Levitsky S (eds):.A Textbook of Cardioplegia for Difficult Clinical Problems. Mount Kisco, NY: Futura Publishing Company, Inc. 1992; 71–81.

12. Myocardial preservation in the immature heart

JOHN E. MAYER, Jr.

Introduction

The repair of most congenital intra-cardiac defects in neonates and infants requires a period of myocardial ischemia to provide satisfactory operating conditions for the conduct of the repair. Extensive efforts have been made to improve the preservation of the heart during these periods of surgically induced ischemia, but there is still a need for further improvements in this area. The majority of the experimental efforts have involved 'mature' heart models, but there are reasons to believe that myocardial ischemia may have different effects on the 'immature' heart from the 'mature' heart. Therefore different strategies for myocardial preservation might be desirable for the immature heart. This discussion will focus primarily on preservation of the 'immature' heart although it must be understood that the precise definition of the term 'immature' remains unclear. Further, the crossover point from 'immature' to 'mature' for the human species is unknown as well.

Tolerance of the immature heart to hypoxia/ischemia

The question of whether the immature heart is less sensitive or more sensitive to the effects of hypoxia/ischemia and reperfusion remains unsettled despite numerous investigations. On the theoretical grounds of a greater glycolytic capacity [1], it has been thought that the immature heart would have a better tolerance of hypoxia and/or ischemia than the mature heart. Studies in rabbits [2–6] rats [7,8] and puppies [9] have shown an increased tolerance to either normothermic hypoxia or ischemia when compared to the mature animal. A second potential mechanism involved in improved ischemic tolerance may be better preservation of intracellular high energy phosphates [2,9–11]. The higher levels of high energy phosphates may be related to lower levels of 5′nucleotidase in the immature heart [9]. This enzyme catalyzes the breakdown of adenosine monophosphate to adenosine, and lower levels of this enzyme would be expected to result in higher end-ischemic levels of AMP, which would then be available for rephosphorylation to ATP during reperfusion [9]. Others have noted that the neonatal rabbit heart had less calcium uptake during ischemia than the adult [12]. Julia [13] has also demon-

H.M. Piper and C.J. Preusse (eds): Ischemia-reperfusion in cardiac surgery, 279–291.

strated an increased ability of the puppy heart to utilize amino acids as substrate during normothermic ischemia when compared to the adult dog. These studies demonstrate that a variety of mechanisms may be involved in the tolerance of the neonatal heart to ischemia.

In contrast, experiments in rats [14,15] and pigs [16] have shown a reduced tolerance to ischemia in the neonatal heart, particularly when assessed by the time to ischemic contracture under normothermic conditions. Greater intracellular accumulation of lactic acid as a result of anaerobic (i.e., glycolytic) metabolism has been hypothesized as the injurious mechanism [15]. The most widely quoted clinical study regarding the effects of ischemia on the 'immature' myocardium is that by Bull [17] who found that myocardial ischemic times which seem to be well tolerated in adults with adjunctive hypothermic cardioplegia were associated with a significant mortality risk despite the use of cardioplegia. A subsequent ultrastructural study by Sawa *et al.* has found more mitochondrial injury in human neonates undergoing cardiac repairs than in older children. Thus, the basic issue of the relative susceptibilities of immature vs. mature myocardium to ischemia/reperfusion remains unsettled, but there are sufficient data to suggest that the immature myocardium has certain characteristics which distinguish it from mature myocardium and which may have an important effect on its response to ischemia.

Experimental data on preservation of the immature heart and current clinical applications

Pre-ischemic interventions

Relatively little information is available on the effects of pre-ischemic interventions on the outcome of a subsequent period of ischemia. Experiments in lambs and rabbits have suggested that augmentation of myocardial glycogen improved the tolerance of the neonatal heart to anoxia, and other experiments in mature dogs and rats have suggested that myocardial function is better preserved during normothermic anoxia when myocardial glycogen stores had been augmented prior to the insult [19]. More recently, experiments in puppies have suggested that the provision of aspartate and glutamate just prior to ischemia as part of a warm 'induction' cardioplegic solution results in better tolerance to a subsequent ischemic insult [20]. Clinically, we attempt to metabolically 'resuscitate' neonatal patients prior to operative interventions by use of PGE_1 to restore ductal patency and reverse 'shock', and by liberal use of glucose-amino acid parenteral nutrition.

Interventions during ischemia

Hypothermia

Since the time of Bigelow's experiments in the 1950s demonstrating that hypothermia improved the tolerance of the entire organism to ischemia [21], this physical intervention of reducing the temperature of the tissue during ischemia has remained the mainstay of almost all strategies of myocardial protection. A number of studies have shown that 1 to 2 hours of ischemia can be followed by nearly complete recovery of function in immature hearts protected by hypothermia alone [3,4,22]. Although it has generally been assumed that this protection results from the reduced metabolic demand of the tissues produced by hypothermia, it is not completely clear that this metabolic effect is the only mechanism of action of hypothermia. There is a large body of evidence which suggests that ischemia causes alterations in sarcolemmal permeability to ions such as sodium, potassium, and calcium [23], and it has been shown that one effect of hypothermia is to reduce the accumulation of calcium in the mitochondria during ischemia, presumably through effects on the mitochondrial membrane [24]. It has been hypothesized that hypothermia induces physical changes in the sarcolemma which alter the effects of ischemia on membrane permeability to ions such as sodium and calcium and thereby reduces the likelihood of cell death following a period of ischemia [25]. Nishioka *et al.* [12] have found that newborn rabbit hearts exposed to hypothermic global ischemia had less accumulation of calcium during ischemia and reperfusion than adult rabbit hearts and that post-ischemic ATP levels were inversely related to intracellular calcium accumulation. This same group found improved recovery of mechanical function with hypothermic protection when compared to an adult rabbit heart preparation [11].

Recently, the potential for a deleterious effect of hypothermia prior to the onset of ischemia has been suggested by the report of Reybeka *et al.* [26]. In this experiment in neonatal rabbit hearts, hypothermia prior to the onset of cardioplegia protected ischemia resulted in worse recovery of function than if the heart was kept warm up to the time of the onset of ischemia and then the cardioplegia itself was used to both cool and arrest the heart. The proposed mechanism of this cold-induced exacerbation of an ischemic injury is hypothermia-induced calcium accumulation in the myocardial cells prior to the onset of ischemia [26,27], and there is data from isolated papillary muscle experiments which suggests that hypothermia has a positive inotropic effect through an increase in intracellular calcium. Williams and coworkers [28] have reported clinical data to support this hypothesis by comparing a group of patients in whom hypothermia preceded ischemia with a group in which normothermic conditions were maintained prior to the infusion of cold cardioplegic solution. Improved patient survival and better myocardial function were reported in the group in which pre-ischemic hypothermia was avoided. These findings were in marked contrast to our usual practice of perfusion cooling on bypass prior to the application of the aortic cross clamp without recognizing any significant incidence of the 'cold contracture' phenomenon. Stimulated by this discrepancy, a series of experiments have recently been completed which suggest that in the isolated neonatal lamb heart, reduced ionized calcium levels during preischemic cooling (by the addition of citrate to the perfusion circuit) results in improved recovery of mechanical function after protected ischemia when St. Thomas cardioplegia is utilized [29]. Interestingly, the use of an acalcemic glucose-potassium cardioplegia also prevented the deleterious effects of preischemic hypothermia despite normal calcium levels during cooling (Aoki *et al.*, unpublished data). The precise explanation for these differences remains unclear, but likely involves calcium accumulation during ischemia. Clinically, we continue to use preischemic hypothermia prior to myocardial ischemia. We have measured the ionized calcium concentrations during the preischemic cooling phase of bypass in a series of patients and have found that the ionized calcium concentrations are quite low (0.2–0.3 mM/l). These low calcium concentrations are likely due to the use of an acalcemic crystalloid priming solution and also due to the practice of not 'correcting' the calcium concentration of the citrated blood which is added to the bypass prime. It remains unclear, however, if this relative hypocalcemia during preischemic hypothermia is the only explanation for the differences between our experience and that in Toronto.

Cardioplegia

Debate continues regarding the efficacy of cardioplegia in addition to hypothermia in enhancing the protection of the immature myocardium. Our own study [22] and that of Laks [30] in neonatal lambs and the studies of Baker *et al.* [4,31] in neonatal rabbits all suggest that in the normal heart there may be no additional benefit of adding cardioplegia to hypothermia. Clark *et al.* [32] have reported similar results in the neonatal piglet. Other studies, however, have shown that the addition of cardioplegia to hypothermia is beneficial in neonatal rabbits [33,34]. Two other experiments suggest that in a 'stressed' neonatal heart subjected to an ischemic insult, a beneficial effect of cardioplegia can be demonstrated which may not be apparent in an otherwise normal neonatal heart. Bove and coworkers [35] demonstrated an additive effect of cardioplegia over hypothermia alone in rabbit hearts undergoing ischemia at moderate levels of hypothermia (28°C). Our laboratory [36] showed that in the hearts of neonatal lambs with pre-existing cyanosis, cardioplegia did provide additional protection compared to hypothermia (15]C) alone. The importance of species variation in the interpretation of these types of experiments is demonstrated by the findings of Baker *et al.* [31] who found worse recovery when St. Thomas cardioplegia was added to hypothermia in neonatal rabbits, but found a significant benefit in the neonatal piglet. Unfortunately, no clinical studies comparing hypothermia with hypothermic cardioplegia have been reported, other than that of Bull *et al.*

[17], nor is it clear whether the immature human heart more closely resembles the rabbit, the lamb, or the piglet in its response to ischemia/reperfusion. We have found in our laboratory that excessively cold cardioplegia (<2°C) result in depressed recovery of mechanical and endothelial function in the neonatal lamb heart [37].

Cardioplegia additives
1) *Blood.* Although there are multiple studies in the mature heart regarding blood vs. crystalloid solutions, there are few studies in the immature heart. Our laboratory [22] found no benefit of blood cardioplegia over crystalloid cardioplegia or hypothermia in the normal neonatal lamb, but Corno and coworkers found that in the neonatal piglet model, blood cardioplegia was associated with improved recovery of function compared to crystalloid cardioplegia or hypothermia alone [38]. More recently, Kofsky and coworkers have reported complete recovery of mechanical function and high-energy phosphate levels after two hours of hypothermic ischemia with blood cardioplegia enriched with aspartate and glutamate [20]. *In vitro* studies have shown that the amount of oxygen delivered by deeply hypothermic oxygenated crystalloid solutions and hypothermic oxygenated blood do not differ significantly [39]. Other evidence suggests that the presence of red blood cells in these solutions may provide better perfusion at the microcirculatory level during hypothermic perfusion [40] but this issue has not been addressed in the immature heart. There are other mechanisms by which the addition of blood to cardioplegic solutions may be beneficial including provision of free radical scavenging capacity through the catalase in red blood cells and provision of buffering capacity by blood proteins. We have not used blood cardioplegia in the neonate, but we do use dilute blood cardioplegia in some infants >6 kg (surgeon preference).

2) *Oxygen.* There are convincing data in mature heart systems that the oxygenation of crystalloid cardioplegia solutions is associated with significant improvements in the recovery of post-ischemic function [41,42]. No studies on the effects of oxygenation of cardioplegia solutions in the immature heart have been carried out although Baker *et al.* have reported experimental data which suggests that the level of preischemic oxygenation can influence the outcome of a period of hypothermic ischemia in Krebs-Henseleit perfused rabbit hearts [41]. Clinically, we have oxygenated all cardioplegic solutions over the last 5 years, based primarily on the work by Daggett's group [41,42].

3) *Calcium content.* The 'optimal' concentration of calcium in various cardioplegic solutions remains unresolved. Since the intracellular accumulation of calcium during ischemia and reperfusion has been associated with cellular injury, an argument can be made for minimizing the calcium in the extracellular environment during ischemia to reduce intra-cellular calcium accumulation. However, the occurrence of the 'calcium paradox' phenomenon of

massive calcium accumulation and rapid cell death after perfusion with acalcemic solutions in normothermic rat hearts has been described [25], and therefore there is a theoretical potential for this phenomenon to occur with acalcemic cardioplegic solutions. Subsequently, it has been shown that hypothermia prevents this phenomenon from occurring in some models [25], but Hendren *et al.* have shown that in the adult rat heart, highly alkaline acalcemic cardioplegic solutions can cause ischemic contracture while solutions with lower pH do not [43]. A rigorous study of the question of optimal calcium concentration was carried out for St. Thomas solution where a nearly normal calcium concentration was determined to be 'optimal' when the ischemia was induced at normothermic levels in the adult rat heart [44]. Recently, Robinson *et al.* [45] have found that a reduced calcium concentration (0.6 mM) provided optimal recovery after hypothermic ischemia (20°C) in the adult rat heart. An important point to consider, however, is that there are high magnesium concentrations in St. Thomas cardioplegia which likely completes with calcium at entry points through the cell membrane. Therefore, an optimal calcium concentration determined for a solution containing magnesium may not be applicable if the magnesium is not present. In the adult dog heart normal levels of calcium in non-magnesium containing cardioplegic solutions have been found to adversely affect high energy phosphates and to induce ventricular contraction during ischemia [46]. The recovery of function after ischemia with 'normal' calcium content cardioplegic solutions (1.2 mM) has been markedly worse in some experiments [47,48] but not in others [49]. Other studies have shown that the presence of minimal amounts of calcium is associated with excellent recovery of function after prolonged ischemic intervals [42]. Two studies of calcium concentrations in blood cardioplegia in neonatal piglets have reached opposite conclusions. Caspi and coworkers [50] found better recovery of post-ischemic function when a hypocalcemic blood cardioplegic solution was used while Corno *et al.* [38] found that normal calcium levels were associated with better recovery. The recent report of Kofsky *et al.* [20] supported the use of hypocalcemic blood cardioplegia in the puppy. A study which provides correlative evidence for a deleterious effect of calcium during ischemia is that by Konishi and Apstein who showed that exposure of the neonatal heart to ouabain prior to hypothermic ischemia was associated with significantly worse recovery of function, presumably due to the effect of ouabain to raise the intracellular calcium concentration through inhibition of Na^+/K^+ ATPase [51]. As noted in the discussion of hypothermia above, we have found that there are significant interactions between preischemic hypothermia and the calcium content of cardioplegia solutions (Aoki *et al.*, unpublished data).

4) *Magnesium.* There is no direct data on variations in magnesium concentration in cardioplegic solutions for the immature myocardium. The only direct comparison between magnesium free and magnesium containing solutions in the immature heart was reported by Konishi and Apstein [33] in an isolated

blood perfused rabbit heart system. In this study two magnesium containing crystalloid cardioplegia solutions (St. Thomas solution vs. a magnesium, potassium, glutamate solution used at Hoptial Lariboisiere) were found to provide better recovery of function than an acalcemic glucose potassium solution [33]. Similar results showing added benefit of the addition of magnesium to cardioplegic solutions have been reported for the adult rat heart [46,47]. In a normothermic neonatal rat model, Yano and coworkers have provided data to suggest that the magnesium-containing St. Thomas solution provided good protection of the neonatal and immature heart [7].

Clinically, we have (relatively arbitrarily) chosen to use single-dose oxygenated St. Thomas cardioplegia for most neonatal operations and for many operations in the infant group. In some cases, (by surgeon preference) an oxygenated, dilute blood-glucose cardioplegic solution is used (Hct <5%). Determination of which solution is preferable has been limited by the lack of load and geometry independent methods of determining ventricular contractility in the clinical situation.

Dosing regimens for cardioplegia

In hypothermic models of ischemia in immature hearts, four separate studies all suggest that single dose rather than multiple doses of cardioplegia are associated with improved recovery of function after ischemia. Bove *et al.* found no additional protection of multi-dose St. Thomas cardioplegia compared to single dose in the neonatal rabbit [35], while Baker *et al.*, working with a similar neonatal rabbit heart model found a worse recovery of function with multiple rather than single dose St. Thomas cardioplegia [4]. Sawa and coworkers also found worse outcomes after multi-dose potassium cardioplegia than after single dose [52], and Clark *et al.*, found the best recovery of function after a single dose of 4°C potassium cardioplegia in the newborn piglet heart [32]. DeLeon and coworkers have reported no advantage to multiple doses of blood cardioplegia in children undergoing arterial switch operations [53]. These studies seem to indicate that as long as the heart remains arrested and hypothermic, additional doses of cardioplegia seem to be unnecessary and perhaps even detrimental.

Reperfusion

There is increasing evidence that events occurring during reperfusion may be equally important as those during ischemia in determining the ultimate outcome of an episode of ischemia/reperfusion. Interventions in the areas of substrate enhancement, free radical scavenging, control of perfusion pressure, and control of the introduction of oxygen have all been reported to enhance the recovery of function during reperfusion after ischemia.

Substrate enhancement

Ischemia clearly reduces the level of high energy phosphates in the myocardial cell, and there is some correlation between the levels of ATP and subsequent recovery during the reperfusion period both experimentally [2,9,32,54] and clinically [17,55]. Therefore, it has seemed logical to attempt to enhance the levels of high-energy phosphate precursors so that ATP levels can be readily restored or to provide metabolic substrates from which the high energy phosphates can be generated. The approach of preserving high energy phosphate precursors such as adenosine monophosphate or adenosine has not been evaluated in the immature heart, although there is evidence that adenosine monophosphate (AMP) levels are better preserved during ischemia in the immature heart compared to - the adult heart [9]. This better preservation of AMP during ischemia has been associated with the finding of a lower level of 5′nucleotidase, the enzyme which catalyzes the conversion of AMP to the much more diffusible metabolite adenosine, which can then be lost from the cell into the interstitial space. In mature hearts, there is some evidence that addition of adenosine to cardioplegia solutions [56,57] or its administration during reperfusion [58] may result in better recovery of ATP levels and function during post-ischemic recovery. Recently, we have found that an infusion of adenosine during the first 20 min of reperfusion in isolated neonatal lamb hearts subjected to two hours of hypothermic ischemia resulted in a marked improvement in both coronary blood flow and recovery of mechanical function (Nomura *et al.*, abstract accepted, American Heart Association meeting, 1992). An alternative approach which has been reported in a mature heart model is the provision of ribose and adenine during the post-ischemic period to serve as the substrate from which adenine nucleotides can be re-synthesized through the *de novo* pathway [59–61]. The rationale for the use of glucose in many cardioplegic solutions was to provide substrate which could be utilized by the ischemic cell, but as pointed out previously, multiple dose cardioplegia has been associated with either no improvement or worse outcome in the immature heart, despite providing more substrate for metabolism during ischemia. The approach of providing metabolic substrates which can then be metabolized to generate ATP has not been well studied in the immature heart until recently. Experiments in which the amino acids glutamate and aspartate have been added to the initial reperfusate after normothermic hypoxia in puppies have shown improvement in high energy phosphate levels and mechanical function [62], and the addition of glutamate and aspartate to hypothermic blood cardioplegia during 2 hours of ischemia has also been found to improve post-ischemic recovery [20]. These amino acids enter into the tricarboxylic acid (Krebs) cycle and ATP is then generated through oxidative phosphorylation.

Free radical scavengers

The observation that highly reactive oxygen species (free radicals), which have destructive effects on the cellular membrane, are generated during reperfusion after ischemia has led to experiments in which free radical formation is prevented or in which free radical 'scavenger' interventions are used. No experiments have been reported in which these types of interventions have been employed in the neonatal heart subjected to hypothermic ischemia. However, Otani *et al.* [16] have reported experiments in the neonatal piglet heart subjected to 60 min of normothermic ischemia which suggest that free radical formation was an important factor in the injury which occurred after this type of ischemia/reperfusion insult. The source of the free radicals in ischemia/reperfusion injury is also not completely resolved, and there has been recent interest in both white blood cells and the endothelium in this regard. The role of any or all of these free radical reducing strategies on the outcome of ischemia/reperfusion in the immature heart remains uncertain.

Oxygen

It is clear that oxygen must be re-introduced after ischemia in order to make the transition back into an oxidative metabolic state. In most clinical situations of surgically induced myocardial ischemia in which cardiopulmonary bypass is used, the restoration of blood flow to the heart after ischemia is accompanied by hyperoxia since the gas provided to the oxygenator of the cardiopulmonary bypass circuit is generally 95–100% oxygen. A recent set of experiments in our laboratory have raised concerns about reperfusion under these conditions of hyperoxia [63]. Isolated blood perfused neonatal lamb hearts underwent two hours of deeply hypothermic ischemia with cardioplegia and then were reperfused either with normoxic ($P_{02} = 200$ torr) or hyperoxic ($P_{02} = 540$ torr) blood for the first 10 min after ischemia. The hearts reperfused with normoxic blood achieved remarkably better recovery of mechanical function and, interestingly, also showed much better recovery of endothelial function as assessed by the vasodilator response to acetylcholine. The mechanisms underlying these effects of varying oxygen tension during reperfusion are not clear, but potential mechanisms may involve free radical formation by the myocytes or leukocytes or a direct vascular effect of hyperoxia, which is known to have a vasoconstrictor effect on systemic arteries. The potential clinical significance of this finding remains to be investigated.

Perfusion pressure

Stimulated by anecdotal clinical observations that high initial reperfusion pressures may be deleterious to the recovery of function after ischemia, a series of experiments in our laboratory have shown that in the isolated, blood-perfused neonatal lamb heart model, a protocol of low initial reperfusion pressure (20 mmHg for the first 10 min) followed by a gradual increase of pressure up to 60 mmHg during the remainder of reperfusion was associated with significant improvement in the recovery of mechanical function [64] and of coronary endothelial function [65]. Interestingly, this phenomenon of 'high' pressure reperfusion mechanical dysfunction could be blocked by the administration of either nitroglycerine or nifedipine during the early reperfusion period [64]. This observation along with the finding that the coronary blood flow was extremely high in the first few minutes of high pressure reperfusion [65] raise the possibility that the deleterious effect of high reperfusion pressure was related to excessive shear forces on the endothelium made 'vulnerable' by the period of ischemia. The use of vasodilator agents could possibly offset this effect by inducing maximal vasodilation and thereby reducing shear stress at the arteriolar and microcirculatory level. It is of interest that a number of pharmacologic agents which have been reported to improve the recovery of mechanical function after ischemia also have vasodilator activity. The mechanisms involved in this high pressure reperfusion injury remain under investigation, but it seems likely that the preservation of the vascular bed in general and the endothelium in particular will be important issues in the future.

Calcium

Although no studies have been carried out in the immature heart, an interesting study on 'calcium-induced reperfusion injury' was reported by Hamasaki and coworkers [66]. After 90 min of hypothermic arrest in isolated adult rat hearts, reperfusion at 37°C with normal calcium levels resulted in depressed functional recovery and significant creatine kinase losses. These effects were offset by initial reperfusion with hypocalcemic perfusate or by lowering the temperature of the reperfusate.

Clinically, we apply some, but not all, of these post-ischemic interventions. Perfusion pressures are kept low during the initial 5–10 min of reperfusion by use of phentolamine for alpha adrenergic blockade and by reducing the bypass flows until the heart resumes spontaneous contraction. Calcium concentration is not normalized until well into rewarming (rectal temperatures >28–30°C).

Summary

Although primary surgical repair of a variety of defects is now routinely carried out in neonates and infants, our understanding of the mechanisms of ischemic injury and its prevention in the immature heart remains incomplete. The advances in the preservation of the adult heart, especially hypothermic cardioplegic arrest, have provided remarkable improvement in the results of adult cardiac surgery, and we have all adopted them, in one form or another, for use in the immature heart. However, as our pediatrician colleagues are fond of saying, "The child is not a small adult". We must continue our effort to understand the effects of ischemia on the immature heart and to understand the effects of the interventions that we use in attempting to protect it during periods of surgically induce ischemia.

References

1. Haray I. Biochemistry of cardiac development. In Berne RM (ed): Handbopk of physiology, Section 2 – the cardiovascular system, Volume 1 – The Heart. Baltimore: Williams and Wilkins, 1979; 43–60.
2. Jarmakani JM, Nakazawa M, Nagatomo T *et al.* Effect of hypoxia on mechanical function in the neonatal mammalian heart. Am J Physiol 1978; 235(5): H469–H474.
3. Bove EL, Stammers AH. Recovery of left ventricular function after hypothermic global ischemia: Age-related differences in the isolated working rabbit heart. J Thorac Cardiovasc Surg 1986; 91: 115–22.
4. Baker JE, Boerboom LE, Olinger GN. Age-related changes in the ability of hypothermia and cardioplegia to protect ischemic rabbit myocardium. J Thorac Cardiovasc Surg 1988; 96: 717–24.
5. Bove EL, Gallahger KP, Drake DH *et al.* The effect of hypothermic ischemia on recovery of left ventricular function and preload reserve in the neonatal heart. J Thorac Cardiovasc Surg 1988; 95: 814–8.
6. Grice WN, Konishi T, Apstein CS *et al.* Resistance of neonatal myocardium to injury during normothermic and hypothermic ischemic arrest and reperfusion. Circulation 1987; 76(Suppl V): V150–V155.
7. Yano Y, Braimbridge MV, Hearse DJ: Protection of the pediatric myocardium. J Thorac Cardiovasc Surg 1987; 94: 887–96.
8. Avkiran M, Hearse DJ. Protection of the myocardium during global ischemia: Is crystalloid cardioplegia effective in the immature myocardium? J Thorac Cardiovasc Surg 1989; 97: 220–8.
9. Murphy CE, Salter DR, Morris JJ *et al.* Age-elated differences in adenine ‘ nucleotide metabolism during in vivo global ischemia. Surgical Forum 1986; 37: 288–90.
10. Young HH, Shimizu T, Nishioka K *et al.* Effect of hypoxia and reoxygenation on mitochondrial function in neonatal myocardium. Am J Physiol 1983; 245: H998–H1006.
11. Nishioka K, Jarmakani JM. Effect of ischemia on mechanical function and high-energy phosphates in rabbit myocardium. Am J Physiol 1982; 242: H1077–H1083.
12. Nishioka K, Nakanishi T, Jarmakani JM. Effect of ischemia on calcium exchange in the rabbit myocardium. Am J Physiol 1984; 247: H177–H184.
13. Julia PL, Kofsky ER, Buckberg GD *et al.* Studies of myocardial protection in the immature heart. J Thorac Cardiovasc Surg 1990; 100: 879–87.
14. Wittnich C, Peniston C, Ianuzzo D *et al.* Relative vulnerability of neonatal and adult hearts to ischemic injury. Circulation 1987; 76(Suppl V): V156–V160.
15. Chiu CJ, Bindon W. Why are newborn hearts vulnerable to global ischemia? Circulation 1987; 76(Suppl V): V146–V149.
16. Otani H, Engelman RM, Rousou JA *et al.* The mechanism of myocardial reperfusion injury in neonates. Circulation 1987; 76(Suppl V): V161–V167.
17. Bull CM, Cooper J, Stark J. Cardioplegic protection of the child's heart. J Thorac Cardiovasc Surg 1984; 88: 287–93.
18. Sawa Y, Matsuda H, Shimazaki Y *et al.* Ultrastructural assessment of the infant myocardium receiving crystalloid cardioplegia. Circulation 1987; 76(Suppl V): V141–V145.
19. Hewitt RL, Lolley DM, Adrouny GA *et al.* Protective effect of myocardial glycogen on cardiac function during anoxia. Surgery 1973; 73: 444–53.
20. Kofsky ER, Julia P, Buckberg GD *et al.* Studies of myocardial protection in the immature heart V. Safety of prolonged aortic clamping with hypocalcemic glutamate/aspartate blood cardioplegia. J Thorac Cardiovasc Surg 1991; 101: 33–43.
21. Bigelow WG, Callaghan JC, Hopps JA. General hypothermia for experimental intracardiac surgery. Ann Surg 1950; 132: 531–9.
22. Fujiwara T, Heinle J, Britton L *et al.* Myocardial Preservation in Neonatal Lambs: Comparison of Hypothermia with Crystalloid and Blood Cardioplegia. J Thorac Cardiovasc Surg 1991; 101: 703–12.

23. Buja LM, Chien KR, Burton KP *et al.* Membrane damage in schemia. Adv Exp Med Biol 1982; 161: 421–31.
24. Ferrari R, Raddino R, DiLisa F *et al.* Effects of temperature on myocardial calcium homeostasis and mitochondrial function during ischemia and reperfusion. J Thorac Cardiovasc Surg 1990; 99: 919–28.
25. Rich TL, Langer GA. Calcium depletion in rabbit myocardium: calcium paradox protection by hypothermia and cation substitution. Circ Res 1982; 51: 131–41.
26. Rebeyka IM, Diaz RJ, Augustine JM *et al.* Effect of rapid cooling contracture on ischemic tolerance in immature myocardium. Circulation 1991; 84(Suppl III): III-389–III-393.
27. Rebeyka IM, Hanan SA, Borges MR *et al.* Rapid cooling contracture of the myocardium. J Thorac Cardiovasc Surg 1990; 100: 240–9.
28. Williams WG, Rebeyka IM, Tibshirani RJ *et al.* Warm induction blood cardioplegia in the infant. J Thorac Cardiovasc Surg 1990; 100: 896–901.
29. Aoki M, Nomura F, Kawata H *et al.* Effect of calcium and preischemic hypothermia on recovery of myocardial function after cardioplegic ischemia in neonatal lambs. J Thorac Cardiovasc Surg 1993; 105: 207–13.
30. Laks H, Milliken J, Haas G *et al.* Myocardial protection in the neonatal heart. In Marcelletti C (ed): Pediatric cardiology. Edinburgh: Churchill Livingstone 1986: 13–26.
31. Baker JE, Boerboom LE, Olinger GN. Is protection of ischemic neonatal myocardium by cardioplegia species dependent?. J Thorac Cardiovasc Surg 1990; 99: 280–7.
32. Clark III BJ, Woodford EJ, Malec EJ *et al.* Effects of potassium cardioplegia on high-energy phosphate kinetics during circulatory arrest with deep hypothermia in the newborn piglet heart. J Thorac Cardiovasc Surg 1991; 101: 342–9.
33. Konishi T, Apstein CS. Comparison of three cardioplegic solutions during hypothermic ischemic arrest in neonatal blood-perfused rabbit hearts. J Thorac Cardiovasc Surg 1989; 98: 1132–7.
34. Diaco M, DiSesa VJ, Sun SC *et al.* Cardioplegia for the immature myocardium. J Thorac Cardiovasc Surg 1990; 100: 910–3.
35. Bove EL, Stammers AH, Gallagher KP. Protection of the neonatal myocardium during hypothermic ischemia: Effect of cardioplegia on left ventricular function in the rabbit. J Thorac Cardiovasc Surg 1987; 94: 115–23.
36. Fujiwara T, Kurtts T, Anderson W. Myocardial protection in cyanotic neonatal lambs. J Thorac Cardiovasc Surg 1988; 96: 700–10.
37. Aoki M, Kawata H, Mayer JE Jr. Coronary endothelial injury by cold crystalloid cardioplegic solution in neonatal lambs. Circulation 1992; 86: II-346–II-352.
38. Corno AF, Bathencourt DM, Laks H *et al.* Myocardial protection in the neonatal heart. J Thorac Cardiovasc Surg 1987; 93: 163–72.
39. Digerness SB, Vanini V, Wideman FE. *In vitro* comparison of oxygen availability from asanguinous and sanguinous cardioplegic media. Circulation 1981; 64(Suppl II): II80–II83.
40. Suaudeau J, Shaffer B, Daggett WM *et al.* Role of procaine and washed red cells in the isolated dog heart perfused at 5 degrees C. J Thorac Cardiovasc Surg 1982; 84: 886–96.
41. Bodenhamer RM, DeBoer WV, Geffin GA *et al.* Enhanced myocardial protection during ischemic arrest. J Thorac Cardiovasc Surg 1983; 85: 769–80.
42. Randolph JD, Toal KW, Geffin GA *et al.* Improved myocardial preservation with oxygenated cardioplegic solutions as reflected by on-line monitoring Qf intramyocardial pH during arrest. J Vasc Surg 1986; 3: 216–25.
43. Hendren WG, Geffin GA, Love TR *et al.* Oxygenation of cardioplegic solutions. J Thorac Cardiovasc Surg 1987; 94: 614–25.
44. Yamamoto F, Braimbridge MV, Hearse DJ *et al.* Calcium and cardioplegia: The optimal calcium content for the St. Thomas' Hospital cardioplegic solution. J Thorac Cardiovasc Surg 1984; 87: 908–12.
45. Robinson LA, Harwood DL. Lowering the calcium concentration in St. Thomas' Hospital cardioplegic solution improves protection during hypothermic ischemia. J Thorac Cardiovasc Surg 1991; 101: 314–25.

46. Torchiana DF, Love TR, Hendren WG *et al.* Calcium-induced ventricular contraction during cardioplegic arrest. J Thorac Cardiovasc Surg 1987; 94: 606–13.
47. Gerrin GA, Love TR, Hendren WG *et al.* The effects of calcium and magnesium in hyperkalemic cardioplegic solutions on myocardial preservation. J Thorac Cardiovasc Surg 1989; 98: 239–50.
48. Boggs BR, Torchiana DF, Geffin GA *et al.* Optimal myocardial preservation with an acalcemic crystalloid cardi oplegic solution. J Thorac Cardiovasc Surg 1987; 93: 838–46.
49. Bing OHL, LaRaia PJ, Franklin A *et al.* Myocardial protection utilizing calcium containing and calcium free perfusates. Basic Res Cardiol 1985; 80: 399–406.
50. Caspi J, Herman SL, Coles JG *et al.* Effects of low perfusate Ca^{2+} concentration on newborn myocardial function after ischemia. Circulation 1990; 82, (Suppl IV): IV-371–IV-379.
51. Konishi T, Apstein CS. Deleterious effects of digitalis on newborn rabbit myocardium after simulated cardiac surgery. J Thorac Cardiovasc Surg 1991; 101: 337–41.
52. Sawa Y, Matsuda H, Shimazaki Y *et al.* Comparison of single dose versus multiple dose crystalloid cardioplegia in neonate: Experimental study with neonatal rabbits from birth to 2 days of age. J Thorac Cardiovasc Surg 1989; 97: 229–34.
53. DeLeon SY, Idriss FS, Ilbawi MN *et al.* Comparison of single versus Multidose blood cardioplegia in arterial switch procedures. Ann Thorac Surg 1988; 45: 548–53.
54. Starnes VA, Hammon Jr JW, Lupinetti FM *et al.* Functional and metabolic preservation of immature myocardium with Verapamil following global ischemia. Ann Thorac Surg 1982; 34: 58–65.
55. Hammon Jr JW, Graham Jr TP, Boucek Jr RJ *et al.* Myocardial Adenosine triphosphate content as a measure of metabolic and functional myocardial protection in children undergoing cardiac operation. Ann Thorac Surg 1987; 44: 467–70.
56. Bolling SF, Bies LE, Gallagher KP *et al.* Enhanced myocardial protection with Adenosine. Ann Surg 89; 47: 809–15.
57. De Jong JW, VanderMeer P, van Loon H *et al.* Adenosine as adjunct to potassium cardioplegia: Effect on function, energy metabolism, and electrophysiology. J Thorac Cardiovasc Surg 1990; 100: 445–54.
58. Pitarys CJ, Virmani R, Vildibill HD *et al.* Reduction of myocardial reperfusion injury by intravenous adenosine administered during the early reperfusion period. Circulation 1991; 83: 237–47.
59. StCyr JA, Bianco RW, Schneider JR *et al.* Enhanced high energy phosphate recovery with ribose infusion after global myocardial ischemia in a canine model. J Surg Res 1989; 46: 157–62.
60. Foker JE, Einzig S, Wang T *et al.* Adenosine metabolism and myocardial preservation. J Thorac Cardiovasc Surg 1980; 80: 506–16.
61. Ward HB, StCyr JA, Cogorgan JA *et al.* Recovery of adenine nucleotide levels after global myocardial ischemia in dogs. Surgery 1984; 248–55.
62. Julia P, Young HH, Buckberg GD *et al.* Studies of myocardial protection in the immature heart IV. Improved tolerance of immature myocardium to hypoxia and ischemia by intravenous metabolic support. J Thorac Cardiovasc Surg 1991; 101: 23–32.
63. Sawatari K, Kawata H, Assad RS *et al.* Effects of PO_2 level during initial reperfusion after hypothermic cardioplegia in neonatal lambs. Circulation 1990; 82(Suppl III): III-146.
64. Fujiwara T, Kurtts T, Silvera M *et al.* Physical and pharmacological manipulation of reperfusion conditions in neonatal myocardial preservation. Circulation 1988; 78(Suppl II): II-444.
65. Sawatari K, Kadoba K, Bergner KA *et al.* Influence of reperfusion pressure after hypothermic cardioplegia on endothelial modulation of coronary tone in neonatal lambs: impaired coronary vasodilator response to Acetycholine. J Thorac Cardiovasc Surg 1991; 101: 777–82.
66. Hamasaki T, Duroda H, Mori T. Temperature dependency of calcium-induced reperfusion injury in the isolated rat heart. Ann Thorac Surg 1988; 45: 306–10.

PART FOUR

Evaluation of cardioplegic methodology

13. High-energy phosphates and their catabolites

JAN WILLEM DE JONG, TOM HUIZER, MAARTEN JANSSEN, ROB KRAMS, MONIQUE TAVENIER, and PIETER D. VERDOUW

"Energy is Eternal Delight"
William Blake (1757–1827)
The Voice of the Devil

Introduction

In this chapter we put emphasis on the use of high-energy phosphates and their breakdown products to characterize the metabolic status of the heart before, during and after cardiac surgery. We address the relationship between these compounds and cardiac function, e.g. during stunning. In addition we describe their role for cardioprotection, e.g. during cardioplegia.

Energy metabolism

High-energy phosphates are energy-rich molecules such as phosphoenolpyruvate, phosphoglyceroyl phosphate, phosphocreatine, ATP and ADP. The free energy, ΔG, liberated from these molecules by hydrolysis of an anhydride bond, supports energetically unfavorable reactions. Dependent on the standard-free-energy change ΔG^0, these compounds release more or less energy. As discussed below, ATP, phosphocreatine and phosphoenolpyruvate are useful for therapeutic and/or diagnostic purposes. Figure 13.1 shows the formation and breakdown of purine and pyrimidine 5′-triphosphates. Adenine nucleotides play an important role storing and transferring metabolically available energy. ATP is the most important carrier of free energy ($\Delta G^0 = -7.3$ kcal mol^{-1}). Phosphocreatine, with a higher standard-free-energy change (-10.3 kcal mol^{-1}), can transfer its phosphoryl group to ADP, generating ATP. In this way ATP shuttles between the mitochondria, where it is synthesized from ADP by oxidative phosphorylation, and the myofibrils, where it delivers energy for contraction.

Anaerobic metabolism can also generate ATP, but it produces only 3 moles of ATP for every mole of glucose metabolized, compared with 38 moles generated by aerobic metabolism. The heart uses its ATP at a rapid rate. Mechanically quiescent hearts consume approximately 10 μmol ATP min^{-1} g wet weight^{-1} to maintain ionic homeostasis. A heart rate of 75 beats min^{-1} requires another 23 μmol min^{-1} g^{-1}. Thus, per beat the heart uses

H.M. Piper and C.J. Preusse (eds): Ischemia-reperfusion in cardiac surgery, 295–315.

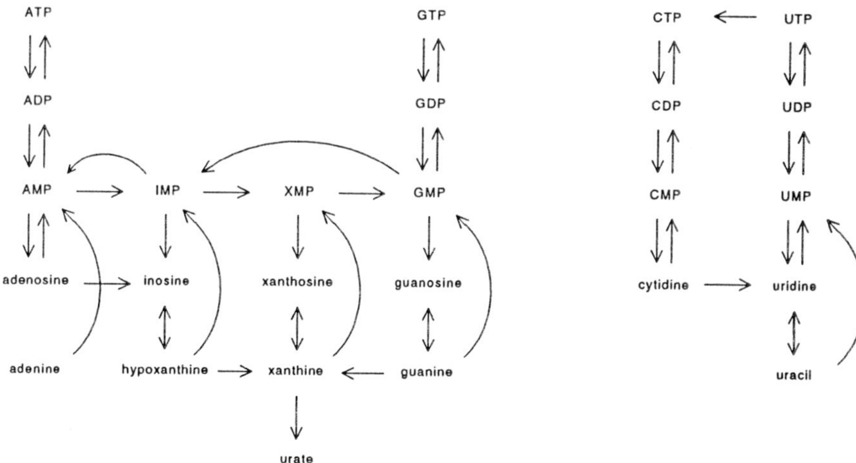

Figure 13.1. Formation and breakdown of high-energy phosphates. Cardiac AMP formation from IMP takes places via adenylosuccinate. Direct GMP formation from guanosine by adenosine kinase or (low activity) guanosine kinase is not unlikely [1].

about 5% of its energy stores. (This organ can store up to 5–6 μmol g^{-1}.) Some energy reserve is available from phosphocreatine but this suffices only for a few minutes [2].

Other high-energy compounds, such as GTP, UTP and CTP, drive several biosynthetic reactions; their concentration is $\leqslant$5% of that of ATP. UTP is the immediate phosphate donor for many reactions leading to polysaccharide synthesis. CTP is the energy donor in lipid biosynthesis. We were unable to locate any literature data on cardiac XTP and ITP.

Catabolism

During hypoxia, abundant myocardial ATPase activity ensures the rapid breakdown of ATP to ADP, with subsequent catabolism to AMP by the myokinase reaction. Adenosine 5′-monophosphate is not a high-energy phosphate because its dephosphorylation by 5′-nucleotidase to the regulatory metabolite adenosine produces relatively little energy ($\Delta G^0 = -3.4$ kcal mol^{-1}). The alternative pathway, deamination to IMP (see Figure 13.1), is relatively inactive in heart muscle, but its postulated role is preservation of the purine ring inside myocytes (as nondiffusable IMP) [3]. Breakdown of adenosine depends on the ubiquitous adenosine deaminase. Little is known about 5′-nucleotidase and adenosine deaminase in human myocardium; their cardiac activities vary considerably among species [4]. The activity of 5′-nucleotidase is lower in ventricles than in atria accompanied with a transmural distribution across the left ventricle wall, with the highest values in the subepicardial and the subendocardial regions [5]. During ischemia 5′-nucleotidase activity decreases, whereas adenosine deaminase activity increases [6]. Purine nucleoside phosphorylase provides hypoxanthine, the substrate for the xanthine oxidoreductase reaction, which catalyzes the breakdown of hypoxanthine to xanthine and urate. Histochemical studies of xanthine oxidoreductase in human, bovine and rat myocardial tissue have revealed its localization in the endothelial cells [7,8]. During ischemia and reperfusion, proteases convert the native form of the enzyme, xanthine dehydrogenase, to the oxyradical-generating oxidase form. Reported activities in human myocardium vary from high [7,9] to very low [10–13]. Various tissue sources and assay techniques, as well as self-inactivation [14], could explain these large differences. In patients undergoing coronary angioplasty, we observed urate release [15], an indication of active xanthine oxidoreductase. However, our group found also that explanted (diseased) human hearts, perfused with hypoxanthine, released little urate [16]. Urate production during angioplasty and heart surgery might come from extracardiac factors like neutrophils or other blood components. This could explain the difference found between clinical studies [13,15] and ex vivo studies with blood-free solutions [16]. Although the sum of the literature data suggests that human myocardium is almost devoid of xanthine oxidoreductase, we cannot exclude the possibility that a desulpho form – which is inactive with hypoxanthine and xanthine – generates oxyradicals (cf. [17]).

High-energy phosphates as markers of ischemia

In animal studies, but also in clinical work, high-energy phosphates have been used to characterize the metabolic status of the heart. Analysis of ATP and phosphocreatine takes place in biopsies frozen immediately in liquid nitrogen. The presence of blood makes it difficult to distinguish between myocardial and erythrocyte adenine nucleotides. In deproteinized samples the compounds of interest can be determined with HPLC, phospholuminescence, and other sensitive techniques. Usually the data are expressed on a non-collagen protein basis. Magnetic resonance spectroscopy (see next subsection) offers an alternative to the chemical analysis of high-energy phosphates.

In anesthetized dogs, circumflex occlusion gives rise to myocardial adenine nucleotide breakdown and accumulation of nucleosides and bases [18]. ATP depletion is more rapid in the endocardial layers. Quite a few authors measured myocardial high-energy phosphates to study the efficacy of calcium antagonists as adjuncts to cardioplegia (for review, see [19]). In coronary-bypass patients, the adenylate and phosphocreatine contents decrease substantially in the infarcting heart; in patients without infarction, severe stenosis of the left anterior descending coronary artery results in myocardial dysfunction associated with adenylate pool depletion, but mitochondrial function remains intact [20].

Magnetic resonance spectroscopy

Slowly nuclear magnetic resonance (NMR) spectroscopy finds its way into the heart clinic. The technique has the advantage of *non-invasive* assessment of high-energy phosphates, inorganic phosphate and pH, but it is insensitive and expensive. In addition, blood contribution to cardiac NMR spectra, e.g. from the ventricular cavities, is a potential problem. Using surface-coils on rat and dog hearts, various investigators [21–23] showed that changes in high-energy phosphate metabolism could predict rejection of heterotopic cardiac allografts. Bottomley *et al.* [24] found that patients with heart transplants had a 20% lower ratio of anterior myocardial phosphocreatine to ATP compared with that of healthy control subjects. Ratios of phosphocreatine to inorganic phosphate also appeared lower whenever detectable. The authors concluded, however, that ^{31}P-NMR spectroscopy did not permit reliable identification of patients who required augmented therapy for rejection. Nevertheless regular monitoring post-transplantation, using patients as their own control, might be useful. The same group demonstrated that resting humans with ischemic and idiopathic dilated cardiomyopathy have also reduced myocardial phosphocreatine/ATP ratios [25]. The investigators corrected their ^{31}P-spectra for contaminating blood components.

Purines as markers of ischemia

One can measure the catabolites of high-energy phosphates in biopsies or in myocardial effluent. In patients undergoing bypass grafting, Flameng *et al.* [20] observed that nucleosides, in particular inosine, accumulated in the infarcting heart. During heart surgery, Smoleński *et al.* [13,26] measured substantial increases in adenosine, inosine and hypoxanthine in coronary effluent collected during subsequent infusions of cardioplegic fluid into the coronary root. They did not detect xanthine, and attributed the release of urate to washout of this oxypurine accumulated in the myocardium [13]. The much higher release of purines (and lactate as well as phosphate) in children as opposed to adults provides evidence for more severe metabolic injury during cardioplegic arrest to the juvenile heart [26].

Inhibitors of purine catabolism/uptake

Adenosine deaminase inhibitors

Prevention of adenosine catabolism is insufficient for adequate (rat) ventricular recovery unless tissue [ATP] remains above about 1.0 μmol g^{-1}. Erythro-9-(2-hydroxy-3-nonyl)adenine (EHNA) + adenosine (low Ca^{2+}) conserve ATP, improve functional recovery of hearts markedly, and thus may play a role to play in myocardial preservation during elective cardiac arrest [27] (cf. Table 13.1).

Table 13.1. "Purine blockers" used adjunctive to potassium cardioplegia.

Compound	Mode of action	Effect	Reference
EHNA Deoxycoformycin	ADA inhibition	>Function recovery; (>ATP)	[28–30]
Allopurinol Oxypurinol	XO inhibition; radical scavenging?	<CK release; >function recovery	[31–35]
R75231 Dipyridamole NBMPR Mioflazine Lidoflazine Dilazep	Nucleoside transport inhibition (anti-platelet aggregation; Ca^{2+}-entry blockade; vasodilation?)	>Heart transplantation; <ventricular fibrillation; >function recovery	[36–40]

Abbreviations: ADA, adenosine deaminase; CK, creatine kinase; EHNA, erythro-9-(2-hydroxy-3-nonyl)adenine; NBMPR, 6-[(4-nitrobenzyl)-mercapto]purine ribonucleoside; XO, xanthine oxidase.

Xanthine oxidase inhibitors

Allopurinol and its catabolite oxypurinol are xanthine oxidase inhibitors, useful to prevent damage by free radicals. Table 13.1 shows that these inhibitors, administered during potassium cardioplegia, improve function and metabolism. Addition of allopurinol to blood cardioplegia increases function in severely ischemic dog ventricles [41]. Allopurinol and oxypurinol also improve function when given during reperfusion of rabbit hearts [42], with varying results in rat hearts [32,43]. This is surprising, because rabbit (and human) hearts seem devoid of xanthine oxidoreductase, in contrast to rat hearts [16]; allopurinol may be effective, because it is a weak radical scavenger. Allopurinol pretreatment of donor dogs diminishes malondialdehyde production, which is an indicator of free radical generation; concomitantly function of the transplanted hearts improves [44] (cf. [45]). The drug is present in the University of Wisconsin cardioplegic solution (see below). In patients undergoing coronary artery bypass grafting, allopurinol as adjunct to cardioplegia reduces the number of chromosomal aberrations found after crossclamping by 60% [46]. In some studies pretreatment with the drug decreases drastically enzyme release and the incidence of cardiac complications in heart surgery [47–49]. However, the effect of allopurinol and oxypurinol on infarct size is variable (for review, see [50]), and may depend on the efficiency of myocardial protection with cardioplegia and cooling [51] Allopurinol increases hyperemic flow after embolization [52]. The literature data leave the overall impression that allopurinol is useful for cardioprotection during heart surgery.

Nucleoside transport blockers

Dipyridamole blocks the (re)uptake of adenosine. By raising local plasma concentrations of this nucleoside, it reduces arrhythmias due to ischemia and reperfusion in dogs [53]. It also reduces platelet activation and depletion during bypass surgery [54]. Another blocker, 6-[(4-nitrobenzyl)-mercapto]-purine ribonucleoside (NBMPR), in combination with EHNA, protects against ATP depletion and heart function loss due to ischemia in a canine model [55]. Yet other blockers, including R75231, appear useful as adjunct to potassium cardioplegia (Table 13.1). Using dogs, Flameng *et al.* [36] assessed the effect of nucleoside transport inhibition with R75321 in the cardioplegic fluid on 24 hour's preservation of donor hearts for transplantation. Serial transmural left-ventricular biopsies revealed moderate ATP catabolism during cold storage in the control group. On reperfusion ATP content declined further, accompanied with washout of the accumulated nucleosides. In the treated group, ATP breakdown was similar during cold storage and continued up to 1 hour after reperfusion. The nucleosides adenosine and inosine, however, did not wash out. ATP content recovered completely after 2 hours of reperfusion. Nucleoside transport blockers as cardioprotectants deserve more attention.

Pyrimidines as markers of ischemia

Much more is known about purine metabolism than about pyrimidine metabolism. Pyrimidine nucleotide breakdown in ischemic myocardium seems to parallel degradation of adenylates [56,57]. We reported recently that during heart transplantation procedures the uridine content in human donor myocardium increases during cold storage; during reperfusion, after aorta declamping, the implanted heart also releases uridine. During corrections of congenital or acquired heart defects, we observed a continuous degradation of uridine nucleotides in the ischemic myocardium [58]. Isolated, perfused human hearts release uridine, rat hearts uracil, as the end product of ischemic pyrimidine nucleotide breakdown. It follows that uridine phosphorylase activity in human heart is very low compared to rat heart. This agrees with the activity of the enzyme measured in homogenates of rat and human heart, 153 and 2.7 mU g wet weight^{-1}, respectively [58]. The opposite is true for another catabolic enzyme, cytidine deaminase, which is responsible for the production of uridine. Its activity is 14 mU g^{-1} in human heart and <1.0 mU g^{-1} in rat heart [59]. In rat and human heart, release of uracil and uridine is a potential marker for ischemia, respectively.

Cardiac energetics and function

Correlation between ATP content and function

During prolonged ischemia, myocardial high-energy phosphate content will decrease. The extent of this reduction depends on the duration of ischemia. Several studies show a good correlation between myocardial ATP content

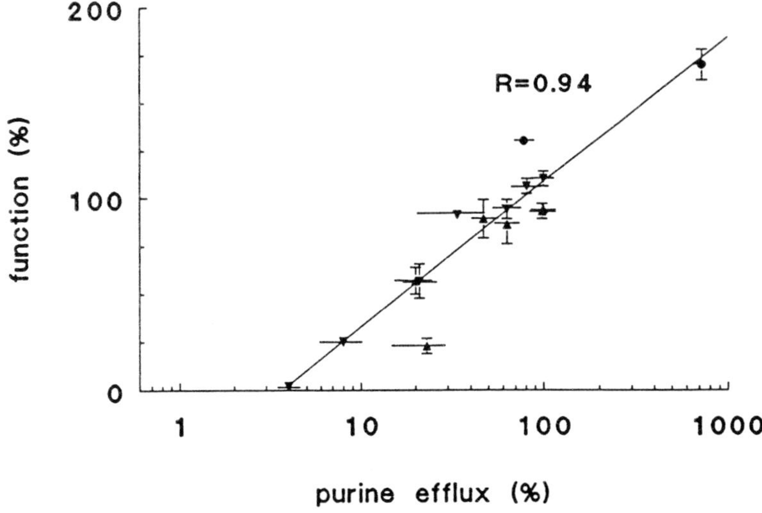

Figure 13.2. Correlation between *normoxic* function and *ischemic* energy metabolism. Data were obtained in rat hearts perfused according to Langendorff [66,67]. The figure shows that cardioprotection before ischemia is imperative. Closed dots: 5.0 and 1.4 mM $CaCl_2$ in perfusion medium. ▲ and ▼: various concentrations of bepridil and nisoldipine in the perfusion medium, respectively. Each point shows the mean of 4–6 observations; vertical and horizontal lines indicate s.e.m. Function 100% = function of untreated hearts; purine efflux 100% = efflux of untreated hearts. From [68].

and cardiac function [60–62]. However, in some experimental models, an acceptable myocardial performance takes place at seriously deprived [ATP] [63–65]. Until the early eighties, biochemical recovery from myocardial ischemia was assumed to be complete within a short period. However, Reimer *et al.* [62] demonstrated that it takes at least a week to regenerate myocardial nucleotides lost during ischemia. The phenomenon 'myocardial stunning', the temporary incomplete recovery of function in reperfused heart, seems to confirm the importance of metabolic recovery (see next subsection).

Figure 13.2 shows that myocardial function *before* ischemia determines ATP breakdown *during* ischemia. We calculated whether decreased purine efflux from the heart reflected better preservation of myocardial ATP or resulted from reduced membrane permeability. The close correlation between ATP loss and purine efflux confirmed a lower ATP breakdown. We speculate that during heart surgery hypothermia and chemical arrest contribute to the efficacy of cardioplegic solutions through the phenomenon described in Figure 13.2.

Cardiac function and ATP during stunning

After brief periods of ischemia cardiac function remains depressed for hours to days, while tissue necrosis is undetectable [69]. This is a clinical entity often observed after coronary angioplasty, silent ischemia and cardioplegia. To explain the relatively long depression of cardiac function, obtained after one occlusion in animal experiments, Heyndrickx *et al.* [70] postulated that the decreased ATP synthesis rate became the rate-limiting step in ATP delivery to the contractile machinery. They based this hypothesis on the relationship between depression in intracellular [ATP] and duration of occlusion; the former changes in concert with severity of cardiac dysfunction [61]. Furthermore, regeneration of nucleotides from purines and de novo synthesis is slow (for review, see [71]), which could account for the slow return of cardiac function. Some fundamental, theoretical arguments do not support this hypothesis: (1) The [ATP] not necessarily reflects the ATP-turnover rate (balance between ATP-synthesis and hydrolysis), but merely the cellular outward diffusion of catabolites from ATP like adenosine, inosine and hypoxanthine (see section on Catabolism). (2) The myofibrils have a low K_m-value for ATP [72], which implies that the [ATP] has to decrease to very low values before it becomes the rate-limiting step in cross-bridge cycling and therefore in cardiac function. Literature estimates indicate that developed left-ventricular pressure is independent of the [ATP] unless it falls to values <50% of normal [64,73]; such low values are rare during brief periods of ischemia and subsequent reperfusions. In addition a considerable body of evidence also argues against a role of a decreased rate of ATP synthesis as a cause of myocardial stunning. Phosphocreatine increases immediately and transiently upon reperfusion, indicating the quickly restored capability of the mitochondria to rephosphorylate creatine after reinstitution of blood supply [74]. Several authors have challenged the stunned myocardium by inotropic stimulation [75–79]. They showed invariably that inotropic stimulation can recruit cardiac function, thereby indirectly confirming that the ATP-synthesis rate is not the rate-limiting step. Cardiac function did not deteriorate after withdrawal of the inotropic agent and the [ATP] did not decrease during stimulation, suggesting that the increase of ATP-synthesis rate during inotropic stimulation matches the myofibrillar ATP-hydrolysis rate [75].

Since these arguments are rather qualitative, there was a need for further support. A modified ^{31}P-NMR technique, which enabled the simultaneous measurement of the net ATP production rate [80] and myocardial O_2-consumption (MVO_2), provided non-invasively data on phosphorylation efficacy in the post-ischemic myocardium. These were similar to those in control hearts, indicating unchanged efficiency of the Krebs-cycle, despite a 50% reduction in [ATP] [80]. However, in that study MVO_2 was normal, notwithstanding depressed cardiac function. The relatively high MVO_2 indicates a high ATP turnover, whereby conversion to mechanical energy fails to take place (see below). Unfortunately during most of the *in vivo* experiments, MVO_2 has not been measured during inotropic stimulation. Furthermore, *in vivo*, cardiac function is often assessed by systolic segment-length shortening or systolic wall thickening. These indexes of cardiac function are highly

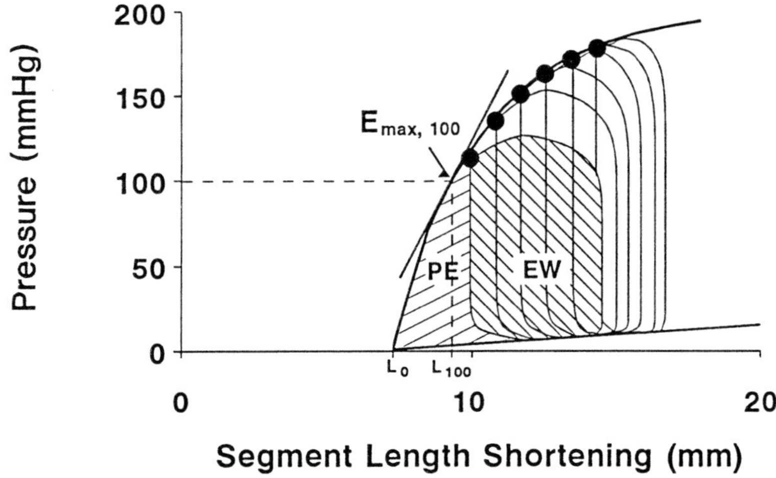

Figure 13.3. Theoretical graph illustrating the calculations possible by applying the time-varying elastance concept [81]: PLA = PE + EW and EET = EW/PLA (see section on Purines as markers of ischemia). $E_{max,100}$ (mmHg min^{-1}) is the index of contractility at 100 mmHg. Together with segment shortening at 0 and 100 mmHg (L_0 and L_{100}, respectively), it describes the end-systolic pressure-length relation ESPLR. PE is the area of the triangle below the ESPLR. Abbreviations: PLA, pressure-length area; PE, potential energy; EW, external work; EET, efficiency of energy transfer.

load-dependent. Coupling of inotropic recruitment and ATP-turnover are therefore debatable.

These combined theoretical and experimental arguments strongly suggest a relationship between decreased function of post-ischemic myocardium and defective ATP-utilization [74], rather than impaired ATP synthesis.

To avoid load-dependent indexes of myocardial contractile function, we have applied the time-varying elastance concept, introduced by Suga and Sagawa for the whole heart [81], to regionally stunned myocardium of open-chest pigs. This approach allows, besides the determination of a load-independent index of contractility (E_{max}), also the calculation of external work (EW), potential energy (PE, see Figure 13.3) together with the pressure-length area (PLA = EW + PE) and the efficiency of energy transfer (EET = EW/PLA*100%). E_{max}, PLA and basal metabolism are the major determinants of MVO_2 [81,82]. Myocardial stunning does not affect the basal metabolic rate, which implies that changes in E_{max} and PLA are responsible for alterations in MVO_2. By relating changes in these compounds to those in MVO_2 before and after inotropic stimulation with dobutamine, we obtained a better insight into the mechanism underlying the disturbance of ATP-utilization. The stunned myocardium, induced by 2 periods of 10–min occlusion and 30 min of reperfusion, showed decreased contractility (50% decrease of E_{max}) in accordance with the postulated decrease of myofibrillar

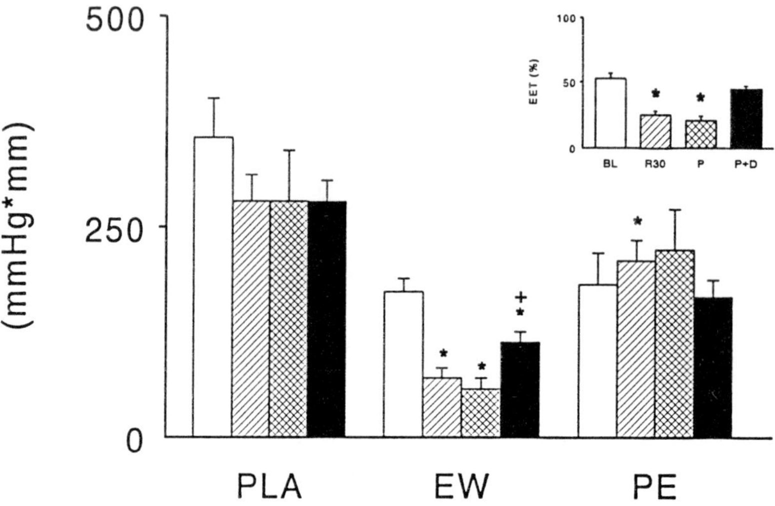

Figure 13.4. Results of the mechanical determinants, pressure-length area (PLA), external work (EW), potential energy (PE); and the resulting efficiency of energy transfer (EET, inset) in stunned swine myocardium. Open bars: baseline (BL); hatched bars: after 30 min of reperfusion (R30); crosshatched bars: after atrial pacing (P); filled bars: after pacing plus inotropic stimulation with dobutamine (P + D). $^{*}p < 0.05$ vs baseline; $^{+}p < 0.05$ vs pacing. The difference between pacing alone and pacing plus dobutamine is due to pure inotropic effects of the drug. Mean ± s.e.m., n = 10.

Ca^{2+}-sensitivity [83], and decreased MVO_2 (a 33% drop). Due to the decrement in contractility, external work decreased [81,82]. Because of the regional nature of the stunning protocol, end-systolic pressure changed little, however. Consequently end-systolic segment length increased. As a result PE rose, thereby counterbalancing the decrease in EW (Figure 13.4). Since PE is not used for pump function and PE eventually degrades to heat, the efficiency of energy transfer fell from 55% to 25% (Figure 13.4, inset). Thus, not only MVO_2 and therefore ATP-utilization decreased, but also ATP proved to be converted less efficiently. During dobutamine infusion contractility (E_{max}) of the stunned myocardium recovered, in addition to a return to baseline of PLA and its distribution in EW and PE (and thus EET). In concert with these mechanical parameters, MVO_2 normalized, indicating that ATP-utilization and mechanical function were still matched during inotropic stimulation of the stunned myocardium. One must keep in mind, however, that dobutamine induced a 20% drop in peripheral vascular resistance, possibly contributing to the beneficial effects.

Nevertheless, our data indicate that in the stunned myocardium contractility and EW are reduced to lower MVO_2, thereby redistributing its available cellular energy to processes that keep cellular integrity intact [74]. As a consequence, however, PE increases, offsetting the benefit of decreased contractility plus EW and reduced efficiency of energy transfer. The balance

Table 13.2. High-energy phosphates used adjunctive to potassium cardioplegia.

Compound	Mode of action	Effect	Reference
ATP Phosphocreatine (Phosphoenol- pyruvate)	Membrane stabilization; energy donor??	>Function recovery; >ATP; >phosphocreatine; <CK release; >birefringerence	[38,87–104]

Abbreviation: CK, creatine kinase.

between the decrease of contractility plus EW and the increase of PE determines whether MVO_2 changes; it potentially explains the variability of MVO_2 in stunned myocardium reported [84–86]. Reversibility of the process was confirmed by the short-lasting inotropic stimulation with dobutamine. Apparently inotropic stimulation with dobutamine overrides the energetic down-regulation of the contractile machinery, without an extra need for energy requirements. Inotropic stimulation up to 1 hour is without unwanted side effects [74]; it is questionable whether longer periods of stimulation do not induce tissue necrosis.

Anabolism

High-energy phosphates

The alleged protective properties of extracellular high-energy phosphates are controversial [38]. Table 13.2 lists the effects seen after the use of ATP, phosphocreatine and phosphoenolpyruvate for cardioprotection. ATP and phosphocreatine seem to be useful for post-ischemic recovery [87,91,105], the latter possibly also in man [88,90,94,99] (but see [89,106]). Their mechanism of action remains to be elucidated, but it is unlikely that direct uptake of these compounds by the cardiomyocyte takes place. The effect of phosphoenolpyruvate is unclear [102,107–109]. Exogenous ATP suppresses supraventricular tachycardias in patients [110].

High-energy precursors

Adenosine. Figure 13.5 depicts the role of (endogenous) adenosine in the energy demand/supply balance. Adenosine given during normoxic perfusion in Langendorff rat hearts increases tissue ATP and phosphocreatine but does not affect post-ischemic functional recovery or ATP [112]. Adenosine alone or adjunctive to high potassium cardioplegia arrests rat hearts quicker [29,113], which seems advantageous. It is, however, ineffective in arresting fibrillating baboon hearts [114]. Recently, we observed that adenosine, added to St. Thomas' Hospital cardioplegic solution at concentrations of 0.05, 0.5 and 5 mM did not improve high-energy phosphate metabolism in working

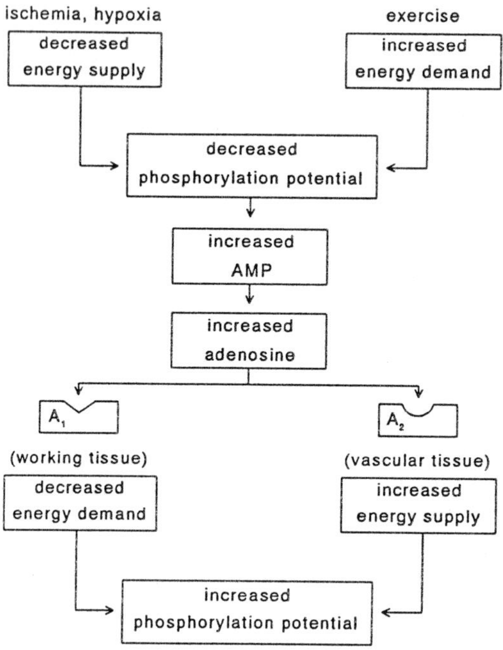

Figure 13.5. Role of (endogenous) adenosine in the energy demand/supply balance. A_1 and A_2 depict adenosine receptors. Adapted from [111].

rat hearts. However, the lower two concentrations improved recovery of function (Huizer *et al.*, unpublished observations). Table 13.3 shows that the nucleoside, given adjunctive to potassium cardioplegia, improves functional recovery under various experimental conditions. Concomitant inhibition of adenosine deamination could be beneficial [28].

Adenosine is one of the many ingredients of the University of Wisconsin cardioplegic solution. It has provided excellent preservation for the pancreas, kidney, and liver after extended cold ischemic storage times [119]. The solution may be useful for heart transplantation as well [119–121] (but see [122]); studies are underway to determine whether adenosine (and other components) are essential for its cardioprotective action [123]. Adenosine administration during reperfusion increases rabbit- and canine-heart ATP content, without concomitant improvement in contractility [124,125]. The opposite is true in rat heart [126]. Through receptor activation, the nucleoside may play a role in "preconditioning" [127–130]. It reduces infarct size and improves regional ventricular function in the ischemic zone in dogs [131–133]. A raised local plasma adenosine concentration reduces the incidence and severity of the life-threatening ischemia/reperfusion arrhythmias [110]. However, the intravenous infusion of adenosine in man provokes angina-like chest pain [134,135].

Table 13.3. ATP-precursors used adjunctive to potassium cardioplegia.

Compound	Mode of action	Effect	Reference
Adenosine	Hyperpolarization; nucleotide synthesis; vasodilation; adrenergic modulation	Quicker arrest; >function recovery; >ATP	[28,29,38,114,115]
Inosine	Salvage pathway; vasodilation??	>Function recovery; >ATP	[116]
AICAr	De novo nucleotide synthesis? adenosine production	>Function recovery; >ATP	[117]
Ribose (+purines)	Through PRPP?	>ATP	[118]

Abbreviations: AICAr, 5-amino-1-β-D-ribofuranosylimidazole-4-carboxamide riboside; PRPP, α-5-phosphoribosyl-1-pyrophosphate.

Adenosine catabolites. Inosine enhances reperfusion ATP [136,137]. Addition of inosine to the reperfusion fluid as well as the cardioplegic solution further improves nucleotide levels and recovery of cardiac output [116] (Table 13.3). Urate, produced by the heart of many species [16], is a radical scavenger [138]; it protects against reperfusion damage. Of course its plasma concentration in man is already very high, in comparison to that of other species.

De novo synthesis of purines. Post-ischemic administration of acadesine (AICAr = 5-amino-1-β-D-ribofuranosylimidazole-4-carboxamide riboside, see Figure 13.6), which can be metabolized to ATP and GTP via IMP, does not increase rabbit-heart ATP or contractility [124]. AICAr pretreatment augments adenosine release from ischemic canine heart nearly 10-fold, accompanied by increased collateral blood flow and decreased arrhythmias [139,140]. In a similar set-up, AICAr does not change cardiac adenine nucleotide, but it increases IMP content 13– to 25-fold, concomitant with early recovery of regional function [141]. In earlier work, AICAr administration during reperfusion proved to be detrimental for heart function [125], although nucleotide synthesis rate increased [142]. In cat heart AICAr improved post-ischemic function, but not ATP [143]. It may decrease infarct size [144] and myocardial ischemia in coronary microembolization [145]. We conclude that AICAr deserves further attention as an agent for cardioprotection.

Ribose stimulates the rate of myocardial ATP synthesis during reperfusion after coronary artery occlusion in the dog, although to a (much) smaller extent than adenosine or AICAr [142]. Using NADH fluorometry to monitor rat myocardial metabolism, Horvath *et al.* [146] observed that a ribose-

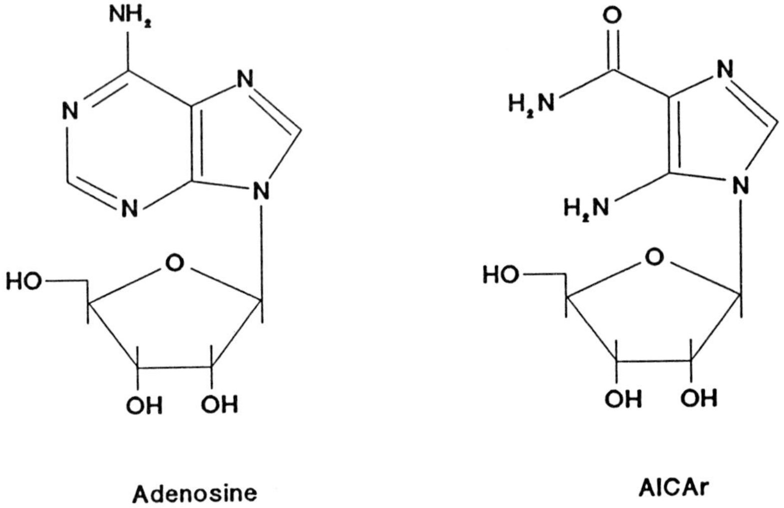

Figure 13.6. Structural relationship between adenosine and acadesine (AICAr = 5-amino-1-β-D-ribofuranosylimidazole-4-carboxamide riboside). Although initially used for de novo synthesis of purines/nucleotides, the latter may be useful for cardioprotection through a rise in endogenous adenosine.

enriched perfusate improved glycogen content and myocardial function, but not high-energy phosphates levels.

Conclusions

The measurement of myocardial high-energy phosphates (especially ATP and phosphocreatine) with biopsy or NMR spectroscopic techniques provides information about the metabolic status of the heart. They could predict rejection of heart transplants. Breakdown products of high-energy phosphates, such as purines and pyrimidines, seem useful as markers of cardiac ischemia. They can be measured in the cardiac efflux. The correlation between energy content and function is often poor. Decreased function of post-ischemic myocardium seems related to defective ATP utilization rather than decreased ATP synthesis. Adenosine and related compounds could play a role in cardioprotection. Such agents often protect heart function and ATP content against the ill effects of ischemia/reperfusion, if used, e.g. adjunct to potassium cardioplegia.

Acknowledgements

We are grateful for the secretarial assistance of Ms. C.D.M. Poleon-Weghorst and the financial support of The Netherlands Heart Foundation (Grants 88.253, 89.096 and 90.272).

References

1. Geisbuhler TP, Rovetto MJ. Guanosine metabolism in adult rat cardiac myocytes: ribose-enhanced GTP synthesis from extracellular guanosine. Pflügers Arch 1991; 419: 160–5.
2. Jennings RB, Schaper J, Hill ML *et al.* Effect of reperfusion late in the phase of reversible ischemic injury. Changes in cell volume, electrolytes, metabolites and ultrastructure. Circ Res 1985; 56: 262–78.
3. Skladanowski AC. On the role of myocardial AMP-deaminase. In De Jong JW (ed): Myocardial Energy Metabolism. Dordrecht: Martinus Nijhoff 1988; 53–65.
4. Meghji P, Middleton KM, Newby AC. Absolute rates of adenosine formation during ischaemia in rat and pigeon hearts. Biochem J 1988; 249: 695–703.
5. De Tata V, Gini S, Simonetti I *et al.* The regional distribution of adenosine-regulating enzymes in the left and right ventricle walls of control and hypertrophic heart. Basic Res Cardiol 1989; 84: 597–606.
6. Choong YS, Humphrey SM. Differences in the regional distribution and response to ischaemia of adenosine-regulating enzymes in the heart. Basic Res Cardiol 1987; 82: 576–84.
7. Jarasch E-D, Bruder G, Heid HW. Significance of xanthine oxidase in capillary endothelial cells. Acta Physiol Scand 1986; 548 (Suppl): 39–46.
8. Samra ZQ, Oguro T, Fontaine R *et al.* Immunocytochemical localization of xanthine oxidase in rat myocardium. J Submicros Cytol Pathol 1991; 23: 379–90.
9. Wajner M, Harkness RA. Distribution of xanthine dehydrogenase and oxidase activities in human and rabbit tissues. Biochim Biophys Acta 1989; 991: 79–84.
10. Eddy LJ, Stewart JR, Jones HP *et al.* Free radical-producing enzyme, xanthine oxidase, is undetectable in human hearts. Am J Physiol 1987; 253: H709–H711.
11. Grum CM, Gallagher KP, Kirsh MM *et al.* Absence of detectable xanthine oxidase in human myocardium. J Mol Cell Cardiol 1989; 21: 263–7.
12. Podzuweit T, Beck H, Müller A *et al.* Absence of xanthine oxidoreductase activity in human myocardium. Cardiovasc Res 1991; 25: 820–30.
13. Smoleński RT, Skladanowski AC, Perko M *et al.* Adenylate degradation products release from the human myocardium during open heart surgery. Clin Chim Acta 1989; 182: 63–73.
14. Terada LS, Beehler CJ, Banerjee A *et al.* Hyperoxia and self- or neutrophil-generated O_2 metabolites inactivate xanthine oxidase. J Appl Physiol 1988; 65: 2349–53.
15. Huizer T, De Jong JW, Nelson JA *et al.* Urate production by human heart. J Mol Cell Cardiol 1989; 21: 691–5.
16. De Jong JW, Van der Meer P, Nieukoop AS *et al.* Xanthine oxidoreductase activity in perfused hearts of various species, including humans. Circ Res 1990; 67: 770–3.
17. Abadeh S, Killacky J, Benboubetra M *et al.* Purification and partial characterization of xanthine oxidase from human milk. Biochim Biophys Acta 1992; 1117: 25–32.
18. Reimer KA, Jennings RB. Myocardial ischemia, hypoxia, and infarction. In Fozzard HA, Haber E, Jennings RB *et al.*(eds): The Heart and Cardiovascular System, second edition. New York: Raven Press 1992; 1875–1973.
19. De Jong JW. Cardioplegia and calcium antagonists: A review. Ann Thorac Surg 1986; 42: 593–8.
20. Flameng W, Vanhaecke J, Van Belle H *et al.* Relation between coronary artery stenosis and myocardial purine metabolism, histology and regional function in humans. J Am Coll Cardiol 1987; 9: 1235–42.
21. Canby RC, Evanochko WT, Van Barrett L *et al.* Monitoring the bioenergetics of cardiac allograft rejection using *in vivo* P-31 nuclear magnetic resonance spectroscopy. J Am Coll Cardiol 1987; 9: 1067–74.
22. Fraser CD, Chacko VP, Jacobus WE *et al.* Early phosphorus 31 nuclear magnetic resonance bioenergetic changes potentially predict rejection in heterotopic cardiac allografts. J Heart Transpl 1990; 9: 197–204.

23. Haug CE, Shapiro JI, Chan L *et al.* P-31 Nuclear magnetic resonance spectroscopic evaluation of heterotopic cardiac allograft rejection in the rat. Transplantation 1987; 44: 175–8.
24. Bottomley PA, Weiss RG, Hardy CJ *et al.* Myocardial high-energy phosphate metabolism and allograft rejection in patients with heart transplants. Radiology 1991; 181: 67–75.
25. Hardy CJ, Weiss RG, Bottomley PA *et al.* Altered myocardial high-energy phosphate metabolites in patients with dilated cardiomyopathy. Am Heart J 1991; 122: 795–801.
26. Smoleński RT, Swierczynski J, Narkiewicz M *et al.* Purines, lactate and phosphate release from child and adult heart during cardioplegic arrest. Clin Chim Acta 1990; 192: 155–63.
27. Humphrey SM, Seelye RN. Improved functional recovery of ischemic myocardium by suppression of adenosine catabolism. J Thorac Cardiovasc Surg 1982; 84: 16–22.
28. Bolling SF, Bies LE, Bove EL *et al.* Augmenting intracellular adenosine improves myocardial recovery. J Thorac Cardiovasc Surg 1990; 99: 469–74.
29. De Jong JW, Van der Meer P, Van Loon H *et al.* Adenosine as adjunct to potassium cardioplegia: Effect on function, energy metabolism and electrophysiology. J Thorac Cardiovasc Surg 1990; 100: 445–54.
30. Zhu QY, Chen S, Zou C. Protective effects of an adenosine deaminase inhibitor on ischemia-reperfusion injury in isolated perfused rat heart. Am J Physiol 1990; 259: H835–H838.
31. Bergsland J, LoBalsomo L, Lajos P *et al.* Allopurinol in prevention of reperfusion injury of hypoxically stored rat hearts. J Heart Transpl 1987; 6: 137–40.
32. Chambers DJ, Braimbridge MV, Hearse DJ. Free radicals and cardioplegia: Allopurinol and oxypurinol reduce myocardial injury following ischemic arrest. Ann Thorac Surg 1987; 44: 291–7.
33. Myers CL, Weiss SJ, Kirsh MM *et al.* Effects of supplementing hypothermic crystalloid cardioplegic solution with catalase, superoxide dismutase, allopurinol, or deferoxamine on functional recovery of globally ischemic and reperfused isolated hearts. J Thorac Cardiovasc Surg 1986; 91: 281–9.
34. Périer P, Fabiani JN, Bocher M *et al.* Protection myocardique pendant l'arrêt cardiaque ischémique: Étude hémodynamique des effects de l'allopurinol dans un soluté cardioplégique. Arch Mal Coeur 1980; 73: 713–8.
35. Stewart JR, Crute SL, Loughlin V *et al.* Prevention of free radical-induced myocardial reperfusion injury with allopurinol. J Thorac Cardiovasc Surg 1985; 90: 68–72.
36. Flameng W, Sukehiro S, Möllhoff T *et al.* A new concept of long-term donor heart preservation: Nucleoside transport inhibition. J Heart Lung Transplant 1991; 10: 990–8.
37. Guvendik L, Hynd J, Drake-Holland A *et al.* Myocardial protective effects of lidoflazine during ischemia and reperfusion. Thorac Cardiovasc Surg 1990; 38: 15–9.
38. Hearse DJ, Stewart DA, Braimbridge MV. Cellular protection during myocardial ischemia. The development and characterization of a procedure for the induction of reversible ischemic arrest. Circulation 1976; 54: 193–202.
39. Masuda M, Demeulemeester A, Chang-Chun C *et al.* Cardioprotective effects of nucleoside transport inhibition in rabbit hearts. Ann Thorac Surg 1991; 52: 1300–5.
40. Van Belle H, Janssen PAJ. Comparative pharmacology of nucleoside transport inhibitors. Nucleos Nucleot 1991; 10: 975–82.
41. Vinten-Johansen J, Chiantella V, Faust KB *et al.* Myocardial protection with blood cardioplegia in ischemically injured hearts; reduction of reoxygenation injury with allopurinol. Ann Thorac Surg 1988; 45: 319–26.
42. LoBalsamo L, Bergsland J, Lajos P *et al.* Prevention of reperfusion injury in ischemic-reperfused heart by oxypurinol and allopurinol. Transpl Int 1989; 2: 218–22.
43. Thompson-Gorman SL, Zweier JL. Evaluation of the role of xanthine oxidase in myocardial reperfusion injury. J Biol Chem 1990; 265: 6656–63.
44. Bando K, Tago M, Teramoto S. Prevention of free radical-induced myocardial injury by allopurinol. Experimental study in cardiac preservation and transplantation. J Thorac Cardiovasc Surg 1988; 95: 465–73.

45. Godin DV, Garnett ME. Altered antioxidant status in the ischemic/reperfused rabbit myocardium: Effects of allopurinol. Can J Cardiol 1989; 5: 365–71.
46. Emerit I, Fabiani J-N, Ponzio O *et al.* Clastogenic factor in ischemia-reperfusion injury during open-heart surgery; protective effect of allopurinol. Ann Thorac Surg 1988; 46: 619–24.
47. Johnson WD, Kayser KL, Brenowitz JB *et al.* A randomized controlled trial of allopurinol in coronary bypass surgery. Am Heart J 1991; 121: 20–4.
48. Rashid MA, William-Olsson G. Influence of allopurinol on cardiac complications in open heart operations. Ann Thorac Surg 1991; 52: 127–30.
49. Tabayashi K, Suzuki Y, Nagamine S *et al.* A clinical trial of allopurinol (Zyloric) for myocardial protection. J Thorac Cardiovasc Surg 1991; 101: 713–8.
50. Werns SW, Grum CM, Ventura A *et al.* Xanthine oxidase inhibition does not limit canine infarct size. Circulation 1991; 83: 995–1005.
51. Bochenek A, Religa Z, Spyt TJ *et al.* Protective influence of pretreatment with allopurinol on myocardial function in patients undergoing coronary artery surgery. Eur J Cardiothorac Surg 1990; 4: 538–42.
52. Hori M, Gotoh K, Kitakaze M *et al.* Role of oxygen-derived free radicals in myocardial edema and ischemia in coronary microvascular embolization. Circulation 1991; 84: 828–40.
53. Wainwright CL, Parratt JR. An antiarrhythmic effect of adenosine during myocardial ischaemia and reperfusion. Eur J Pharmacol 1988; 145: 183–94.
54. Teoh KH, Christakis GT, Weisel RD *et al.* Dipyridamole preserved platelets and reduced blood loss after cardiopulmonary bypass. J Thorac Cardiovasc Surg 1988; 96: 332–41.
55. Abd-Elfattah AS, Jessen ME, Hanan SA *et al.* Is adenosine 5′-triphosphate derangement or free-radical-mediated injury the major cause of ventricular dysfunction during reperfusion? Circulation 1990; 82 (Suppl IV): IV-341–50.
56. Manfredi JP, Holmes EW. Purine salvage pathways in myocardium. Annu Rev Physiol 1985 47: 691–705.
57. Swain JL, Sabina RL, McHale PA *et al.* Prolonged myocardial nucleotide depletion after brief ischemia in the open-chest dog. Am J Physiol 1982; 242: H818–H826.
58. Smoleński RT, De Jong JW, Janssen M *et al.* Formation and breakdown of uridine in ischemic hearts of rats and humans. J Mol Cell Cardiol 1993; 25: 67–74.
59. Smoleński RT, Kochan Z, Janssen M *et al.* Different catabolism of myocardial pyrimidines in human and rat heart. J Mol Cell Cardiol 1993; 25 (Suppl I): S.132 (abstr).
60. De Boer LWV, Ingwall JS, Kloner RA *et al.* Prolonged derangements of canine myocardial purine metabolism after a brief coronary artery occlusion not associated with anatomic evidence of necrosis. Proc Natl Acad Sci USA 1980; 77: 5471–5.
61. Jennings RB, Steenbergen Jr C. Nucleotide metabolism and cellular damage in myocardial ischemia. Annu Rev Physiol 1985; 47: 727–49.
62. Reimer KA, Hill ML, Jennings RB. Prolonged depletion of ATP and of the adenine nucleotide pool due to delayed resynthesis of adenine nucleotides following reversible myocardial ischemic injury in dogs. J Mol Cell Cardiol 1981; 13: 229–39.
63. Ichihara K, Neely JR. Recovery of ventricular function in reperfused ischemic rat hearts exposed to fatty acids. Am J Physiol 1985; 249: H492–H497.
64. Neely JR, Grotyohann LW. Role of glycolytic products in damage to ischemic myocardium. Dissociation of adenosine triphosphate levels and recovery of function of reperfused ischemic hearts. Circ Res 1984; 55: 816–24.
65. Rosenkranz ER, Okamoto F, Buckberg GD *et al.* Biochemical studies: Failure of tissue adenosine triphosphate levels to predict recovery of contractile function after controlled reperfusion. J Thorac Cardiovasc Surg 1986; 92: 488–501.
66. De Jong JW, Huizer T, Tijssen JGP. Energy conservation by nisoldipine in ischaemic heart. Br J Pharmacol 1984; 83: 943–9.
67. Huizer T, De Jong JW, Achterberg PW. Protection by bepridil against myocardial ATP-

catabolism is probably due to negative inotropy. J Cardiovasc Pharmacol 1987; 10: 55–61.
68. Huizer T. Myocardial ATP catabolism and its pharmacological prevention. Rotterdam: Acad Thesis 1991; 29.
69. Heyndrickx GR, Millard RW, McRitchie RJ *et al.* Regional myocardial functional and electrophysiological alterations after brief coronary artery occlusion in conscious dogs. J Clin Invest 1975; 56: 978–85.
70. Heyndrickx GR, Baig H, Nellers P *et al.* Depression of regional blood flow and wall thickening after brief coronary occlusions. Am J Physiol 1978; 234: H653–H659.
71. De Jong JW, Achterberg PW. ATP-metabolism in normoxic and ischemic heart. In De Jong JW (ed): Myocardial Energy Metabolism. Dordrecht: Martinus Nijhoff 1988; 3–7.
72. Katz AM. Contractile proteins of the heart. Physiol Rev 1970; 50: 63–158.
73. Taegtmeyer H, Roberts AFC, Raine AEG. Energy metabolism in reperfused heart muscle: metabolic correlates to return of function. J Am Coll Cardiol 1985; 6: 864–70.
74. Schaper W, Schott RJ, Kobayashi M. Reperfused myocardium: Stunning, preconditioning, and reperfusion injury. In Heusch G (ed): Pathophysiological and Rational Pharmacotherapy of Myocardial Ischemia. New York: Springer-Verlag 1990; 175–97.
75. Ambrosio G, Jacobus WE, Bergman CA *et al.* Preserved high energy phosphate metabolic reserve in globally "stunned" hearts despite reduction of basal ATP content and contractility. J Mol Cell Cardiol 1987; 19: 953–64.
76. Becker LC, Levine JH, Dipaula AF *et al.* Reversal of dysfunction in postischemic stunned myocardium by epinephrine and postextrasystolic potentiation. J Am Coll Cardiol 1986; 7: 580–9.
77. Buda AJ, Zotz RJ, Gallagher KJ. The effect of inotropic stimulation on normal and ischemic myocardium following coronary occlusion. Circulation 1987; 77: 163–72.
78. McFalls EO, Duncker DJ, Sassen LMA *et al.* Dobutamine restores oxygen consumption but not lactate utilization in regionally stunned porcine myocardium. Circulation 1991; 84 (Suppl II): II-658 (abstr.).
79. McFalls EO, Duncker DJ, Krams R *et al.* Right ventricular stunning in swine. Eur Heart J 1991; 12 (Abstr Suppl): 310 (abstr.).
80. Sako EY, Kingsley-Hickman PB, From AHL *et al.* ATP synthesis kinetics and mitochondrial function in the postischemic myocardium as studied by ^{31}P-NMR. J Biol Chem 1988; 263: 10600–7.
81. Suga H. Total mechanical energy of a ventricular model and cardiac oxygen consumption. Am J Physiol 1979; 236: H498–H505.
82. Suga H. Ventricular energetics. Physiol Rev 1990; 70: 247–77.
83. Kusuoka H, Porterfield JK, Weismann HF *et al.* Pathophysiology and pathogenesis of stunned myocardium. Depressed Ca^{2+} activation of contraction as a consequence of reperfusion-induced cellular calcium overload in ferret hearts. J Clin Invest 1987; 79: 950–61.
84. Bavaria JE, Furukawa S, Kreiner G *et al.* Myocardial oxygen utilization after reversible global ischemia. J Thorac Cardiovasc Surg 1990; 100: 210–20.
85. Dean EN, Schlafer M, Nicklas JM. The oxygen consumption paradox of "stunned myocardium" in dogs. Basic Res Cardiol 1990; 85: 120–31.
86. Laxson DD, Homans DC, Dai X-Z *et al.* Oxygen consumption and coronary reactivity in postischemic myocardium. Circ Res 1989; 64: 9–20.
87. Bricco G, Piacenza G, Borgoglio R *et al.* La fosfocreatina nella protezione del miocardio in corso di arresto cardioplegico, aspetti biochimici funzionali nel cane. Cardiologia 1986; 31: 509–14.
88. Ceriana P, Pagnin A, Locatelli A *et al.* Role of creatine phosphate in myocardial protection in heart surgery. Minerva Anest 1989 55: 341–7.
89. Chambers DJ, Braimbridge MV, Kosker S *et al.* Creatine phosphate (Neoton) as an additive to St. Thomas' Hospital cardioplegic solution (Plegisol). Results of a clinical study. Eur J Cardiothorac Surg 1991; 5: 74–81.

90. D'Alessandro LC, Cini R, Stazi G *et al.* Creatin fosfato: un additivo alla soluzione cardioplegic. Studio clinico. Cardiologia 1987; 32: 307–13.
91. Konorev EA, Medvedeva NV, Jaliashvili IV *et al.* Participation of calcium ions in the molecular mechanism of cardioprotective action of exogenous phosphocreatine. Basic Res Cardiol 1991; 86: 327–39.
92. Kopf GS, Chaudry I, Condos S *et al.* Reperfusion with ATP-$MgCl_2$ following prolonged ischemia improves myocardial performance. J Surg Res 1987; 43: 114–7.
93. Kupriianov VV, Shteinshneider Al, Lakomkin VL *et al.* Study of the protective effect of phosphocreatine on the ischemic myocardium during cardioplegia using the P-31 NMR method. Biull Vses Kardiol Nauchn Tsent AMN-SSR 1985; 8: 14–9.
94. Mogilevskii GM, Sharov VG, Saks VA *et al.* Structural and biochemical characteristics of the effectiveness of intraoperative protection of the myocardium. Arkh Patol 1985; 47: 24–9.
95. Popov IV, Saprygin DB, Egorova IF *et al.* Effectiveness of protecting the myocardium against ischemia with a normothermic cardioplegic solution and creatine phosphate. Biull Eskp Biol Med 1985; 99: 108–10.
96. Robinson LA, Braimbridge MV, Hearse DJ. Enhanced myocardial protection with high-energy phosphates in St. Thomas' Hospital cardioplegic solution. Synergism of adenosine triphosphate and creatine phosphate. J Thorac Cardiovasc Surg 1987; 93: 415–27.
97. Robinson LA, Braimbridge MV, Hearse DJ. Creatine phosphate: an additive myocardial protective and antiarrhythmic agent in cardioplegia. J Thorac Cardiovasc Surg 1984; 87: 190–200.
98. Ronca-Testoni S, Galbani P, Ronca G. Effect of creatine phosphate administration on the rat heart adenylate pool. J Mol Cell Cardiol 1985; 17: 1185–8.
99. Semenovsky ML, Shumakov VI, Sharov VG *et al.* Protection of ischemic myocardium by exogenous phosphocreatine. II. Clinical, ultrastructural, and biochemical evaluations. J Thorac Cardiovasc Surg 1987; 94: 762–9.
100. Severin ES, Alakhov Vl, Kondrat'ev AD *et al.* Mechanisms of the conduction of cellular regulatory signals. Vestn Akad Med Nauk SSSR 1989 12: 63–70.
101. Sharov VG, Saks VA, Kupriyanov VV *et al.* Protection of ischemic myocardium by exogenous phosphocreatine. I. Morphologic and phosphorus 31-nuclear magnetic resonance studies. J Thorac Cardiovasc Surg 1987; 94: 749–61.
102. Thelin S, Hultman J, Ronquist G *et al.* Enhanced protection of rat hearts during ischemia by phosphoenolpyruvate and ATP in cardioplegia. Thorac Cardiovasc Surg 1986; 34: 104–9.
103. Thelin S, Hultman J, Ronquist G *et al.* Improved myocardial protection by creatine phosphate in cardioplegic solution. An *in vivo* study in the pig during normothermic ischemia. Thorac Cardiovasc Surg 1987; 35: 137–42.
104. Thelin S, Hultman J, Ronquist G *et al.* Metabolic and functional effects of creatine phosphate in cardioplegic solution. Studies on rat hearts during and after normothermic ischemia. Scand J Thorac Cardiovasc Surg 1987; 21: 39–45.
105. Zucchi R, Poddighe R, Limbruno U *et al.* Protection of isolated rat heart from oxidative stress by exogenous creatine phosphate. J Mol Cell Cardiol 1989; 21: 67–73.
106. Thorelius J, Thelin S, Ronquist G *et al.* Biochemical and functional effects of creatine phosphate in cardioplegic solution during aortic valve surgery – a clinical study. Thorac Cardiovasc Surg 1992; 40: 10–3.
107. Thelin S, Hultman J, Jakobson S *et al.* Functional effects of phosphoenolpyruvate and ATP on pig hearts in cardioplegia and during reperfusion. An *in vivo* study with cardiopulmonary bypass. Eur Surg Res 1987; 19: 348–56.
108. Thelin S, Hultman J, Ronquist G *et al.* Myocardial high-energy phosphates, lactate and pyruvate during moderate or severe normothermic ischemia in rat hearts perfused with phosphoenolpyruvate and ATP in cardioplegic solution. Scand J Thorac Cardiovasc Surg 1987; 21: 245–9.
109. Thelin S, Hultman J, Ronquist G *et al.* Interrelated effects of nucleoside mono- and

triphosphates and phosphoenolpyruvate on rat hearts subjected to cardioplegic arrest at normothermia. Scand J Thorac Cardiovasc Surg 1987–21: 33–8.
110. Rankin AC, Oldroyd KG, Chong E *et al.* Adenosine or adenosine triphosphate for supraventricular tachycardias – comparative double-blind randomized study in patients with spontaneous or inducible arrhythmias. Am Heart J 1990; 119: 316–23.
111. Bruns RF. Adenosine receptors – Roles and pharmacology. Ann NY Acad Sci 1990; 603: 211–26.
112. Hohlfeld T, Hearse DJ, Yellon DM *et al.* Adenosine-induced increase in myocardial ATP: Are there beneficial effects for the ischaemic myocardium? Basic Res Cardiol 1989; 84: 499–509.
113. Schubert T, Vetter H, Owen P *et al.* Adenosine cardioplegia. Adenosine versus potassium cardioplegia; effects on cardiac arrest and postischemic recovery in the isolated rat heart. J Thorac Cardiovasc Surg 1989; 98: 1057–65.
114. Boehm DH, Human PA, Reichenspurner H *et al.* Adenosine and its role in cardioplegia – Effects on postischemic recovery in the baboon. Transpl Proc 1990 22: 545–6.
115. Bolling SF, Bies LE, Gallagher KP *et al.* Enhanced myocardial protection with adenosine. Ann Thorac Surg 1989; 47: 809–15.
116. DeWitt DF, Jochim KE, Behrendt DM. Nucleotide degradation and functional impairment during cardioplegia: Amelioration by inosine. Circulation 1983; 67: 171–8.
117. Galiñanes M, Mullane KM, Hearse DJ. Acadesine (AICAr) affords sustained protection against injury during ischemia and reperfusion in the transplanted rat heart. Circulation 1991; 84: II-305 (abstr.).
118. Wyatt DA, Ely SW, Lasley RD *et al.* Purine-enriched asanguineous cardioplegia retards adenosine triphosphate degradation during ischemia and improves postischemic ventricular function. J Thorac Cardiovasc Surg 1989; 97: 771–8.
119. Swanson DK, Pasaoglu I, Berkoff HA *et al.* Improved heart preservation with UW preservation solution. J Heart Transpl 1988; 7: 456–67.
120. Jeevanandam V, Auteri JS, Sanchez JA *et al.* Improved heart preservation with University of Wisconsin solution: Experimental and preliminary human experience. Circulation 1991; 84 (Suppl 3) III-324–III-328.
121. Möllhoff T, Sukehiro S, Van Aken H *et al.* Long-term preservation of baboon hearts. Effects of hypothermic ischemic and cardioplegic arrest on high-energy phosphate content. Circulation 1990; 82 (Suppl IV): IV-264–IV-268.
122. Möllhoff T, Sukehiro S, Flameng W *et al.* Katabolismus energiereicher Phosphate während der Langzeitpräservierung explantierter Donor-Herzen im Hundemodell. Anästh Intensivther Notfallmed 1990; 25: 399–404.
123. Wicomb WN, Hill JD, Avery J *et al.* Optimal cardioplegia and 24–hour heart storage with simplified UW solution containing polyethylene glycol. Transplantation 1990; 49; 261–4.
124. Ambrosio G, Jacobus WE, Mitchell MC *et al.* Effects of ATP precursors on ATP and free ADP content and functional recovery of postischemic hearts. Am J Physiol 1989; 256: H560–H566.
125. Hoffmeister HM, Mauser M, Schaper W. Effect of adenosine and AICAR on ATP content and regional contractile function in reperfused canine myocardium. Basic Res Cardiol 1985; 80: 445–58.
126. Ledingham SJ, Katayama O, Lachno DR *et al.* Beneficial effect of adenosine during reperfusion following prolonged cardioplegic arrest. Cardiovasc Res 1990; 24: 247–53.
127. Kitakaze M, Hori M, Takashima S *et al.* Augmentation of adenosine production during ischemia as a possible mechanism of myocardial protection in ischemic preconditioning. Circulation 1991; 84 (Suppl II): II-306 (abstr.).
128. Liu GS, Thornton J, Van Winkle DM *et al.* Protection against infarction afforded by preconditioning is mediated by A1 adenosine receptors in rabbit heart. Circulation 1991; 84: 350–6.
129. Murphy E, London RE, VanderHeide R *et al.* Role of adenosine in preconditioning in rat heart. Circulation 1991; 84 (Suppl II): II-306 (abstr.).

130. Van Winkle DM, Davis RF. Ischemic preconditioning of myocardium: Effect of the adenosine agonist phenylisopropyl adenosine (PIA). Circulation 1991; 84 (Suppl II): II-305 (abstr.).
131. Homeister JW, Hoff PT, Fletcher DD *et al.* Combined adenosine and lidocaine administration limits myocardial reperfusion injury. Circulation 1990; 82: 595–608.
132. Olafsson B, Forman MB, Puett DW *et al.* Reduction of reperfusion injury in the canine preparation by intracoronary adenosine: importance of the endothelium and the no-reflow phenomenon. Circulation 1987; 76: 1135–45.
133. Pitarys II CJ, Virmani R, Vildibill Jr HD *et al.* Reduction of myocardial reperfusion injury by intravenous adenosine administered during the early reperfusion period. Circulation 1991; 83: 237–47.
134. Crea F, Pupita G, Galassi AR *et al.* Role of adenosine in pathogenesis of anginal pain. Circulation 1990; 81: 164–72.
135. Lagerqvist B, Sylveń C, Hedenström H *et al.* Intravenous adenosine but not its 1st metabolite inosine provokes chest pain in healthy volunteers. J Cardiovasc Pharmacol 1990; 16: 173–6.
136. Harmsen E, De Tombe PP, De Jong JW *et al.* Enhanced ATP and GTP synthesis from hypoxanthine or inosine after myocardial ischemia. Am J Physiol 1984; 246: H37–H43.
137. Yoshiyama M, Sakai H, Teragaki M *et al.* The effect of inosine on the post ischemic heart as bio-energy recovering factor in ^{31}P-MRS. Biochem Biophys Res Commun 1988; 151: 1408–15.
138. Becker BF, Reinholz N, Leipert B *et al.* Role of uric acid as an endogenous radical scavenger and antioxidant. Chest 1991; 100: 176S-81S.
139. Engler R. Consequences of activation and adenosine-mediated inhibition of granulocytes during myocardial ischemia. Fed Proc 1987; 46: 2407–12.
140. Gruber HE, Hoffer ME, McAllister DR *et al.* Increased adenosine concentration in blood from ischemic myocardium by AICA riboside. Effects on flow, granulocytes, and injury. Circulation 1989; 80: 1400–11.
141. Glower DD, Spratt JA, Newton JR *et al.* Dissociation between early recovery of regional function and purine nucleotide content in post-ischaemic myocardium in the conscious dog. Cardiovasc Res 1987; 21: 328–36.
142. Mauser M, Hoffmeister HM, Nienaber C *et al.* Influence of ribose, adenosine, and "AICAR" on the rate of myocardial adenosine triphosphate synthesis during reperfusion after coronary artery occlusion in the dog. Circ Res 1985; 56: 220–30.
143. Mitsos SE, Jolly SR, Lucchesi BR. Protective effects of AICAriboside in the globally ischemic isolated cat heart. Pharmacology 1985; 31: 121–31.
144. McAllister D, Engler R, Laikind P *et al.* Experimental infarct size reduction by a new mechanism: augmented adenosine release. Clin Res 1987; 35: 303A (abstr.).
145. Hori M, Sato H, Koretsune Y *et al.* AICA-riboside (5–amino-4–imidazole carboxamide riboside), a novel adenosine potentiator, attenuates myocardial ischemia in coronary microembolization. Circulation 1991; 84 (Suppl II): II-305 (abstr.).
146. Horvath KA, Torchiana DF, Daggett WM *et al.* Monitoring myocardial reperfusion injury with NADH fluorometry. Lasers Surg Med 1992; 12: 2–6.

14. Lactate monitoring during and after cardiopulmonary bypass: an approach implicating a perioperative measure for cardiac energy metabolism

ERNST-GEORG KRAUSE, DOROTHEA PFEIFFER, ULLA WOLLENBERGER, and HANS-GEORG WOLLERT

Introduction

The beating warm-blooded heart cannot tolerate ischemia and a reduction of oxygen delivery for more than a short time – one minute at most – without serious impairments of its function. From the point of view of the needs of energy of the muscle, this is not so much because the myocardial energy reserves (i.e., glycogen) may become exhausted, but rather because the rate of glycogenolysis is not high enough in mammalian heart muscle to compensate for this deficiency, in face of a continued utilization of high energy phosphate (HEP) and of low efficacy of the glycolysis, by an adequate synthesis of adenosine triphosphate (ATP) in the mitochondria. As well known, the majority (>90%) of myocardial ATP is produced aerobically by oxidative phosphorylation in the normal heart [1].

Cardiac energy metabolism at limited oxygen supply

Under conditions of limited oxygen supply (e.g., ischemia and/or cardioplegia) the production of ATP is mainly or exclusively accounted for by glycolysis, which may be important in order to compensate, in part, for the ATP demand of the heart [2,3]. Even with optimal conditions (high coronary perfusion rates, near maximal rate of substrate transport) anaerobic glycolysis cannot provide the energy required for a reduced cardiac metabolism, such as under the conditions of cardioplegia and hypothermia [4–9]. Although blood cardioplegia provides better protection than crystalloid cardioplegia, a depletion in HEP and an activation of anaerobic metabolism have been demonstrated. The state of energy of the chronically diseased human heart may be even more in jeopardy. There is evidence for an impairement of ATP synthesis resulting in a lower level of HEP, especially of ATP, as well as of the amount of total adenine nucleotides (TAN) in transmural bioptic samples of the left ventricle muscle of patients with chronic myocardial diseases [6]. A loss in the level of ATP has been found to be related to the degree of coronary artery stenosis [6]. However, for the cardiac ATP as

H.M. Piper and C.J. Preusse (eds): Ischemia-reperfusion in cardiac surgery, 317–333.

Table 14.1. Potent chemical and biochemical parameters for monitoring the energy state in reperfused pre-ischemic and cardioplegic heart muscle.

Origin/sources	
Myocardium, blood	Myocardial oxygen consumption
Ditto	Venoarterial pCO_2 gradient
Myocardium	Intramyocardial pH
Ditto	^{31}P-NMR imaging of HEP and pH (indirectly)
Ditto	$NADH^+/NADPH^+$ fluorescence
Venous blood from coronary sinus	K^+ concentration; P_i concentration
Ditto	purine
Ditto	lactate
Blood	proteins

well as TAN assayed from endomyocardial biopsies of patients with dilated cardiomyopathy such a deficit in HEP may not exist [10].

For cardiac bypass surgery the combination of an inadequate ATP synthesis in the early phase of the aerobic reperfusion in combination with a substantial deficit in cardiac HEP in general [4,7] may be deleterious during the rewarming of the organ. It can result in a non-optimal resuscitation of the cation gradients and of the efficacy of the contractile properties of the heart as a pump. It may be possible for the cardiac surgeon, however, to influence the imbalance between cardiac energy supply and energy demand if he could monitor the energy stateof the heart muscle during surgery. By the use of such data the weaning from the bypass, which can lead to a very abrupt restoration of cardiac work, can be optimized. The discontinuation of cardio-pulmonary bypass seems to be a crucial point in terms of an adequate energy supply [4,6,8,9]. Disarrangements at the level of HEP may represent important causal factors for the observed transient biventricular dysfunction leading to a low outcome which may require administration of catecholamines to patients in the postoperative phase [11,12]. A plethora of data show that the degradation of ATP in cardiac tissue is accompanied by an accumulation of adenosine monophosphate (AMP), inorganic phosphate, adenosine, inosine, hypoxanthine as well as lactate [4,7,8].

Biochemical parameter of energy state in the post-cardioplegic heart

Several cardiac metabolites, which are released into the coronary sinus blood, are candidates for an assessment of energy metabolism. Up to now a great number of clinical studies investigating the energy state of the myocardium during cardiopulmonary bypass surgery had to be performed in a retrospective manner, since the analytic procedures of the chosen metabolic parameters were very time-consuming. Table 14.1 lists more recently developed techniques for obtaining data that are related directly or indirectly to the energy state of the heart. Some of these techniques, as ^{31}P-NMR-measurements can be employed in chronically diseased patients to monitor HEP and intracellular pH continuously and non-invasively [13,14]. However, the application of NMR imaging during heart surgery is, practically not possible for technical reasons, at this time and in the near future. Also the superficial NADH/NADPH-fluorescence pattern, which is a sensitive indicator directly related to cardiac energy metabolism [15,16], is presently not feasible under surgical conditions. Apart from classic assay of myocardial oxygen consumption, the coronary venoarterial pCO_2 gradient [17] as well as the intramyocardial pH [18–20] have been employed for evaluating anaerobic metabolism during cardiopulmonary resuscitation and reflow after coronary bypass surgery.

During bypass surgery and cardioplegia with or without hypothermia it has been observed that the imbalance between energy utilization and energy supply results in an acceleration of glycolysis accompanied with a production of lactate, which is released into the venous blood [21–29]. For monitoring myocardial lactate release during bypass surgery the coronary sinus has to be catheterized for taking venous blood samples in short time intervals. For using blood lactate as a metabolic parameter for the assessment of cardiac energy metabolism, its measurement has to be performed in less than one-minute intervals during bypass surgery. The recent development of a biosensor for lactic acid [30,50] now allows the ultra-rapid assay of this end product of glycolysis. To employ successfully such a metabolic measurement, which was recently used in the operation theatre [26,31], one depends on its sensitivity and practicability (see below). The possibility to assess the state of energy metabolism during heart surgery may allow the surgeon and the anaesthesiologist to judge, continuously, the energetic state of the myocardium.

Coronary sinus lactate release as an index of transient myocardial anaerobiosis – a way for detecting perioperatively deficits in myocardial energetics

In fasting patients at rest, carbohydrates make up only a small fraction of myocardial metabolic substrate. Glucose has a fractional uptake of 2.6%, lactate one of 15.7%, whereas plasma free fatty acids represent the principal substrates [32]. The use of radioactive, ^{14}C- or ^{3}H-labelled lactate has facilitated the study of substrate utilization and extraction. Using this technique it was shown that the primary fate of lactate in the myocardium is its oxidation [33]. If the lactate concentration raised in the blood, there is a preference for lactate utilization in the heart in comparison to free fatty acids and glucose [34]. The entry into the myocytes is mediated by a transport mechanism, i.e., the lactate permease. Intra-cellularly lactate is oxidised, even though the equilibrium constant for lactate dehyrogenase is in the direction of lactate formation, because (i) the lactate dehydrogenase isoenzyme found in heart

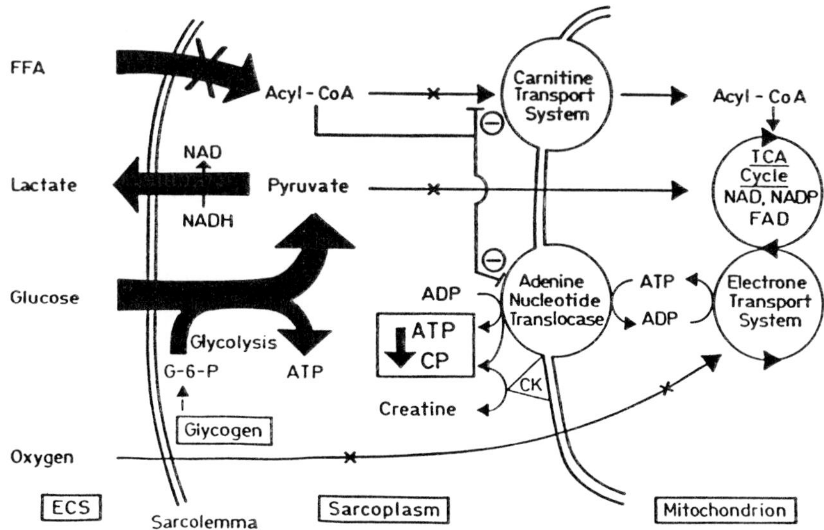

Figure 14.1. Energy supply and ATP synthesis in myocardial ischemia. Under ischemic conditions there is an inhibition of oxidative phosphorylation, of tricarboxylic acid cycle (TCA), of carnitine transport system as well as of adenine nucleotide translocase in the mitochondria, followed by a loss in cytosolic ATP and creatine phosphate (CP). FFA utilization is therefore stopped: the anaerobic utilization of glucose and glucosyl residues of glycogen leads to a moderate synthesis of ATP and lactate. The end product of glycolysis is released into the extracellular space (ECS) and the venous blood in the coronary sinus (see also text).

has a low affinity for pyruvate and (ii) the reaction is forced in the direction of the formation of pyruvate by a rapid removal of the reaction products via the malate-aspartate shuttle into the mitochondria. Therefore, in the aerobic heart little or no pyruvate will be converted to lactate. Only if the oxygen supply becomes limited – as during bypass surgery – net lactate is produced, when the levels of NADH become very high in the myocytes. This is followed by a release of the lactate into the extracellular space, signalling the transition from lactate consumption to lactate production (see Figure 14.1; [28,29]). Therefore this classic metabolite of anaerobic glycolysis represents a very prominent and sensitive marker for the switching from the aerobic to the anaerobic pathway of ATP synthesis in the myocardium as well as vice versa. There is no doubt that lactate release from the ischemic myocytes and its appearance in the cardiac venous blood is considered as an index of anaerobiosis.

The release of lactate from the myocardium is beneficial because it allows an oxidation of accumulating NADH and reduces the development of intracellular acidosis which would inhibit glycolytic flux, ATP synthesis [2,34,35] and calcium-triggered contractile activity [37].

The increase in lactate concentration in coronary sinus blood after reperfusion of the cardioplegic heart (i) is the consequence of the anaerobic energy metabolism during crossclamping and (ii) reflects the re-established coronary flow and a washout of accumulated metabolites. However, there is an increased incidence of local injuries at the level of the microvasculature and changes in extravascular resistance due to extracellular edema after cardioplegic arrest, which can impaire the washout of the accumulated metabolite(s) [38]. Nevertheless, the normalization in coronary sinus blood lactate levels is an indicator of the reinstatement of aerobic ATP synthesis in the mitochondria, at least in large parts of ventricular muscle. The time point at which the coronary sinus lactate concentration falls below the arterial levels can be determined as a 'cross-over point', which indicates that myocardial muscle tissue now starts to use lactate as a substrate via oxidative phosphorylation. There are theoretical considerations concerning the relevance of such a transition point in cellular metabolic regulation (cross-over theorem;[39]). Based on such considerations the so-called 'cross-over-point' (COP) was introduced for theinterpretation of changes in arterio-coronary venous lactate concentration to assess the cardiac energy state perioperatively [26]. In these studies [26,40] the blood lactate was monitored by a biosensor which allowed the measurement of the metabolite within 30s (see below). Taking blood samples from the coronary sinus and the periphery (A. radialis) in 2 min-intervals a metabolic-energy state monitoring of the myocardium was done during open heart surgery for the first time ([26]; see below).

Detection of lactate

Classic enzymatic methods

Usually lactate is determined using photometric monitoring of NADH produced during the lactate dehydrogenase (LDH, EC 1.1.1.27) catalyzed pyruvate conversion:

$$\text{L-lactate} + \text{NAD}^+ \underset{}{\overset{\text{LDH}}{\rightleftharpoons}} \text{NADH} + \text{pyruvate} + \text{H}^+ \qquad (1)$$

The increasing amount of NADH, measured at 340 nm, corresponds to the lactate concentration directly. As the equilibrium of reaction (1) is far toward lactate and NAD^+ ($K = 2.76 \times 10^{-5}$ mol/l at pH 7.0) conditions have to be chosen to change the equilibrium. Applying NAD^+ in excess the equilibrium is shifted completely to the right. Pyruvate is trapped by alanine aminotransferase (GPT, EC 2.6.1.2)

$$\text{pyruvate} + \text{L-glutamate} \overset{\text{GPT}}{\rightleftharpoons} \text{L-alanine} + \alpha\text{-ketoglutarate} \qquad (2)$$

or pyruvate oxidase (PO, EC 1.2.3.3)

$$\text{pyruvate} + O_2 + \text{phosphate} + H_2O \overset{\text{PO}}{\rightleftharpoons} \text{acetylphosphate} + H_2O_2 + CO_2 \qquad (3)$$

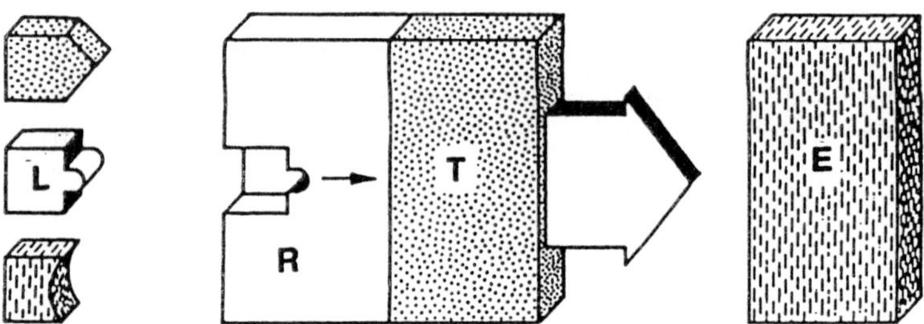

Figure 14.2. Configuration of a lactate biosensor. L: lactate; R: receptor (lactate converting enzyme); T: transducer; E: electronics.

The measurement of whole blood needs more than 20 min including the required deproteinization. Parallel determination of a blank value is recommended because of the slight instability of NAD^+ at alkaline conditions as well as turbidity caused by lipemia. This traditional method has been mainly used in retrospective studies concerning heart metabolism (see above; [52]).

Biosensors for lactate analysis

Biosensors are characterized by the direct coupling of a matrix-bound bioactive recognition substance and a transducer. For the specific recognition isolated enzymes, organelles, cells, tissue slices, immunocomponents, and receptors can be employed. The transformation of the biochemical/biophysical signal into an electrically detectable one can be achieved by electrochemical electrodes, field effect transistors, thermistors, optoelectronic and piezoelectric detectors. Finally, an electronic device is used for signal amplification and display (Figure 14.2).

The predominant feature of this kind of analytical system is the simple handling with coloured solutions and rapid response within seconds. The drastic reduction in cost per analysis based on the re-use of the immobilized biocomponent for up to more than 10,000 times during a period of longer than 30 days is a further advantage compared to the photometric method. Thus, biosensors are very well suited for emergency analysis in the operation theatre and otherwise.

Today, amperometric enzyme membrane electrodes, combining an enzyme for recognition with an amperometric electrode separated by a dialysis membrane from the real sample, represent the highest developed type of biosensors [40]. They are based on heterogeneous electron transfer reactions, i.e. the oxidation of H_2O_2 and the reduction of O_2, both joined in oxidase catalyzed reactions. Since the rate of the overall process is controlled by mass transfer, the diffusion current I_2 is proportional to the concentration of the substance to be determined (S_0):

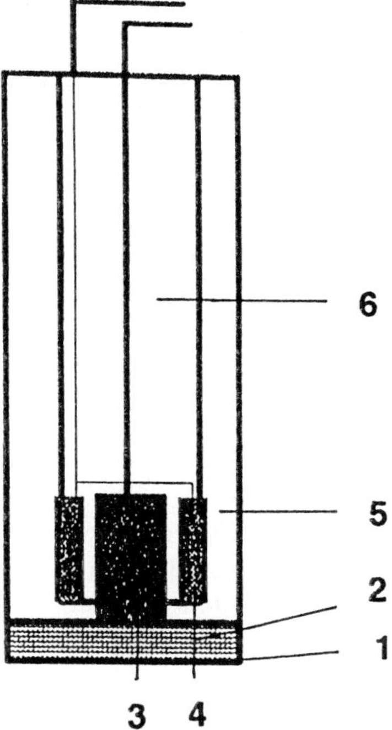

Figure 14.3. Amperometric lactate enzyme electrode. 1: semipermeable dialysis membrane; 2: enzyme membrane; 3: platinum anode; 4: Ag/AgCl reference electrode; 5: electrolyte solution; 6: electrode body.

$$I_d = nAFD_sS_0/d \qquad (4)$$

d = thickness of the diffusion layer
n = number of exchanged electrons
A = electrode surface area
F = Faraday constant
D_s = diffusion coefficient

Figure 14.3 presents the scheme of an amperometric lactate sensor based on a CLARK-type electrode, the most widely used amperometric electrode. It consists of a platinum working and an Ag/AgCl reference electrode, both positioned in an electrolyte solution. The electrode is covered by a piece of enzyme membrane consisting of about 5 U lactate converting enzyme entrapped in an appropriate matrix. The enzyme membrane is separated from the substrate-containing measuring solution and the electrode surface by identical cellulose dialysis membranes. The contact of the enzyme electrode with a lactate containing sample causes the substrate diffusion into the enzyme layer, the enzyme reaction is initiated and the electrode active species is sensed by the electrode resulting in a current output.

Four different enzymes are applicable in biosensors for lactate determination: Lactate dehydrogenase, cytochrome b_2 (cyt b_2, EC 1.1.2.3), lactate monooxygenase (LMO, EC 1.13.12.4); and lactate oxidase (LOD, EC 1.1.3.2).

$$\text{L-lactate} + NAD^+ \xrightleftharpoons{\text{LDH}} \text{pyruvate} + NADH + H^+ \tag{5}$$

$$\text{L-lactate} + 2[Fe(CN)_6]^{3-} \xrightleftharpoons{\text{cyt } b_2} \text{pyruvate} + 2[Fe(CN)_6[^{4-} + 2H^+ \tag{6}$$

$$\text{L-lactate} + O_2 \xrightleftharpoons{\text{LMO}} \text{acetate} + CO_2 + H_2O \tag{7}$$

$$\text{L-lactate} + O_2 \xrightleftharpoons{\text{LOD}} \text{pyruvate} + H_2O_2 \tag{8}$$

The LDH reaction can be coupled to redox electrodes by anodic oxidation of NADH, either directly [41] or via electron mediators such as N-methylphenazinium [42]. They are not suited for routine application to biological samples.

A cytochrome b_2 electrode was first described in 1970 [43], using the anodic detection of the hexacyanoferrat (II) formed during enzymatic reaction. LMO based electrodes have been described since 1981 [44] and Mascini *et al.* [45] have reported a good correlation with the established photometric method using reconstituted human sera and detecting the oxygen consumption. However, problems may arise from differences in the oxygen content of buffer and sample solution. Only carefully air-saturated solutions allow analysis with high precision and accuracy. Weigelt *et al.* [46] have described a highly precise working sensor (measuring frequency 60/h, serial imprecision below 1%) with a functional stability of more than 55 d for diluted plasma.

The lactate converting enzyme used most successfully, lactate oxidase, is the only one producing hydrogen peroxide during lactate oxidation. Because of potential disturbances caused by changes in oxygen concentration the detection of hydrogen peroxide at +600 mV is the method of choice of most of the lactate sensors [40,47] and of the enzyme electrode based lactate analyzers that are on the market at present (Table 14.2).

Two types of lactate analyzing systems based on lactate oxidase electrodes offered for the application to cardiological research will be explained in detail. Both are based on lactate oxidase isolated from Pediococcus species (Boehringer Mannheim, Germany) and entrapped in a polyurethane matrix [48]. The addition of different semipermeable and perforated gas permeable membranes results in enzyme sandwich membranes of different diffusion behaviour. They are applicable to highly diluted (method A; [49]) or undiluted blood samples (method B; [50,51]). All the lactate oxidase membranes are developed and commercialized by BST Bio Sensor Technology (Berlin-Buch, Germany).

Table 14.2. Lactate analyzer based on enzyme electrodes.

Company	Model	Sample frequency (h^{-1})	CV* (%)	Functional stability (d)
Application of Highly Diluted Whole Blood/Serum:				
La Roche (Switzerland)	LA 640	20–30	<5	30
YSI (USA)	23 L	42	3	30
PGW Medingen (Germany)	ESAT 6661	100–120	<2	14
Eppendorf (Germany)	EBIO	100–120	<2	14
Application of Undiluted Whole Blood/Serum				
NOVA (USA)	STAT-Profile 5	25–38	<4.1	7
EKF (Germany)	BIOSEN	>30	<5	10

* Coefficient of Variation.

Method A

A hypotonic phosphate buffer solution, pH 7.0, with the following composition is neccessary for sample dilution (1:50) as well as for rinsing the sensor (buffer A): 3 mmol/l KH_2PO_4, 10 mmol/l Na_2HPO_4, 30 mmol/l KCl, 1 ml/l Kathon WT (purchased from Fa. Rohm & Haas, Frankfurt/M, Germany). The buffer provides hemolysis and complete inhibition of glycolysis. Method A is applied to the analyzer ESAT 6661 (Prüfgeräte-Werk Medingen, Germany) and EBIO (Eppendorf Hamburg, Germany). Sensors are calibrated with solutions of 3, 6, 12, and 24 mmol/l lactate. These solutions are diluted 1:50 with the buffer A. The diluted standard solutions and buffer A solution are sold by the companies producing the ESAT 6661 and EBIO, respectively.

For assaying lactate concentration in the coronary blood as well as in samples from A. radialis 20 μl blood samples have to be diluted in 1 ml buffer A solution immediatly after withdrawal. The analyzer, which has to be pre-calibrated with 20 μl of a 12 mmol lactate/l containing standard solution, assayed the blood sample within 40 s with an imprecision below 2% using a measuring frequency of 120/h. The automatically calculated concentration of lactate is monitored digitally and can be screened together with other monitored parameter within the operation theatre. The comparison of results obtained by the ESAT 6661 (PGW Medingen, Germany) with those of the established photometric method [52] demonstrates the high accuracy of this lactate oxidase electrode based analyzer (Figure 14.4). Comparable results of high quality have been obtained with the EBIO system (Eppendorf) based on the same lactate oxidase membrane.

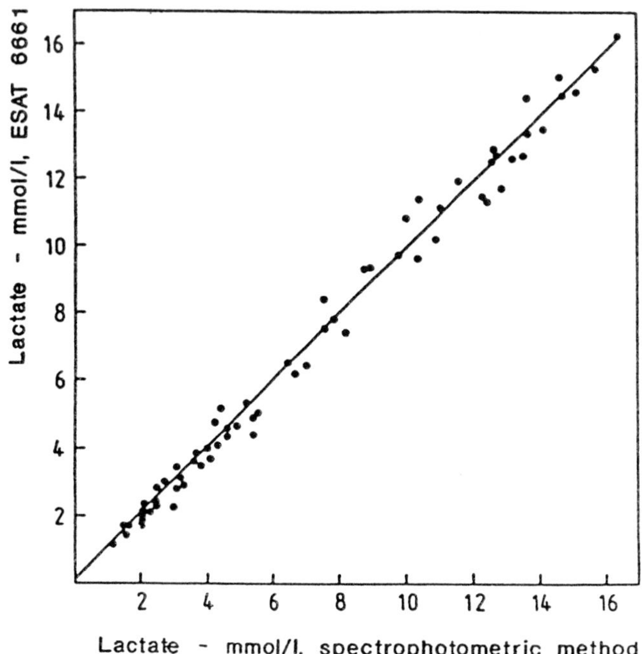

Figure 14.4. Comparison of lactate concentrations in highly diluted whole blood samples as measured with the Enzyme Chemical Analyzer ESAT 6661 and the spectrophotometric method: y = 0.9907x + 0.166; r = 0.9923; n = 71.

Method B

Method B is applied to the portable lactate device BIOSEN as shown in Figure 14.5. In contrast to Method A, undiluted whole blood without any preanalytics is used. Thus, the procedure is more simplified and faster in comparison to method A, providing the user with reliable lactate results without delay in time.

For sensor rinsing an isotonic phosphate buffer, 0.16 M, pH 7.0, containing 0.5 ml/l heparine (5000 IU/ml) and 1 ml/l Kathon WT is incorporated in the device. The rinsing as well as calibration solution of 5, 10, 15, and 20 mmol/l lactate are sold by the company EKF Magdeburg (Germany).

For assaying lactate concentration the unprepared whole blood (or serum) sample is put in the BIOSEN by the insertion of a capillary; the rinsing procedure is controlled by a microcomputer. A measuring chamber below 20 μl allows flow rates of less than 0.3 ml/min.

Simple handling and prompt results make this method a device ideally suited for use in the operating theatre. The application field of the portable device BIOSEN, however, can be extended up to the physician's consulting room and intensive care units. Furthermore, the analytical performance is of high quality: The response time of less than 10 s results in measuring

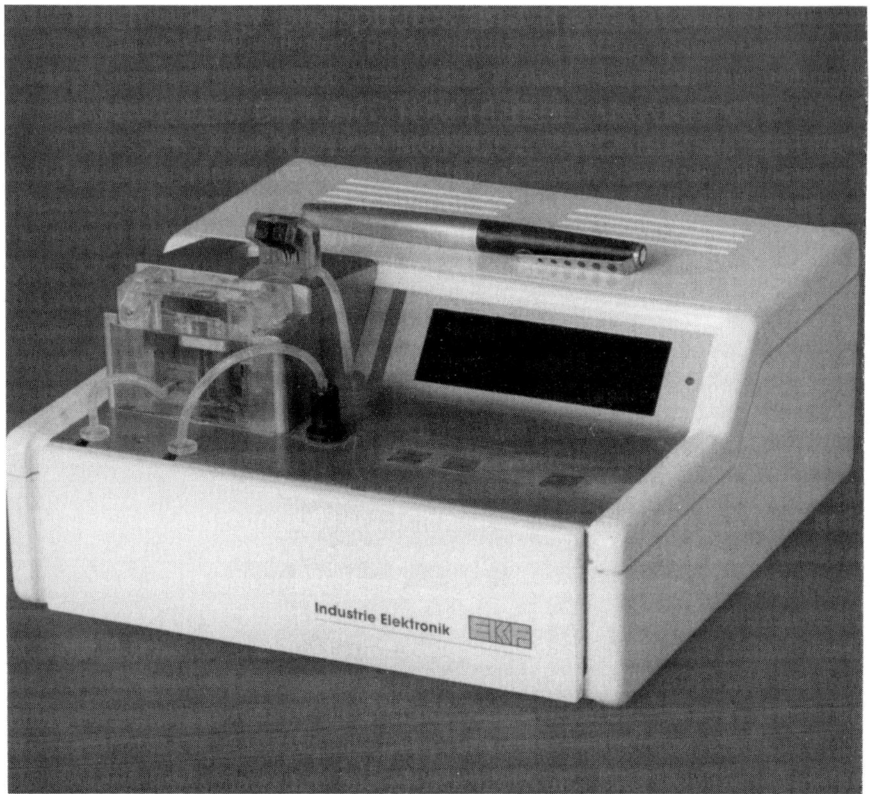

Figure 14.5. Portable lactate analyzing device BIOSEN-Lactate based on a lactate oxidase electrode. The BIOSEN device enables the user the measurement of lactate concentration in the whole blood within 10 s. We thank EKF Industrial Electronics Magdeburg (Germany) for providing a photograph of the newly developed device.

frequencies of more than 30/h with a serial imprecision below 5% for whole blood and serum [50]. The accuracy is demonstrated by comparison with the established analyzer ESAT 6661 as described by the following correlation equation:

$$y = 1.012x - 0.212 \text{ mmol/l}; \quad r = 0.987; \quad n = 35. \tag{9}$$

Due to the easy handling of the BIOSEN its application will probably be extended in the near future to intensive care units as well as to the physician's consulting room.

Application of the lactate biosenor for the assessment of cardiac energy metabolism

Coronary sinus lactate release during heart surgery

The intraoperative monitoring of the energy state of the human heart by means of arterio-coronary venous difference in lactate concentration during the rewarming of the cardioplegic organ before, during, and after cardiopulmonary bypass was performed for the first time using the lacate oxidase electrode based ESAT 6661 by Wollert *et al.* [26]. In this study forty-three patients undergoing heart surgery were subject to extended metabolic monitoring. In 95% of investigated patients a significant increase in the coronary sinus lactate concentration above the arterial concentration was estabilshed, as had been demonstrated earlier by conventional technique [21–29]. It showed no dependence on the indication for heart surgery (NYHA II to III), on the age and sex as well as on the aortic cross clamping time (CCT) of the individual patients. According to the data obtained [26], it is remarkable that the transient rise in coronary sinus lactate is characterized in 27 patients (63%) by an early 'cross-over-point'. On the average in two-thirds of the described heart surgery cases, using Bretschneider-HTK solution for the cardioplegic cardiac arrest, the reperfusion time (RT) for obtaining the COP was <10 min (7 ± 1 min) after starting reperfusion (patient group with early COP = ECOP). The individual measurements on these types of patients are given in Figure 14.6. In a smaller group of patients (n = 16) the coronary sinus lactate release persisted (see Figure 14.6B) and was found to be normalized only after >15 min 42 ± 5 min; patient group with late COP: LCOP), which in some cases occurred after weaning from the cardiopulmonary bypass [26].

Based on the role of lactate release into the coronary sinus [35] as a parameter of the energy metabolism of the heart (see above) one can assume that an only transient increase of lactate in the coronary sinus blood (group with ECOP) reflects the washout of the accumulated metabolite during cardioplegia and a rapid re-established aerobic ATP supply via oxidative phosphorylation in the mitochondria. A prolongation of high lactate concentration in the venous cardiac blood during cardiopulmonary bypass (patient group with LCOP) indicates, on the other hand, a delay in the normalization of aerobic ATP synthesis. This must have consequences for the re-establishment of the pump function of the heart, particularly in the case of a too early weaning from the assist device. Indeed, as can be seen in Table 14.3, the intra- and postoperative need for catecholamines in patients belonging to the socalled ECOP- and LCOP-groups, respectively, was found to be significant different. In the LCOP group, i.e. the one with an impaired cardiac energy metabolism in the period of re-animation of the postcardioplegic heart, supporting therapy by catecholamines was needed with higher dosages and for longer time [26].

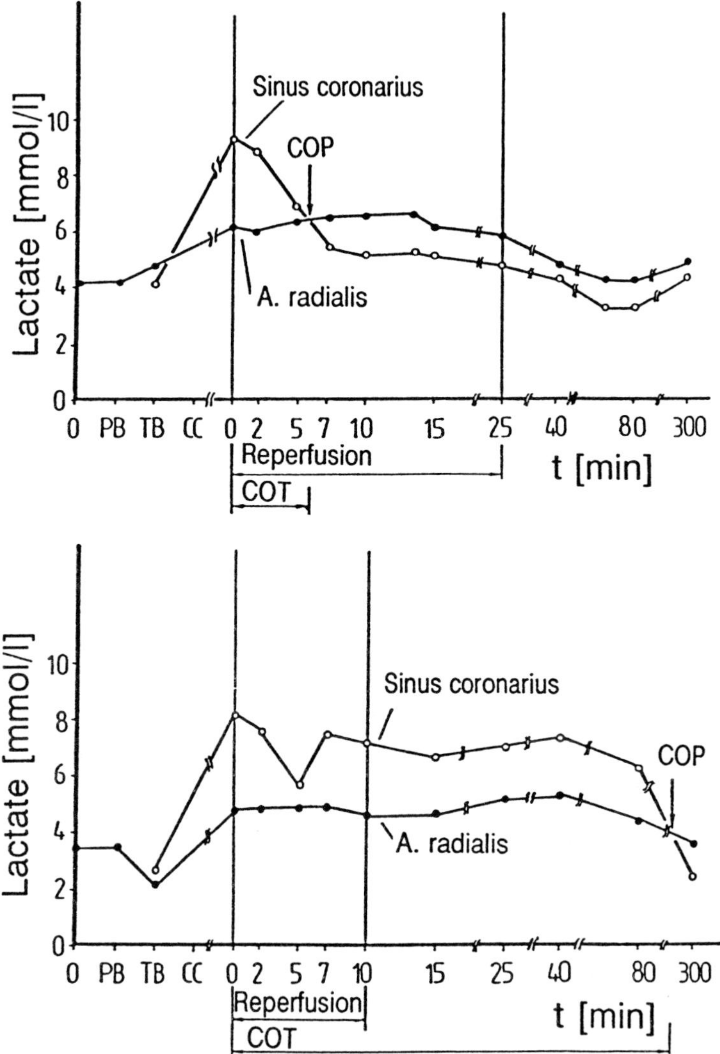

Figure 14.6. Metabolic energy-state assessment during cardiopulmonary bypass heart surgery by lacate monitoring. The time course of arterial and coronary venous concentration of lactate was followed by the lactate biosensor technique in 2 min and later in 20–30 min intervals. The dynamic changes in lactate consumption and lactate production and release, respectively, are defined by the cross-over-point (COP), indicating the reestablishment or at least the partial normalization of cardiac aerobic energy metabolism. The time of cardiopulmonary bypass is indicated (Reperfusion) as well as the time for obtaining COP (COT). Upper: patient R.K, male, 50 years old; mitral valve replacement (cross clamping time: 100 min). Lower: patient H.L., male, 35 years old; aortic valve replacement (cross clamping time: 75 min). Data modified and taken from [53].

Table 14.3. Necessity for supporting heart function after cardiac surgery by cardiotonics. Data modified from [26].

Group	n	CT-Score	Necessity for therapy (number of patients)	
			+	−
ECOP	27	$1.2 \pm 0.3^{a)}$	$11^{b)}$	$16^{b)}$
LCOP	16	$5.2 \pm 1.1^{a)}$	$13^{c)}$	$3^{c)}$

The intra- and postoperative catecholamines used were dopamine, adrenaline (Germed) and Dobutamin (Eli Lilly GmbH). For semi-quantitative judgement of catecholamine therapy, Wollert *et al.* [26] devised a score according to which 1 score point per day was allocated for a single drug administration of 3 μg/kg body weight per h and 1 score point per day for each additional cadioactive drug.

[a)] Significant differences in CT-score values according t-test: $p < 0.005$;

[b,c)] Differences in the necessity of therapy and CHI^2-test was used ($p < 0.005$).

ECOP; LCOP: patients with early cross-over-point and late cross-over-point, respectively, after reperfusion of the postcardioplegic heart (see also text).

Thus, with the aid of metabolic monitoring by coronary sinus lactate measurements in the operation theatre a new and sensitive diagnostic and prognostic parameter is now available. By this means a cardiac exhaustion at the levels of energy reserve and energy supply becomes detectable before hemodynamic parameters can be firmly assessed. It remains to be seen whether parameters like pH or pCO_2 as well as oxygen consumption are as sensitive as lactate, which represents the real end product of anaerobic energy metabolism and one of the real substrates for aerobic ATP synthesis in the heart.

Whether this parameter can be used to optimize the perioperative outcome due to a correct timing of the discontinuation of the bypass, especially in selected patients (NYHA III/IV, re-operation, high-risk operation [26]), needs further clinical studies. Of course, a lactate monitoring is excluded if the circuit fluid for cardiopulmonary bypass is substituted by high concentration of lactate [24].

Coronary sinus lactate during exercise catheter investigation

The developed biosenor for lactate can be employed also for identifying ischemic episodes during exercise catheter investigations, as was done recently [50]. The simple handling of the portable device BIOSEN for measuring lactate, together with the rapidity of the assay and requirement of only 20 μl blood may further extend the usage of this very classic parameter in cardiology.

References

1. Kobayashi K, Neely JR. Control of maximum rates of glycolysis in rat cardiac muscle. Circ Res 1979;44: 166–75.
2. Wollenberger A, Krause EG. Metabolic control characteristics of the acutely ischemic myocardium. Am J Cardiol 1968, 22: 349–59.
3. Olsson RA. Changes in content of purine nucleoside in canine myocardium during coronary occlusion. Circ Res 1970; 26: 301–6.
4. Bretschneider HJ. Überlebenszeit und Wiederbelebenszeit des Herzens bei Normo- und Hypothermie. Verh Dtsch Ges Kreisl-Forsch 1964; 30: 11–34.
5. Preusse CJ, Bretschneider HJ, Gebhard MM. Comparison of cardioplegic methods of Kirklin, Bretschneider, and St. Thomas' Hospital by means of biochemical and functional analyses during the postischemic aerobic recovery period. In Isselhard E (eds): Myocardial protection for cardiac surgery. Pharmaz. Verlagsgesell mbH München: 1981; 184–193.
6. Flameng W, van Haecke J, van Belle H *et al.* Relation between coronary artery stenosis and myocardial purine metabolism, histology and regional function in humans. J Am Coll Cardiol 1987; 9: 1235–42.
7. Vusse van der GJ, Coremans WA, Veen van der E *et al.* ATP, creatine phosphate and glycogen content of human myocardial biopsies: markers for the efficacy of cardioprotection during aorto- coronary bypass surgery. Vasc Res 1984;18: 127–34.
8. Veen van der FH, Vusse van der GJ, Flameng W *et al.* Metabolic and haemodynamic changes in the heart during the early phase of cardiopulmonary bypass: I. Clinical observations. Cardiovasc Res 1989; 22: 468–71.
9. Veen van der FH, Vusse van der GJ, Kruger RTI *et al.* Metabolic and haemodynamic changes in the heart during the early phase of cardiopulmonary bypass: II. Animal experiments. Cardiovasc Res 1989; 23: 472–7.
10. Regitz V, Fleck E. Adenine nucleotide metabolism and contractile dysfunction in heart failure – Biochemical aspects, animal experiments, and human studies. Basic Res Cardiol 1992; 187 (Suppl 1): 321–9.
11. Fremes SE, Weisel RD Mickle DAG *et al.* Myocardial metabolism and ventricular function following cold potassium cardioplegia. J Thorac Cardiovasc Surg 1985; 89: 531–46.
12. Philips HR, Carter JE, Okada RD *et al.* Serial changes in left ventricular ejection fraction in the early hours after aortocoronary bypass grafting. Chest 1983; 83: 28–34.
13. Schaefer S, Gober J, Valenza M *et al.* Nuclear magnetic resonance imaging-guided phosphorus-31 spectroscopy of the human heart. J Am Coll Cardiol 1988; 12: 1449–55.
14. Hardy JH, Weiss RG, Bottomley PA *et al.* Altered myocardial high-energy phosphate metabolites in patients with dilated cardiomyopathy. Am Heart J 1991; 122: 795–801.
15. Barlow CH, Harken AH, Chance B. Evaluation of cardiac ischemia by NADH fluorescence photography. Science 1976; 193: 909–10.
16. Simon MB, Harden WR, Barlow CH *et al.* Epicardial ischemia as delineated with epicardial S-T segment mapping and nicotinamide adenine dinucleotide (NADH) fluorescence photography. Am J Cardiol 1979; 44: 263–9.
17. Gudipati CV, Weil MH, Gazmuri RJ *et al.* Increases in coronary vein CO_2 during cardiac resuscitation. J Appl Physiol 1990; 68: 1405–8.
18. Preusse CJ, Gebhard MM, Bretschneider HJ. Interstitial pH value in the myocardium as indicator of ischemic stress of cardioplegically arrested hearts. Basic Res Cardiol 1982; 77: 372–87.
19. Frombach R, Reil G-H, Hiltermann G *et al.* Kontinuierliche pH-Registrierungen im Koronarsinus in vivo bei ischämischer und normoxischer Laktazidose mittels eines ISFET-Katheters. Z Kardiol 1989; 78: 253–61.
20. Khuri SF, Marston WA, Josa M *et al.* Observations on 100 patients with continuous intraoperative monitoring of intramyocardial pH. J Thorac Cardiovasc Surg 1985; 89: 170–82.
21. Apstein CS, Deckelbaum L, Müller M *et al.* Graded global ischemia and reperfusion. Cardiac function and lactate metabolism. Circulation 1977; 55: 864–71.

22. Engelman RM, Rousou JH, Lemeshow S *et al*. The metabolic consequences of blood and crytalloid cardioplegia. Circulation 1981; 64 (Suppl. II) 67–74.
23. Kaijser L, Jansson E, Schmidt W *et al*. Myocardial energy depletion during profound hypothermic cardioplegia for cardiac operation. Thorac Cardiovasc Surg 1985; 90: 869–900.
24. Teoh KH, Mickle DAG, Weisel RD *et al*. Improving myocardial metabolic and functional recovery after cardioplegic arrest. J Thorac Cardiovasc Surg 1988; 95: 788–98.
25. Jalonen J, Heikkila H, Arola *et al*. Myocardial oxygen balance and cardiopulmonary bypass in patients undergoing coronary artery bypass grafting. J Cardiothorac Anesth 1989; 3: 311–20.
26. Wollert HG, Müller W, Fischer D *et al*. Perioperative assessment of cardiac energy metabolism by means of arterio-coronary venous difference in lactate concentration (acDL). Eur J Cardio-thorac Surg 1990; 4: 278–83.
27. Gunnicker M, Freund U, Hirche H *et al*. Hemodynamics and myocardial energy balance in coronary surgery patients during high-dose fentanyl-pancuronium anesthesia and modified neurolept-pancuronium anesthesia. Anaesthesist 1990; 39: 406–11.
28. Smolenski RT, Swierczynski J, Narkiewicz M *et al*. Purines, lactate and phosphate release from child and adult heart during cardioplegic arrest. Clin Chim Acta 1990; 192: 155–64.
29. Yau TM, Weisel RD, Mickle DA *et al*. Optimal delivery of blood cardioplegia. Circulation 1991; 84 (Suppl 5): III 380–8.
30. Schubert F, Pfeiffer D, Wollenberger U *et al*. Enzyme-chemical Analyzer ECA 20/ESAT 6660. In Schmid RD, Scheller F (eds): GBF Monographs 1990; 15: 11–5.
31. Pfeiffer D, Setz K, Kliemes N *et al*. Enzyme electrodes for medical applications. In Scheller FW, Schmid RD (eds): GBF Monographs 1992; 17: 11–8.
32. Bergmann G, Atkinson L, Metcalf J *et al*. Beneficial effect of enhanced myocardial carbohydrate utilization after oxfenicine (L-hydroxyphenylglycine) in angina pectoris. Eur Heart J 1980; 7: 247–52.
33. Griggs DM, Nagano S, Lipana JG *et al*. Myocardial lactate oxidation in situ, and the effects thereon of reduced coronary flow. Am J Physiol 1966; 68: 295–303.
34. Bing JR, Siegel A, Vitale A *et al*. Metabolic studies on the human heart in vivo. I. Studies on carbohydrate metabolism of the human heart. Am J Med 1953; 15: 284–96.
35. Ferrari R, Agnoletti G, Ciampalini G *et al*. Coronary sinus lactate release as an index of myocardial anaerobiosis: Effect of interventions. Adv Cardiol 1986; 35: 115–26.
36. Opie LH. Role of Metabolism in ischemia. In: Abe H, editor. Regulation of cardiac function. Japan Sci Soc Press, Tokyo/VNU Sci Press, Utrecht 1984, 129–51.
37. Langer GA. The effect of pH on cellular and membrane calcium binding and contraction of myocardium. Circ Res 1985; 57: 374–82.
38. Schaper J, Walter P, Scheld H *et al*. The effects of retrograde perfusion of cardioplegic solution in cardiac operations. J Thorac Cardiovasc Surg 1985; 90: 882–7.
39. Chance B, Higgins J, Holmes W *et al*. Localization of interaction sites in multicomponent transfer systems: Theorem derived from analogues. Nature 1958; 182: 1190–2.
40. Scheller FW, Schubert F (eds). Biosensors. Amsterdam-London-New York-Tokyo: Elsevier, 1992; 1–325.
41. Blaedel WJ, Engstrom RC. Reagentless enzyme electrodes for ethanol, lactate, and malate. Anal Chem 1980; 52: 1691–7.
42. Malinauskas A, Kulys JJ. Alcohol, lactate and glutamate sensors based on oxidoreductases with regeneration of nicotinamide adenine dinucleotide. Analyt Chim Acta 1978; 98: 131–9.
43. Williams DL, Doig AR, Korosi A. Electrochemical – enzymatic analysis of glucose and lactate. Anal Chem 1970; 42: 118–21.
44. Schindler JG, von Gülich M. L-Lactat-Durchflußelektrode mit immobilisierter Lactatoxidase. Fresenius Z Anal Chem 1981; 308: 434–6.
45. Mascini M, Moscone D, Palleschi G. A lactate electrode with lactate oxidase immobilized on nylon net for blood serum samples in flow systems. Analyt Chim Acta 1984; 157: 45–51.

46. Weigelt D, Schubert F, Scheller F. Enzyme sensor for the determination of lactate and lactate dehydrogenase activity. Analyst 1987; 112: 1155–8.
47. Mullen WH, Churchhouse SJ, Keedy FH *et al.* Enzyme electrode for the measurement of lactate in undiluted blood. Clin Chim Acta 1986; 157: 191–7.
48. Nentwig J, Scheller F, Weise H *et al.* Laminierte Membran und Verfahren zu ihrer Anwendung. DD patent 1986; 2778–884.
49. Pfeiffer D, Scheller FW, Setz K *et al.* Amperometric enzyme electrodes for lactate and glucose analysis in highly diluted and in undiluted media. Analyt Chim Acta 1993; in press.
50. Pfeiffer D, Setz K, Schulmeister T *et al.* Development and characterization of an enzyme based lactate probe for undiluted media. Biosensors & Bioelectronics 1992; 7: 661–71.
51. Scheller F, Seyer I, Scheller O *et al.* Sterilisierbare Enzymelektrode. DD-Patent 1977; 131 414.
52. Hohorst HJ, Kreutz FH, Bücher T. Über Metabolitgehalte und Metabolitkonzentrationen der Leber der Ratte. Biochem Z 1959; 332: 118–46.
53. Fischer D. Die arterio-koronarvenöse Differenz der Laktatkonzentration während herzchirurgischer Eingriffe. Dissertation, Martin-Luther Univ. Halle-Wittenberg 1990.

15. Myocardial tissue pH in the assessment of the extent of myocardial ischemia and the adequacy of myocardial protection

MICHAEL B. TANTILLO and SHUKRI F. KHURI

Introduction

In almost every cardiac surgical operation, the aorta is cross-clamped and the myocardium is deprived of its blood and nutrient supply. A compendium of methodologies have been devised under the umbrella of 'myocardial protection' aimed at avoiding the damage caused by the ischemic and reperfusion injuries that can be elicited by aortic clamping and at extending as long as possible the 'safety' of this period. Unfortunately, to date, there are no dependable clinically applicable methods which would allow the surgeon to monitor the efficacy of these protective methodologies *during* the vulnerable period of aortic clamping. Measurement of myocardial temperature can only reflect the adequacy of the delivery of the cardioplegia solution during the initial period following aortic clamping. Furthermore, temperature is no indication of the metabolic viability of the myocardium since one can cool even a dead heart!

Research in our laboratory over the past thirteen years has been directed towards the development of a technique which would monitor the metabolic viability of the heart in the course of cardiac surgery, and particularly during the period of aortic clamping. We theorized that such a technique, if validated, would allow for intraoperative intervention to improve the metabolic protection of the heart, and will also provide a tool and an end-point for the evaluation of the various myocardial protective methods and techniques. Research in the field of myocardial protection to date has been markedly hampered by the lack of such a definable end-point.

Based on original work in which myocardial tissue pCO_2, measured with a mass spectrometer, was demonstrated to be quantitatively reflective of the tissue hydrogen ion concentration and of regional myocardial ischemia, we developed a tissue pH electrode and a system for intraoperative on-line metabolic monitoring of the heart with the hypothesis that the hydrogen ion is a reliable metabolic indicator of the magnitude of myocardial ischemia and of the adequacy of myocardial protection from ischemic damage. The first part of this chapter addresses the basis of this hypothesis by reviewing the role of the hydrogen ion in myocardial ischemia and the evidence which justifies its use in the quantitation of the magnitude of regional ischemic injury. The second part of this chapter addresses the clinical application

H.M. Piper and C.J. Preusse (eds): Ischemia-reperfusion in cardiac surgery, 335–352.

of the method developed in our laboratory for the on-line intraoperative measurement of myocardial tissue pH in the course of cardiac surgery.

Basic considerations

Sources of hydrogen ion in myocardial cells

The myocardium extracts approximately seventy percent of arterial oxygen, the highest fractional oxygen extraction of any organ in the body, and approximately ten percent of the arterial carbon substrate [1]. Therefore, it is not surprising that myocardial metabolism is critically dependent on oxygen supply and is almost entirely aerobic [1]. In the healthy, non-ischemic heart, oxidation of free fatty acids and carbohydrates provide the energy for ATP production [1,2]. The relative importance of each carbon source varies with the physiological state of the body. During a fasted state lipids provide the major carbon source and are transported across the sarcolemma into the cytosol. Lipids are then transported across the mitochondrial membrane via the acyl-carnitine transport mechanism in order to undergo beta-oxidation within the mitochondria. Each molecule of palmitate which is fully oxidized yields 130 molecules of ATP [2]. Following a high carbohydrate meal when glucose and insulin concentrations in the blood are high, glucose transport across the sarcolemma is enhanced and glucose is oxidized to pyruvate by glycolysis in the cytosol. Pyruvate is then oxidized in the citrate cycle within the mitochondria. Each molecule of fully oxidized glucose yields 38 molecules of ATP [2]. During glycolysis NAD, rather than oxygen, serves as the reducing substance; therefore, the oxidation of glucose to pyruvate (or lactate) is an oxygen independent process [2]. During exercise the rate of glycolysis and glycogenolysis can be rapidly increased, and lactate uptake from the bloodstream is increased. Each molecule of lactate which is fully oxidized via conversion to pyruvate and then the citrate cycle yields 18 molecules of ATP [2]. Because the myocyte is able to use a variety of carbon substrates for energy supply, and since normal extraction of carbon substrate is quite low, carbon substrate supply does not limit ATP production; oxygen is the limiting metabolite for ATP production [1].

Many metabolic reactions produce hydrogen ion in the myocardial cells. In the normally perfused myocardium, hydrogen production and washout are in equilibrium. The hydrolysis of ATP, the synthesis of triglycerides from palmitate, the hydrolysis of triglycerides, glycolysis, and glycogenolysis are all major sources of hydrogen ion production in the myocardial cell [3]. Carbon dioxide retention from decarboxylative oxidation of substrate might also serve to acidify the cell [3]. During total global ischemia the oxidative production of ATP falls to zero and the anaerobic glycolysis is the major source of ATP production. An intracellular decrease in high energy phosphates and increase in inorganic phosphate initially promote and sustain anaerobic glycolysis via the Pasteur effect; however, with increasing severity of ischemia, lactate and hydrogen ion will inhibit glycolysis [2]. Catecholamine release activates the phosphorylase which begins glycogenolysis, thus increasing substrate for glycolysis. Anaerobic glycolysis is able to proceed rapidly for 60–120 seconds, then slows to a plateau for approximately 90 minutes, and finally ceases [4]. Myocardial contractility decreases, thus preserving ATP. Thus, the hydrogen ions accumulate in the ischemic myocardial tissue as a result of two distinct processes. An increased production of hydrogen ion production from glycogenolysis, anaerobic glycolysis, and ATP hydrolysis; and a decreased wash-out of hydrogen ions secondary to a reduction or cessation of blood flow [5,6]. Due to the presence of bicarbonate and carbonic anhydrase, this acidosis results in the production of CO_2 and H_2O. Like hydrogen ion, CO_2 accumulates in the ischemic myocardium, and its concentration is also determined by a balance between continued production and decreased washout [5].

During regional ischemia oxygen is still available to the myocyte, although in reduced concentrations. Nonetheless, anaerobic ATP production is only a fraction of the total ATP production in the cell, and glycolytic ATP production is maintained at a lower but significant rate [6]. The metabolic changes which lead to myocardial acidification during regional ischemia are a presence of a limited oxygen supply enabling ATP production to persist albeit at a decreased rate, the continued production of carbon dioxide, ATP hydrolysis, and the decreased washout of metabolites [6]. Therefore the intracellular metabolism of functional but ischemic myocardial cells actively produces hydrogen ions which will accumulate in the myocardial cell and interstitium if the rate of washout does not exceed the rate of production.

The intracellular hydrogen ion concentration is regulated primarily by two cellular ion pump systems. The pump system of primary importance in reducing an increase in intracellular hydrogen ion is the Na^+/H^+ exchange pump located on the plasma membrane [7]. The Na^+/H^+ exchange pump is a 1:1 exchange with a greater than first order dependence on the intracellular hydrogen ion concentration which extrudes hydrogen from the intracellular space to the interstitium and pumps Na^+ into the cell [8]. In addition to regulating intracellular pH and mediating cell recovery from an acid load, this pump also plays an important role in the regulation of cell volume and metabolic responses to hormones such as insulin [8]. The plasma membrane Na^+/Ca^{++} exchanger also plays an important role in the regulation of intracellular pH. This pump is reversible, although throughout most of the cardiac cycle it functions to pump calcium from the cytosol to the interstitium in exchange for sodium [2]. The intracellular calcium concentration and intracellular pH move in opposite directions. As calcium is pumped out of the cell, the intracellular calcium ion concentration decreases and intracellular hydrogen ion then exchanges with calcium at intracellular buffer sites, thereby, at least partially replacing the cytosolic free calcium and increasing the intracellular pH. The precise Ca^{++}/H^+ buffer sites are as yet not fully defined; although the sarcoplasmic reticulum and the mitochondria are likely to play a role [7,9]. The importance of such Na^{+}/Ca^{++}, exchange at the plasma membrane followed by Ca^{+}/H^{+} exchange intracellularly in regulating intracellular pH has been demonstrated in mammalian cardiac muscle [9]. Anion transport, specifically that of chloride and bicarbonate, does not play a role in the regulation of intracellular pH [7]. Following an intracellular acid load, hydrogen ions are buffered within the cell and actively extruded from the cytosol to the interstitium. Therefore, under ischemic conditions, one would expect extracellular pH to fall more than intracellular pH. Simultaneous measurements of intracellular and extracellular pH in the intact heart, however, have been scarce.

Acidosis is associated with depressed myocardial function [10–15]. The mechanisms by which acidosis depresses contractility are complex and not completely understood. A comprehensive review article by Orchard and Kentisk [16] describes the potential mechanisms by which acidosis might alter the intracellular calcium concentration. Calcium delivery to myofilimants may be reduced by inhibition of the inward calcium current, resulting in a reduction of the amount of calcium released from the sarcoplasmic reticulum, and a shortening of the action potential as sometimes occurs. On the other hand, acidosis may enhance calcium delivery to the myocyte by prolonging the action potential and by a rise in calcium influx during diastole which leads to increased uptake and subsequent release of calcium by the sarcoplasmic reticulum. The rise of diastolic calcium influx may be due to increased sodium entry into the cell via the sodium-hydrogen exchange which subsequently leads to increased calcium in the cell via the calcium-sodium exchange. Acidosis might increase mitochondrial release of calcium as well as displacement of calcium from intracellular buffers; both actions would also increase the calcium concentration during diastole [16]. However, regardless of the net effect on intracellular calcium concentration by the mechanisms described above, acidosis does seem to decrease sensitivity of the myocyte contractile proteins to calcium [16–18] probably by decreasing the binding of calcium to troponin-c [16]. Furthermore the hydrogen ion itself may act directly on the actin-myosin cross bridges decreasing the maximum force of contraction [16]. Hydrogen ions can also depress gap junction conductance, regulate ATPase activity, and depress the rate of cardiac energy metabolism [19]. Therefore hydrogen ions can depress myocardial contractility through direct actions on the myocyte as well as through interactions with intracellular calcium.

Myocardial tissue pCO_2, which has been shown to correlate well with myocardial tissue hydrogen ion concentration [5], has been shown to decrease myocardial contractility as well [20]. Since tissue acidosis results in increased CO_2 production through the carbonic anhydrase reaction, the relative contribution of the increased hydrogen ion concentration versus that of increased pCO_2 to the ischemic decrease in myocardial contractility remains unclear.

Methods of measuring tissue acidosis

Various methods of measurement of myocardial pH have been utilized to date; however, most have been fraught with significant limitations [4]. For the measurement of extracellular tissue pH, both epicardial/surface [21–23] and intramyocardial/plunge [24–33] electrodes have been used. Surface glass electrodes were used briefly [21–23], but were abandoned because of their poor reproducibility and their failure to measure pH in the deeper layers of the heart which are more vulnerable to ischemic changes [4]. Glass tipped electrodes, polymer tipped electrodes, and fiberoptic probes have all been used as part of a plunge probe in order to measure extracellular tissue pH [4]. The electrode developed in our laboratory over the past decade is the only electrode which has been shown to be reproducible and clinically applicable in patients undergoing hypothermic cardiopulmonary bypass. It differs from polymer and other plunge electrodes by not incorporating the reference electrode in the sensing tip along with the pH electrode. The reference electrode is placed in extracorporeal KCl and connected to the subcutaneous tissues of the periphery with a salt bridge, allowing for accurate calibration to be made in the face of discordant myocardial and systemic temperatures [34]. The assumptions used in the calibrations of this tissue electrode are currently being verified in our laboratory because they borrow from known relationships between blood (not tissue) pH and temperature. Separating the reference electrode from the pH electrode has markedly improved the reproducibility and performance of this system without interfering with its accuracy and sensitivity. In the canine under baseline conditions, the myocardial pH measured with various types of glass electrodes of varying reliability has been reported to range from 6.80 to 7.50; it has been reported to range from 7.21 to 7.39 with Polymer-tipped electrodes and fiberoptic probes [35]. In a large number of canine studies in our laboratory, the average baseline myocardial pH obtained is 7.31 ± 0.095, and the average baseline myocardial pH in a large number of isolated rabbit heart studies is 7.23 ± 0.095.

Measurement of intracellular myocardial pH has been most consistently achieved by the use of ^{31}P nuclear magnetic resonance (NMR) spectroscopy [4]. With this experimental technique, resonance peaks which correspond with high energy phosphates (HEP), phosphocreatine (PCr), and inorganic phosphate (Pi) are readily identifiable. The position of the Pi peak is dependent on the intracellular pH, and the intracellular pH can be calculated from the relationship of the Pi peak to the PCr peak [37]. However, the accuracy of the intracellular pH measurement is subject to several factors. The signal to noise ratio largely determines the accuracy of the baseline peak Pi and PCr position assignments; and therefore, the accuracy of the Pi shift. Baseline fluctuations, peak overlap, and calibration uncertainty can also contribute to errors in pH calculations [38]. Another potential shortcoming of NMR spectroscopy is that of intracellular compartmentation, that is the potential metabolic differences between the cytoplasm and intracellular organelles. To date a heterogeneity of intracellular myocardial pH has not been reported, although, an intracellular pH gradient of 0.5–1.0 has been reported in hepatocytes, kidney cells, skeletal muscle, and E. coli [37]. A transthoracic surface NMR coil has been utilized for myocardial ^{31}P NMR spectroscopy clinically [39–42]. HEP and PCr peaks have been defined by this technique but intracellular pH measurements have not been reported with it.

Electrode-derived myocardial pH as a measurement of regional ischemia

Myocardial tissue pH, as measured with our glass electrode, has been shown to reflect the extent of regional myocardial ischemia in several experimental studies. Under ischemic conditions, it correlated highly with myocardial tissue pCO_2 [5] which, in turn, had been shown to correlate with intramyocardial ST segment changes on the electrocardiogram [30]. It also correlated with the magnitude of fall in myocardial blood flow, and with the magnitude of the ischemic process as assessed by ultrastructural analyses [5]. The electrode was also highly specific and sensitive in depicting ischemic events in the conscious chronically instrumented canine [28], and in reflecting the degree of myocardial protection in the canine subjected to global ischemia during cardiopulmonary bypass [32]. Recently, measurements of electrode-derived myocardial tissue pH in the intact open chest canine, were obtained simultaneously, for the first time, with measurements of intracellular pH obtained by NMR spectroscopy [24]. A baseline gradient of 0.2 pH units was observed between the more acidic intracellular pH and the electrode-derived tissue pH. During ischemia, however, the correlation coefficient between the two pH measurements exceeded 0.95 (see Figure 15.1A). More importantly, the fall in electrode-derived myocardial pH during ischemia correlated, to the same degree, with the fall in myocardial ATP (see Figure 15.1B), underscoring the ability of the electrode to quantify the extent of metabolic ischemic changes [24].

During prolonged regional ischemia (3 hours) in the canine model, the extracellular pH within the ischemic region progressively falls to a nadir then begins to rise despite persistent ischemia and no change in regional myocardial blood flow. The late rise in myocardial pH during the occlusion parallels a fall in tissue pCO_2 and is indicative of progressive cellular dysfunction with a decreased production of hydrogen ion [5]. The ability of the myocardial cell to produce hydrogen ion is in all probability indicative of its cellular viability.

With relatively short (less than 25 min) periods of successive regional ischemia with 45 min of reperfusion in between, the amount of hydrogen ion produced during the first ischemic period is significantly more than the amount of hydrogen ion produced during the subsequent ischemic periods (see Figure 15.2) [36]. As the severity of the experimental ischemic insult

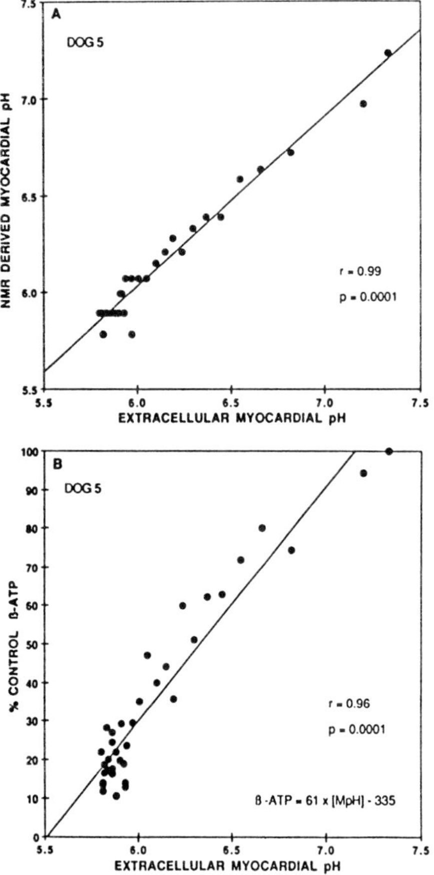

Figure 15.1. Data acquired from an open chest canine subjected to 3 h of LAD occlusion. A 2 cm two-turn surface coil was sutured to the epicardium for acquisition of phosphorus-31 NMR spectroscopy from a region of the ischemic midmyocardium. A pH electrode was plunged into the midmyocardium adjacent to the coil for extracellular pH measurement. 1A: A linear regression plot of extracellular pH versus NMR-derived intracellular pH in one representative animal during 3 h of ischemia. 1B: A linear regression plot of extracellular myocardial pH versus myocardial ATP content (expressed as percent control) from one representative animal during three hours of ischemia. From Axford TC, Dearani JA, Khait I *et al.* Electrode-derived myocardial pH measurements reflect intracellular myocardial metabolism assessed by phosphorus 31-nuclear magnetic resonance spectroscopy during normothermic ischemia. J Thorac Cardiovasc Surg 1992, 103. 902–7, used with permission.

is increased by increasing the duration of coronary artery occlusion, the difference between the amount of hydrogen ion produced during the first and the second occlusions becomes greater, and the amount of contractile dysfunction present during reperfusion, as measured by myocardial regional

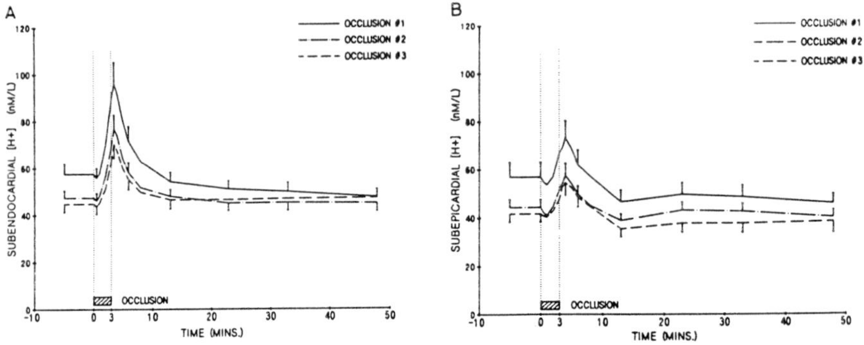

Figure 15.2. Cumulative data obtained from fifteen open chest canines, each subjected to three serial three-minute occlusions of the LAD with each occlusion separated by a forty-five minute period of reperfusion. Myocardial pH was measured with two pH electrodes, one placed with the tip in the subendocardium and one placed with the tip in the subepicardium. Figure 15.1A shows the hydrogen ion accumulation in the subendocardium, and Figure 15.1B shows the hydrogen ion accumulation in the subepicardial region. The patterns of hydrogen ion accumulation were similar in both regions; although, the subendocardium was more acidic than the subepicardium. The hydrogen ion accumulation was greatest during the first occlusion, and the accumulation during the second and third occlusions were similar. From Warner KG, Khuri SF, Marston W *et al.* Significance of the transmural dimunition in regional hydrogen ion production after repeated coronary artery occlusions. Circ Res 1989; 64: 616–28 used by permission of the American Heart Association, Inc.

systolic shortening, also worsens [36]. Hence, the changes in myocardial tissue pH following the first of a series of coronary artery occlusions has been interpreted as a form of 'metabolic stunning' [36].

Under physiologic conditions, hypothermia elicits a rise in tissue pH which has been assumed to be parallel to that of the pH of blood or water [43–45]. It is estimated that for every one-degree change in myocardial temperature, the tissue pH changes by 0.015–0.017 pH units. Thus, failure of the tissue pH to rise in the face of a fall in myocardial temperature is indicative of relative tissue acidosis. These relationships are paramount in the interpretation of myocardial pH changes during the period of aortic occlusion and immediate reflow in the course of cardiac surgery. Cold alkaline cardioplegia solutions administered during this period should elicit a significant rise in myocardial pH. This rise is primarily due to hypothermia and is independent of the alkalinity of, or the increased washout elicited by, the cardioplegia solution [46].

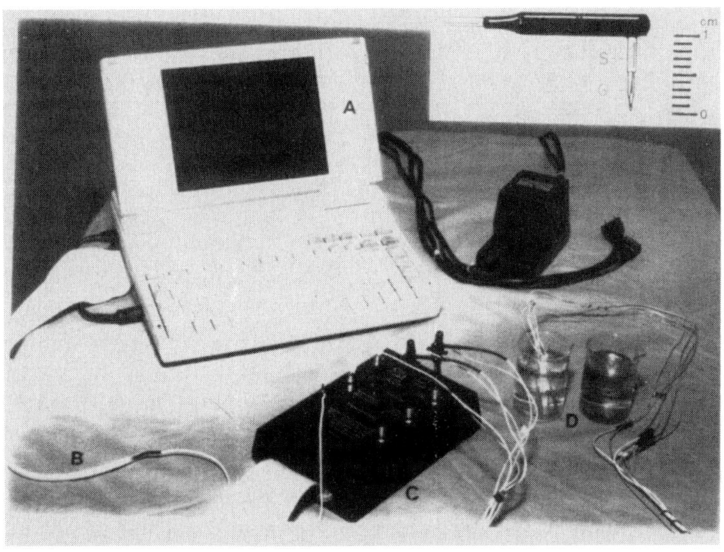

Figure 15.3. The myocardial pH monitor currently in use in the operating room at our institution. A. Laptop computer for display and storage of on-line myocardial pH and temperature corrected myocardial pH. B. Agar bridge which completes the circuit from the patient's subcutaneous tissue to the reference beaker of KCl. C. The probe junction box which interfaces the laptop computer with the tissue pH electrodes and tissue temperature probes. D. pH and temperature probes submerged in reference buffer. Inset: the pH electrode currently used at our institution. It is 10 mm in length and composed of a 4 mm glass sensing tip (G), and a steel jacket (S).

Clinical applications

Methodology

Myocardial tissue pH is commonly monitored at our institution in patients undergoing complex cardiac surgical procedures. The electrode is 10 mm long, 1 mm in outside diameter, glass tipped and steel jacketed with a completely shielded coaxial cable (Figure 15.3). The stabilization time is two to five minutes and the *in vitro* 95% response time is two to three seconds. The pH drift after six hours in tissue is less than 0.01 units. A separate reference electrode is placed outside the body and connected to the subcutaneous tissue in the forearm via a salt bridge. The electrode is inserted into the midmyocardium and affixed with a fine epicardial suture. A separate temperature plunge electrode is also inserted within a few millimeters of the pH electrode. Signals from both the pH electrode and the corresponding temperature probe are directed into a laptop computer (Figure 15.3) for processing, calibration, and temperature correction. On-line pH and temperature data are continuously displayed on the screen and stored permanently on disk, and can be exported into a variety of PC software applications for further analysis. In the majority of cases, temperature and pH are monitored in the anterior (or anterolateral) and the inferior (or posterolateral) walls of the left ventricle.

Assessment of adequacy of preservation

Myocardial pH, as measured by the system described above, has been shown to provide a reliable on-line assessment of the adequacy of myocardial preservation. In the first forty patients at our institution in whom myocardial pH was measured intraoperatively, a clinical scoring system was devised to assess the adequacy of intraoperative myocardial protection. This preservation score was based on the patient's need for intraoperative inotropic support, the need for intraaortic balloon counterpulsation, the postoperative electrocardiograms, the postoperative CPKs and MB bands, the postoperative radioventriculogram, and the need for postoperative inotropic support. A high score was indicative of clinical evidence of poor myocardial protection while a low score was indicative of good protection. The mean myocardial pH during the period of aortic clamping correlated well with the clinical assessment of myocardial preservation; the higher the mean myocardial pH the lower was the score. The duration of the period of aortic clamping also correlated with the preservation score; the longer the period, the higher the score. Myocardial temperature, in contrast, did not correlate with the preservation score [30].

Figure 15.4A displays the intraoperative myocardial pH and temperature plots in an example of good myocardial protection. The patient was a 67-year-old man who underwent a mitral valve replacement with a double coronary artery bypass graft. A pH electrode and a temperature probe were each placed in the anterior and postero-lateral walls of the left ventricle. At the time of cardioplegia delivery and topical cooling, the temperature in both walls of the left ventricle fell and the myocardial pH in both walls rose. The myocardial pH and temperature remained relatively stable throughout the period of aortic clamping. Upon reperfusion the myocardial temperature rose and, as expected, the myocardial pH fell to its pre-clamping level. Figure 15.4B displays the pH data in both walls assuming a constant temperature of 37°C throughout the course of the operation. This display corrects for the physiologic effect of temperature on pH and allows a direct appreciation of the acid-base status of the myocardium. Note that during the course of the operation the temperature-corrected pH remained mostly over 7.0 in both walls, indicating adequate myocardial protection. This patient was weaned from cardiopulmonary bypass with no significant inotropic support and had a smooth and uneventful postoperative course.

Figure 15.5 is an example of inadequate myocardial protection of the posterior wall of the left ventricle. This 70-year-old man had not been known to have coronary artery disease and underwent a complex aortic valve re-

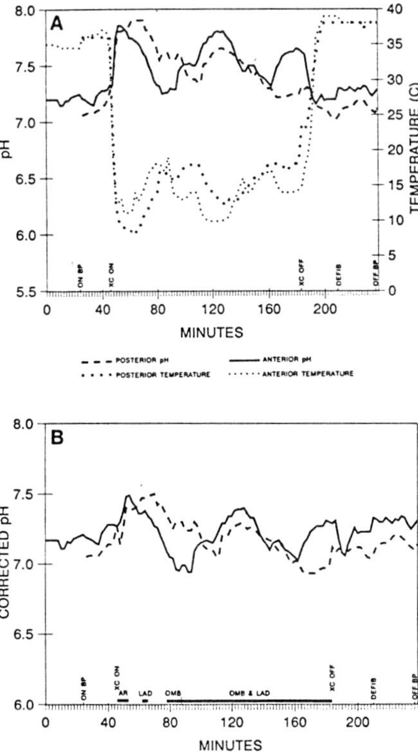

Figure 15.4. Myocardial pH and temperature tracings from a 67–year-old man who underwent mitral valve replacement and two-vessel coronary artery revascularization. Figure 15.4A shows the actual pH and temperature tracings throughout the case. Figure 15.4B shows the pH corrected to 37°C. In Figure 15.4B the times and routes of cardioplegia delivery are displayed by horizontal bars. A pH, anterior wall pH; P pH, posterior wall pH; AT, anterior wall temperature, PT, posterior wall temperature; BP, cardiopulmonary bypass; XC, aortic cross clamp; Defib, defibrillation; AR, aortic root; LAD, left anterior descending coronary artery; OMB, obtuse marginal coronary artery.

placement procedure. Despite the continuous administration of cold blood cardioplegia, initially through the aortic root and subsequently through the orifice of the left main coronary artery, and despite the fact that a low myocardial temperature was achieved equally in the anterior and the posterior left ventricular walls, adequate myocardial pH was achieved only in the anterior wall. In the posterior wall, the myocardial pH during the period of aortic clamping fell progressively to a very low ischemic level, indicating inadequate metabolic protection of the posterior wall. Following uneventful weaning from cardiopulmonary bypass and chest closure, the patient de-

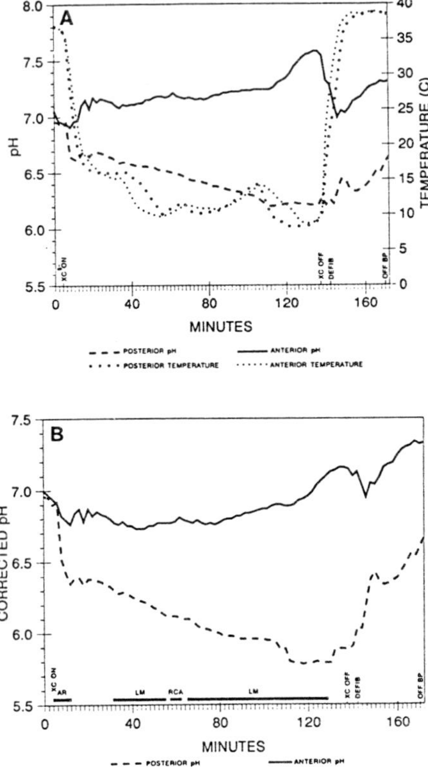

Figure 15.5. Myocardial pH and temperature tracings from a 70–year-old man who underwent aortic valve replacement. Figure 15.5A shows the actual pH and temperature tracings throughout the case. Figure 15.5B shows the pH corrected to 37°C. In Figure 15.5B the times and routes cardioplegia delivery are noted. A pH, anterior wall pH; P pH, posterior wall pH; AT, anterior wall temperature, PT, posterior wall temperature; BP, cardiopulmonary bypass; XC, aortic cross clamp; Defib, defibrillation; AR, aortic root; LM, left main coronary artery; RCA, right coronary artery.

veloped a ventricular fibrillation arrest. He was resuscitated and an intraortic balloon was placed. The patient subsequently had an uneventful recovery but both the postoperative ECG and the CPK isoenzymes indicated a large posterior myocardial infarction and confirmed the intraoperative myocardial pH data.

Lessons learned

To date we have monitored myocardial pH intraoperatively in more than 300 patients undergoing aortocoronary bypass grafting and/or valve replacement.

Experience with these patients has shown that it is sufficient to monitor the myocardial pH at two left ventricular sites (the anterior and posterior walls) to obtain a reasonable assessment of the adequacy of metabolic protection of the left ventricle as a whole. Furthermore, metabolic preservation seems to be adequate if myocardial pH, corrected to 37°C, remains above 6.8 throughout the period of aortic clamping. The major determinants of myocardial pH during the period of aortic clamping are the pH at the onset of the clamping, the type of disease (reflecting the duration of aortic clamping), the left ventricular mass, and the type of cardioplegia delivered [47]. The myocardial pH at the onset of aortic cross clamping is reflective of the underlying disease as well as of myocardial management prior to application of the aortic clamp. Expeditious surgery reduces the period of aortic clamping and achieves a higher mean myocardial pH during this period. Avoidance of ventricular fibrillation also prevents a fall in myocardial pH [31]. A hypertrophied LV is inherently more difficult to protect due to its large mass, and is therefore more vulnerable to acidosis during the period of aortic clamping [48]. Continuous cold blood cardioplegia has been shown to maintain a higher myocardial pH than either crystalloid cardioplegia or intermittent cold blood cardioplegia [49,50].

Myocardial temperature alone is a poor indicator of the metabolic viability of the underlying myocardium. This is clearly demonstrated in Figure 15.5 which shows the temperature in the anterior and posterior walls to fall equally, yet also shows a discrepancy in the metabolic protection of these walls. The metabolic response of the diseased heart to hypothermia can vary widely, and no correlation exists between mean myocardial pH and mean myocardial temperature during the period of aortic clamping. Optimal myocardial management during cardiac surgical procedures is more likely to be achieved by monitoring myocardial pH and myocardial temperature rather than myocardial temperature alone [51].

Continuous metabolic monitoring of the myocardium at times may allow for intraoperative intervention to improve the metabolic protection of the heart. A case in point is shown in Figure 15.6 which depicts the myocardial pH and temperature tracings obtained with two sets of pH electrodes and thermistor probes in a 70-year-old man with three vessel coronary artery disease, including a completely occluded circumflex coronary artery, and significant aortic stenosis. This patient underwent coronary artery bypass grafting to an obtuse marginal artery and a diagonal artery as well as aortic valve replacement with a St. Jude valve. Cold blood cardioplegia was initially delivered through a Sarnes cardioplegia needle placed into the aortic root. Although the heart was arrested immediately, the myocardial pH of the posterior wall fell precipitously despite adequate cooling. This fall in myocardial pH was accompanied by a return of electrical ventricular activity prompting the surgeon to shift the cardioplegia delivery site from the aortic root to a catheter which had been previously placed in the coronary sinus. This intervention (arrow A in Figure 15.6B) resulted in a marked rise in the

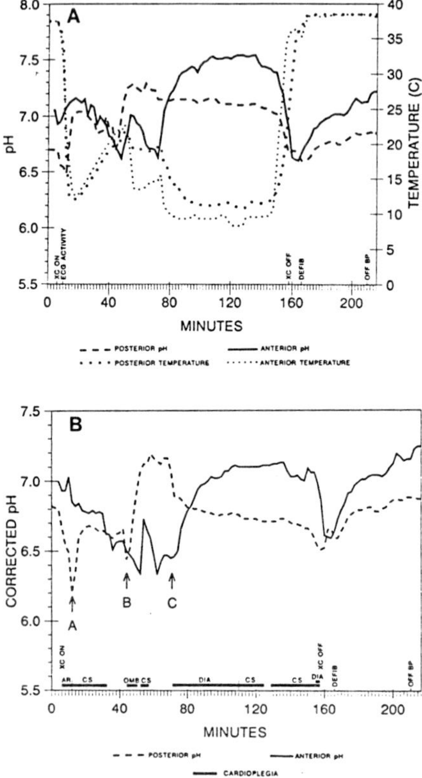

Figure 15.6. Myocardial pH and temperature tracings from a 70–year-old man who underwent aortic valve replacement and two vessel coronary revascularization. Figure 15.6A shows the actual pH and temperature tracings throughout the case. Figure 15.6B shows the pH corrected to 37°C. In Figure 15.6B the times and routes cardioplegia delivery are noted. A pH, anterior wall pH; P pH, posterior wall pH; AT, anterior wall temperature, PT, posterior wall temperature; BP, cardiopulmonary bypass; XC, aortic cross clamp; Defib, defibrillation; AR, aortic root; CS, coronary sinus; OMB, obtuse marginal coronary artery, DIA, diagonal coronary artery.

corrected myocardial pH from 6.2 to 6.6. Recognizing that this level of myocardial pH was still suboptimal, the surgeon constructed first the distal anastomosis of the obtuse marginal graft and then delivered cold blood cardioplegia through the proximal end of the graft effecting a further increase in the posterior wall myocardial pH to optimal levels (arrow B in figure 15.6B). The distal anastomosis of the graft to the diagonal artery was then performed. When cardioplegia was delivered through this graft (arrow C in Figure 15.6B the myocardial pH in the anterior wall rose progressively from 6.45 to 7.1. Thereafter the route of cardioplegia delivery was varied in order to keep the corrected myocardial pH above 6.7 in both the anterior and posterior walls. This patient was weaned from cardiopulmonary bypass with no inotropic support and had a smooth and uneventful operative and perioperative course. Clearly, in this case, myocardial management during the period of aortic clamping was guided by the myocardial pH data with the aim of avoiding acidosis in the anterior and posterior walls of the left ventricle.

Summary

Accumulation of the hydrogen ion in the extracellular tissue space during myocardial ischemia results from two processes: an anaerobic increase in the production of hydrogen ion and a flow-dependent decrease in its washout. The resultant acidosis, when measured with a glass electrode developed in our laboratory, is a reliable metabolic quantifier of the magnitude of regional myocardial ischemia. On-line intraoperative measurement of myocardial pH in more than 300 patients undergoing cardiac surgery at our institution has demonstrated the utility of this technique in the assessment of the adequacy of myocardial protection during the period of aortic clamping, taught us several lessons in regard to our current myocardial management techniques, and underscored the failure of myocardial temperature to adequately reflect the degree of metabolic protection of the heart. On-line measurement of myocardial pH in both the anterior and posterior walls of the left ventricle should enhance myocardial management in the course of cardiac surgery and should provide a valuable end-point with which newer myocardial protection philosophies and techniques can be evaluated.

Acknowledgements

The authors would like to acknowledge with gratitude the administrative and technical assistance of Nancy A. Healey, B.S. and Michael A. Zolkewitz, B.S.

This work was funded by the Richard Warren Surgical Research and Educational Fund, Westwood, Massachusetts.

References

1. Morgan HE, Neely JR. Metabolic regulation and myocardial function.In Hurst JW, Schlant RC, Rackley CE *et al.* (eds): The heart, arteries and veins. New York: McGraw-Hill Information Services Company 1990; 91–105.
2. Opie LA. The heart physiology and metabolism. 2nd ed. New York: Raven Press, 1991.
3. Gevers W. Generation of protons by metabolic processes in heart cells. J Mol Cell Cardiol 1977; 9: 867–74.
4. Siouffi SY, Kwasnik EM, Khuri SK. Methods for the metabolic quantification of regional myocardial ischemia. J Surg Res 1987; 43: 360–78.

5. Khuri SF, Kloner RA, Karaffa SA *et al.* The significance of the late fall in myocardial pCO_2 and its relationship to myocardial pH after regional coronary occlusion in the dog. Circ Res 1985; 56: 537–47.
6. Opie LH. Effects of regional ischemia on metabolism of glucose and fatty acids. Circ Res 1976; 38: I52–I68.
7. Aickin CC. Intracellular pH regulation by vertebrate muscle. Ann Rev Physiol 1986; 48: 349–61.
8. Aronson PS. Kinetic properties of the plasma membrane Na^+-H^+ exchanger. Ann Rev Physiol 1985; 47: 545–60.
9. Vaughn-Jones RD, Lederer WJ, Eisner DA. Ca^{++} ions can affect intracellular pH in mammalian cardiac muscle. Nature 1983; 301: 522–4.
10. Cingolani HE, Koretsune Y, Marban E. Recovery of Contractility and pHi during respiratory acidosis in ferret hearts: role of Na^+-H^+ exchange. Am J Physiol 1990; 258: H843–H848.
11. Clarke K, O'Connor AJ, Willis RJ. Temporal relation between energy metabolism and myocardial function during ischemia and reperfusion. Am J Physiol 1987; 253: H412–H421.
12. Jeffery FMH, Malloy CR, Radda GK. Influence of intracellular acidosis on contractile function in the working rat heart. Am J Physiol 1987; 253: H1499–H1505.
13. Schaefer S, Schwartz GG, Gober JR *et al.* Relationship between myocardial metabolites and contractile abnormalities during graded regional ischemia. J Clin Invest 1990; 85: 706–13.
14. Teplinsky K, O'Toole M, Olman M *et al.* Effect of lactic acidosis on canine hemodynamics and left ventricular function. Am J Physiol 1990; 258: H1193–H1199.
15. Williamson JR, Schaffer SW, Ford C *et al.* Contribution of tissue acidosis to ischemic injury in the perfused rat heart. Circulation 1976; 53: I3–I14.
16. Orchard CH, Kentish JC. Effects of changes of pH on the contractile function of cardiac muscle. Am J Physiol 1990; 258: C967–C981.
17. Orchard CH, McCall E, Kirby MS *et al.* Mechanical alterations during acidosis in ferret heart muscle. Circ Res 1991; 68: 69–76.
18. Poole-Wilson PA. Regulation of intracellular pH in the myocardium; relevance to pathology. Mol Cel Biochem 1989; 89: 151–5.
19. Jacobus WE, Pores IH, Lucas SK *et al.* The role of intracellular pH in the control of normal and ischemic myocardial contractility: a ^{31}P nuclear magnetic resonance and mass spectrometry study. In Intracellular pH: its measurement, regulation, and utilization in cellular functions. New York: Alan R. Liss, 1982: 537–65.
20. Walley KR, Lewis TH, Wood LDH. Acute respiratory acidosis decreases left ventricular contractility but increases cardiac output in dogs. Circ Res 1990; 67: 628–35.
21. Cohn LH, Fujiwara Y, Collins JJ. Mapping of ischemic myocardium by surface pH determinations. J Surg Res 1974; 16: 210.
22. Deauvaert FE, Cohn LH, Collins JJ. The detection of ischemic myocardium by surface pH measurements. Surgery 1973; 74: 437.
23. Knoll D, Kirchhoff PG, Nordbeck H *et al.* Comparison of tolerance to ischemia in human and animal myocardium during various forms of induced cardiac arrest. Thoraxchirurgie 1975; 23: 313.
24. Axford TC, Dearani JA, Khait I *et al.* Electrode-derived myocardial pH measurements reflect intracellular myocardial metabolism assessed by phosphorus 31-nuclear magnetic resonance spectroscopy during normothermic ischemia. J Thorac Cardiovasc Surg 1992; 103: 902–7.
25. Khabbaz KR, Krisanda J, Wolfe JA *et al.* Simultaneous *in vivo* measurements of intracellular and extracellular myocardial pH during repeated episodes of ischemia. Current Surg 1989; 46: 399–400.
26. Krisanda J. Simultaneous measurement of intracellular and extracellular pH. Circulation (Supp II): 1988.
27. Takach TJ, Glassman LR, Ribakove GH *et al.* Continuous measurement of intramyocardial

pH: correlation to functional recovery following normothermic and hypothermic global ischemia. Anal Thorac Surg 1986; 42: 31–6.
28. Wolfe JA, Khabbaz KR, Marquardt CA *et al.* Postoperative metabolic monitoring of myocardial ischemic events in the conscious canine. Submitted for publication.
29. Hicks GL, Hill A, DeWeese JA. Monitoring of midmyocardial and subendocardial pH in normal and ischemic ventricles. J Thorac Cardiovasc Surg 1976; 7252–6.
30. Khuri SF, Josa M, Martson W *et al.* First report of intramyocardial pH in man. J Thorac Cardiovasc Surg 1983; 86: 667–8.
31. Khuri SF, Marston WA, Josa M *et al.* Observations on 100 patients with continuous intraoperative monitoring of intramyocardial pH. J Thorac Cardiovasc Surg 1985; 89: 170–82.
32. Lange R, Kloner RA, Zierler M *et al.* Time course of ischemic alterations during normothermic and hypothermic arrest and its reflection by on-line monitoring of tissue pH. J Thorac Cardiovasc Surg 1983; 86: 418–34.
33. Randolph JD, Toal KW, Geffin GA *et al.* Improved myocardial preservation with oxygenated cardioplegic solutions as reflected by on-line monitoring of intramyocardial pH during arrest. J Vasc Surg 1986; 3: 216–25.
34. Khuri SF, Marston W, Josa M *et al.* First report of intramyocardial pH in man: I. Methodology and initial results. Med Instrum 1984; 18: 167–71.
35. Khuri SK, Warner KG. Intraoperative pH monitoring for the detection of progressive myocardial ischemia. In Roberts AJ (ed): Myocardial protection in cardial surgery. New York: Marcel Dekker Inc 1987; 399–412.
36. Warner KG, Khuri SF, Marston W *et al.* Significance of the transmural dimunition in regional hydrogen ion production after repeated coronary artery occlusions. Circ Res 1989; 64: 616–28.
37. Ingwall JS. Phosphorus nuclear magnetic resonance spectroscopy. Am J Physiol 1982; 242: H729–H744.
38. Madden A, Leach MO, Sharp JC *et al.* A quantitative analysis of the accuracy of in vivo pH measurements with ^{31}P NMR spectroscopy: assessment of pH measurement methodology. NMR in Biomed 1991; 4: 1–11.
39. Bottomley PA. Human *in vivo* NMR spectroscopy in diagnostic medicine: clinical tool of research probe? Radiology 1989; 170: 1–15.
40. Bottomley PA, Weiss RG, Hardy CJ *et al.* Myocardial high-energy phosphate metabolism and allograft rejection in patients with heart transplants. Radiology 1991; 181: 67–75.
41. Hardy CJ, Weiss RG, Bottomley PA *et al.* Altered myocardial high-energy phosphate metabolites in patients with dilated cardiomyopathy. Am Heart J 1991; 3: 795–801.
42. Weiss RG, Bottomley PA, Hardy CJ *et al.* Regional myocardial metabolism of high-energy phosphates during isometric exercise in patients with coronary artery disease. N Eng J Med 1990; 323: 1593–600.
43. Rahn H, Reeves RB, Howell BJ. Hydrogen ion regulation, temperature and evolution. Am Rev Respir Dis 1975; 112: 65.
44. Reeves RB, Malan A. Model studies of intracellular acid base temperature responses in ectoderms. Respir Physiol 1976; 28: 49.
45. White FN. A comparative physiological approach to hypothermia. J Thorac Cardiovasc Surg 1981; 82: 821–31.
46. Lange R, Cavanaugh AC, Zierler M *et al.* The relative importance of alkalinity, temperature, and the washout effect of bicarbonate-buffered, multidose cardioplegic solution. Circ 1984; (Supp I): I75–I83.
47. Butler M, Warner KG, Lavin P *et al.* Predictors of myocardial tissue acidosis during the period of aortic clamping in man. Submitted for publication.
48. Warner KG, Khuri SF, Kloner RA *et al.* Structural and metabolic correlates of cell injury in the hypertrophied myocardium during valve replacement. J Thorac Cardiovasc Surg 1987; 93: 741–54.
49. Khuri SK, Warner KG, Josa M *et al.* The Superiority of continuous cold blood cardioplegia

in the metabolic protection of the hypertrophied human heart. J Thorac Cardiovasc Surg 1988; 95: 442–54.
50. Warner KG, Josa M, Marston W *et al*. Reduction in myocardial acidosis using blood cardioplegia. J Surg Res 1987; 42: 247–56.
51. Dearani JA, Axford TC, Patel MA *et al*. Routine measurement of myocardial temperature is not reflective of myocardial metabolism during cardial surgery. Surg Forum 1990; XLI: 228–30.

16. Morphology of the acute and chronic ischemic myocardium in man

MARCEL BORGERS and WILLEM FLAMENG

Introduction

The outcome of protective measures in cardiac surgery depends on a number of aspects which are related to the nature of the interventions used (controllable) and to the condition of the myocardium at the moment of surgery (not controllable).

There are only limited measures available to assess the effects of acute ischemia or reperfusion on the heart. Besides functional and some metabolic parameters, the morphologic examination of heart muscle prior to and after surgical intervention can be a valuable tool in judging the degree of protection afforded by cardioplegia and/or pharmacological interventions. Moreover, the morphologic approach may be of help in elucidating the variable outcome of recovery of ventricular function (immediate, delayed or none) after cardiac surgery. Examination of biopsies obtained from a large number of coronary artery bypass graft (GABG) patients, revealed the existence of a variety of structural alterations which might be held responsible for the observed variation in functional recovery [1–8].

Patients undergoing cardiac surgery for coronary bypass grafting cannot be put into one defined group. Indeed, the underlying substructure of the myocardium represents a plethora of cellular and extracellular characteristics which vary in quality and quantity from patient to patient.

Admittedly, the tolerance to an acute ischemic episode of a heart (imposed during CABG) highly depends on whether the underlying structure is (1) normal; (2) remodelled as a consequence of a previous acute ischemic event (stunning or infarction); (3) changed during chronic exposure to a low oxygen environment (hibernation); (4) adapted as a consequence of underlying pathology (cardiomyopathies with different etiology).

This makes it difficult to employ uniform protective measures which could be optimal in every situation. Studying the detailed morphology of biopsies obtained from this plethora of alterations may not be of immediate help to find a way to optimize such interventions, but it allows us to understand why interventions such as cardioplegia result in a variable outcome of ventricular function after cardiac surgery.

H.M. Piper and C.J. Preusse (eds): Ischemia-reperfusion in cardiac surgery, 353–375.

Morphology in perspective

Changes in ultrastructure which occur during and after an ischemic insult have been extensively reported for the heart. Using pure morphological criteria, alterations can be divided into categories ranging from minor reversible changes to damage beyond repair.

The severity of the changes largely depends on the degree and duration of ischemia. In animals, the time-related injury after complete ischemia and post-ischemic reperfusion is well documented in a series of reviews [2,9–11] and will be only briefly commented upon in this paper.

Changes which are currently used to appreciate the degree of injury after acute ischemia in animals concern the following subcellular organelles and are given in increasing order of severity:

1. Mitochondria: swelling with loss of intramatricial granules; clarification of the matrix; disorientation and disruption of cristae; blebbing and disruption of the outer membrane, presence of flocculent densities (Jennings granules).
2. Cytosol: depletion of glycogen stores; increased intracellular water content, reflected by increased volume of cells.
3. Nucleus: margination of chromatin; pyknosis.
4. Sarcoplasmic reticulum: swelling.
5. Sarcolemma: fuzzy appearance of the sarcolemma-glycocalyx complex; blebbing and discontinuities of sarcolemma; swelling of T-tubular invaginations; loss of cytoskeletal-sarcolemma connections.
6. Sarcomeres: irregularities and deletion of Z-lines; contraction bands; overt myolysis.

Cytochemistry in perspective

Since some of the above descriptive criteria of morphologic changes are arbitrarily chosen it is likely that some confusion could rise in the comparative interlaboratory evaluations, especially concerning the stages before irreversible damage becomes apparent. In these cases auxiliary techniques such as cytochemistry of enzymes and ions can offer valid complementary information. A cytochemical aid is perhaps less essential to judge severe ischemic injury, although hard proof, such as loss of pivotal enzymes and loss of membrane integrity as appreciated by permeation of tracer molecules, may be very useful to quantify the degree of irreversible damage. More essential may be the role of cytochemical techniques in the identification of subtle, reversible alterations, which are usually observed after CABG procedures.

Among the subfields of cytochemistry most apt to fulfil these purposes are assays of enzyme activities and localization of cations [12]. Since enzymes and cations may undergo drastic quantitative or redistributional changes during a prolonged ischemic insult they lend themselves very well to topographical quantification of the degree of injury.

Enzyme cytochemistry

The main cytochemical markers of irreversible myocardial injury are those that demonstrate the loss of enzymes such as dehydrogenases, cytochrome c oxidase, calcium ATPase, aspartate aminotransferases and creatine kinases [13–18]. The findings usually coincide with overt structural damage, so that no real advantage is offered over classic histological staining procedures such as stains for lipids, cellular proteins, carbohydrates and extracellular matrix.

The assessment of enzyme cytochemistry to detect subtle changes in the early phase of ischemia may be more relevant for predicting the final outcome after an ischemic event. For the heart it has been demonstrated that as early as 15 min after coronary artery ligation, acid phosphatase activity increases in the enlarged lysosomes of the ischemic myocardial cells. This activity begins to decrease after 30 min ligation and is greatly reduced 1–3 hours after ischemia. The enzyme which leaks from lysosomes, is scattered in the sarcoplasm and this is accompanied by structural changes indicating irreversible injury [19]. It has been described that the aggregation and enlargement of lysosomes and the activation of enzymes such as cathepsin D, b-glucuronidase and acid phosphatase takes place 15–30 min after coronary ligation [20–22]. The subsequent leakage of enzymes into the sarcoplasm occurs simultaneously with ultrastructural signs of irreversible injury.

In the last years, much attention has been focused on free radicals and hydrogen peroxide in mediating early ischemic cell injury [23–26]. Recently an exogenous NADH-oxidase, an enzyme that uses NADH and molecular oxygen to produce hydrogen peroxide, was shown to be a potent free radical generator in heart mitochondria [27]. Since ischemia depresses enzymes of the respiratory chain, the oxidation of NADH and the reduction of molecular oxygen is inhibited making both substrates available for the cyanide insensitive NADH-oxidase. Furthermore, a direct inhibition of the ATPase synthase complex can be obtained when mitochondria are exposed to hydrogen peroxide [28]. The major biological function of this enzyme in intact mitochondria is to produce ATP from ADP and Pi. On the other hand, it is known that under non-energized conditions, such as ischemia, the ATPase-synthase complex hydrolyses ATP to ADP and Pi (proton translocating ATPase). Furthermore, low ATP levels have also been proposed as a causal factor for ischemic damage [9]. Therefore, the hypothesis that hydrogen peroxide produced by NADH oxidase activity during ischemia may be involved in reversing the ATP synthase to the ATPase activity may be envisaged. Cytochemical localization procedures have been described to demonstrate proton translocating ATPase as well as NADH oxidase activity [29–31]. Using these procedures it has been demonstrated that in control non-ischemic myocardium the ATPase and NADH oxidase activation is weak or absent [32–34].

In slightly altered ischemic cells ATPase activity is prominent in mitochondria which also show an activation of the enzyme NADH oxidase. In the infarcted areas, severely damaged mitochondria are devoid of both enzyme activities. These cytochemical studies indicate that hydrogen peroxide, produced in the mitochondria by a high NADH-oxidase activity, may contribute not only to ischemic damage but also to a disturbance in mitochondrial respiratory activity by increasing ATP hydrolysis. Activation of these enzymes occurs very early during ischemia, preceding overt signs of ultrastructural cell damage. Therefore, the cytochemical procedures mentioned may represent very sensitive methods to determine early myocardial ischemic injury induced during cardiac surgery.

Ion cytochemistry

The role of calcium in ischemia is intensively investigated and its redistribution and accumulation often used as markers for both irreversible and reversible injury [35–37]. Its usefulness in determining changes at the edge of irreversibility has been highlighted recently [11,38,39].

In normal myocardium calcium deposits, visible as 20 nm particles, are confined to the inner leaflet of the sarcolemma, the transverse tubules and intercalated discs [40]. This sarcolemma-bound calcium has been suggested to play an important role in cell viability [11,38]. At the gap junctions, the deposits are clearly visible in pairs. Single deposits are sometimes observed in the mitochondria, whereas all other organelles are completely devoid of calcium precipitate. During ischemia and after post-ischemic reperfusion a redistribution of calcium has been observed which is directly related to the duration of ischemia [11]. After short ischemic periods a decrease in the amount of sarcolemma-associated calcium deposits is seen and this amount remains low upon reperfusion. Longer periods of ischemia result in a further decrease of sarcolemma-bound calcium and in an accumulation of single calcium deposits in the mitochondria upon reperfusion. Finally, the plasma membrane becomes completely devoid of calcium precipitate. Reperfusion at this stage results in a marked exacerbation of injury to most subcellular organelles and mitochondria avidly accumulate calcium deposits varying from single spots to clusters. The most severely affected cells show no mitochondrial calcium accumulation but contain flocculent densities. The sarcolemma of such cells is always devoid of calcium precipitate and often presents discontinuities. The cytochemical calcium localization suggests that the loss in the ability of the sarcolemma to bind calcium is a change that occurs at the edge of irreversibility [39]. Indeed, in areas which become irreversibly damaged upon reperfusion, cells no longer contain calcium deposits prior to reperfusion.

Vulnerability of human myocardium to acute ischemia

Limitations of evaluating human myocardial structure

An obvious limiting factor in doing morphologic work on human cardiac biopsies is the sample size. This is well recognized by pathologists who have to rely on a very small endocardial biopsy for diagnostic purpose.

It is possible to take transmural biopsies during the CABG procedure from a given region of the LV wall with known functional parameters. Biopsies can be divided into a subendocardial and a subepicardial part and prepared for combined morphologic-cytochemical examination. Semi-thick (2 μm) sections can be used for quantification of the ischemic changes through the whole subendo- and subepicardial parts, whereby an overview of the degree and extent of the injury is provided. Areas of interest can then be selected for detailed electron microscopic and cytochemical examination. Despite such optimal usage of the entire biopsy, the sample under examination might not be representative for the whole ventricular area involved.

Another aspect that limits morphologic examination and interpretation of the myocardial structure in a biopsy is the damage induced by the biopsy procedure. The cells at the periphery of the biopsy undergo mechanical disruption which may cause contraction of the whole biopsy. Especially at the cutting edges, severe contracture can occur thereby artificially producing bands which can be mistaken, at least at the light microscopical level, for contraction band necrosis. Therefore, the peripherally located cell layers of a biopsy have to be neglected.

Furthermore, due to the inherent procedure of fixing the biopsy by immersion, the preservation of the ultrastructure is not ideal because the fixative penetrates slowly which in addition might pose problems for enzyme and ion localization studies.

Differences in vulnerability to ischemia between human and animal myocardium

Electron microscopic investigations of human myocardium related to preservation during cardiopulmonary bypass have been extensively reported previously [1,2,42–51].

The vulnerability to ischemia of various organelles in human myocardium differs considerably from that reported in animals. The reason is that in animals the observed changes reflect alterations of acute ischemia in normal tissue, whereas in man they often reflect ischemic alterations in tissue that has been exposed to reduced blood flow for weeks to years. The main factors in animals which determine the structural outcome after ischemia are time and temperature of the ischemic episode, species and age of the animal. In man, another factor, which is at least as important, is the condition of the myocardium at the moment of cardiac surgery. In the large majority of patients the myocardium has been subjected to either intermittent or chronic ischemic insults and therefore has undergone adaptive changes. These can be classified in graded order of severity as preconditioning, stunning, hibernation, infarction, myopathy or any combination of the above.

Preconditioned and stunned myocardium

The structural adaptations of preconditioning and stunning have not been documented in man, but pictures resembling the subtle changes as seen in stunned myocardium of animals [32–34] are frequently seen in human biopsies prior to and after repeated short ischemic periods when the intermittent aorta cross clamping procedure is used for CABG.

As described in animals, a characteristic change of stunning was the loss of intramatricial granules in mitochondria and the occurrence of clumped cristae, a picture never seen in normal myocardium. Clumping of cristae was the earliest sign of deterioration noticed and was shown to be accompanied by activation of proton translocating ATPase and the intramitochondrial formation of harmful oxygen species [34]. As the structural equivalent of stunned myocardium is unknown in man, it is impossible to say whether the stunned myocardium is more or less vulnerable for structural deterioration, for example in states of acute ischemia during cardiac surgery. The same holds true for the preconditioned state, although one would tend to believe, from experimental studies with animals, that preconditioning is a protective intervention. If this was the case, one should envisage the intermittent aorta cross clamping technique to have the inherent advantage of selfprotection.

Hibernating myocardium

At the most recent symposium on myocardial viability during the annual sessions of the American College of Cardiology, Rahimtoola pointed out that hibernating myocardium is not a single entity of cardiac dysfunction but consists of subsets with different underlying pathologies which may be held responsible for the fact that after revascularization the functional recovery is rapid, slow or very slow. The structural changes seen in asynergic but non-infarcted segments have been reported [7,8] and consist of a typical adaptive cellular remodelling which can be well appreciated with light microscopy, especially when the tissues are stained with a polychrome or a PAS (Periodic Acid Schiff) stain. The degree of structural change might be directly related to the speed of recovery after restoration of blood flow. In the light microscope, two important qualitative changes distinguish asynergic non-infarcted myocardium from healthy myocardium. First of all, myocardial cells in the former become gradually depleted of contractile material however, without a reduction in cell volume (Figure 16.1). The loss of contractile material always starts around the nucleus and spreads concentrically towards the periphery, leaving only few or no sarcomere bands opposed to the sarco-

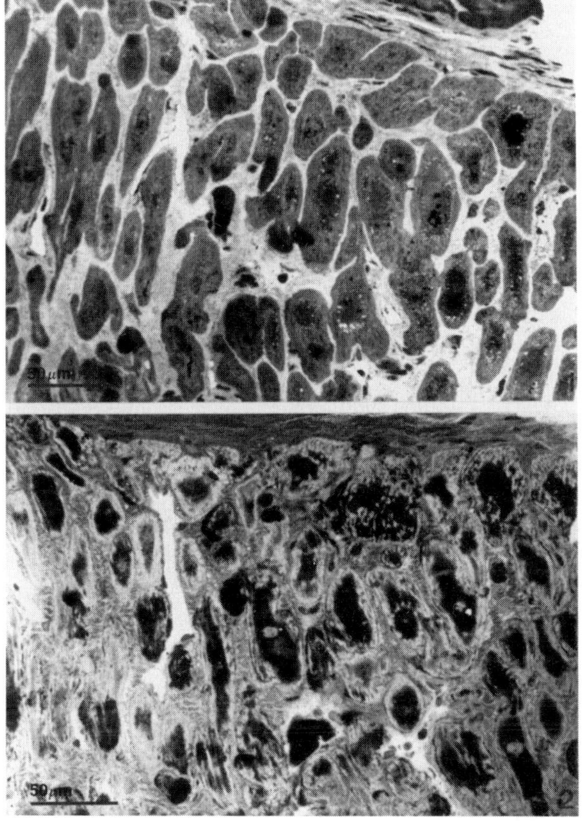

Figure 16.1 (*top*) *and 16.2* (*bottom*). Light microscopy of asynergic, non-infarcted myocardium showing cells with myolytic changes. 1. Toluidine blue stained section. In most of the cells the central area is devoid of myofibrils (sarcomeres). 2. Periodic Acid Schiff (PAS) stained section. The cell centres are PAS positive (densely stains zones) indicative for high glycogen content.

lemma. The space left by the dissoluted myofilaments (area of myolysis) is occupied by an amorphous, strongly PAS positive material (stain for glycogen) (Figure 16.2). Events of pure degenerative nature such as acute necrosis of myocytes, abnormal storage of lipids and phospholipids in the form of droplets or multilamellar bodies, gross intracellular edema and the presence of inflammatory cells, as described in acute myocardial infarction, congestive heart failure and in various forms of cardiomyopathies, are only rarely seen. Secondly, a feature that is consistently present in areas where structurally affected myocardial cells prevail, is a limited increase in connective tissue in between the cells.

In the electron microscope, the most striking feature is the gradual depletion of contractile material and its replacement by huge plaques of glycogen.

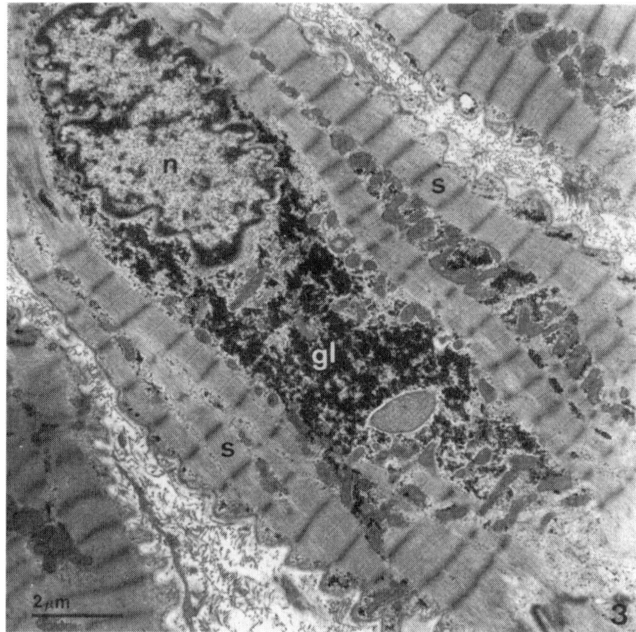

Figure 16.3. Electron microscopy of asynergic, non infarcted myocardium. Early stage of loss of sarcomeres starting in the perinuclear zone. Glycogen (gl) occupies the centre. n = nucleus: s = sarcomeres.

The depletion of sarcomeres is always seen in the perinuclear area and progresses towards the cell periphery (Figures 16.3–16.5). Unlike in the condition of typical cell atrophy, the peripherally located sarcomere strands often remain well organised (Figure 16.6), suggesting that a limited but orderly and unidirectional contractile ability might be preserved.

Another characteristic feature is the presence of lots of small mini-mitochondria (Figure 16.7) in the areas adjacent to the glycogen rich perinuclear zones. They are often found intermingled with glycogen. In some fortuitous sections the mitochondria are linearly arranged and have a spaghetti-like appearance.

A third change concerns the nuclei which have lost their normal smoothly stretched contour, but instead have a tortuous appearance projecting numerous extensions into the surrounding cytosol (Figures 16.3 and 16.4). The nuclear chromatin is evenly distributed. The sarcoplasmic reticulum is virtually absent, instead a network of disorganised profiles of reticular membranes remained present in the myolytic areas. The sarcolemma no longer projects protrusions (T-tubules) into the cytoplasm. Very often, the sarcolemma presents numerous pynocytotic vesicles, resembling those of endo-

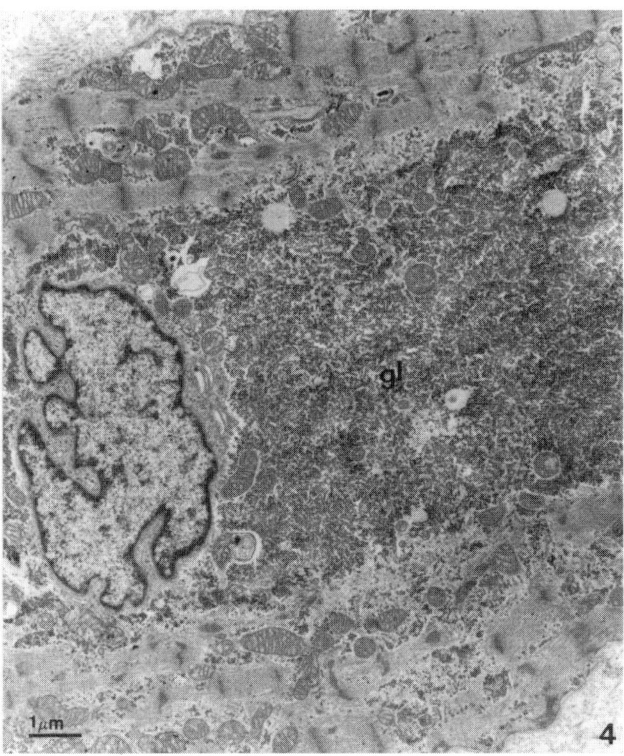

Figure 16.4. Electron microscopy of asynergic, non infarcted myocardium. More advanced stage of myolysis with massive accumulation of glycogen (gl).

thelial and smooth muscle cells. The number of microperoxisomes in the perinuclear space is also elevated.

Remarkably, degenerative changes such as cytoplasmic vacuolization, cytosolic edema, mitochondrial swelling, membrane disruption, accumulation of secondary lysosomes, membranous whorls and lipid droplets are virtually absent. The general impression is that the substructures present in the affected cells of asynergic segments are perfectly healthy.

As far as the intracellular space is concerned, apart from an increased amount of collagen fibres, no other striking abnormalities are noticed. Microvascular endothelium, pericytes and interstitial mesenchymal cells are present in usual number and display well preserved substructures.

Susceptibility of hibernating myocardium to acute ischemia

Examination of biopsies from asynergic LV segments taken at the end of CABG reveals that the adapted or 'hibernating' cells are much less suscep-

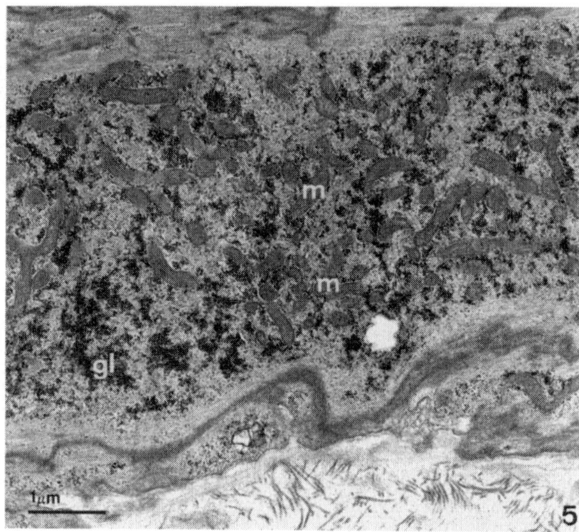

Figure 16.5. Electron microscopy of asynergic, non infarcted myocardium. Almost complete loss of sarcomeres. The cytoplasm is filled with glycogen (gl) intermingled with numerous small mitochondria (m).

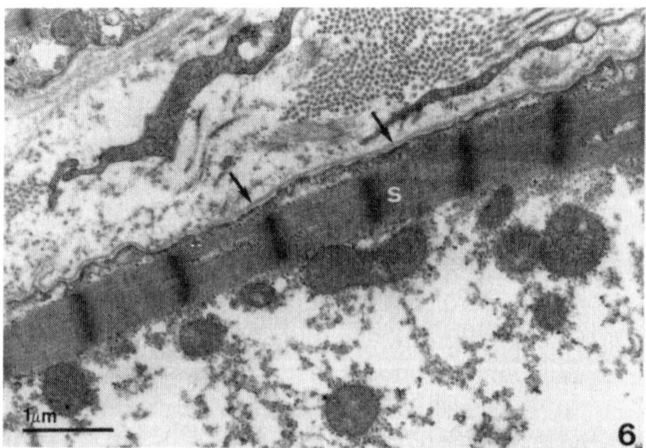

Figure 16.6. Electron microscopy of asynergic, non infarcted myocardium. Periphery of a cell affected by myolysis. A single strand of sarcomeres (s) remains. Note the intactness of the sarcolemma-glycocalyx complex (arrows).

tible to acute ischemia than the adjacent cells which have a normal ultrastructure. The most pronounced differences are seen at the level of mitochondria, nuclei and the sarcolemma-glycocalyx complex. Firstly, the numerous mini-mitochondria in adapted cells are not or only slightly swollen (Figure 16.8)

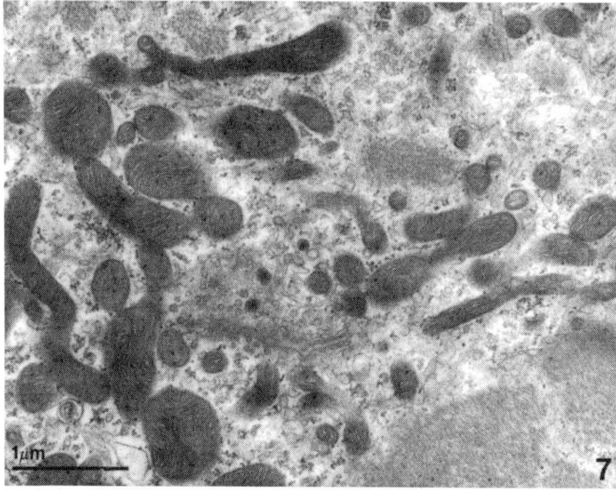

Figure 16.7. Electron microscopy of asynergic, non infarcted myocardium. Centre of a myolytic cell showing variously sized mitochondria, many of them smaller than usual.

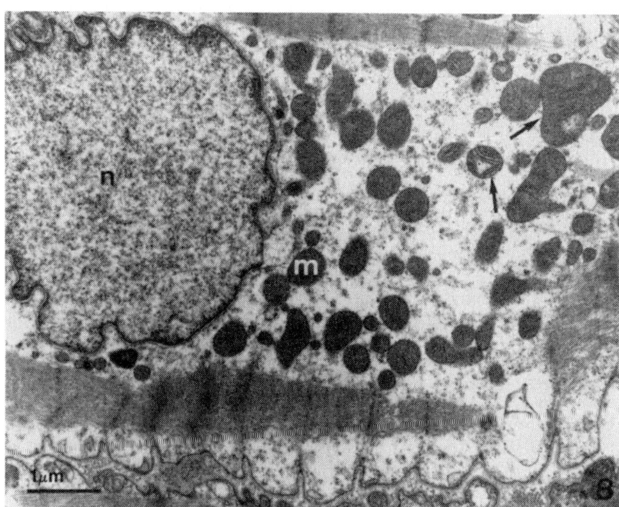

Figure 16.8. Hibernating (myolytic) cell from a post CABG biopsy. Note the absence of characteristic ischemic changes at the level of the mitochondria (m) and the nucleus (n). At the left of this cell is a normally structured cell which shows mitochondria (arrows) with typical ischemic changes such as matrix swelling and cristae abnormalities.

when compared to those in the pre-CABG biopsy. In adjacent normally structured cells mitochondria show a more marked clarification of the matrix (Figure 16.8). Such swelling of the mitochondrial matrix and interruptions of the cristae can be considered as reversible changes. Because the preservation of the tissue occurs by immersing the biopsy into the fixative, the phenomenon of swelling and disruption of mitochondria might represent an exaggerated replica of what really happens. It cannot be excluded that slight osmotic imbalance in mitochondria brought about by ischemia, results in breakage of membranes during the fixation procedure. The picture is completely different in the case of evolving infarction where clear signs of irreversible damage are manifest such as mitochondria with flocculent densities and overt disruption of the sarcolemma and nuclear pyknosis (Figures 16.9 and 16.10).

Secondly, no difference in the substructure of sarcolemma-glycocalyx complex of adapted cells is seen between pre- and post-CABG biopsies. The intimate association of the external lamina of the glycocalyx with the sarcolemma is preserved and no discontinuities in the lipid bilayer are seen (Figure 16.11). In contrast, clear abnormalities of the sarcolemma-glycocalyx complex are observed in cells possessing normal substructures (Figure 16.12).

Thirdly, the nuclei of adapted cells show no chromatin margination or chromatin clumping as do nuclei of normal cells in the post-CABG biopsies. When calcium localization is compared between pre-and post-CABG biopsies containing a mixture of normal and adapted cells, it is obvious that redistribution of calcium is much less pronounced in the adapted cells. Signs of calcium overload in mitochondria of such cells are seldom seen (Figure 16.13). This is in contrast to normal cells where mitochondria accumulate more calcium in the post- than in the pre-CABG biopsies (Figure 16.14). Moreover, the calcium precipitate of the sarcolemma of adapted cells remains unaltered in the post-CABG sample (Figure 16.15), in contrast to what is often seen in normally structured cells which lose sarcolemmal calcium, especially when the sarcolemma becomes dissociated from the cytoskeleton (Figure 16.16).

In summary, a clear distinction in substructural vulnerability towards acute ischemia is seen between normally structured and adapted cells of myocardium derived from asynergic segments. It is postulated that the adapted cells might remodel after revascularization and contribute to an increased contractile behavior of the ventricular wall. However, it is proposed that segments in which these hibernating cells prevail, will not recover immediately after revascularization but might show a delayed recovery because the structural remodelling to rebuilt sufficient contractile material needs time [8,52].

Age-related differences in susceptibility to ischemia

The information available in the literature on the differences in susceptibility of young versus adult myocardium is very scanty [53]. In biopsies of patients with tetratology of Fallot, normally structured cells show a greater vulnerabil-

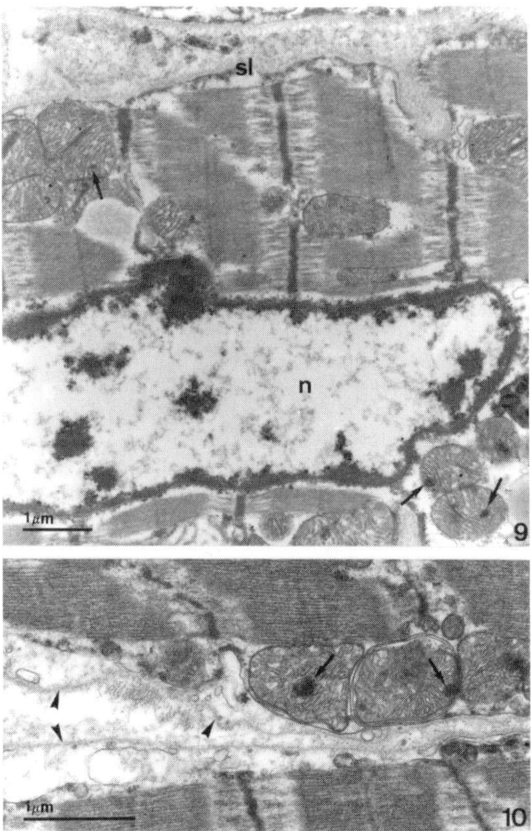

Figure 16.9 (top) and 16.10 (bottom). Irreversible degenerative changes in myocardial cells from an area of evolving infarction. A pyknotic nucleus (n), disrupted sarcolemma (sl), flocullent densities in mitochondria (arrows), and loss of close apposition of the glycocalyx outer lamina to the sarcolemma (arrowheads) are characteristic features.

ity to ischemia than cells which have undergone adaptive changes (Figure 16.17 and 16.18), like those seen in asynergic segments of adult myocardium.

The same holds true for tissue derived from children with ALCAPA (left coronary system originating from the pulmonary artery). These patients' myocardium contains a large number of 'hibernating' cells, a number of degenerated cells (Figure 16.19), and infarcted scar tissue [54].

Infarction

The detailed morphology of acute myocardial infarction and healed infarction (scar or fibrotic tissue) is described before. An interesting aspect however, which is not well documented concerns the immediate surroundings of a

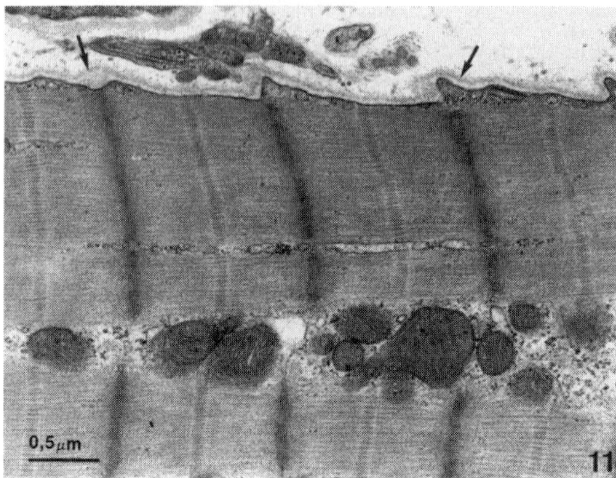

Figure 16.11. Periphery of a hibernating cell obtained from a biopsy at the end of CABG. Note the intactness of the sarcolemma-glycocalyx complex (arrows).

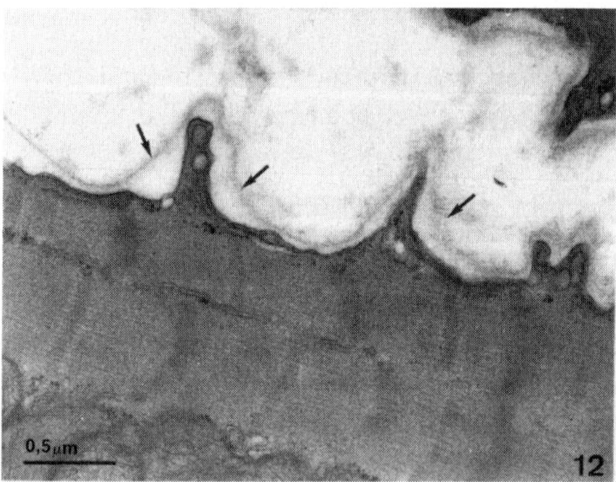

Figure 16.12. Periphery of a normally structured cell obtained from a biopsy at the end of CABG. In this cell the external lamina of the glycocalyx clearly dissociates from the sarcolemma at spots indicated by arrows.

healed infarct. Cells which border the fibrotic scar are usually of the 'hibernating' type. Again such cells have a higher tolerance to acute ischemic injury than normally structured cells.

Cardiomyopathic myocardium

In an important number of the biopsies obtained from cardiomyopathic patients 'hibernating' cells are found intermingled with cells which clearly

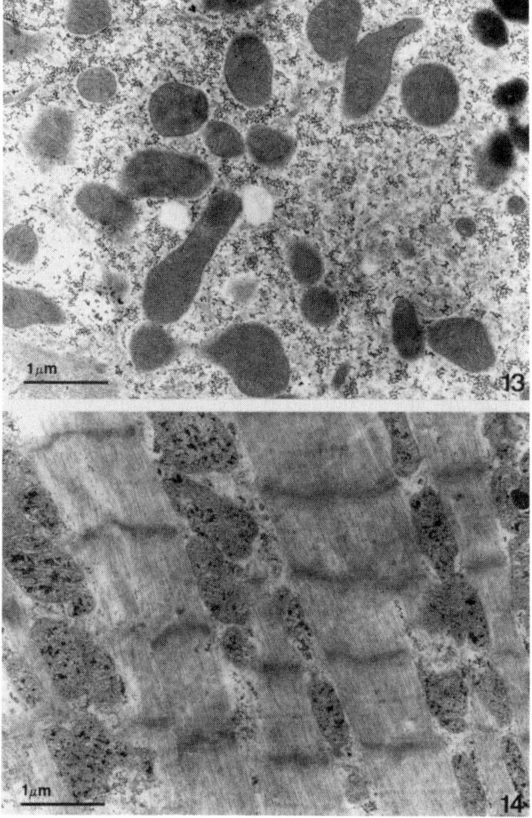

Figure 16.13 (top) and 16.14 (bottom). Calcium localization in mitochondria of hibernating (Figure 16.13) and normally structured (Figure 16.14) cells from post CABG biopsies. Notice the considerably higher content of calcium precipitate in the normally structured cell, indicative for greater susceptibility to ischemic injury.

show signs of degeneration (Figure 16.20). In the latter cells the most common changes are the presence of myolysis, tortuous nuclei, mega-mitochondria (the size of nuclei) (Figure 16.21) sometimes presenting lipid-like inclusions and intramatricial glycogen clumps, and whorl-like myelin structures (a common sign of membrane degeneration) [55–61]. The content of calcium as assessed with cytochemical or microprobe methods is markedly elevated in such degenerated cells (De Nollin *et al.*, unpublished results). It has been shown recently that the pleomorphic mitochondria as seen in a patient with ventricular tachychardia, resembling those seen in cardiomyopathy, are virtually devoid of cytochrome c oxidase [62].

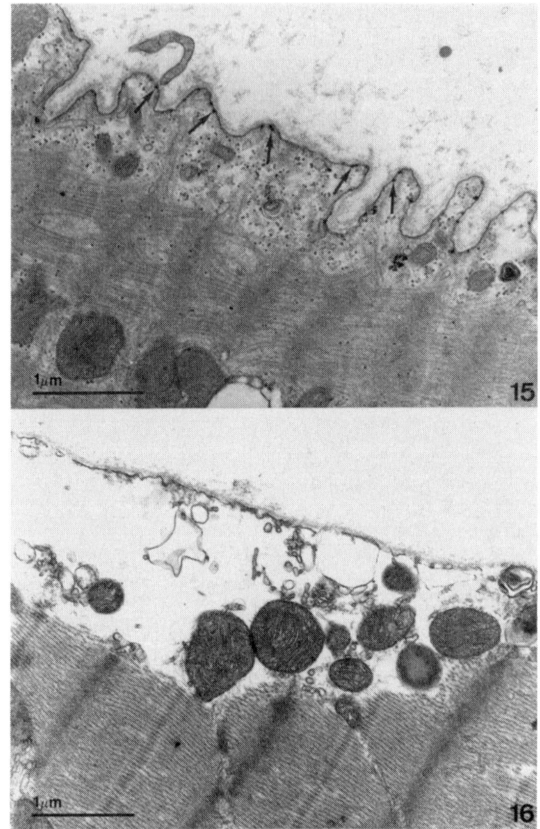

Figure 16.15 (top) and 16.16 (bottom). Calcium localization at the sarcolemma of a hibernating cell (Figure 16.15) and a normally structured but damaged cell (Figure 16.16) obtained from post CABG biopsies. Single deposits of calcium precipitate (arrows) are only present in the well preserved hibernating cell.

Morphologic assessment of protective interventions in cardiac surgery

A detailed account of the ultrastructural changes in the human heart using cardiac arrest with the Kirsch cardioplegic solution in relation to time of arrest is given by Schaper [2]. She alluded in extenso to the validity of the use of mitochondrial, nuclear and sarcomere changes as hall-marks of reversible and irreversible changes during ischemia and postischemic reperfusion. She reported a general agreement between data obtained in dogs and man as far as the different degree of tolerance to ischemia of the various subcellular organelles is concerned. The data pertain, however, only to cardiac arrest for periods ranging from 20 min to >60 min, followed by reperfusion. The same author reported on the tolerance to ischemia of hyper-

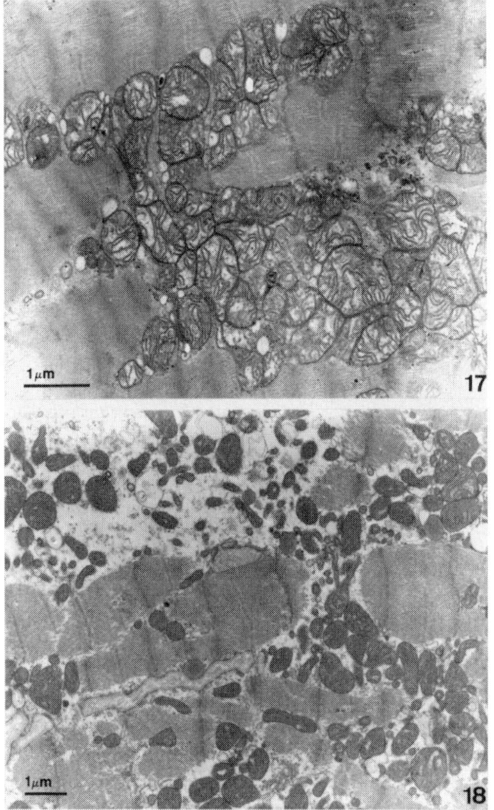

Figure 16.17 (top) and 16.18 (bottom). Tetralogy of Fallot. Myocardial cells from a normally structured (Figure 16.17) and a "hibernating" cell of post-operative biopsies. The damage due to the acute ischemic insult is more pronounced in mitochondria of the normally structured cell.

trophic myocardium in patients with aortic valvular disease and concluded that the tolerance to ischemia appeared to decrease with increasing cardiac hypertrophy. This observation was attributed to an elevated level of cardiac metabolism and oxygen consumption in hypertrophic hearts [63].

The morphologic outcome of the myocardium using other cardioplegic solutions in combination with the intermittent aorta cross-clamping technique has been reported by Flameng and his group. They compared St. Thomas cardioplegic solution with topical cooling of the heart [49], the effect of St. Thomas's solution versus intermittent aortic cross-clamping at 25°C and 34°C [51] and intermittent aortic cross clamping at 32°C [50]. The structural correlate of chronic heart failure was investigated by assessing myocardial tissue obtained from patients undergoing cardiac transplantation because of end-stage dilated cardiomyopathy [61,63]. Besides a number of clear degenerative changes, adaptive alterations were observed which resembled those seen

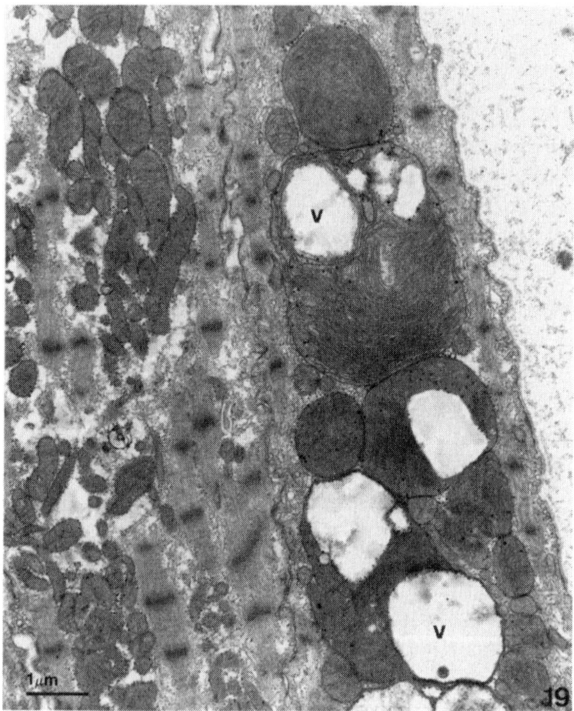

Figure 16.19. Post-CABG biopsy derived from an ALCAPA patient. The cell at the left is of the 'hibernating' type and underwent only marginal ischemic damage whereas the cell at the right is of the degenerative type and shows signs of severe damage such as vacuolizations (v) in mega-mitochondria.

in hibernating myocardium. The authors, however, made little distinction between these changes and the pure degenerative ones. The same view was held by Thiedemann [64] in his extensive review describing the structural features of chronic ischemic myocardium in man. Other features of pathological changes in human myocardium are dealt with in several other reports [55,56,61,65].

Besides the above methods of preservation which use energy conservation by hypothermia, potassium-induced cardiac arrest or their combination, there are a number of pharmacological interventions that aim at limiting the jeopardized ion homeostatic mechanisms by blocking specific channels such as the L-type slow calcium channel by nifedipine [66], by preventing calcium overload by primarily counteracting sodium overload [67], by preventing the uptake and breakdown of nucleotides [68–70], or by a combination of inhibition of calcium overload and nucleotide breakdown such as lidoflazine [71–73] The latter drug has been administered in conjunction with the intermittent aortic cross clamping technique for CABG or in addition to cold cardioplegia in valvular surgery in over 10,000 patients, operated in various Belgian

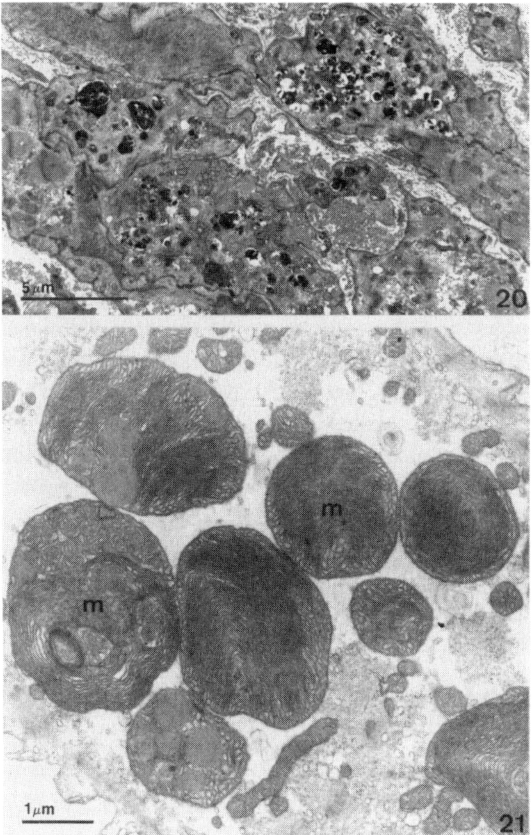

Figure 16.20 (top) and 16.21 (bottom). Biopsies derived from congestive cardiomyopathy patients. Note the severe generalized damage in Figure 16.20 and a detail of mega-mitochondria (m) in Figure 16.21.

cardiac surgery units. The morphologic correlate of its protective activity has been documented both in animal studies [71] and in man [72,73]. Most pronounced were the effects seen at the level of the sarcolemma-glycocalyx where it prevented the dissociation of the close apposition between sarcolemma and the external lamina of the glycocalyx. The labile and exchangeable calcium binding to the sarcolemmal lipid bilayer was also found to be stabilized under these conditions [74,75].

Preservation of donor hearts for transplantation

This is a an important challenge for the cardiac surgeons, where morphologic evaluation could have an important guiding role in order to determine more optimal preservation procedures. Up to date, with the current methods of cold storage after cardioplegic arrest the storage time is limited to 3–4 hours because of the risk of postoperative low cardiac output which restricts the distant procurement of donor hearts. For this reason, extension of the preservation period and improvement in the donor heart preservation procedures would increase the donor pool and the final transplantation success rate.

A new concept of long-term donor heart preservation, namely through nucleoside transport inhibition has been proposed recently [68–70]. These studies show that the combined intervention of cold cardioplegia and nucleoside transport inhibition, aimed at the preservation of high levels of adenosine at the site of production thereby preventing its breakdown and wash out of its metabolites during reperfusion, improved the outcome after transplantation. The concept has been tested in animals [69,76] and man [70]. Preliminary morphologic studies, taking all of the above described substructural criteria into account, confirm the better preservation during prolonged storage with the combined treatment and functional recovery after transplantation.

Acknowledgements

The authors are indebted to F. Thoné, L. Leyssen, G. Jacobs and Mrs I. Gevers for skilful assistance and to Dr. B. Shivalkar for critical reading of the manuscript.

References

1. Schaper J, Hehrlein F, Schlepper M *et al.* Ultrastructural alterations during ischemia and reperfusion in human hearts during cardiac surgery. J Mol Cell Cardiol 1977; 9: 175.
2. Schaper J. Ultrastructure of the myocardium in acute ischemia. In Schaper W (ed): The pathophysiology of myocardial perfusion. North-Holland: Elsevier, 1979: 581–673.
3. Flameng W, Suy R, Schwarz F *et al.* Ultrastructural correlates of left ventricular contraction abnormalities in patients with chronic ischemic heart disease: determinants of reversible segmental asynergy postrevascularization surgery. Am Heart J 1981; 102: 846–57.
4. Slezak J, Geller SA, Litwak RS *et al.* Long-term study of the ultrastructural changes of myocardium in patients undergoing cardiac surgery, with more than 10 years follow-up. Int J Cardiol 1983; 4: 153–68.
5. Unverferth DV, Fetters JK, Unverferth BJ *et al.* Human myocardial histologic characteristics in congestive heart failure. Circulation 1983; 68: 1194–200.
6. Schaper J. Effects of multiple ischaemic events on human myocardium -an ultrastructural study. Eur Heart J 1988; 9: 141–9.
7. Flameng W, Wouters L, Sergeant P *et al.* Multivariate analysis of angiographic, histologic, and electrocardiographic data in patients with coronary heart disease. Circulation 1984; 70: 7–17.
8. Borgers M, Flameng W. Structural correlates of hibernating myocardium in man. J Am Coll Cardiol 1992; 19: 285A.

9. Jennings RB, Hawkins JK, Lowe JE *et al.* Relation between high energy phosphate and lethal injury in myocardial ischaemia in the dog. Am J Pathol 1978; 92: 187–214.
10. Borgers M. The role of calcium in the toxicity of the myocardium. Histochem J 1981; 13: 839–48.
11. Borgers M, Guo Shu L, Xhonneux R *et al.* Changes in ultrastructure and Ca^{2+} distribution in the isolated working rabbit heart after ischemia. A time-related study. AJP 1987; 126: 92–102.
12. Borgers M, Vandeplassche G, Van Reempts J. Cytochemical markers of ischaemia in the heart and brain. Histochem J 1990; 22: 125–33.
13. Okuda M, Lefer AM. Lysosomal hypothesis in the evolution of myocardial infarction. Subcellular fractionation and electron microscopic cytochemical study. Jpn Heart J 1979; 20: 643.
14. Fishbein MC, Meerbaum S, Rit J *et al.* Early phase acute myocardial infarct size quantification: validation of the triphenyl tetrazolium chloride tissue enzyme staining technique. Am Heart J 1981; 101: 593–600.
15. Chopra P, Sabherwal U. Histochemical and fluorescent techniques for detection of early myocardial ischaemia following experimental coronary artery occlusion: a comparative and quantitative study. Angiology 1988; 39: 132–40.
16. Siegel RJ, Edwalds G, Ref R *et al.* Distribution of cytosolic and mitochondrial asparatate aminotransferase in normal, ischaemic and necrotic myocardium. An immunohistochemical study. Lab Invest 1984a; 51: 648–54.
17. Siegel RJ, Said JW, Shell WE *et al.* Identification and localization of creatine kinase B and M in normal, ischaemic and necrotic myocardium. An immunohistochemical study. J Mol Cell Cardiol 1984b; 16: 95–103.
18. Fukuhara T, Kawashima T, Kubota I *et al.* Changes of calcium ATPase and cytochrome oxidase activity of myocardial cell under early and late ischaemia comparison with ultrastructural changes. Jpn Circ 1987; 51: 403–10.
19. Nakamura N, Sasai Y, Takeyama Y *et al.* Electron microscopic cytochemical studies on acid phosphatase activity in acute myocardial ischaemia. Jpn Heart J 1983; 24(4): 595–606.
20. Decker RS, Poole AR, Griffin EE *et al.* Altered distribution of lysosomal cathepsin D in ischaemic myocardium. J Clin Invest 1977; 59: 911.
21. Decker RS, Wildenthal K. Sequential lysosomal alterations during cardiac ischaemia. Ultrastructural and cytochemical studies. Lab Invest 1978; 38: 662.
22. Decker RS, Wildenthal K. Lysosomal alterations in hypoxic and reoxygenated hearts. Ultrastructural and cytochemical studies. Am J Pathol 1980; 98: 425.
23. Hess ML, Manson NH, Okabe E. Involvement of the radicals in the pathophysiology of ischaemic heart tissue. Can J Physiol Pharmacol 1982; 60: 1382–9.
24. McCord JM. Oxygen derived free radicals in postischaemic tissue injury. N Engl J Med 1985; 312; 159–64.
25. Downey JM, Miura T, Eddy L *et al.* Xanthine oxidase is not a source of free radicals in the ischaemic rabbit heart. J Mol Cell Cardiol 1987; 19: 1053–60.
26. Shlafer M, Meyers C, Adkins S. Mitochondrial hydrogen peroxide generation and activities of glutathione peroxidase and superoxide dismutase following global ischaemia. J Mol Cell Cardiol 1987; 19: 1195–206.
27. Nohl F. A novel superoxide generator in heart mitochondria. FEBS Lett 1987; 214: 269–73.
28. Hyslop PA, Hinshaw DB, Halsey WA *et al.* Mechanisms of oxidant-mediated cell injury. J Biol Chem 1988; 263(4): 1665–75.
29. Borgers M, Schaper J, Schaper W. Localization of specific phosphatase activities in canine blood vessels and heart muscle. J Histochem Cytochem 1971; 19: 526–39.
30. Borgers M, De Nollin S, Thoné F *et al.* Cytochemical localization of NADH-oxidase in *Candida albicans*. J Histochem Cytochem 1977; 25: 193–9.
31. Briggs RT, Drath DB, Karnovsky ML *et al.* Localization of NADH-oxidase on the surface

of human polymorphonuclear leucocytes by a new cytochemical method. J Cell Biol 1975; 67: 566–86.
32. Vandeplassche G, Hermans C, Thoné F *et al.*Mitochondrial hydrogen peroxide generation by NADH oxidase activity following regional myocardial ischaemia in the dog. J Mol Cell Cardiol 1989; 383–92.
33. Vandeplassche G, Thoné F, Borgers M. Cytochemical evidence of NADH-oxidase activity in the isolated working rabbit heart subjected to normothermic global ischaemia. Histochem J 1989; 22: 11–7.
34. Vandeplassche G, Hermans C, Thoné F *et al.* Stunned myocardium has increased mitochondrial NADH oxidase and ATPase activities. Cardioscience 1991; 2: 47–53.
35. Katz AM, Reuter H. Cellular calcium and cardiac cell death. Am J Cardiol 1979; 44: 188–90.
36. Poole-Wilson PA, Harding DP, Bourdillon PDV *et al.* Calcium out of control. J Mol Cell Cardiol 1984; 16: 175–87.
37. Cheung J, Bonventre J, Malis CD *et al.* Calcium and ischaemic injury. N Engl J Med 1986; 314: 1670–6.
38. Borgers M, Thoné F, Ver Donck L. Sarcolemma-bound calcium. Its importance for cell viability. Basic Res Cardiol 1985; 80(Suppl. I) 31–5.
39. Borgers M, Piper M. Calcium shifts in anoxic cardiac myocytes. A cytochemical study. J Mol Cell Cardiol 1986; 18: 439–48.
40. Borgers M, Thoné F, Verheyen A *et al.* Localization of calcium in skeletal and cardiac muscle. Histochem J 1984; 16: 295–309.
42. Björk VO. Safety factors in open-heart surgery. J Thorac Cardiovasc Surg 1967; 54: 161–70.
43. Walter P, Schwarz F, Becker V *et al.* Morphology of poorly contracting ventricle in patients with coronary artery disease. Thor Cardiovasc Surg 1980; 28: 177–83.
44. Schachner A, Schimert G, Lajos T *et al.* Selective intracavitary and coronary hypothermic cardioplegia for myocardial preservation – Clinical, physiologic and ultrastructural evaluation. Arch Surg 1976; 111: 1197–206.
45. Nasseri M, Bücherl ES, Herbst R. Praktische Erfahrungen mit Procain-Magnesium-Aspartat in der offenen Herzchirurgie. Thoraxchirurgie 1973; 21: 67–77.
46. DeGasperis C, Miani A, Donatelli R. Ultrastructural changes in human myocardium associated with ischemic arrest. J Mol Cell Cardiol 1970; 1: 169–76.
47. Vitali-Mazza L, Anversa P, Tedeschi F *et al.* Ultrastructural basis of acute left ventricular failure from severe acute aortic stenosis in the rabbit. J Mol Cell Cardiol 1972; 4: 661–74.
48. Flameng W, Borgers M, Daenen W *et al.* Ultrastructural and cytochemical correlates of myocardial protection by cardiac hypothermia in man. J Thorac Cardiovasc Surg 1980; 79: 413–24.
49. Flameng W, Borgers M, Daenen W *et al.* St. Thomas cardioplegia versus topical cooling: ultrastructural and biochemical studies in humans. Ann Thorac Surg 1981; 31: 339–46.
50. Flameng W, van der Vusse GJ, Borgers M *et al.* Intermittent aortic crossclamping at 32°C, a safe technique for multiple aortocoronary bypass grafting. Thorac Cardiovasc Surg 1981; 29: 216–22.
51. van der Vusse GJ, van der Veen FH, Flameng W *et al.* A biochemical and ultrastructural study on myocardial changes during aorto-coronary bypass surgery: St. Thomas hospital cardioplegia versus intermittent aortic cross-clamping at 34 and 25°C. Eur Surg Res 1986; 18: 1–11.
52. Schelbert HR. Myocardial scar of hibernating myocardium? The role of positron emission tomography. In Bulla N, Henderson A, Krayenbühl HP (eds): LV function in stunned and hibernating myocardium. Proc. Symp. 13th Congress Eur Soc Cardiol, Amsterdam: Exerpta Medica 1991; 56–68.
53. Murashita T, Borgers M, Hearse DJ. Developmental changes in tolerance to ischemia in the rabbit heart: disparity between interpretations of structural enzymatic and functional indices of injury. 1991. Submitted.

54. Shivalkar B, Herijgers P, Borgers M *et al.* Is the hibernating myocardium dedifferentiating? Circulation 1991; 84(Suppl): 2895.
55. Maron BJ, Ferrans VJ, Roberts WC. Ultrastructural features of degenerated muscle cells in patients with cardiac hypertrophy. Am J Pathol 1975; 76: 387–434.
56. Maron BJ, Ferrans VJ. Intramitochondrial glycogen deposits in hypertrophied human myocardium. J Mol Cell Cardiol 1975; 7: 697–702.
57. Krayenbuhl HP, Hess OM, Schneider J *et al.* Physiologic or pathologic hypertrophy. Eur Heart J 1983; 4 (Suppl A): 29–34.
58. Fleischer M, Warmuth H, Backwinkel KP *et al.* Ultrastructural morphometric analysis of normally loaded human myocardial left ventricles from young and old patients. Virch Arch (Abt A) 1978; 380: 123–33.
59. Fleischer M, Wippo W, Themann H *et al.* Ultrastructural morphometric analysis of human myocardial left ventricles with mitral insufficiency. Virc Arch (Abt A) 1980; 389: 205–10.
60. Hess OM, Schneider J, Koch R *et al.* Diastolic function and myocardial structure in patients with myocardial hypertrophy. Circulation 1981; 63: 360–71.
61. Olivetti G, Melissari M, Capasso JM *et al.* Cardiomyopathy of the aging human heart. Circ Res 1991; 68: 1560–8.
62. Schwartzkopff B, Zierz S, Frenzel H *et al.* Ultrastructural abnormalities of mitochondria and deficiency of myocardial cytochrome c oxidase in a patient with ventricular tachycardia. Virchows Archiv A Pathol Anat 1991; 419: 63–8.
63. Schaper J, Froede R, Hein St *et al.* Impairment of the myocardial ultrastructure and changes of the cytoskeleton in dilated cardiomyopathy. Circulation 1991; 83: 504–14.
64. Thiedemann K-U. Ultrastructure in chronic ischemia studies in human hearts. In Schaper W (ed): The pathophysiology of myocardial perfusion. North-Holland: Elsevier 1979; 675–716.
65. Maron BJ, Ferrans VJ, Roberts WC. Myocardial ultrastructure in patients with chronic aortic valve disease. Am J Cardiol 1975; 35: 725–39.
66. Clark RE, Ferguson TB, Marbarger JP. The first American clinical trial of nifedipine in cardioplegia. J Thorac Cardiovasc Surg 1981; 82: 848–59.
67. Ver Donck L, Borgers M. Myocardial protection by R 56865: a new principle based on prevention of ion channel pathology. Am J Physiol 1991; 261: H1828–H1835.
68. Flameng W, Sukehiro S, Mollhoff T *et al.* A new concept of long-term donor heart preservation: nucleoside transport inhibition. J Heart Lung Transpl, 1991; 10: 990–8.
69. Masuda M, Demeulemeester A, Chang-Chun C *et al.* Cardioprotective effects of nucleoside transport inhibition in ischemia-reperfused rabbit hearts. A role of endogenous adenosine. J Mol Cell Cardiol 1991; 23(Suppl V): S127.
70. Masuda M, Flameng W. Effects of nucleoside transport inhibition on ischemic human myocardium. J Mol Cell Cardiol 1991; 23(Suppl V): S127.
71. Flameng W, Daenen W, Borgers M *et al.* Cardioprotective effects of Lidoflazine during 1-hour normothermic global ischemia. Circulation 1981; 64: 796–807.
72. Flameng W, Borgers M, van der Vusse G *et al.* Cardioprotective effects of Lidoflazine in extensive aorta-coronary bypass grafting. J Thorac Cardiovasc Surg 1983; 85: 758–68.
73. Kirklin JW, Akins CW, Blackstone EH *et al.* Guidelines and indications for coronary artery bypass graft surgery. A report of the American College of Cardiology/American Heart Association task force on assessment of diagnostic and therapeutic cardiovascular procedures (Subcommittee on Coronary Artery Bypass Graft Surgery). J Am Coll Cardiol 1991; 17(3): 543–89.
74. Borgers M. The role of the sarcolemma-glycocalyx complex in myocardial cell function. In De Bakey ME, Gotto AM (eds): Factors influencing the course of myocardial ischemia. Amsterdam: Elsevier Science Publishers 1983; 56–67.
75. Borgers M. Loss of sarcolemmal integrity in ischemic myocardium. In Piper HM (ed): Pathophysiology of severe ischemic myocardial injury, Vol. 104. Dordrecht: Kluwer Academic Publishers 1990; 69–89.
76. Van Belle H, Janssen PAJ. Comparative pharmacology of nucleoside transport inhibitors. Nucleosides & Nucleotides 1991; 10: 975–82.

17. Muscle birefringence

SALLY DARRACOTT-CANKOVIC

Introduction

Quantitative birefringence measurements (QBM) are a valuable means of assessing myocardial protection during open heart surgery because they provide an index of myocardial contractility at a cellular level [1]. Most importantly they can be done on small needle biopsies and can measure changes in myocardial function even when the heart is arrested and conventional hemodynamic assessment is impossible.

More than 2000 patients from several centers undergoing cardiac investigation [2,3], various types of cardiac surgery [4–12] and heart transplantation [13–16] have been monitored by QBM. The results of these clinical series showed that QBM not only successfully monitored myocardial protection during surgery, but that they also predicted the postoperative outcome of the patients.

Routine biopsy monitoring of patients during open heart surgery is no longer relevant due to the efficacy of cardioplegic arrest and topical hypothermia as methods of myocardial protection. This success also means that it is now more difficult to evaluate clinically the benefit of any proposed changes in operative technique or additives to cardioplegic solutions, since several hundred patients may have to be studied before a significant difference is observed [17–19]. However our studies and those of other workers have identified where specific problems remain and this chapter highlights these areas.

Methodology

Explanation of the muscle birefringence response to ATP-calcium buffer

Myosin micelles are anisotropic and possess form birefringence which depends quantitatively on the degree of orientation of the myosin micelles. Current theories of the structure and function of muscle assume that the degree of orientation of myosin remains constant with the actin filaments sliding over them [20,21]. However, in 1965 Chayen and co-workers [1] observed that freshly thawed myocardial fibers in cryostat sections viewed

H.M. Piper and C.J. Preusse (eds): Ischemia-reperfusion in cardiac surgery, 377–402.

under a polarizing microscope exhibited little birefringence, but if a drop of buffer containing ATP and calcium was placed on the section the muscle birefringence increased threefold. This anomaly was explained by the fact that most workers studying muscle contraction used glycerinated muscle fibers for such investigations [22]. When we treated our cryostat sections similarly, by immersing them in 20% glycerine, there was an increase in birefringence indicating increased orientation of the myosin micelles. Additionally if ATP and calcium buffer was added to the glycerine solution there was a slight further increase in birefringence of the fibers. However the addition of buffer containing carnosine, a relaxant of cardiac muscle [23], to sections previously exposed to the ATP-calcium medium, caused a decrease in birefringence to the values initially recorded in air.

In their studies on muscle contraction Huxley and Hanson [24] showed that the sarcomere length decreased to 80% of its initial length and we recorded a similar decrease (to 83%) in cryostat sections of normal dog myocardium before and after the addition of glycerine containing ATP and calcium [1]. Pretreatment of sections with each of two selective inhibitors of myosin ATPase, tripropyl tin and p-chloromercuribenzoate, markedly depressed the response of the fibers to ATP-calcium buffer. These studies (and others described elsewhere) [1,25] indicated that the effect of ATP-calcium medium on myocardial fibers depended on the activity of myosin ATPase to induce a change in the actual birefringent properties of the myosin micelles. This implies that the effect of such ATPase activity, in the presence of calcium ions, increases the degree of orientation of the myosin. The process of 'flash-drying' cryostat sections onto the microscope slide leaves them relatively immobilised. Consequently the changes which we observe in the muscle cells in response to ATP and calcium are assumed to be related to isometric contraction.

Biopsy procedure

Full-thickness biopsies are taken from the apex of the left ventricle (LV) by means of an air powered drill or a Tru-cut biopsy needle. The biopsies are either: (1) immediately frozen by precipitate immersion in n-hexane at –70°C for 20 seconds and then transferred and stored in cold tubes in a thermos flask packed with solid carbon dioxide at –70°C; or (2) placed in specimen tubes, immediately frozen in liquid nitrogen and then stored at –70°C. The specimens remain viable for periods up to 3 months.

Mounting and sectioning

All biopsies from each patient are processed together so that the specimens from the beginning of bypass can serve as controls for those obtained during the course of or at the end of bypass.

The biopsies are mounted on metal chucks pre-cooled to –70°C in a constant freezing mixture of alcohol and solid CO_2. A drop of water placed on top of the chuck freezes rapidly, and when a thin film of water is left approximately the same size as the specimen, the biopsy is quickly picked up with cold forceps and placed in the film of water. The residual water freezes the tissue to the drop of ice on the chuck. The biopsy specimens are then oriented so as to give a large proportion of longitudinal fibers and sectioned at 8 μm in a cryostat with the cabinet temperature at –30°C.

Apparatus required for quantitative polarization microscopy

The following are needed: a polarizing microscope (e.g., Zeiss Universal) fitted with special polarized light objectives (×10, 0.22 NA and ×25, 0.60 NA), a strain-free condenser suitable for polarized light (1.3 Pol), a sub-stage polarizer and an analyzer set into the tube of the microscope. The microscope tube also has a slot, set at 45° to the normal axes of the microscope, into which a Brace-Kohler rotatable lambda/30 compensator can be inserted. The illumination is provided by a 100 watt halogen lamp.

Measurement of birefringence

The freshly cut cryostat sections may be stored for up to three hours in the cabinet of the cryostat or for several days in a freezer at –70°C. The section, mounted on a microscope slide, is rapidly air-dried and placed on the stage of the microscope with the longitudinal muscle fibers in the center of the field. The analyzer and polarizer are then crossed to give complete extinction of the background. The microscope stage is then rotated so that the fibers are lying at 45° to the N-S, E-W axes and appear maximally bright. The lambda/30 rotating compensator is then inserted between the specimen and the analyzer and rotated until the background between the muscle fibers is maximally black (Figure 17.1A). The graduated scale on the compensator is read and gives the initial value e.g., 11.5°. The compensator is then rotated until the muscle fibers *just* appear to go black, and this value is noted, e.g., 7.5°. (If the compensator is rotated further the fibers get darker, but for accurate measurements it is important to take the reading when the fibers *just* achieve uniform darkness.) Therefore for this specimen the optical angle of rotation ψ from a maximally dark background to dark fibers is 11.5°-7.5° = 4.0°.

A drop of barbitone-sodium buffer (pH 7.8) containing 2 mmol ATP and 36 mmol calcium chloride is placed on the section still lying on the microscope stage and there is an immediate increase in birefringence due to increased orientation of the myosin micelles (Figure 17.1B). A coverslip is placed on the section and the same muscle fibers measured again, e.g., maximally black background at 11.6°, fibers just dark at 1.3°, giving an optical angle of rotation ψ of 11.6°-1.3° = 10.3°.

The optical angles of rotation measured with the compensator are then

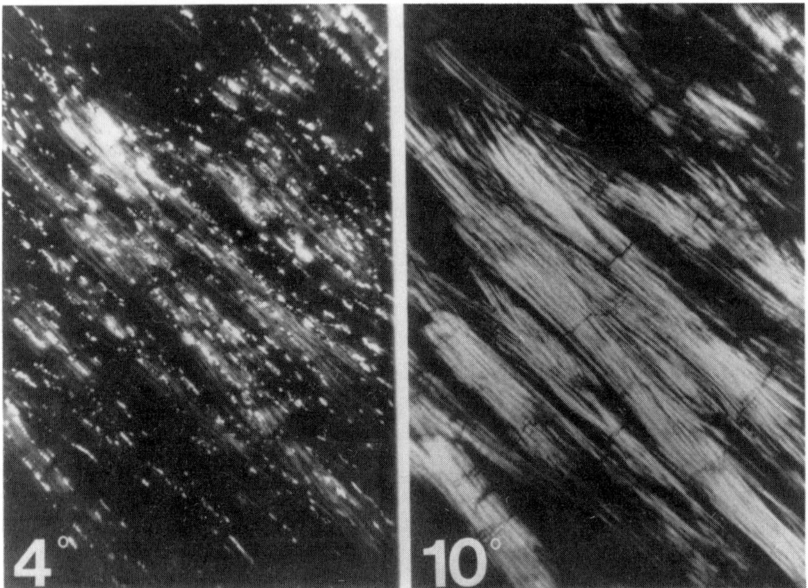

Figure 17.1. Fibers of normally functioning myocardium viewed under crossed polars (A) before and (B) after immersion in the ATP-calcium medium (birefringence values of the muscle fibers measured 4° and 10° respectively). Thus the ATP calcium medium caused an increase in birefringence of 6° (converted to linear units of optical path difference, incremental birefringence = 4.5 nm).

converted into linear optical path difference (Ro, in nm) in the fibers by means of the expression Ro = Rc sin 2 ψ where Rc is a constant for the particular compensator used, and is supplied by the manufacturer. For example, if Rc for the compensator is 21.25, then the angle of rotation 10.3° is converted into linear optical path difference by Ro = 21.25 × sin (2 × 10.3°)

$$= 21.25 \times \sin 20.6°$$
$$= 21.25 \times 0.3518$$
$$= 7.48 \text{ nm}$$

Thus the incremental birefringence of the muscle fibers shown in Figures 17.1.A and 17.1B, i.e., the change in birefringence in response to the addition of ATP and calcium, expressed in linear units of optical path difference =

$$7.48 - 2.96 = 4.52 \text{ nm}$$

In contrast the ischemic muscle fibers shown in Figure 17.2 had a higher value in air 5.0° (3.69 nm), a diminished response to ATP and calcium 10.0° (7.27 nm) and an incremental birefringence of only 3.58 nm. Post mortem muscle shows virtually no change in birefringence in response to ATP and calcium.

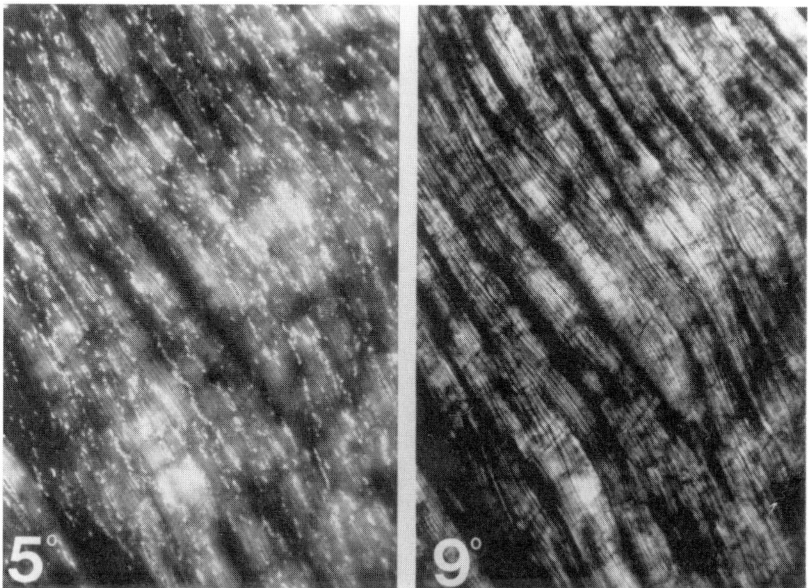

Figure 17.2. Fibers of poorly functioning myocardium viewed under crossed polars. In contrast with Figure 17.1A there is an appreciable birefringence in the muscle fibers in air (A) (birefringence value 5°). (B) The same fibers mounted in ATP – calcium medium are shown (birefringence value 9°). Incremental birefringence = 4° (converted to linear units o.p.d. = 0.97).

As birefringence = optical path difference ÷ thickness, and as the same muscle fibers are measured before and after the application of ATP and calcium, the thickness of the fibers, at least as regards the concentration of myosin measured, is constant. Consequently the optical path difference measured is directly proportional to birefringence.

Validation of birefringence measurements – correlation with physiological measurements of cardiac function

In a blind study two hundred fifty patients were fully investigated by physiological measurements at cardiac catheterization. At the same time birefringence measurements were made on LV endomyocardial biopsy specimens taken with a bioptome. The hemodynamic status of the patient was assessed by left ventricular end-diastolic pressure and volume; cardiac index; ejection rate and fraction; peak ventricular circumferential fiber shortening; KV max and post-ectopic KV max. The patients were then assigned into groups of physiological function: good, intermediate and bad [26]. Of these, 19 patients were assessed normal by all physiological criteria and 51 were poor. The QBM assessments of normal hearts were significantly higher than those with poor myocardial function (mean incremental birefringence 4.22 ± 0.10 nm

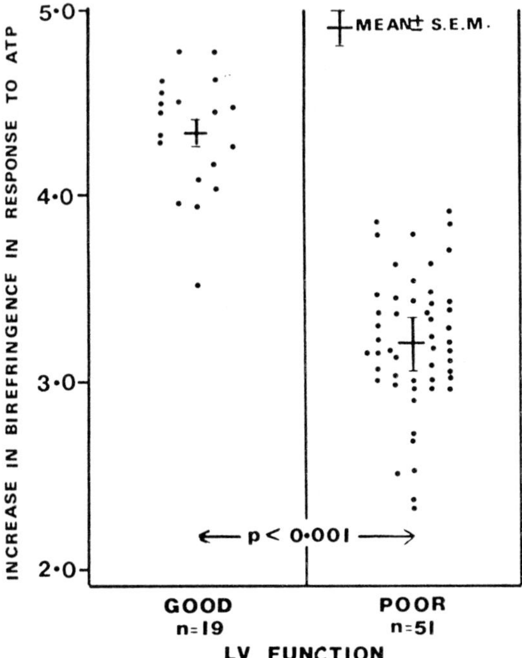

Figure 17.3. The relation between the change in birefringence, induced by the ATP-calcium medium, and the physiological assessment of cardiac function. The difference between the group with good left ventricular (LV) function and the group with bad LV function is highly significant: $p < 0.001$ (Students t test).

and 3.29 ± 0.16 nm respectively, $p < 0.001$, Figure 17.3) [1,7,8]. Thus birefringence measurements give an assessment of myocardial function and can provide valuable information at times when it is not possible to do the usual physiological tests of function, e.g. *during* cardiopulmonary bypass and heart transplantation.

Grading of biopsy specimens

(1) During routine open heart surgery with relatively short ischemic times, myocardial deterioration during cardiopulmonary bypass was found to be the most significant factor in assessing the prognosis during the immediate post-operative period. Thus, a diminished incremental birefringence (ATP – air figure) during bypass greater than 0.4 nm was strongly indicative of a low cardiac output in the immediate post-operative period [4–12].

(2) During heart transplantation, which necessitates extended periods of ischemia, biopsy assessment of myocardial function at the beginning of

the procedure was found to be an equally significant prognostic indicator [13–16]. Also muscle birefringence both in air and ATP was found to be more variable during protracted ischemia and so a ratio (incremental birefringence divided by the air figure) was used to assess changes during transplantation. Donor hearts with either (i) an initial birefringence ratio of 1.15 or less, or (ii) a decrease greater than 0.21 during transplantation were classed as having a poor prognosis.

Clinical studies: immediate problems: experimental model to clinical trial – rigorous monitoring protects the patient

Stringent clinical evaluation is always required when a technique of myocardial protection, developed and tested in an animal model, is transferred to the operating theatre, so that any unsuspected inadequacies in the technique can be rapidly identified and corrected. When the St Thomas' Hospital Cardioplegic Solution No. 1 (McCarthy's) which was developed by Hearse and associates based on their studies in the isolated rat heart model [27], and later solution No. 2 tested in the rat and dog heart [28,29] were first used clinically, biopsy assessments quickly detected problems which had not been apparent experimentally.

The need for topical cooling

One advantage of assessment by QBM in full thickness needle biopsies is that they facilitate comparison of endo- and epimyocardial protection. This proved important during clinical testing of cold cardioplegic arrest. With our previous method of protection, continuous coronary perfusion of a beating heart at 32°C, assessment of full thickness biopsies taken at the beginning and end of cardiopulmonary bypass had shown that the endomyocardium was most vulnerable to damage. However when we compared results of the last 16 consecutive patients undergoing AVR with this method and the first 16 protected with cold cardioplegic arrest, it was apparent that the situation had reversed and the epimyocardium was now at risk (Figure 17.4). With continuous coronary perfusion, endomyocardial deterioration occurred in 10 (63%) patients and epimyocardial in one (6%), but with cardioplegic arrest epimyocardial deterioration occurred in 5 (31%, p = NS) patients and there was no incidence of isolated endomyocardial injury ($p < 0.001$).

This emphasised the vulnerability of the surface of the heart (particularly those with hypertrophy) to rewarming during cardioplegic arrest. Because of this finding, in the next 50 patients the surface of the heart was irrigated continuously with cold Hartmann's solution and the incidence of epimyocardial deterioration fell to 8%. As overall myocardial protection improved, the incidence of postoperative low CO fell from 25% to 12.5% and 8% in the three groups respectively. (Figure 17.4).

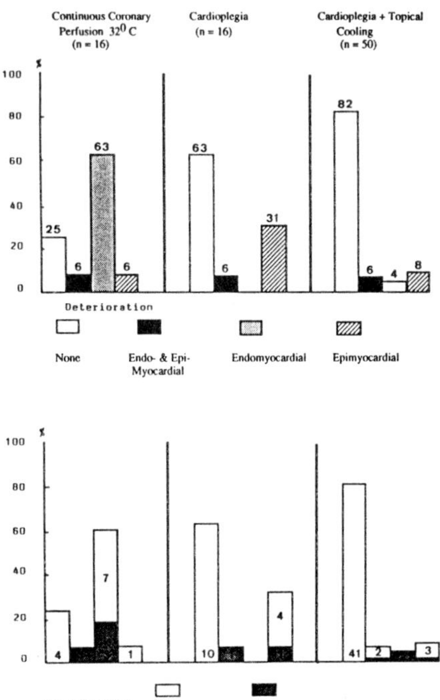

Figure 17.4. QBM assessment of endo- and epimyocardial protection during cardiopulmonary bypass. In the upper histograms each column refers to the percentage of patients in each particular group showing good or poor protection. The lower histograms show the postoperative clinical outcome of the same patients.

The need for multidose cardioplegia

The necessity for multiple infusions of the cardioplegic solution was demonstrated in the early aortic and mitral valve experience. With a single infusion of cardioplegic solution (mean A'Cl 129 ± 5 min) QBM detected myocardial deterioration in 3 of 9 (33%) patients studied; 2 had low CO postoperatively.

These results alerted the surgeon to the possibility that noncoronary collateral flow was causing washout of the cardioplegic solution allowing resumption of myocardial activity and consequent depletion of myocardial energy stores. In subsequent patients the cardioplegic infusion was repeated at 45–60 min intervals. This resulted in improved myocardial protection in 14 patients studied sequentially (mean A'Cl 126 ± 8 min), since deterioration was observed in 2 only (14%).

The need for filtration of the cardioplegic solution

Following experimental testing in the rat and dog model [28] a randomized clinical study comparing the newly formulated St Thomas' Hospital cardio-

Table 17.1. Pilot study comparing myocardial protection with St. Thomas' hospital cardioplegic solutions Nos. 1 and 2.

Aetiology		Infusions	Deterioration			Low CO
			LV endo	LV epi	RV	
Soln. 1	CABG	1	–	–	+	0
	CABG	1	–	–	–	0
	CABG	2	–	–	–	0
	CABG	2	–	–	–	0
	CABG	3	–	–	–	0
	CABG	3	–	–	–	0
	AVR, CABG	3	+	–	–	0
Soln. 2	CABG	1	–	+	–	0
	CABG	1	–	+	–	0
	CABG	2	+	+	+	+
	CABG	3	–	–	+	+
	CABG	3	–	+	–	0
	AVR	3	+	+	+	*
	MVR	3	+	+	+	+

*Ventricular ectopics

plegic solution No. 2 with solution No. 1 began in 1981. Solution 2 differed from No. 1 in that procaine was omitted as experimentally it had been shown to have little protective effect [29] and the calcium content had been lowered to 1.2 mmoles/L since this had been shown to improve protection [30]. The solution was buffered to pH 7.8 with sodium bicarbonate immediately prior to use.

It rapidly became apparent that the new solution had a deleterious effect on the myocardium since QBM showed deterioration in each of the first seven hearts arrested with it (Table 17.1). Three had biventricular deterioration and 3 patients had low cardiac output postoperatively (1 balloon pump). Protection was superior in seven control patients arrested with Solution No. 1 and all recovered uneventfully.

The clinical trial was halted and further tests showed that particulate contamination in the unfiltered cardioplegic solution caused coronary vasoconstriction and impaired recovery of contractility in isolated rat hearts [31.32]. Since a microfilter had been routinely employed in the experimental infusion apparatus, this problem did not become manifest until the new solution was tested clinically in the absence of a microfilter. (The incorporation of procaine in Solution No. 1 had been shown experimentally to have vasodilatory properties which mitigated the effects of this contamination.) The use of a microfilter then became standard clinical practice and St Thomas' Hospital cardioplegic solution No. 2 (Plegisol) was reintroduced clinically with success [33].

None of these clinical problems could have been predicted on the basis of the experimental studies employed during optimization of the individual components of the St Thomas' Hospital cardioplegic solutions. Rigorous screening by QBM during the introductory phase minimized the deleterious consequences to the patients, since rapid identification of the problems prompted technical adjustments which ensured the success of the technique.

Long-term monitoring for identification of limitations of the preservation technique

After careful monitoring of the efficacy of any new method of myocardial protection and the correction of any immediate technical inadequacies, only painstaking longer-term monitoring will identify any more subtle limitation of the technique, e.g. is it time dependent, does it provide uniform protection throughout the heart, and is it effective during the correction of all cardiac defects?

The effect of ischemic time

Various studies have shown that ischemic times up to 180 min are well tolerated during multidose cardioplegia [11,34–38]. Engelman [35] comparing patients with arrest times above and below 120 min duration found no difference in serum enzyme generation, incidence of perioperative myocardial infarction, utilization of inotropic agents or postoperative mortality. However he did find that with ischemic times greater than 120 min, postoperative CPK-MB levels were significantly elevated in patients following valve replacement compared with those undergoing coronary revascularisation [35,36] and suggested that in patients with hypertrophic valvular disease ischemic times above 3 hours duration were not commensurate with optimal preservation.

During the period 1975–86 biopsy assessment of myocardial protection was performed on one third of the 1464 patients undergoing routine open heart surgery, during cardioplegic arrest at St Thomas' Hospital. With single-dose cardioplegia in 113 patients the incidence of LV myocardial deterioration was similar in hearts arrested for less, or more than 120 min (17% and 21% respectively, Table 17.2). However with multidose cardioplegia a time-limiting effect became apparent. Of 372 patients studied, the incidence of myocardial deterioration was 23/304 (8%) for those arrested <120 min; 6/50 (12%) for those arrested between 120–150 min ($p = NS$), and this increased significantly to 8/18 (44%) for periods over 150 min ($p < 0.001$, Table 17.2).

This poor myocardial protection during prolonged ischemia correlated with a poorer clinical outcome of the patients since 2/18 (11%) had low CO and 8 (44%) died. This patient group comprised 2 undergoing AVR; 3 CABG; 3 A & MVR and 10 CABG & VR. The causes of death were: (A & MVR) 2 from low CO and 1 from pulmonary emboli; (CABG & VR) 1 from low CO, 1 graft spasm, 1 calcium emboli and 2 from hepato-renal failure.

Table 17.2. Effect of duration of ischemia on myocardial protection and clinical outcome of 485 patients undergoing routine open heart surgery.

Duration of ischemia (mins)	Biopsy assessment		Clinical outcome		
	Good %	Deteriorated %	Good %	Low CO %	Mort %
Single dose Cardioplegia*					
<120 (n = 99)	83	17	87	9	4
>120 (n = 14)	79	21	65	21	14
Multidose Cardioplegia					
<120 (n = 304)	92	8[b]	92	6	2[b]
120–150 (n = 50)	88	12[a]	90	6	4[b]
>150 (n = 18)	56	44	45	11	44

*No patient in this group had an ischemic time >150 mins.
Incidence significantly less ([a]$p < 0.01$, [b]$p < 0.001$) compared with that of patients arrested >150 mins.

These results indicated that for complex corrective surgical procedures necessitating >150 min of ischemia, myocardial protection with the St Thomas' Hospital cardioplegic solution No. 1 was inadequate.

A comparison of right and left ventricular protection

Since effective protection of the left heart has been achieved with multidose cardioplegic arrest and topical hypothermia, interest has focussed on the problem of protecting the thin walled right heart. The right heart is superficially more exposed to warming by the operating theatre lights, less protected by the cooling bath of fluid maintained within the pericardial cavity [39] and subjected to rewarming by the return of blood from pulmonary bronchial and mediastinal noncoronary collaterals during surgery [40,41]. The atria are particularly vulnerable to ischemia since they only receive approximately half as much cardioplegic solution per gram tissue as the ventricles do [42] and inadequate atrial protection has been implicated in the increased incidence of postoperative supraventricular arrhythmias, conduction disturbances and atrial transport functional abnormalities reported following cardioplegic arrest [42,43].

Studies showing non-uniform cooling of the heart [44–46] have stimulated measures to ensure more effective cooling [39,47–49] and to assess accurately right ventricular protection during surgery. Chen [50] compared protection in the LV, RV, and RA of 20 patients during surgery and reported that ultrastructurally the LV was the best protected and that the RA was the worst. Teoh [51] and Christakis [52] found that ATP levels decreased significantly in both ventricles during cardioplegic arrest for CABG.

We have compared right and left ventricular protection in 306 patients protected by multidose cardioplegia during open heart surgery for a variety

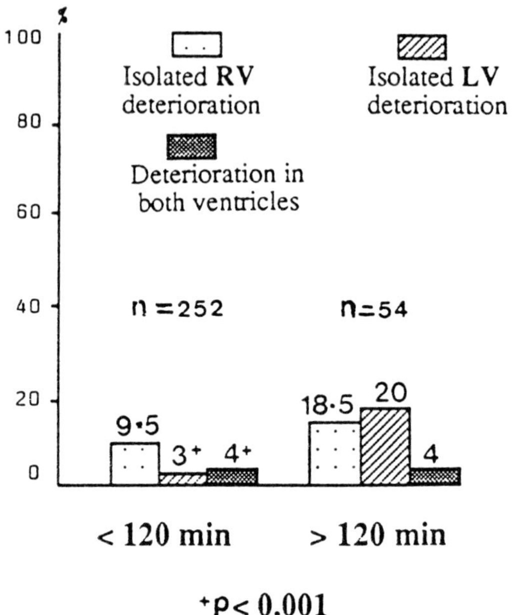

Figure 17.5. A comparison of right and left ventricular myocardial protection (assessed by QBM) during open heart surgery. Each column refers to the percentage of patients in each particular group showing poor protection (results of hearts arrested <120 mins and >120 mins are shown separately).

of lesions. Meticulous care was taken to ensure effective right heart cooling with a catheter spraying 4°C Hartmann's solution over the ventricle and another inserted into the right atrium delivering cold solution. The results of this study were interesting because significant differences in right and left ventricular protection were only apparent in hearts arrested <120 min, the time period during which LV protection had been shown to be adequate. Of 252 hearts studied 9.5% showed only RV deterioration and 3% had LV deterioration ($p < 0.001$). In addition 4% of hearts had both RV and LV deterioration (Figure 17.5). This study showed that the RV was more vulnerable to ischemic damage during cardioplegic arrest and that more stringent measures are needed to ensure uniformity of myocardial protection.

During prolonged ischemia (>120 min) the incidence of isolated RV or LV deterioration increased significantly to 18.5% ($p = 0.05$) and 20% ($p < 0.001$) respectively in the 54 hearts studied. Again 4% had biventricular deterioration. The incidence of postoperative supraventricular dysrhythmias was not affected by the duration of ischemia and was 16% and 17% for both groups. The importance of achieving adequate myocardial protection in both ventricles is emphasised by the fact that during this study three patients had right ventricular failure following CABG: 2 died. QBM showed that 2 of these patients had both right and left ventricular deterioration during surgery

(A'Cl 140 and 102 min) and the third had very poor RV myocardium throughout the bypass period (A'Cl 108 min).

Do coronary artery stenoses impair cardioplegic protection of the heart?

The difficulties of achieving uniform distribution of the cardioplegic solution and uniform cooling of the myocardium in patients with stenosed or occluded coronary arteries have been well documented [53–56]. However, in our biopsy series QBM indicated that with multidose cardioplegia and topical cooling, LV myocardial protection in 147 patients undergoing CABG was comparable with that during aortic or mitral valve replacement since 94%, 94% and 91% respectively were assessed as well protected.

However, the efficacy of myocardial protection during CABG was affected by the duration of ischemia. QBM assessment of 132 patients with ischemic times <120 min showed a 5% incidence of left ventricular myocardial deterioration compared with 12% of 17 patients arrested >120 min. Right ventricular biopsies studied in 120 and 16 patients from each group respectively showed that the incidence of RV deterioration rose significantly from 8% to 25% following prolonged ischemia ($p < 0.05$). Once again poorer myocardial protection correlated with poorer patient outcome since results of the larger clinical series showed that the incidence of postoperative low CO rose from 4% in 701 patients arrested < 120 min to 15% in 95 patients arrested >120 min ($p < 0.001$). Postoperative mortality was also increased from 2% to 9% ($p < 0.001$).

The results of our large clinical series also showed that the frequency of cardioplegic infusion did not affect the clinical outcome of the patients. Twenty five received singledose cardioplegia, 191 had infusions repeated at 45–60 min intervals; and 605 were reinfused every 30 min. 92%, 90% and 92% of patients in each group had an uncomplicated postoperative recovery.

Thus the results of this longer-term monitoring of patients during routine heart surgery for the correction of various defects (valve replacement, CABG etc) showed that the incidence of myocardial deterioration fell from 18% with singledose cardioplegia to 10% with multidose cardioplegia. This was reflected by improved clinical outcome of the patients since the incidence of postoperative low cardiac output was halved from 12% to 6%. However QBM highlighted two areas where improvements were needed since myocardial protection was sub-optimal in the right ventricular myocardium and also in hearts arrested for prolonged periods during correction of complex defects.

Assessment of myocardial protection during congenital heart surgery

In 1984 Bull [9] reviewed the results of 200 children undergoing correction of various congenital defects with the myocardium protected by multidose (20 min) cardioplegia. She reported a 15% mortality rate and observed that this mortality rose sharply when hearts were arrested >85 min. Myocardial protection was monitored by QBM in RV biopsies obtained from 129 of these children and showed that approximately 50% of perioperative deaths were due to inadequate protection.

Does Nifedipine improve hypothermic cardioplegic protection?

Since the correction of congenital heart defects often necessitate prolonged operating times, a study was undertaken at the Hospital for Sick Children, to see whether the addition of Nifedipine, a calcium channel blocker shown to have cardioprotective properties in some experimental and clinical studies [57–59], would enhance myocardial protection during congenital heart surgery. Forty-four children aged 6 months – 14 years (mean 5 ± 3 years) were randomized into two groups. There was no difference in cyanosis, age or weight between the groups. Patients received multidose cardioplegia ± Nifedipine every 30 min, their hearts were maintained <20°C by means of topical cooling. QBM on RV biopsies taken before, after 45 min of, and 20 min following aortic cross-clamping showed no beneficial effect of Nifedipine since 32% of those treated with Nifedipine deteriorated compared with 36% of those receiving cardioplegic solution alone (Figure 17.6). The postoperative outcome of the patients was similar since 14% and 18% respectively required moderate or high dose catecholamine support postoperatively.

These results were at variance with a previous study in which dog hearts were maintained at 20°C without topical hypothermia during 200 min ischemic arrest [58]. In this series both QBM and hemodynamic parameters had shown a significant benefit of Nifedipine as an additive to the St Thomas' Hospital cardioplegic solution. However other studies in isolated rat hearts [60] arrested for 150 min had shown that the extra protection which Nifedipine conferred during normothermic arrest was lost with hypothermia. Since the hearts in our pediatric series received continuous topical cooling, presumably achieving effective hypothermia, this may have abolished the action of Nifedipine.

Are hearts from cyanotic patients more vulnerable to ischemia?

Some experimental and clinical studies [61–63] have suggested that cyanotic hearts are more susceptible to ischemic damage during cardioplegic arrest. We compared the biopsy assessments of cyanotic and acyanotic patients in our series to see whether this factor accounted for the high incidence of perioperative deterioration which we had observed. Of 29 cyanotic patients, 11 (38%) deteriorated compared with 4/15 (27%) in the acyanotic group ($p = NS$, Figure 17.6). Ischemic times were not significantly different, a mean of 58 ± 5 (range 25–120) min and 49 ± 5 (range 28–98) min in each group respectively. In addition, QBM detected severe myocardial damage in 21% and 33% of cyanotic and acyanotic patients respectively prior to surgery and showed that these hearts remained poor throughout the operation.

The Effect of Nifedipine

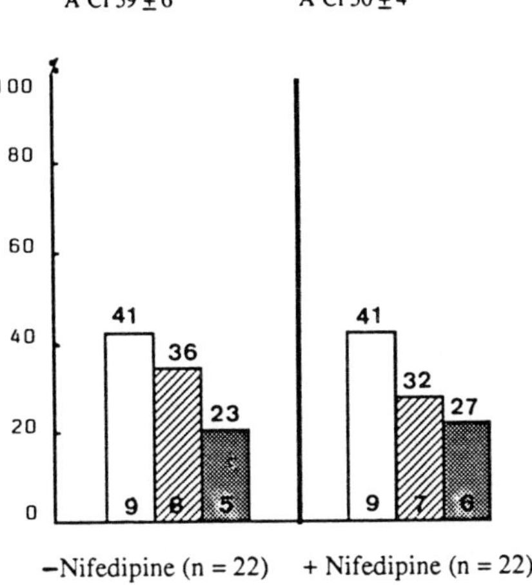

The Effect of Cyanosis

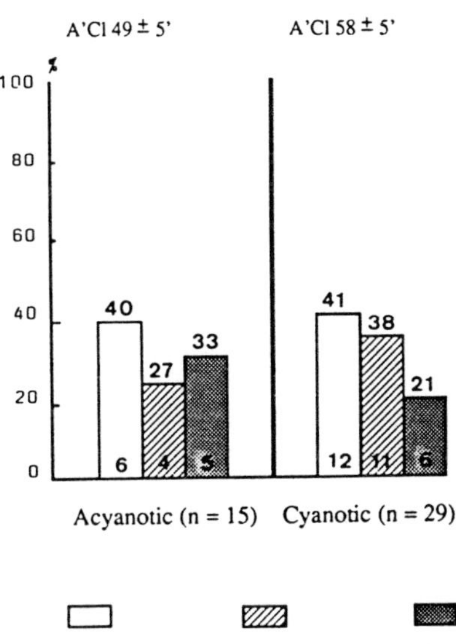

Figure 17.6. The upper group of histograms compare myocardial protection (assessed by QBM) in 22 children protected by cardioplegia and 22 protected by cardioplegia + Nifedipine. In the lower histograms myocardial protection has been studied in the *same* children to assess the effect of pre-existing cyanosis. (Columns refer to the percentage of children whose myocardium was assessed as good, deteriorated or poor during surgery).

This study showed that myocardial protection with the St Thomas' Hospital cardioplegic solution was significantly less effective during congenital heart surgery than in the adult, since RV biopsies indicated that 34% of hearts deteriorated during surgery compared with 9.5% in the adult ($p<0.001$) during similar periods of ischemia (see previous results). Improved methods are needed (i) to protect these hearts during the correction of complex congenital defects and (ii) to enhance the recovery of hearts which have suffered myocardial impairment prior to surgery.

Assessment of myocardial protection during transplantation in 360 human donor hearts

More than 19,000 heart transplants have now been performed worldwide and data gathered by the International Heart Transplant Registry shows that the 30 day mortality has remained between 9 and 10% for several years [64]. Since 23% of these hospital deaths were due to donor organ failure which was unrelated to infection, rejection or right sided heart failure [65], this indicates that current methods do not accurately assess the viability of a donor heart.

Following 2 deaths from graft failure early in the transplant programme at Papworth Hospital, Cambridge, subsequent hearts were monitored routinely by QBM to see whether they were adequately protected (1) before excision and (2) during transplantation.

Full thickness LV biopsies were taken from 360 donor hearts (i) before excision; (ii) after arrest with the St Thomas' Hospital cardioplegic solution; (iii) after storage and transport at 4°C; (iv) before removal of the aortic clamp; (v) shortly before the chest was closed at the end of the procedure [13–16].

Although all of the hearts were judged clinically as suitable for transplantation, at a microscopical level QBM identified significant myocardial injury in 139 (39%) hearts before excision (mean QBM ratio 1.06 ± 0.01 compared with 1.41 ± 0.01, $p < 0.001$ for the remaining 221 hearts, Figure 17.7). A further 126 (35%) hearts deteriorated acutely during the period of ischemia (QBM mean 1.43 ± 0.01 at excision deteriorated to 1.19 ± 0.02, $p < 0.001$ at the end of implantation). Therefore only 95 (26%) of the 360 donor hearts were assessed as satisfactory throughout transplantation by QBM. This indicated the need for improved methods to protect these hearts both before and during transplantation.

Morbidity and mortality of recipients

There was a significantly higher requirement for inotropic support at the end of implantation in hearts assessed by QBM as damaged, compared with those

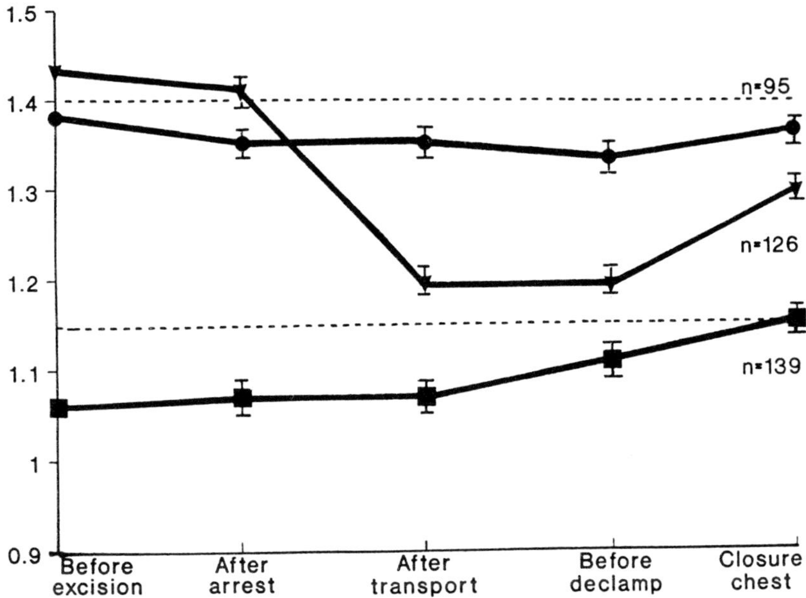

Figure 17.7. Changes in birefringence ratio during transplantation in 360 donor hearts: ■ 139 hearts had an abnormal birefringence ratio throughout. 221 hearts had good initial values. ● 95 remained good throughout the procedure, but ▲ 126 deteriorated during cold storage and implantation. (Bars are standard error of the mean).

assessed as satisfactory (47% and 16%, respectively, $p < 0.001$). Of 8 deaths resulting from donor organ failure, 7 occurred in recipients of hearts which were poor at excision and 1 in the recipient of a heart which deteriorated during transplantation. In addition 1 recipient of a deteriorated donor heart died from a sudden arrhythmia twelve days after transplantation.

The overall 30 day mortality of the 360 recipients was 39 (11%). During this period only 2 recipients died with hearts classed as good throughout transplantation, 2% compared with 16% and 11% respectively in recipients of poor or deteriorated donor hearts (Table 17.3). The current long term mortality (6 months to 8 years after transplantation) of the recipients of good donor hearts is significantly lower than those of poor or deteriorated donor hearts (19% compared with 42% and 44%, respectively, $p < 0.001$, Table 17.4).

Correlation of biopsy assessment of donor heart damage with poorer early and long-term clinical outcome of the recipients emphasises the need for improved protection of the donor heart both (1) before and (2) during transplantation.

Table 17.3. Incidence and cause of postoperative deaths occurring within 30 days of transplantation in 360 donor hearts.

	Poor Donor (n = 139)	Deteriorated During Ischemia (n = 126)	Good Throughout (n = 95)
Donor organ failure	6	1	0
Acute rejection	6	5	0
Infection	3	3	1
Elevated PVR	2	1	1
Sudden cardiac death	0	1	0
Miscellaneous	4	3	0
Unknown	1	0	0
Total	22 (16%)*	14 (11%)*	2 (2%)

Note: The recipients have been assigned to one of three groups according to the biopsy assessment of their donor hearts.
Abbreviation: PVR = pulmonary vascular resistance.
*Incidence significantly greater ($p < 0.01$) compared with that of recipients classed as good throughout transplantation.

Table 17.4. Overall incidence and cause of postoperative death or graft failure in 360 donor hearts transplanted between February 1983 and December 1991.

	Poor Donor (n = 139)	Deteriorated During Ischemia (n = 126)	Good Throughout (n = 95)
Donor organ failure	7	1	0
Acute rejection	13[a]	16[a]	3
Infection	12[a]	15[a]	4
Elevated PVR	2	1	1
Coronary occlusive disease	13 (2)	9 (3)	4
Graft fibrosis	1 (1)	0	0
Sudden cardiac death	1	6	0
Renal failure	1	0	0
Multiorgan failure	1	0	0
Malignancy	1	3	3
Miscellaneous	6	3	3
Unknown	1	1	0
Total	59 (42%)[b]	55 (44%)[b]	18 (19%)

Note: The recipients have been assigned to one of three groups according to the biopsy assessment of their donor hearts. Numbers in brackets refer to recipients who were retransplanted.
[a]Incidence significantly greater ($p < 0.05$) compared with that of recipients classed as good throughout transplantation.
[b]Incidence significantly greater ($P < 0.01$) compared with that of the third group.

Does hormonal pre-treatment improve the viability of the donor heart?

Most organ donors are suffering from head injury or brain hemorrhage. There is extensive clinical and experimental evidence that the 'sympathetic storm' following brain death results in cardiac damage [66–71]. As early as 1954 Smith and Tomlinson [66] demonstrated subendocardial hemorrhage in the myocardium of patients dying from intracranial legions and major electrocardiographic, hemodynamic and histopathologic changes have been demonstrated in numerous animal models including primates. Novitzky and Cooper found that circulating levels of plasma free triiodothyronin (T3), plasma cortisol, glucagon and insulin fell significantly within hours of the onset of brain death in the pig and baboon. They showed that such changes were associated with a reduction in myocardial energy stores and increased tissue lactate [69,70], but replenishment of these hormones resulted in a return to aerobic metabolism and improved myocardial function [71,72]. Having tested the effect of this therapy in a series of potential organ donors [73] they reported improved cardiac function and no early deaths from low output failure.

In an attempt to improve the 1/3 of hearts at Papworth Hospital which already had biopsy evidence of myocardial deterioration prior to explantation, a randomized study of 24 human donor hearts was undertaken to ascertain whether hormonal pretreatment of the donor improved myocardial function before transplantation. Twelve donors were conventionally treated controls and 12 received hourly (range 1–3 hours) hormonal pretreatment (2 mcg T3, 100 mgms cortisol and insulin) as described by Novitzky and Cooper [73]. At excision, QBM in myocardial biopsies detected no difference between the 2 groups of donors (mean ratio 1.31 ± 0.02, Figure 17.8).

In 12 consecutive donors the dose of T3 was therefore increased to a 4 mcg bolus injection followed by a continuous infusion of 4 mcg/hr. QBM indicated a trend towards better myocardial function in these hearts at excision (mean value 1.39 ± 0.05, p = NS, Figure 17.8) and throughout transplantation compared with the 2 mcg group.

In all three groups QBM in endomyocardial biopsies taken 1 week and 1 month after transplantation were not significantly different from the control biopsies taken from the donor heart before excision. Since the mean QBM of hearts pretreated with continuous T3 approximated to the values of normal myocardium defined previously (>1.40), randomized studies are needed to confirm the benefit of this therapy.

A comparison of myocardial protection during heart-lung and heart transplantation

In view of the clinical impression of the surgeons at Papworth Hospital that immediately following transplantation hearts harvested as heart-lung blocks were of better quality than orthotopically transplanted hearts, biopsy assess-

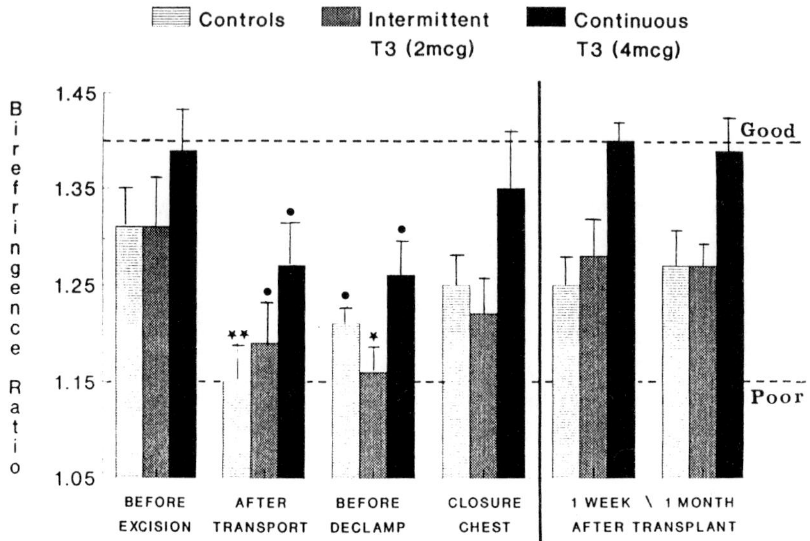

Figure 17.8. Biopsy assessment of the effect of hormonal pretreatment on myocardial function at transplantation. 24 donors were randomized into 2 groups to study the effect of hourly pretreatment with 2 μg T3, 100 mg Cortisol and Insulin. 12 consecutive donors received an initial injection of 4 μg T3 followed by a continuous infusion of 4 μg hourly. In all groups QBM in biopsies taken at excision were similar to those obtained 1 week and 1 month following Tx. All data are expressed as mean ± SEM, · $p < 0.05$, *$p < 0.01$, **$p < 0.001$ in comparison to control biopsies before excision.

ments were performed during 46 heart-lung and 115 heart transplant operations during the period 1989–92. QBM indicated that 87% of heart-lung hearts were satisfactory at excision compared with only 57% of heart transplant hearts ($p < 0.001$). In spite of similar ischemic times during transplantation (193 min, range 106–297, and 196 min, range 89–137, respectively) only 7% of heart-lung hearts deteriorated compared with 27% of heart transplant hearts ($p < 0.02$ Figure 17.9). Thus 80% of heart-lung hearts remained satisfactory throughout transplantation compared with only 30% of the 115 conventional donor hearts transplanted during the same period ($p < 0.001$).

Because all of these hearts were from brain dead donors with no significant differences in their clinical histories, other variables were sought to account for the disparity between the 2 groups. Superior lung function of the heart-lung donors may have enhanced myocardial protection by maintaining normal tissue oxygen levels and with lung function being a more difficult variable to preserve than cardiac function, the hearts of heart-lung donors may have been artificially selected good hearts. Additionally, the clinical practice of infusing prostacyclin (10–20 ng/kg/min) into the pulmonary artery of the heart-lung donors approximately 15–20 min before explantation of the organ

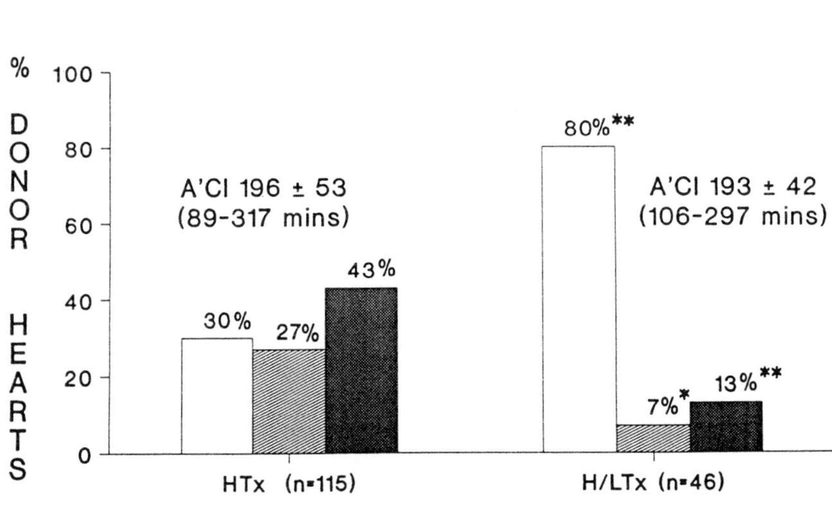

Figure 17.9. Comparison of myocardial protection during heart (n = 115) and heart-lung transplantation (n = 46). All transplant operations were carried out within the same period. Incidence significantly different (*$p < 0.02$, **$p < 0.001$) compared with that of patients undergoing heart transplantation.

[74] may by its vasodilatory effect also have improved perfusion and oxygenation of the tissues. The superior myocardial function detected in the heart-lung group by biopsy assessments prior to excision may explain why these hearts were more resilient during periods of storage and implantation of up to 5 hours duration.

Assessment of serial biopsies by quantitative birefringence measurements has enabled deficiencies in myocardial protection to be identified in donor hearts (1) prior to and (2) during transplantation. Such serial biopsies are the only method presently available for detailed monitoring of the donor heart. Because our studies of orthotopically transplanted hearts have shown a correlation between myocardial injury (as assessed by QBM) at transplantation with increased morbidity and mortality in recipients of these hearts, interventions aimed at (1) improving the management of prospective organ donors and (2) optimizing myocardial protection throughout the transplant period need careful evaluation [16,73,75,76]. The criteria for donor selection have now been broadened in an attempt to increase the pool of donor hearts, and hearts from domino donors, donors over 40 years of age, and hearts stored for prolonged periods are now widely used. A serial and accurate assessment of the viability of the donor heart has therefore become of critical importance.

Summary

Quantitative birefringence measurements on cryostat sections of myocardial biopsies can be made routinely in any pathology laboratory. QBM are particularly useful since they can provide an index of myocardial function even when the heart is arrested and it is not possible to perform any physiological assessment, e.g. during open heart surgery or heart transplantation. Because the amount of tissue required is small, serial biopsies allow comparison of myocardial protection in different regions of the heart. The measurements are cardiospecific (each patient acting as his or her own control) and independent of the correction of the cardiac defect.

An obvious question in the use of biopsy assessments is how representative are the results on a small biopsy in relation to the function of the whole heart? The fact that the results correlate well with the postoperative clinical outcome of the individual patients does indicate that these biopsies are giving a representative reflection of the whole heart. Our experimental observations using multiple biopsies from different regions in dogs support this view.

The improved protection provided by cold cardioplegic arrest during routine open heart surgery has made it possible for careful intraoperative monitoring to pinpoint specific areas where improvements are still needed to optimize the clinical outcome of the patients. These include the need to achieve uniform protection of the heart, and to provide improved protection during prolonged and complex procedures, during congenital heart surgery and during heart transplantation.

Acknowledgements

This work was supported by grants from the British Heart Foundation, the National Heart Research Fund and the St Thomas' Hospital Endowments Trustees. I acknowledge with gratitude the collaboration of my colleagues: L Bitensky, MV Braimbridge, M Cankovic, N Cary, DJ Chambers, J Chayen, F Derome, TAH English, S Gundry, SR Large, J Stark, J Wallwork, FC Wells, DR Wheeldon.

References

1. Chayen J, Bitensky L, Braimbridge MV *et al.* Increased myosin orientation during muscle contraction: a measure of cardiac contractility. Cell Biochem Funct 1985; 3: 101–14.
2. Webb-Peploe MM. Apport de la biopsie myocardique au diagnostic et au traitement des myocardiopathies primitives. Ann Cardiol Angiol 1978; 27: 579–88.
3. Malcolm AD, Cankovic-Darracott S, Chayen J *et al.* Biopsy evidence of left ventricular myocardial abnormality in patients with mitral leaflet prolapse and chest pain. Lancet 1979; 8125: 1052–5.
4. Cankovic-Darracott S, Braimbridge MV, Williams BT *et al.* Myocardial preservation during

aortic valve surgery. Assessment of 5 techniques by cellular chemical and biophysical methods. J Thorac Cardiovasc Surg 1977; 73: 699–706.

5. Braimbridge MV, Chayen J, Bitensky L *et al.* Cold cardioplegia or continuous coronary perfusion? J Thorac Cardiovasc Surg 1977; 74: 900–6.
6. Cankovic-Darracott S, Braimbridge MV, Bitensky L *et al.* Evaluation of perfusion conditions in cardiopulmonary bypass. In Kobayashi T, Ito Y, Rona G (eds): Recent advances in studies on cardiac structure and metabolism, Vol 12. Cardiac adaptation. New York: University Park Press 1978; 593–6.
7. Braimbridge MV, Cankovic-Darracott S. Quantitative polarization microscopy and cytochemistry in assessing myocardial function. In Pattison JR, Bitensky L, Chayen J (eds): Quantitative cytochemistry and its application. London: Academic Press 1979; 221–30.
8. Darracott-Cankovic S. Methods for assessing preservation techniques – invasive methods (enzymatic, cytochemical). In Engelman RM, Levitsky, L (eds): A handbook of clinical cardioplegia. New York: Futura Publishing Co 1982; 43–61.
9. Bull C, Cooper J, Stark J. Cardioplegic protection of the child's heart. J Thorac Cardiovasc Surg 1982; 88: 287–93.
10. Pepper JR, Lockey E, Cankovic-Darracott S *et al.* Cardioplegia versus intermittent ischaemic arrest in coronary bypass surgery. Thorax 1982; 37: 887–92.
11. Chambers DJ, Darracott-Cankovic S, Braimbridge MV. Clinical and quantitative birefringence assessment of 100 patients with aortic clamping periods in excess of 120 minutes of hypothermic cardioplegic arrest. Thorac Cardiovasc Surg 1983; 31: 266–72.
12. Braimbridge MV, Darracott-Cankovic S, Chambers DJ *et al.* Biopsy assessment of myocardial protection for valve replacement over the last 24 years. Ann Thorac Surg 1989; 48: 567–8.
13. Darracott-Cankovic S, Cory-Pearce R, Stovin PGI *et al.* Biopsy assessment of 50 hearts during transplantation. J Thorac Cardiovasc Surg 1987; 93: 95–102.
14. Darracott-Cankovic S, Stovin PGI, Wheeldon D *et al.* Effect of donor heart damage on survival after transplantation. Eur J Cardiothorac Surg 1989; 3: 525–32.
15. Darracott-Cankovic S, English TAH, Wallwork J. Assessing damage to the donor heart. In D'Alessandro LC (ed): Heart Surgery 1991. Rome: Casa Editrice Scientifica Internazionale 1991; 459–74.
16. Darracott-Cankovic S. Assessment of myocardial preservation during heart and heart–lung transplantation. Transplant Rev 1992; 6(2): 102–14.
17. Chiu RC-J. Cardioplegia: from the bedside to the laboratory and back again. Ann Thorac Surg 1991; 52: 1209–10.
18. Chambers DJ, Kosker S, Takahashi A *et al.* Comparison of standard (non- oxygenated) vs oxygenated St Thomas' Hospital cardioplegic solution No. 2 (Plegisol). Eur J Cardiothorac Surg 1990; 4 :549–55.
19. Chambers DJ, Braimbridge MV, Kosker S *et al.* Creatine phosphate (Neoton) as an additive to St Thomas' Hospital cardioplegic solution (Plegisol). Eur J Cardio Thorac Surg 1991; 5: 74–81.
20. Huxley AF. Muscle structure and theories of contraction. Prog Biophys 1957; 7: 255–310.
21. Huxley HE. The mechanism of muscular contraction. Science. 1969; 64: 1356–66.
22. Hanson J, Huxley HE. Structural basis of the cross-striations in muscle. Nature 1953; 172: 530–6.
23. Hayashi T. Chemical physiology of excitation in muscle and nerve. Tokyo: Nakayama-Shoten 1956; 92–3.
24. Huxley HE, Hanson J. Changes in the cross-striations of muscle during contraction and stretch and their structural interpretation. Nature 1954; 173: 973–5.
25. Darracott-Cankovic S. PhD Thesis: Cellular biochemical and biophysical studies of myocardial preservation during cardiac surgical procedures. University of London, 1982: 120–258.
26. Kolettis M, Jenkins BS, Webb-Peploe MM. Assessment of left ventricular function by indices derived from aortic flow velocity. Br Heart J 1976; 38: 18–31.
27. Hearse DJ, Stewart DA, Braimbridge MV. Hypothermic arrest and potassium arrest;

metabolic and myocardial protection during elective cardiac arrest. Circ Res 1975; 36: 481–9.
28. Jynge P, Hearse DJ, Feuvray D *et al.* The St Thomas' Hospital cardioplegic solution: a characterization in two species. Scand J Thorac Cardiovasc Surg 1981; 30: 1–28.
29. Hearse DJ, Braimbridge MV, Jynge P. Components of cardioplegic solutions. In: Protection of the ischemic myocardium. New York: Raven Press, 1981; 209–99.
30. Yamamoto F, Braimbridge MV, Hearse DJ. Calcium and cardioplegia. J Thorac Cardiovasc Surg 1984; 87: 908–12.
31. Robinson LA, Braimbridge MV, Hearse DJ. The potential hazard of particulate contamination of cardioplegic solutions. J Thorac Cardiovasc Surg. 1984; 87: 48–58.
32. Hearse DJ, Erol C, Robinson LA *et al.* Particle-induced coronary vasoconstriction during cardioplegic infusion. Characterization and possible mechanisms. J Thorac Cardiovasc Surg 1985; 89: 428–38.
33. Chambers DJ, Sakai A, Braimbridge MV *et al.* Clinical validation of St Thomas Hospital cardioplegic solution No. 2 (Plegisol). Eur J Cardio-thorac Surg 1989; 3: 346–52.
34. Bleese N, Döring V, Kalmar P *et al.* Clinical application of cardioplegia in aortic cross-clamping periods longer than 150 minutes. Thorac Cardiovasc Surgeon 1979; 27: 390–2.
35. Engelman RM, Rousou JH, Vertrees RA *et al.* Safety of prolonged ischemic arrest using hypothermic cardioplegia. J Thorac Cardiovasc. Surg 1980; 79: 705–12.
36. Engelman RM, Gianelly RE, Rousou JH *et al.* The effect of prolonged cardioplegic arrest on long-term ventricular function. Thorac Cardiovasc Surgeon 1981; 29: 223–6.
37. Stapenhorst K. Prolonged safe ischemic cardiac arrest using hypothermic Bretschneider cardioplegia combined with topical cardiac cooling. Thorac Cardiovasc Surgeon 1981; 29: 272–4.
38. Berglin E, Feddersen K, Gatzinsky P *et al.* Aortic cross-clamping for more than 2 hours in open-heart surgery. Early results in 87 patients. Thorac Cardiovasc Surgeon 1983; 31: 273–6.
39. Braimbridge MV, Darracott-Cankovic S. Assessment of right ventricular preservation during cold cardioplegic arrest. In Birks W, Ostermeyer J, Schulte HD (eds): Cardiovascular surgery. Berlin: Springer Verlag 1980; 625–8.
40. Hetzer R, Warnecke H, Wittock H *et al.* Extracoronary collateral myocardial blood flow during cardioplegic arrest. J Cardiovasc Surg 1980; 28: 191–6.
41. Braimbridge MV. Myocardial protection. In Taylor KM (ed): Cardiopulmonary bypass-principle and management. London: Chapman and Hall 1986; 375–98.
42. Smith PK, Buhrman WC, Levett JM *et al.*. Supraventricular conduction abnormalities following cardiac operations: a complication of inadequate atrial preservation. J Thorac Cardiovasc Surg 1983; 85: 105–15.
43. Weisel RD. Intraoperative atrial protection. Can J Cardiol 1986; 2: 261–2.
44. Rosenfeldt FL, Watson DA. Interference with local myocardial cooling by heat gain during aortic cross-clamping. Ann Thorac Surg 1979; 27: 13–6.
45. Fisk RL, Ghaswalla D, Guillbeau EJ. Asymmetrical myocardial hypothermia during hypothermic cardioplegia. Ann Thorac Surg 1982; 34: 318–23.
46. Chiu RC-J, Mulder DS. Complications of cardioplegic preservation. In Engelman RM, Levitsky L (eds): A handbook of clinical cardioplegia. New York: Futura Publishing Co 1982; 391–403.
47. Bonchek LI, Olinger GN. An improved method of topical hypothermia. J Thorac Cardiovasc Surg 1981; 82: 878–82.
48. Velardi AR, Widmer SJ, Cilley JH *et al.* Right ventricular myocardial protection through intracavitary cooling in cardiac operations. J Thorac Cardiovasc Surg 1989; 98: 1077–82.
49. Douville EC, Kratz JM, Spinale FG *et al.* Retrograde versus antegrade cardioplegia: impact on right ventricular function. Ann Thorac Surg 1992; 54: 56–61.
50. Chen YF, Lin YT, Wu SC. Inconsistent effectiveness of myocardial preservation among cardiac chambers during hypothermic cardioplegia. J Thorac Cardiovasc Surg 1991; 102: 684–7.

51. Teoh KH, Mullen JC, Weisel RD *et al.* Right and left ventricular metabolites. J Thorac Cardiovasc Surg 1988: 96: 725–9.
52. Christakis GT, Weisel RD, Mickle DAG *et al.* Right ventricular function and metabolism. Circulation 1990; 82: IV332–40.
53. Hilton CJ, Teubl W, Acker M *et al.* Inadequate cardioplegic protection with obstructed coronary arteries. Ann Thorac Surg 1979; 28: 323–34.
54. Landymore RW, Tice D, Trehan N *et al.* Importance of topical hypothermia to ensure uniform myocardial cooling during coronary artery bypass. J Thorac Cardiovasc Surg 1981; 82: 832–6.
55. Daggett WM, Jacocks MA, Coleman WS *et al.* Myocardial temperature mapping. J Thorac Cardiovasc Surg 1981; 82: 883–8.
56. Robertson JM, Buckberg GD, Vinten-Johansen J *et al.* Comparison of distribution beyond coronary stenoses of blood and asanguineous cardioplegic solutions. J Thorac Cardiovasc Surg 1983; 86: 80–6.
57. Naylor WG. Protection of the myocardium against post ischemic reperfusion damage. The combined effect of hypothermia and Nifedipine. J Thorac Cardiovasc Surg 1982; 84: 897–905.
58. Vanden Baviere HFA, Cankovic-Darracott S, De Rose J *et al.* Enhancement of cardio protective activity during myocardial ischemia using Nifedipine as an additive to crystallod cardioplegia. J Cardiovasc Surg 1983; 24: 407.
59. Clark RE, Magovern GJ, Christlieb IY *et al.* Nifedipine cardioplegia experience: results of a 3 year cooperative clinical study. Ann Thorac Surg 1983; 36: 654.
60. Yamamoto F, Manning AS, Braimbridge MV *et al.* Nifedipine and cardioplegia: rat heart studies with the St Thomas' Hospital cardioplegic solution. Cardiovasc Res 1983; 17: 719–27.
61. Silverman NA, Kohler J, Levitsky S *et al.* Chronic hypoxemia depresses global ventricular function during cardioplegic arrest: implications for surgical repair of cyanotic congenital heart defects. Ann Thorac Surg 1984; 37: 304–8.
62. Fujiwara T, Kurtts T, Anderson W *et al.* Myocardial protection in cyanotic neonatal lambs. J Thorac Cardiovasc Surg 1988; 96: 700–10.
63. Del Nido PJ, Mickle DA, Wilson GJ *et al.* Inadequate myocardial protection with cold cardioplegic arrest during repair of tetralogy of Fallot. J Thorac Cardiovasc Surg 1988; 95: 223–9.
64. Kaye MP. The Registry of the International Society for Heart and Lung Transplantation: Ninth official report – 1992. J Heart Lung Transplant 1992; 11: 599–618.
65. Kriett JM, Kaye MP. The Registry of the International Society for Heart Transplantation: Seventh official report – 1990. J Heart Transplant 1990; 9: 323–30.
66. Smith RP, Tomlinson BE. Subendocardial haemorrhages associated with intracranial lesions. J Path Bact 1954; 68: 327–9.
67. De Pasquale NP, Burch GE. How normal is the donor heart? Am Heart J 1969; 77: 719–20.
68. Samuels MA. Neurogenic heart disease: A unifying hypothesis. Am J Cardiol 1987; 60: 15J–19J.
69. Novitzky D, Wicomb WN, Cooper DKC *et al.* Electrocardiographic, haemodynamic and endocrine changes occurring during experimental brain death in the Chacma baboon. Heart Transplant 1984; 4: 63–9.
70. Wicomb WN, Cooper DKC, Lanza RP *et al.* The effects of brain death and 24 hours storage by hypothermic perfusion on donor heart function in the pig. J Thorac Cardiovasc Surg 1986; 91: 896–909.
71. Novitzky D, Wicomb WN, Cooper DKC *et al.* Improved cardiac function following hormonal therapy in brain dead pigs: relevance to organ donation. Cryobiology 1987; 24: 1–10.
72. Novitzky D, Cooper DKC, Morrell D *et al.* Change from aerobic to anaerobic metabolism

after brain death, and reversal following triiodothyronin therapy. Transplantation 1988; 45(1): 32–6.

73. Novitzky D, Cooper DKC, Reichart B. Haemodynamic and metabolic responses to hormonal therapy in brain-dead potential organ donors. Transplantation 1987; 43: 852–4.
74. Hakim M, Higenbottam T, Bethune D *et al*. Selection and procurement of combined heart and lung grafts for transplantation. J Thorac Cardiovasc Surg 1988; 95: 474–9.
75. Ghosh S, Bethune DW, Hardy I *et al*. Management of donors for heart and heart-lung transplantation. Anaesthesia 1990; 45: 672–5.
76. Buckberg GD. Phases of myocardial protection during transplantation. J Thorac Cardiovasc Surg 1990; 100: 461–2.

18. How to measure cardiac energy expenditure

MIYAKO TAKAKI, TAKETOSHI NAMBA, JUNICHI ARAKI, KAZUNARI ISHIOKA, HARUO ITO, TAKUJI AKASHI, LING YUN ZHAO, DAN DAN ZHAO, MIAO LIU, WAKAKO FUJII, and HIROYUKI SUGA

Summary

Total energy expenditure of the heart can be directly determined by cardiac oxygen consumption (Vo_2) according to the energy equivalence of oxygen in aerobic metabolism (1 ml O_2 = 19–21 J). However, Vo_2 determination of an in situ heart is invasive and not always possible, particularly in clinical settings. To circumvent this problem, various methods to predict Vo_2 have been developed over many years. They include external work, total contractile work, systolic pressure, active tension, tension time integral, V_{max}, etc. They have high correlations with directly measured Vo_2 under limited conditions. Both myocardial tension and contractility have been generally accepted as the primary determinants of Vo_2. However, based on detailed mechanoenergetic studies of canine cardiac contractions, we have recently proposed that the total mechanical energy generated by ventricular contraction can be quantitatively assessed by the ventricular pressure-volume area (PVA) which is a specific area bounded by the end-systolic and end-diastolic pressure-volume relations and the systolic pressure-volume trajectory of the ventricle. Myocardial force-length area (FLA) is a muscle version of PVA. Cardiac Vo_2 has been shown to linearly correlate with PVA and FLA. This linear relation ascends or descends in proportion to contractility (E_{max}). These results have shown that PVA is a physiologically sound and reliable predictor of the energy expenditure of the heart.

Introduction

Cardiac energy expenditure can reasonably be determined by cardiac oxygen consumption because the heart is exclusively (95%) aerobic and the energy equivalence of oxygen consumption is reasonably constant regardless of metabolic substrates (1 ml O_2 = 19–21 J) [1–6].

The chemical energy contained in the metabolic substrates such as glucose, lactate and free fatty acids is restored in ATP by the oxidative phosphorylation [5,6]. Various biological processes utilize the free energy of ATP [5,6]. In the myocardium, crossbridge cycling converts ATP energy into mechanical

H.M. Piper and C.J. Preusse (eds): Ischemia-reperfusion in cardiac surgery, 403–419.

work, and Ca and Na-K pumps actively transport the ions against their concentration gradients. Basal metabolism also consumes ATP.

ATP consumption directly shows the energy expenditure [2,5,6], but its continuous measurement is not always available [5]. Oxygen consumption is the second-best measure of the energy expenditure of the heart [1–5], but its measurement is not always easy either.

For these reasons, many indexes have been proposed to predict cardiac oxygen consumption under various loading and contractile conditions [1–5]. In this brief review, we focus on the PVA concept which Suga proposed 15 years ago and the validity of which has been established under various cardiac conditions [3,4].

Cardiac oxygen consumption

Myocardium consumes ATP not only for mechanical contraction but also for activation (i.e., excitation-contraction coupling) and basal metabolism. Mechanical contraction utilizes energy of ATP hydrolyzed by myosin ATPase. Activation utilizes energy of ATP hydrolyzed by Ca and Na-K pump ATPases. Phosphorylation of proteins also uses ATP energy [5]. The ATP energy, or more correctly the free energy of ATP hydrolysis, is approximately 57 kJ/mol [5]. Note that this energy is much greater than the enthalpy of ATP (48 kJ/mol) [5]. Therefore, when the amount of ATP hydrolyzed is known, one can determine the energy expenditure.

Since the rate of ATP hydrolysis is not easily obtainable [5], oxygen consumption rate has preferably been used under aerobic metabolism [1–5]. ATP is synthesized mostly in the oxidative phosphorylation and secondarily by glycolysis in normal hearts. The amount of ATP produced for a given amount of oxygen consumed is relatively constant regardless of metabolic substrates [5,6]. This ratio is called P:O ratio and considered to be about 3 in general, which means 3 ATP versus one atomic oxygen, although the P:O ratio is known to decrease in malfunctioning mitochondria [7].

The enthalpy of metabolic substrates in aerobic metabolism is almost constant at about 20 J/ml O_2 for lactate, glucose, and free fatty acids with only ±5% error [5,6]. Therefore, the efficiency of aerobic ATP production is calculated to be about 65%. The other 35% is converted into heat. This is the biochemical background to support that oxygen consumption can be used as a measure of the energy expenditure of the heart [1–6].

Determinants of cardiac oxygen consumption

Many determinants of cardiac oxygen consumption (Vo_2) have been proposed over this century [1–5]. Cardiac mechanical work was first considered to be the candidate, but it was proved not to correlate consistently with Vo_2.

By contrast, cardiac afterload was found to better correlate with Vo_2. Along the same line, myocardial force, tension and stress are also shown to correlate with Vo_2. Their time integrals such as tension time integral (TTI) and force time integral (FTI) were also proposed. Since heart rate affects Vo_2 per min, arterial pressure-rate product was proposed as a non-invasive determinant of Vo_2.

In the mean time, contractile state or inotropism was found to affect Vo_2 [1]. Rapid contraction or shortening *per se* was considered to be associated with faster crossbridge cycling and more ATP hydrolysis for a given tension development. Several contractility indexes including V_{max} (maximum unloaded shortening velocity) and dP/dt (maximum pressure rising rate) were combined with pressure or force parameters and proposed as better determinants of Vo_2 [1].

Other Vo_2 determinants include the contractile element work (CEW) combining external work and internal work, pressure-work index, total energy demand, peak contractile power, etc [1–5]. However, none of these has widely been accepted as a reliable determinant of Vo_2.

Total mechanical energy and pressure volume area (PVA)

Based on the time-varying elastance model of a contracting ventricular chamber [8], Suga proposed a new concept to quantify the total mechanical energy generated by each ventricular contraction [9]. Figure 18.1 schematically shows this concept. Figure 18.1A shows the ventricular pressure-volume diagram, which draws three pressure-volume loops obtained in a stable contractile state. Suga *et al.* [8] have shown that the left upper corners of these pressure-volume loops fall on a diagonal straight line with a slope of E_{max} and a positive volume-axis intercept of V_0. This line is the end-systolic pressure-volume relation. E_{max} indicates the maximum or end-systolic volume elastance of the ventricle. V_0 is the dead volume at which systolic pressure is zero.

Figure 18.1A also shows that pressure-volume points at a given time in systole of these contractions fall on a less steep line, which is an instantaneous pressure-volume relation. Figure 18.1B shows a family of such instantaneous pressure-volume relations including the end-systolic relation. These pressure-volume relations mean that the contracting ventricle can be modelled by a time-varying elastance E(t) [8]. Figure 18.1C and D show the ventricle model as a time-varying elastic chamber in diastole and systole, respectively.

In this model, an increment in chamber elastance is considered to be accompanied by an increment in elastic (or mechanical) potential energy (Figure 18.1C) [9]. This energy is analogous to the potential energy stored in a stretched spring or rubber. When the model ventricle ejects its content against its load (or afterload), the ventricle performs mechanical work to the outside (Figure 18.1D). Therefore, the total mechanical energy change of

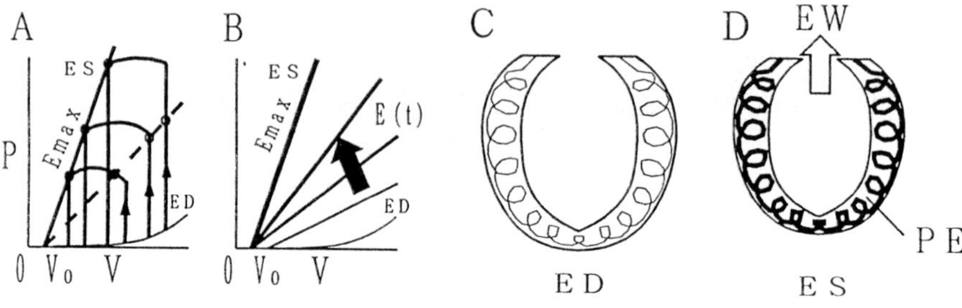

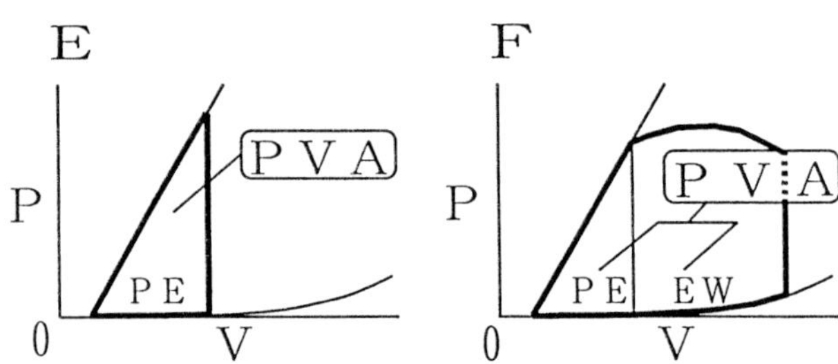

Figure 18.1. How to quantify the total mechanical energy generated by ventricular contraction. Panel A: Ventricular pressure (P)-volume (V) diagram and schematically drawn pressure-volume loops in a stable contractile state. End-systolic pressure-volume relation (ES) passing through the left upper (end-systolic) corners (solid circles) of the pressure-volume loops and one instantaneous pressure-volume relation are also drawn. E_{max} is the slope of the end-systolic pressure-volume relation. ED = end-diastolic pressure-volume relation. Panel B: Schematically drawn family of instantaneous pressure-volume relations of the ventricle, supporting the time-varying elastance model of the ventricle. Heavy arrow indicates the gradual steepening of the instantaneous pressure-volume relation from ED to ES with time in systole. Panel C: End-diastolic (ED) state of the time-varying elastance model of the ventricle. Panel D: End-systolic (ES) state of the time-varying elastance model. The systolic increments in elastance are accompanied by increments in elastic potential energy (PE) and production of external mechanical work (EW). Panel E: Pressure-volume area (PVA) in an isovolumic contraction, consisting only of elastic potential energy (PE). Panel F: Pressure-volume area (PVA) in an ejecting contraction, consisting of elastic potential energy (PE) and external mechanical work (EW).

the contracting model ventricle consists of the end-systolic elastic potential energy (PE) and the mechanical work (EW) performed during systole.

This total mechanical energy corresponds to a specific area in the pressure-volume diagram as shown in Figure 18.1E and F. The total area corresponding to the total mechanical energy generated by ventricular contraction is called 'systolic pressure-volume area' and abbreviated to PVA [9]. It consists of two areas: one representing the external mechanical work and the other the mechanical potential energy.

This can be explained in Figure 18.2 as follows [10,11]. The area in the

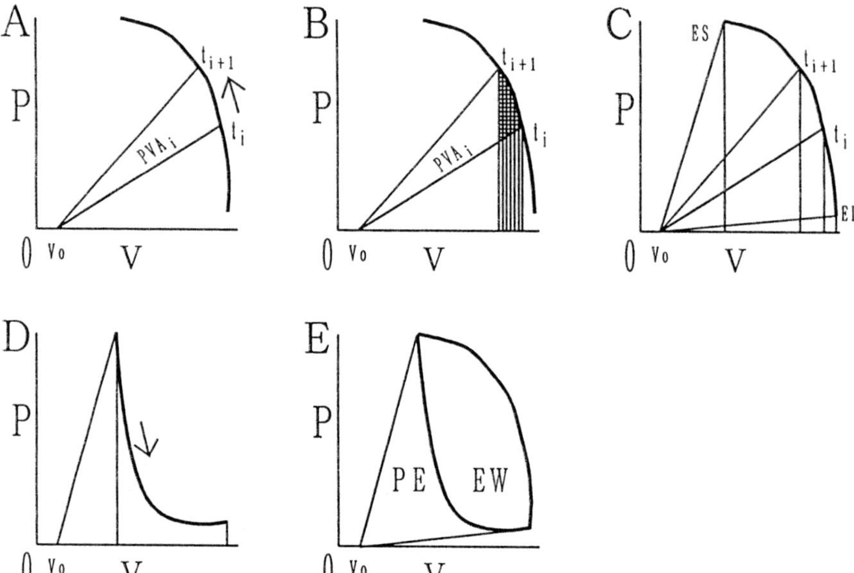

Figure 18.2. Instantaneous increment in mechanical energy in the time-varying elastance model of the ventricle. The solid curve in Panel A is a pressure-volume trajectory during systole. The arrow indicates the direction of the trajectory. t_i and t_{i+1} are two time points. The triangular area (PVA_i) bounded by the pressure-volume segment between t_i and t_{i+1} and two straight lines connecting Vo and these pressure points at t_i and t_{i+1} corresponds to the mechanical (or elastic) energy generated by the time-varying elastance which increases during this time period. Panel B shows that the cross hatched area is the fraction of PVA_i converted into mechanical work. The vertically hatched area is the work converted from the mechanical energy which has been generated until t_i. The sum of these two hatched area corresponds to the mechanical work performed during the period from t_i to t_{i+1}. The other area of PVA_i remains as potential. The vertical lines in Panel C separate mechanical work into the fractions performed between end diastole (ED) and t_i, between t_i and t_{i+1} and between t_{i+1} and end systole (ES). The triangular area on the origin side of these work areas corresponds to the potential energy remaining at end systole. The solid curve in Panel D indicates a pressure-volume trajectory during diastole. The arrow indicates the direction of the trajectory. The area under the curve corresponds to the work given to the heart from outside. Panel E shows a closed pressure-volume trajectory during a cardiac cycle. The area within the loop corresponds to the external work (EW) performed by one contraction. EW is equal to the work performed during systole minus the work given during diastole. The area between the end-diastolic and end-systolic pressure-volume relations on the origin side of the pressure-volume loop corresponds to the elastic potential energy (PE) in one cardiac cycle.

pressure-volume diagram surrounded by the instantaneous pressure-volume relations at two adjacent times (t_i and t_{i+1}) and the pressure-volume trajectory drawn within this time period is equivalent to the energy generated during this period of ventricular contraction in a time-varying elastance model (Figure 18.2A). The area (cross and vertically hatched) directly under the trajectory between t_i and t_{i+1} and above the volume axis is equal to the mechanical work performed during this period (Figure 18.2B). Of this work, the cross hatched area between the last two instantaneous pressure-volume relations is part of the energy generated by the last period, and the other area under the pressure-volume relation at t_i is the work converted from the elastic potential energy generated until t_i after the onset of this contraction. The triangular area between t_i and t_{i+1} other than the area (cross hatched) under the present pressure-volume trajectory is stored as elastic potential energy.

The same holds for every time period during systole. As a whole, the area under the systolic pressure-volume trajectory is equal to the mechanical work performed during systole, and the area under the end-systolic pressure-volume relation is equal to the elastic potential energy which remains as such at the end-systole (Figure 18.2C).

The mechanical work during one cardiac cycle consisting of systole and diastole is not equal to the work performed during systole alone. It depends on the work during diastole. The ventricle is supplied with mechanical work (or performs *negative* work according to the sign convention in muscle physiology) by filling. This work is given by the area under the pressure-volume trajectory during relaxation and diastole (Figure 18.2D). As the net, the area surrounded by the complete pressure-volume loop is equal to the mechanical (or external or stroke) work performed by one contraction (Figure 18.2E). Thus, stroke work varies considerably depending on the end-diastolic pressure-volume relation (or compliance, distensibility or lusitropism) and the speed and extent of relaxation which affect the pressure-volume trajectory during relaxation and diastole.

It is reasonable to assume that the elastic potential energy if not converted to work is degraded into heat, because muscle energetics has shown that heat is generated after isometric contraction [12]. Therefore, the entire area between the end-systolic and end-diastolic pressure-volume relations and the systolic pressure-volume trajectory is equivalent to the total mechanical energy generated by ventricular contraction. We call this entire area 'systolic pressure-volume area' or briefly 'pressure-volume area' and abbreviated it to 'PVA' [3,4,9,10].

The part of PVA other than the area for mechanical work is reasonably considered to be the area for mechanical potential energy because nearly the entire area of PVA can be converted to mechanical work by appropriately releasing ventricular pressure and volume load during relaxation [13]. In other words, a relaxing ventricle can potentially perform external work up to the potential energy area.

Pressure-volume-area (PVA) and cardiac oxygen consumption

We studied whether and how PVA would correlate with oxygen consumption (Vo_2) of the left ventricle [3,4]. We used the excised cross-circulated dog

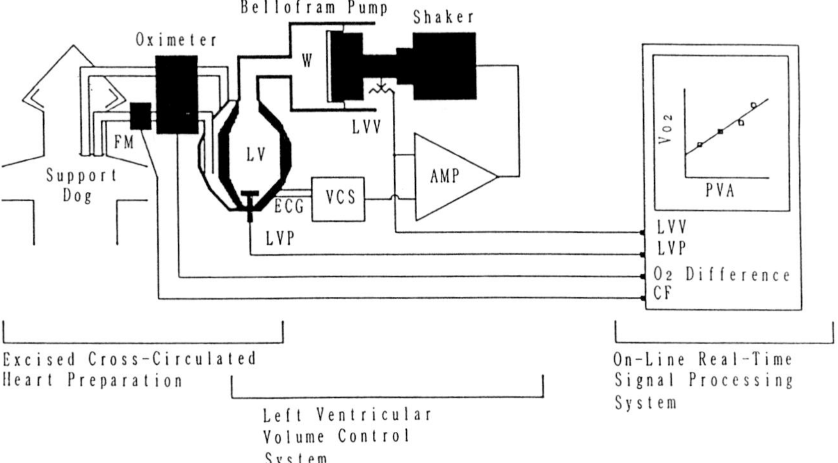

Figure 18.3. Experimental setup of the excised cross-circulated dog heart preparation which has been used in cardiac mechanoenergetic studies. FM = flowmeter. LV = left ventricle. LVP = left ventricular pressure. ECG electrocardiography. W = water. LVV = left ventricular volume. Bellofram = rolling seal diaphragm. VCS = volume command signal. AMP = amplifier. Vo_2 = cardiac oxygen consumption. PVA = pressure-volume area. O_2 difference = coronary arteriovenous oxygen content difference. CF = coronary flow.

heart preparation (Figure 18.3). This preparation can be made without any interruption of coronary flow. The left ventricle was installed with a thin water-filled balloon with a sufficient unstressed volume. Left ventricular volume was measured and controlled with a custom-made servo pump system [14].

The volume command signal was generated by a home-made logic and analog circuit. Left ventricular epicardial electrocardiogram signal triggered the volume signal generator. Left ventricular pressure was measured with a miniature pressure gauge (Konigsberg P-7, USA) placed in the apical end of the balloon. Left ventricular pressure and volume were controlled at our disposal by observing pressure-volume loops on an oscilloscope and manually adjusting end-diastolic and stroke volumes, timings of ejection and filling, and ejection and filling speeds. PVA of each contraction was on-line determined on a 68000-CPU 32-bit signal processor (NEC San-ei, Tokyo, Japan) with a home-made software [10]. Left ventricular PVA was expressed in mmHg ml/beat and normalized for 100 g left ventricle.

Vo_2 was determined as the product of coronary flow and arteriovenous oxygen content difference. Coronary flow was measured with an electromagnetic flowmeter in the coronary venous return tube. Coronary arteriovenous oxygen content difference was measured with a custom-made spectrophotometric PWA-200S oximeter (Erma Inc, Tokyo, Japan) similar in principle to the AVOX analyzer [15]. The oximeter was calibrated against the difference

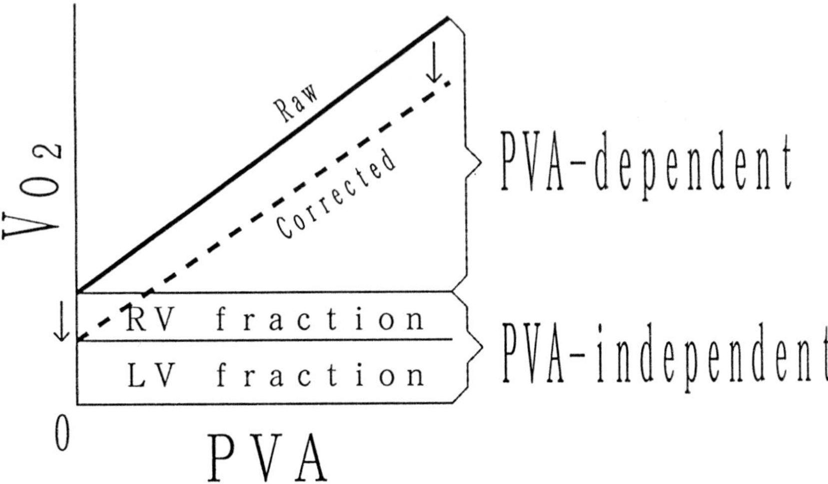

Figure 18.4. Right and left ventricular fractions of cardiac oxygen consumption (Vo_2). Pressure-volume area (PVA)-independent Vo_2 consists of right ventricular (RV) and left ventricular (LV) fractions. PVA-dependent Vo_2 consists of left ventricular fraction only. The raw Vo_2-PVA relation (solid) is the sum of both RV and LV fractions of PVA-independent Vo_2 and LV PVA-dependent Vo_2. After subtracting the RV PVA-independent Vo_2, the corrected Vo_2-PVA relation (dashed) is obtained for LV.

of the oxygen contents of coronary arterial and venous blood samples determined with either a Lex-O_2 Con or an IL-382 CO-Oximeter. Both PVA and Vo_2 were determined in steady state under various loading, heart rate and inotropic conditions.

In our studies, PVA refers only to the left ventricle, but Vo_2 consists of left and right ventricular components. Since the right ventricle was collapsed by continuous drainage of coronary venous return, we assumed that right ventricular PVA was practically zero and hence right ventricular Vo_2 was dependent only on its basal metabolism and activation. Left ventricular Vo_2 should be dependent on all of its PVA, basal metabolism and activation. We assumed that Vo_2 for basal metabolism and activation is homogeneous in the right and left ventricles. Unloaded right ventricular Vo_2 was determined by multiplying unloaded right and left ventricular Vo_2 with the right to total ventricular weight ratio. This was subtracted from total Vo_2 to obtain left ventricular Vo_2 (Figure 18.4). Left ventricular Vo_2 was divided by heart rate and expressed in ml O_2/beat. It was normalized for 100 g left ventricle.

Figure 18.5 shows a representative set of Vo_2-PVA relations in control and enhanced contractile states with either Ca^{2+} or epinephrine in one heart. In either contractile state, both isovolumic and ejecting contractions are pooled. The important findings from the data in Figure 18.5 and similar data in other hearts are summarized as follows [3,4].

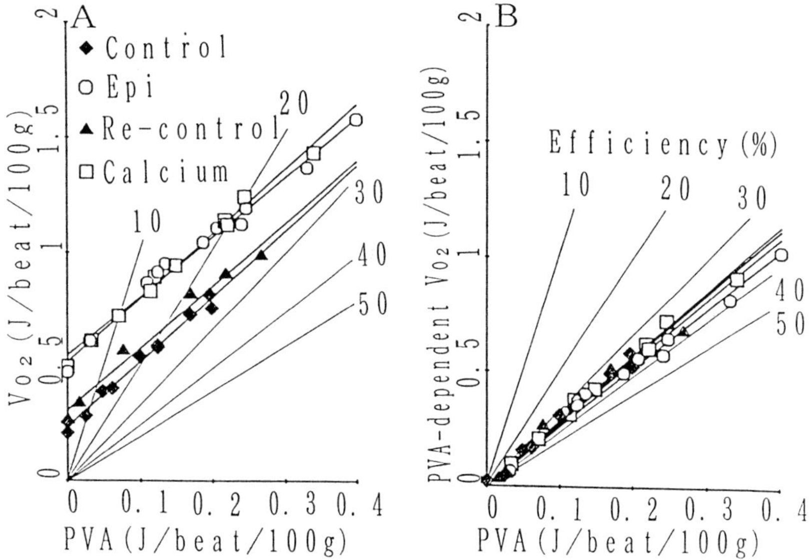

Figure 18.5. Left ventricular oxygen consumption versus PVA relation in control (solid symbols) and enhanced contractile states with Ca^{2+}, and epinephrine (open symbols) in one dog heart (Panel A). When epinephrine and calcium enhanced E_{max} to the same extent, the elevation of the Vo_2-PVA relation was also comparable. Units of both Vo_2 and PVA are J. The family of thin diagonal lines indicate the efficiency of energy conversion from total Vo_2 to PVA. Subtracting PVA-independent Vo_2 (or unloaded Vo_2) from individual Vo_2-PVA relations, Panel B shows the relation between PVA-dependent Vo_2 and PVA. The slopes of these relations are the same as those of the original relations. The efficiency (thin diagonal lines) now indicates the energy conversion efficiency from the PVA-dependent Vo_2 to PVA. This efficiency is called contractile efficiency.

1) Vo_2 correlated linearly with PVA in any stable contractile state whether control, or enhanced by Ca^{2+} or epinephrine in any given heart. The Vo_2 on the ordinate is obtained in unloaded contraction at V_0.
2) The Vo_2-PVA relation has the same slope regardless of the mode of contraction whether isovolumic or ejecting in a given heart.
3) The slope of the Vo_2-PVA relation in a stable contractile state has a relatively constant value in different hearts.
4) The Vo_2-PVA relation is elevated in a parallel manner with an enhanced contractile state by either Ca^{2+} or epinephrine.
5) The magnitudes of the elevation for similar increases in contractility assessed by E_{max} are comparable.

As for the linear Vo_2-PVA relation with a relatively constant slope, we have obtained similar findings whether the pressure-volume loop is normally quasi-rectangular or abnormally distorted in various ways [16] and whether the work is positive or negative [17]. In other words, the contributions of mechan-

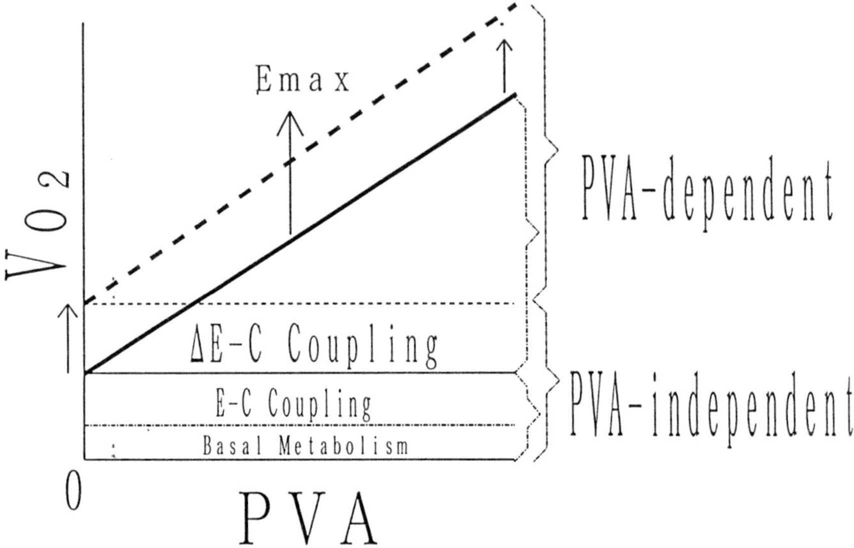

Figure 18.6. Vo_2-PVA relation and PVA-dependent and PVA-independent components of Vo_2. Solid diagonal line is the Vo_2-PVA relation at control E_{max}. Dashed diagonal line is the Vo_2-PVA relation at an enhanced E_{max}. The elevation is equal to the increment in the Vo_2 for excitation-contraction coupling (ΔE-C coupling). PVA-independent Vo_2 consists of basal metabolic Vo_2 and Vo_2 for E-C coupling. PVA-dependent Vo_2 is for generation of PVA.

ical work and potential energy to Vo_2 are always the same, indicating energetic equivalence of the two types of energy in PVA [18].

As for the contractility-dependence of the Vo_2-PVA relation, we have obtained similar findings with other inotropic agents such as other catecholamines (norepinephrine, dobutamine, isoproterenol, denopamine) [3,4], digitalis (ouabain) [19] and so-called new cardiotonic agents (sulmazole, milrinone, OPC-8212 [20], DPI 201–106 [21], UDCG 115 BS). Paired pulse stimulation also elevated the Vo_2-PVA relation in proportion to E_{max} [22].

Negative inotropic agents (propranolol, verapamil) lowered the Vo_2-PVA relation in proportion to E_{max} [3,4]. Decreased coronary flow also lowered the Vo_2-PVA relation [23].

KCl-arrested Vo_2 was not significantly affected by various inotropic agents when KCl was infused directly into coronary circulation at a minimal level enough to cause cardiac arrest in order to prevent calcium overload in myocardial cells [3,4,10]. This result indicates that the fraction of Vo_2 which was changed with E_{max} is related with myocardial activation or excitation-contraction coupling which primarily handles intracellular calcium transport [2,24]. This suggests that the Vo_2 for the activation is independent of PVA. Accordingly, Figure 18.6 shows the components of Vo_2 for three major energy expenditures, i.e. from top down, mechanical contraction, activation and basal metabolism.

The horizontal division between the PVA-dependent and PVA-independent Vo_2 (see below) in Figure 18.6 is based on the assumption that the energy expenditure of calcium handling in the activation is independent of PVA. In fact, we have found that unloaded Vo_2 is independent of whether the unloaded contraction is either isovolumic contraction at V_0 or complete systolic unloaded contraction from a high end-diastolic volume [25].

The linear Vo_2-PVA relation indicates that Vo_2 for mechanical contraction is proportional to PVA. Therefore, it is reasonable to call the Vo_2 above the unloaded Vo_2 'PVA-dependent Vo_2' and the Vo_2 below the unloaded Vo_2 'PVA-independent Vo_2. The Vo_2-PVA relation results in a simple mathematical expression of Vo_2 = PVA-dependent Vo_2 and PVA-independent Vo_2.

Oxygen cost of mechanical energy and contractile efficiency

The slope of the Vo_2-PVA relation means the 'oxygen cost of PVA' or mechanical energy. When the slope is a, PVA-dependent Vo_2 is expressed by aPVA. Then, Vo_2 is given as $Vo_2 = a\text{PVA}$ + PVA-independent Vo_2. From a large number of dog left ventricles, we have obtained an average value of 1.8×10^{-5} ml O_2/(mmHg ml) for the oxygen cost of PVA [3,4]. Since 1 ml O_2 is equivalent approximately to 20 J and 1 mmHg ml PVA to 1.33×10^{-4} J, the a value of 1.8×10^{-5} ml O_2/(mmHg ml) is convertible to 2.5 (dimensionless) [3,4].

The reciprocal of the oxygen cost of PVA, $1/a$, means the efficiency of energy conversion from the PVA-dependent Vo_2 to PVA. This efficiency is called 'contractile efficiency' to be differentiated from other efficiencies such as mechanical work efficiency and crossbridge efficiency [3,4]. The contractile efficiency is 40% on average, ranging between 30 and 50% in different hearts [3,4]. Assuming that the efficiency from Vo_2 to ATP in the oxidative phosphorylation is approximately 65% [5,6], the efficiency from ATP to PVA in the contractile machinery or crossbridge cycling is calculated to be about 62% (=40%/65%). Thus, the introduction of the PVA concept and the contractile efficiency has allowed us to elucidate the stoichiometry in the energy conversion steps from oxygen consumption to the total mechanical energy before mechanical work is generated [3,4].

Oxygen cost of contractility

The activation component of Vo_2 is considered to reflect the energy expenditure by both Na-K and Ca ATPases [5]. Since the total released Ca ions are considered to be increased in an enhanced contractile state, it is easily conceivable that a greater amount of calcium ions is pumped mostly into the sarcoplasmic reticulum by the Ca ATPase consuming more ATP with a stoichiometry of 2Ca:1ATP [24,26]. More calcium ions seem to flow into the myocardial cell through the Ca channel during depolarization in an enhanced contractile state [24,26]. This amount of calcium ions has to be removed out of the cell during repolarization. The Na/Ca exchanger *per se* does not consume ATP to remove Ca in exchange with influx Na (stoichiometry = 3Na:1Ca) [26]. However, this influx Na has to be pumped out by the Na-K pump ATPase with a stoichiometry of 3Na:2K:1ATP. Therefore, the net stoichiometry is 1Ca:1ATP, which is half that of the sarcoplasmic reticulum Ca ATPase. As a whole, enhancement of contractility is associated with an increase in the amount of calcium ions handled in the excitation-contraction-relaxation cycle.

Therefore, our finding of a proportionally increased PVA-independent Vo_2 to increases in E_{max} seems to be based on the stoichiometry between the amount of calcium ions to be handled in the activation and the amount of ATP consumed in the ion pumps [3,4].

We have introduced the oxygen cost of E_{max} to quantify the requirement of PVA-independent Vo_2 for a unit increase in E_{max}. It is expressed by the slope of the relation between PVA-independent Vo_2 and E_{max} obtained while E_{max} is changed by a chosen inotropic agent [3,4]. There are two methods to determine it, as shown in Figure 18.7. One is to obtain the Vo_2-PVA relations at more than two different E_{max} levels and calculate the incremental ratio of their PVA-independent Vo_2 to E_{max} (Figure 18.7A) [27]. Each Vo_2-PVA relation should be obtained by varying loading conditions in a stable E_{max}. This method is liable to have a large estimation error when only two Vo_2-PVA data are taken at each E_{max} [27]. The other method is to fix ventricular volume and change E_{max} in more than one step (Figure 18.7B) [28]. This method does not require changes in ventricular loading conditions, but requires the assumption that the Vo_2-PVA relations at different E_{max} levels are virtually parallel to each other. The parallelism has been validated in many studies using various inotropic agents [3,4]. Figure 18.7C schematically shows a linear relation between thus obtained PVA-independent Vo_2 and E_{max}.

Figure 18.8A schematically shows that the oxygen cost of E_{max} was virtually the same whether E_{max} was increased with Ca^{2+} or epinephrine despite their different pharmacological mechanisms of positive inotropism [10,29]. Ca^{2+} administration into the coronary artery is considered to increase calcium influx and intracellular calcium available in the activation, which in turn increase the total released and removed calcium by consuming ATP. Epinephrine as a β agonist increases intracellular cyclic AMP and phosphorylates (1) sarcolemmal Ca channel, (2) phospholamban, in turn accelerating sarcoplasmic reticulum Ca pumping, and (3) troponin I, in turn decreasing the calcium sensitivity of troponin C [26].

We first expected that epinephrine would have a greater oxygen cost of E_{max} because the decreased calcium sensitivity of the contractile proteins

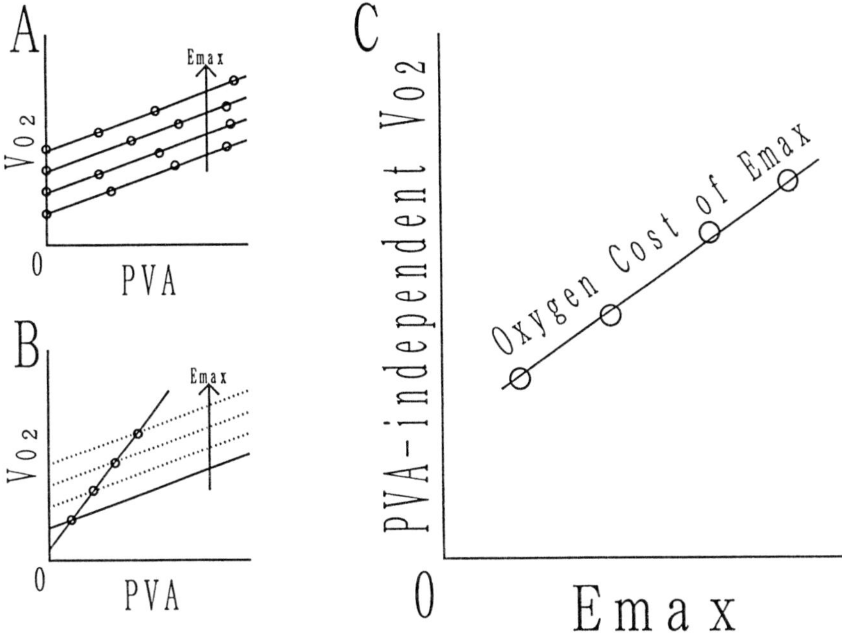

Figure 18.7. Methods to determine the oxygen cost of E_{max}. Panel A: Vo_2-PVA relations are obtained by changing PVA at different E_{max} levels. Panel B: Vo_2-PVA data points are obtained by changing E_{max} at a given volume load. Panel C: PVA-independent Vo_2 values obtained either from Panel A or B are plotted against corresponding E_{max} values. Oxygen cost of E_{max} is obtained as the slope of this relation. Schematic illustration.

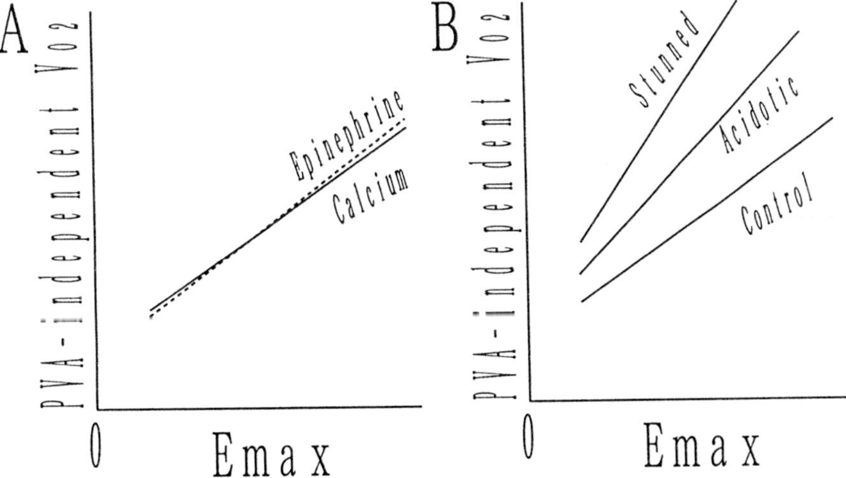

Figure 18.8. Oxygen costs of E_{max} enhanced with calcium (solid) or epinephrine (dashed) in control (Panel A) and acidotic and stunned hearts (Panel B). Schematic illustration.

would require a greater amount of total released calcium to reach a give E_{max} level. However, the result was against our expectation. We studied this mechanism with a computer simulation of calcium kinetics among sarcoplasmic reticulum, contractile proteins and intracellular free calcium. The simulation resulted in only a small increase in total released and removed calcium for a given E_{max} even if the contractile protein calcium sensitivity was halved in normal hearts [24].

The simulation also resulted in only a small saving in total released and removed calcium for a given E_{max} even if the contractile protein calcium sensitivity was doubled in normal hearts [24]. As a whole, changes in the calcium sensitivity of contractile proteins only slightly affect the total released and removed calcium in normal hearts. This seems to underlie the comparable oxygen costs of E_{max} of normal hearts with various positive and negative inotropic agents such as propranolol, verapamil, catecholamines, new cardiotonic agents whether their effects include phosphodiesterase inhibition (activating Ca channel and Ca pump), contractile protein calcium sensitization or desensitization, or activation of Na channel [3,4].

Figure 18.8B schematically shows that both acidotic hearts and post-ischemic reperfused stunned hearts have 1.5–2 times greater oxygen costs of E_{max} than control [29,30]. Two underlying mechanisms can be considered; one is a decreased calcium sensitivity of contractile proteins and the other is an increased calcium leak of sarcoplasmic reticulum [28,30]. The relative importance of these mechanisms remains to be studied.

Interestingly, the simulation also shows that contractile protein calcium sensitization from an abnormally low level would save the oxygen cost of E_{max} [unpublished]. This warrants studies of the effect of calcium sensitizers in failing hearts which have a decreased contractile protein calcium sensitivity.

Final remarks

Evidence supportive of the PVA concept has been accumulating. Hisano and Cooper showed that FLA (force-length area), a linear version of PVA, correlated with Vo_2 in ferret papillary muscles [31]. It shows contractile efficiency of about 40%. Gibbs showed a similar contractile efficiency of 40% in a rabbit myocardium by a thermal method [32]. Mast and Elzinga showed that the elastic potential energy was degraded into heat of the same magnitude in energy [33]. More recently, Gao (a PhD student of Henk ter Keurs) showed that the contractile efficiency was 65% when ATP consumption and FLA were correlated in rat myocardium [34].

However, there are some results which claim the limitation of PVA. Hisano and Cooper showed that an end-systolic quick release curtailed Vo_2 although FLA remained unchanged because it had been determined by the end systole [31]. This observation also hold with PVA [11]. This phenomenon could be accounted for by the consideration that maintenance of force even during relaxation requires some Vo_2 as Monroe had shown earlier [35]. However, as we have shown, addition of the force-time integral term to PVA does not help improve the predictability of Vo_2 from PVA alone [36].

Burkhoff showed that Vo_2 of contractions with ejecting activation was smaller despite increased E_{max} values [37]. Yasumura *et al.* obtained a similar finding [38]. These results indicate that the increase in E_{max} by ejecting activation is different in the mechanism from ordinary positive inotropic interventions and is not caused by an increased total released calcium in the activation process [38].

Significantly steeper Vo_2-PVA relations and hence greater oxygen costs of PVA and smaller contractile efficiency values than the average have been reported in dog hearts [39,40]. We do not understand the mechanism of the lower efficiency. This problem has to be solved as soon as possible. A lower contractile efficiency has been observed in a hyperthyroid heart than a euthyroid heart in the rabbit [41]. This is attributable to a shift of isomyosin from V_3 to V_1 [41].

Acknowledgement

Partly supported by Grants-in-Aid for Scientific Research (04237219, 04454267, 04557041, 04454267, 04557041, 05221224) from the Ministry of Education, Science and Culture, Research Grants for Cardiovascular Diseases (3A-2, 4C-4) from the Ministry of Health and Welfare, and grants from Suzuken Memorial Foundation, Nakatani Electronic Measuring Technology Association, and Shimabara Science Promotion Foundation of Japan.

References

1. Braunwald E. Thirteenth Bowditch Lecture. The determinants of myocardial oxygen consumption. Physiologists 1969; 12: 65–93.
2. Gibbs CL. Cardiac energetics. Physiol Rev 1978; 58: 175–254.
3. Suga H. Ventricular energetics. Physiol Rev 1990; 70: 247–77.
4. Suga H, Goto Y. Cardiac oxygen costs of contractility (E_{max}) and mechanical energy (PVA): new key concepts in cardiac energetics. In Sasayama S, Suga H (eds): Recent Progress in Failing Heart Syndrome. Tokyo. Springer-Verlag 1992, 61–115.
5. Drake-Holland AJ, Noble MIM (eds). Cardiac Metabolism. Chichester: John Wiley and Sons, 1983.
6. Weibel ER. The Pathway for Oxygen. Structure and Function in the Mammalian Respiratory System. Cambridge, Massachusetts: Harvard University Press, 1984.
7. Ugurbil K, Kingsley-Hickman PB, Sako EY *et al.* ^{31}P NMR studies of the kinetics and regulation of oxidative phosphorylation in the intact myocardium. Ann NY Acad Sci 1987; 508: 265–86.
8. Suga H, Sagawa K, Shoukas AA. Load-independence of the instantaneous pressure-volume

ratio of the canine left ventricle and effects of epinephrine and heart rate on the ratio. Circ Res 1973; 32: 314–22.

9. Suga H. Total mechanical energy of a ventricle model and cardiac oxygen consumption. Am J Physiol 1979; 236: H498–H505.
10. Suga H, Hisano R, Goto Y *et al.* Effect of positive inotropic agents on the relation between oxygen consumption and systolic pressure-volume area in canine left ventricle. Circ Res 1983; 53: 306–18.
11. Yasumura Y, Nozawa T, Futaki S *et al.* Time-varying oxygen cost of mechanical energy in dog left ventricle: consistency and inconsistency of time-varying elastance model with myocardial energetics. Circ Res 1989; 64: 763–78.
12. Woledge RC, Curtin NA, Homsher E. Energetic Aspects of Muscle Contraction. London; Academic 1985.
13. Hata K, Goto Y, Suga H. External mechanical work during relaxation period does not affect myocardial oxygen consumption. Am J Physiol 1991; 261: H1778–H1784.
14. Sagawa K, Maughan L, Suga H *et al.* Cardiac Contraction and the Pressure-Volume Relationship. New York: Oxford University Press, 1988.
15. Suga H, Futaki S, Ohgoshi Y *et al.* Arteriovenous oximeter for O_2 content difference, O_2 saturation, and hemoglobin content. Am J Physiol 1989; 257: H1712–H1716.
16. Suga H, Yamada 0, Goto Y *et al.* Oxygen consumption and pressure-volume area of abnormal contractions in canine left ventricle. Am J Physiol 1984; 246: H154–H160.
17. Suga H, Goto Y, Yasumura Y *et al.* Oxygen saving effect of negative work in dog left ventricle. Am J Physiol 1988; 254: H34–H44.
18. Suga H, Hayashi T, Suehiro S *et al.* Equal oxygen consumption rates of isovolumic and ejecting contractions with equal systolic pressure-volume areas in canine left ventricle. Circ Res 1981; 49: 1082–91.
19. Wu D, Yasumura Y, Nozawa T *et al.* Effect of ouabain on the relation between left ventricular oxygen consumption and systolic pressure-volume area (PVA) in dog heart. Heart Vessels 1989; 5: 17–24.
20. Futaki S, Nozawa T, Yasumura Y *et al.* New cardiotonic agent, OPC-8212, elevates the myocardial oxygen consumption versus pressure-volume area (PVA) relation in a similar manner to catecholamines and calcium in canine hearts. Heart Vessels 1988; 4: 153–61.
21. Futaki S, Goto Y, Ohgoshi Y *et al.* Similar oxygen cost of myocardial contractility between DPI 201–106 and epinephrine despite different subcellular mechanisms of action in dog hearts. Heart Vessels 1992; 7: 8–17.
22. Suga H, Futaki S, Tanaka N *et al.* Paired pulse pacing increases cardiac O_2 consumption for activation without changing efficiency of contractile machinery in canine left ventricle. Heart Vessels 1988; 4: 79–87.
23. Suga H, Goto Y, Yasumura Y *et al.* O_2 consumption of dog heart under decreased coronary perfusion and propranolol. Am J Physiol 1988; 254: H292–H303.
24. Suga H, Goto Y, Futaki S *et al.* Calcium kinetics and energetics. simulation study. Jpn Heart J 1991; 32: 57–67.
25. Yasumura Y, Nozawa T, Futaki S *et al.* Minor preload dependence of O_2 consumption of unloaded contraction in dog heart. Am J Physiol 1989; 256: H1289–H1294.
26. Ruegg JC. Calcium in Muscle Activation. Berlin: Springer-Verlag 1988.
27. Burkhoff D, Yue DT, Oikawa RY *et al.* Influence of ventricular contractility on non-work-related myocardial oxygen consumption. Heart Vessels 1987; 3: 66–72.
28. Ohgoshi Y, Goto Y, Futaki S *et al.* New method to determine oxygen cost of contractility. Jpn J Physiol 1990; 40: 127–38.
29. Ohgoshi Y, Goto Y, Futaki S *et al.* Increased oxygen cost of contractility in stunned myocardium of dog. Circ Res 1991; 69: 975–88.
30. Hata K, Goto Y, Kawaguchi O *et al.* Acidosis increases oxygen cost of contractility in dog left ventricle. Circulation 1991; 84(Suppl II) II-94.
31. Hisano R, Cooper G. Correlation of force-length area with oxygen consumption in ferret papillary muscle. Circ Res 87; 61: 318–28.

32. Gibbs CL. Cardiac energetics and the Fenn effect. In Jacob R, Just Hj, Holubarsch Ch (eds):Cardiac Energetics. Basic Mechanisms and clinical Implications. Darmstadt: Steinkopff Verlag 1987; 61–8.
33. Mast F, Elzinga G. Heat released during relaxation equals force-length area in isometric contractions of rabbit papillary muscle. Circ Res 1990; 67: 893–901.
34. Gao WD. The diastolic properties of rat trabeculae during energy deprivation. PhD Thesis. University of Calgary, 1991.
35. Monroe RG. Myocardial oxygen consumption during ventricular contraction and relaxation. Circ Res 1964; 14: 294–300.
36. Suga H, Nozawa T, Yasumura Y *et al.* Force-time integral does not improve predictability of cardiac O_2 consumption from pressure-volume area (PVA) in dog left ventricle. Heart Vessels 1990; 5: 152–8.
37. Burkhoff D, De Tombe PP, Hunter WC *et al.* Contractile strength and mechanical efficiency of left ventricle are enhanced by physiologic afterload. Am J Physiol 1991; 260: H569–H578.
38. Yasumura Y, Nozawa T, Futaki S *et al.* Ejecting activation and its energetics. Circulation 1988; 78(Suppl II): II-225.
39. Nozawa T, Yasumura Y, Futaki S *et al.* Relation between oxygen consumption and pressure-volume area of in situ dog heart. Am J Physiol 1987; 253: H31–H40.
40. Wolff MR, De Tombe PP, Harasawa Y *et al.* Alterations in left ventricular mechanics, energetics, and contractile reserve in experimental heart failure. Circ Res 1992; 70: 516–29.
41. Goto Y, Slinker BK, LeWinter MM. Decreased contractile efficiency and increased non-mechanical energy cost in hyperthyroid rabbit heart: relation between O_2 consumption and systolic pressure-volume area or force-time integral. Circ Res 1990; 66: 999–1011.

19. Cardioplegia and cardiac function

DIETRICH BAUMGART, RAINER SCHULZ, THOMAS EHRING, and GERD HEUSCH

Introduction

Preservation of myocardial integrity and function during cardioplegic arrest has improved steadily in recent years with the widespread use of selective cardiac hypothermia and potassium containing cardioplegia [1–7]. Most operations involving open-heart surgery can now be completed with a cardioplegic arrest of less than 120 minutes duration. Nevertheless, in a number of patients the heart recovering from the surgical trauma and the cardioplegic arrest cannot provide a sufficient peripheral circulation in the immediate postoperative period, although coronary blood flow is restored, and there is no myocardial necrosis. This reversible impairment of postoperative ventricular function represents a form of global myocardial 'stunning' [8]. With the restoration of coronary blood flow, there is a rapid recovery of metabolic parameters. Creatine phosphate is repleted [9,10], lactate production is reversed to consumption [11], and tissue pH is normalized [9]. Changes in myocardial water content occur only to a minor extent during cardioplegia and tissue edema resolves quickly upon reperfusion [12]. Changes of the ST-segment and cardiac rhythm [13–15] are normalized within minutes after reperfusion. Thus, reversibly depressed ventricular function following cardioplegic arrest has no metabolic, electrophysiological or structural correlate and must therefore be assessed as a separate entity. The adequate assessment of cardiac function and its management during the critical postoperative period is essential to the outcome of the operative procedure and the prognosis of patients undergoing cardiac surgery [16,17].

Assessment of cardiac, ventricular, and regional myocardial function

The function of the heart is to provide the transport of blood to and from the peripheral tissues. This *cardiac function* is dependent on a periodic contraction, relaxation, and filling of the right and left ventricle. An inadequate cardiac function, i.e. heart failure, can be attributed to disturbances of ventricular filling (e.g., hypovolemic shock), to disturbances of the contraction frequency (e.g., AV-block), or to an inadequate mechanical function of the ventricles.

H.M. Piper and C.J. Preusse (eds): Ischemia-reperfusion in cardiac surgery, 421–448.

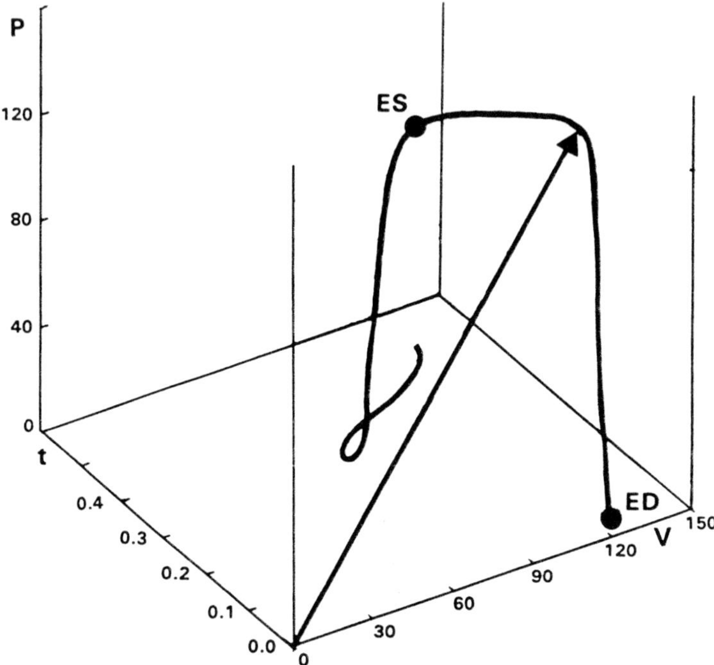

Figure 19.1. Three-dimensional diagram of the pressure-volume-time relationship under resting conditions. Black dots indicate end-diastole (ED) and end-systole (ES). The arrow represents a vector. P: pressure [mmHg]; V: volume [ml]; t: time [s].

Ideally, diastolic and systolic ventricular function are characterized by the simultaneous assessment of ventricular pressure, volume, and time (Figure 19.1) [18]. Assessment of *regional myocardial function* is more complicated, as the arrangement of muscle fibers within a network of collagen requires simultaneous measurements of wall tension and deformation over time. The simultaneous measurement of ventricular pressure and three-dimensional deformation using multiple radiopaque markers within the ventricular wall comes close to meet these ideal requirements (Figure 19.2) [19].

The three-dimensional relationship of ventricular pressure, volume, and time can be quantified by a vector (Figure 19.1). Such an assessment of ventricular function, however, is methodologically difficult in the experimental and even more so in the clinical setting. Reducing the complexity of the analysis, ventricular function is characterized by a two-dimensional approach plotting pressure versus volume but neglecting time. On the regional myocardial level, the pressure-volume relationship is equivalent to a pressure-wall thickness or to a pressure-segment length relationship.

Total cardiac work is the sum of the external work spent for volume displacement and pressure development, for the acceleration of blood during ejection, and for the internal deformation associated with changes in ventricu-

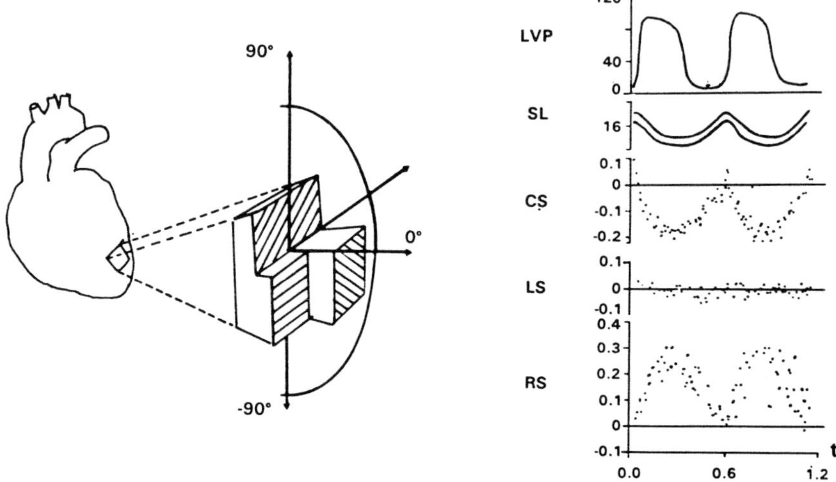

Figure 19.2. Left panel: Three-dimensional fiber orientation of the left ventricular wall. Right panel: Simultaneous recording of left ventricular pressure (LVP, mmHg), segment length (SL, mm), and circumferential (CS), longitudinal (LS) and radial (RS) fiber strain over time (t, s) (modified after Waldman *et al.* [19]).

lar geometry. Under resting conditions the work spent for acceleration and for internal deformation amounts to no more than 10–20% of total cardiac work [20,21]. With increasing heart rate, however, the work spent for acceleration and internal deformation is augmented. The area of the pressure-volume loop accounts only for volume displacement and pressure development, but neglects the work for acceleration and internal deformation.

Determinants of cardiac, ventricular, and regional myocardial function

Preload (PL) relates to the muscle fiber length or the overlap between actin and myosin filaments *before* the muscle contracts. End-diastolic muscle fiber length determines the degree of fiber shortening and force development during the subsequent systole. On the ventricular level, end-diastolic muscle fiber length is represented by end-diastolic volume. On the regional myocardial level, end diastolic segment length or wall thickness may serve as measures of PL. As PL increases along a given end-diastolic pressure-volume curve (assuming the other determinants of ventricular function being constant), the contraction reaches the same end-systolic volume, thus ejecting a larger stroke volume (Frank-Starling mechanism) [22]. Alternatively, the ventricle develops a higher isovolumic pressure starting from a higher PL. The physiological relevance of this mechanism is to adapt stroke volume to

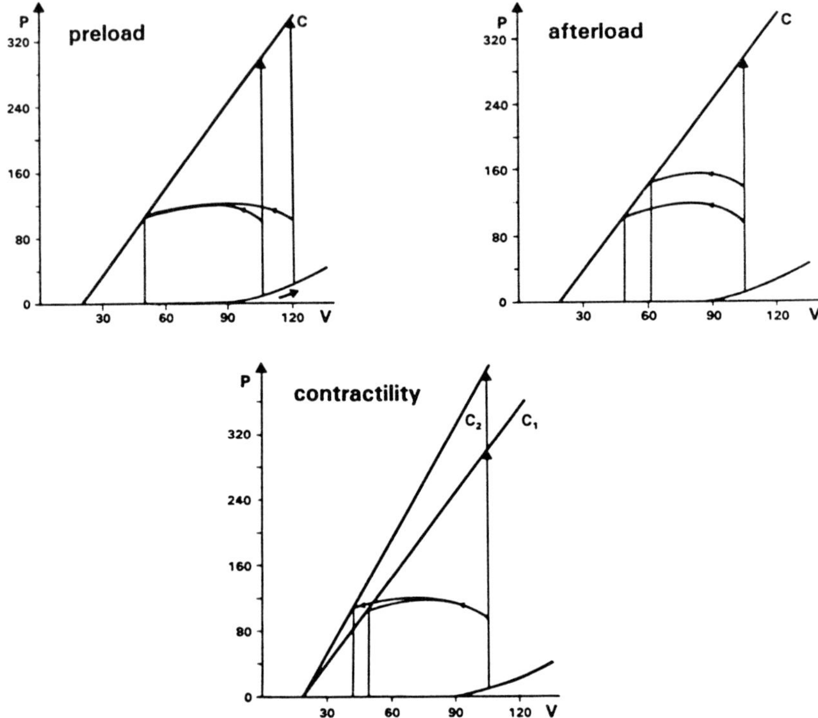

Figure 19.3. Effects of varying PL, AL, and C are displayed in pressure-volume relationships. Upper left panel: As PL increases along a given end-diastolic pressure-volume curve (assuming AL, C, and HR being constant), the contraction reaches the same end-svstolic volume, thus ejecting a larger stroke volume. Alternatively, the ventricle develops a higher isovolumic pressure at a greater PL. Upper right panel: With increasing AL (assuming PL, C, and HR being constant) stroke volume is decreased. Lower panel: Increasing C increases the slope of the end-systolic pressure-volume relationship. The ventricle delivers a larger stroke volume and/or reaches a higher peak isovolumic pressure at a given PL. P: pressure [mmHg], V: volume [ml].

venous return on a beat-to-beat basis and in particular to adjust for respiratory variations in right and left ventricular venous return (Figure 19.3).

Afterload (AL) is the force that opposes the shortening of muscle fibers *during* contraction. In an equilibrium, this force is actively developed by the shortening muscle. When cardiac function is assessed with respect to the peripheral circulation, AL is given by the arterial impedance [23]. Arterial impedance represents the dynamic resistance of the arterial system which opposes the pulsatile outflow of the ventricle. Arterial impedance is properly described by modulus and phase curves derived from frequency domain analyses of pulsatile arterial pressure-flow relationships. Neglecting the functional relevance of the windkessel and the inertia of blood, arterial impedance is reduced to total peripheral or pulmonary vascular resistance, respectively [18]. With respect to ventricular function *per se*, AL is the integral of wall

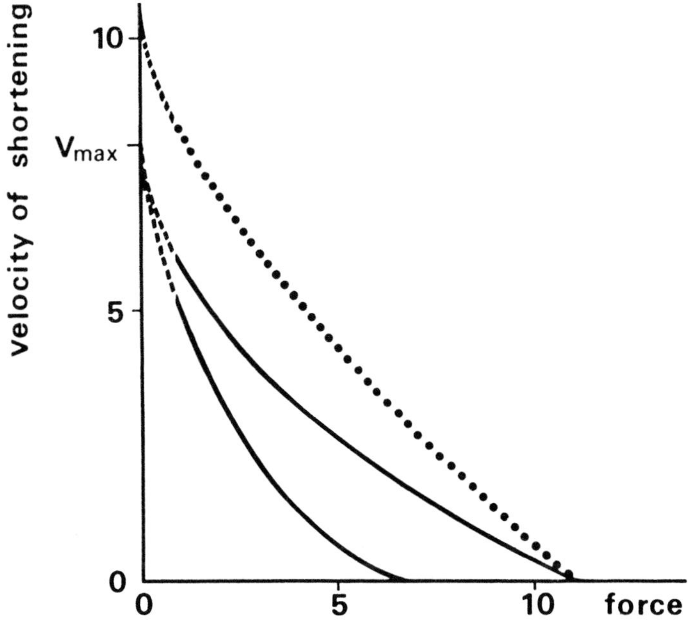

Figure 19.4. Force-velocity curves of an isolated muscle preparation; displayed are increases in PL (from lower to middle solid line) and increases in C (from solid lines to dotted line). At increasing initial fiber length, i.e. PL, the maximal velocity of shortening of the unloaded contractile element (V_{max}) is unchanged. With increases in C, V_{max} is increased. velocity of shortening [mm/s]; force [N].

stress developed in different myocardial regions throughout systole. Wall stress in a given myocardial region is determined by the developed pressure, the wall thickness, and the radius of curvature. Wall stress may therefore differ in different myocardial regions. As an extreme example, in the presence of a ventricular aneurysm wall stress in that particular region is increased, as it is subjected to an unchanged ventricular pressure, but wall thickness in that region is decreased and the radius of curvature increased. Neither arterial impedance nor wall stress can be easily measured. Therefore, using a simplistic approach, AL is often estimated from mean aortic pressure. With increasing AL (assuming PL, contractility, and heart rate being constant) stroke volume is decreased (Figure 19.3).

Contractility (C) relates to the extent and frequency of cross bridge formation between actin and myosin filaments independent of their overlap, and thus relates to the genuine muscle properties. A measure of C can be derived from the force-velocity relationship (Figure 19.4) [24]. At increasing initial fiber length, i.e. PL, the extrapolated maximal velocity of shortening of the unloaded contractile element (V_{max}) remains unchanged. Whereas the developed force is dependent on both PL and muscle mass, V_{max} reflects C only [24]. To use an example, 10 horses can develop 10 times more force than a single horse, but they do not run faster.

End-systolic pressure increases with end-systolic volume or end-systolic muscle fiber length. Experimentally, such relation of end-systolic pressure to end-systolic volume or end-systolic muscle fiber length is generated by systematically varying loading conditions. Using a linear regression, the slope and intercept of such relationship may serve as measures of C which are supposed to be largely independent of loading conditions [18,25]. Increasing C increases the slope of the end-systolic pressure-volume or the pressure-muscle fiber length relationship, respectively. The ventricle delivers a larger stroke volume and/or reaches a higher peak isovolumic pressure at a given PL (Figure 19.3).

PL, AL, and C are related to any single heart beat. *Heart rate* (HR) is, on the one hand, the frequency of heart beats per time unit and, on the other hand, simultaneously impacts on PL, AL, and C. Increasing HR affects the duration of systole and diastole to a different extent and particularly reduces the time for ventricular filling and coronary inflow [26]. Nevertheless, up to a HR of approximately 180 beats/min cardiac output increases. Thereafter, the greatly reduced ventricular PL predominates and cardiac output is decreased. At increasing HR, C is increased, i.e. there is a staircase phenomenon [27,28]. However, this mechanism is probably of minor importance in the non-failing heart *in situ*.

Dynamic interaction between preload, afterload, and contractility

At a given C, a sudden increase in AL will instantaneously result in a decreased stroke volume (Figures 19.3 and 19.5). When venous return is constant, the end-diastolic volume of the subsequent beat is increased; thus, the subsequent contraction is starting from a higher PL. With increased PL, a new steady state develops and the ventricle then ejects its stroke volume against an increased AL (Figure 19.5). The extent of an increase in end-diastolic volume that permits the maintenance of stroke volume in the presence of a higher AL has been termed preload reserve [29]. Preload reserve in a normal ventricle during rest is, however, limited to about 10% [30], since the myocardium already works at a near optimal overlap of actin and myosin filaments. When PL reserve is fully utilized, any further increase in AL results in a decreased stroke volume unless C is increased. Such reduction of stroke volume in response to increased AL at a given C is the expression of a mismatch between AL and C. With a pathological depression of C, stroke volume cannot be maintained even at a normal level of AL [29].

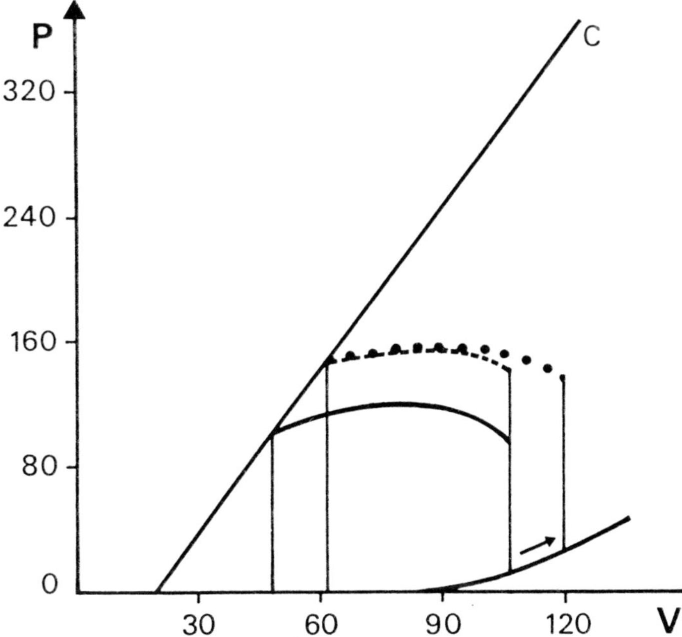

Figure 19.5. Recruitment of PL reserve in response to an increased AL serves to maintain stroke volume. At a given C, a sudden increase in AL will instantaneously result in a decreased stroke volume. When venous return is constant, the end-diastolic volume of the subsequent beat is increased. Thus, the subsequent contraction is starting from a higher end-diastolic volume, i.e. PL. A new steady state develops and the ventricle ejects its stroke volume against an increased AL. P: pressure [mmHg]; V: volume [ml].

Adaptations to chronic increases in volume and pressure

Chronic ventricular volume loading results in dilatation of the myofilament-collagen network and a rightward shift of the end-diastolic pressure-volume curve. With increased end-diastolic volume, a given extent of fiber shortening results in a larger stroke volume at an unchanged C (Figure 19.6). To compensate for the increased wall stress associated with the increased radius of curvature, myocardial hypertrophy develops [31]. Full compensation of chronic volume overload is characterized by myocardial hypertrophy and the delivery of an increased stroke volume by a larger ventricle with an unchanged C. Compensatory mechanisms fail when further increases in ventricular volume induce excessive increases in wall stress and a derangement of muscle fibers.

Acute pressure loading increases end-diastolic volume beyond the limits of PL reserve and therefore reduces stroke volume. However, over several weeks progressive myocardial hypertrophy develops [31], and end-diastolic volume and wall stress return to normal levels. Despite a persistent increase

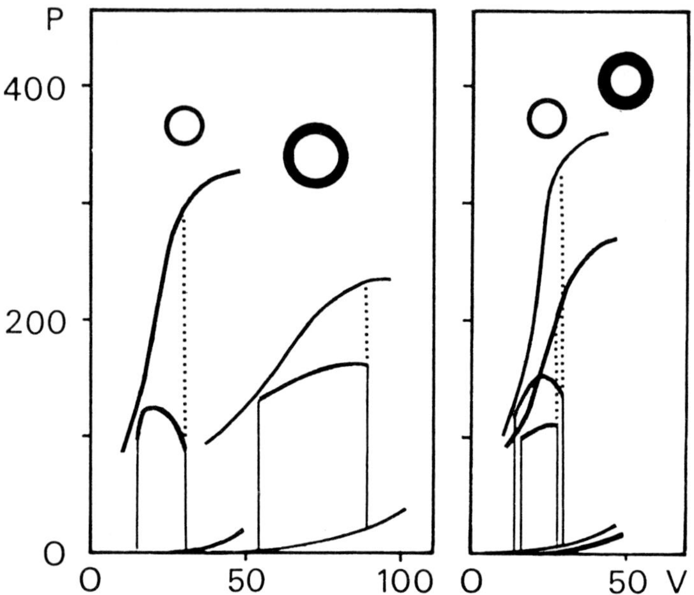

Figure 19.6. Chronic adaptations to pressure and volume loading. Left panel: Chronic ventricular volume loading results in a rightward shift of the end-diastolic pressure-volume curve. With increased end-diastolic volume, a given extent of fiber shortening results in a larger stroke volume at an unchanged C. To compensate for the increased wall stress associated with the increased radius of curvature, myocardial hypertrophy develops. Full compensation of chronic volume load is characterized by myocardial hypertrophy and the delivery of an increased stroke volume by a larger ventricle with unchanged C. Right panel: Chronic pressure loading results in progressive myocardial hypertrophy, and end-diastolic volume and wall stress return to normal levels. Despite a persistent increase in pressure, stroke volume is normal (modified after Jacob and Kissling [153]. P: pressure [mmHg]; V: volume [ml].

in pressure, stroke volume is normalized (Figure 19.6) [32]. The compensatory myocardial hypertrophy is, however, limited, since the coronary vasculature provides adequate nutritive supply only up to a heart weight of about 500 g [33].

Diastolic function

Adequate cardiac function depends not only on systolic contraction but also on isovolumic relaxation and filling during diastole. Isovolumic relaxation is primarily an active energy-dependent process [34] as calcium is actively transported back into the sarcoplasmic reticulum. During the subsequent filling phase, the ventricle is remodeled largely by passive mechanisms [35].

Ventricular or regional myocardial stiffness describes the resistance of the ventricle or a myocardial region to stretch. Ventricular stiffness is defined as the ratio of changes in pressure to changes in volume (dP/dV) during the filling phase. Ventricular and regional myocardial stiffness increase during ventricular filling along a given diastolic pressure-volume or pressure-regional dimension relationship, respectively. To characterize mechanical tissue properties, stiffness is therefore usually determined at end-diastole. Changes in myocardial tissue properties are reflected by displacements of the diastolic pressure-volume or pressure-regional dimension relationship, respectively. Myocardial scar formation increases stiffness; the end-diastolic pressure-volume or the pressure-regional dimension relationship, respectively, is displaced left- and upwards. With a closed pericardium, pericardial scar formation or intrapericardial effusions will also increase stiffness.

Interaction between right and left ventricle

The right ventricle, in comparison to the left ventricle, can handle an increase in volume better than an increase in pressure [36]. Small increments in pulmonary artery pressure are associated with sharp decreases in right ventricular stroke volume [37]. Acute right heart failure occurs with massive pulmonary embolism, and chronic right heart failure develops with chronic lung disease. The normal right ventricle is less stiff than the left ventricle, not because of any intrinsic differences in muscle properties but because of the thinner right ventricular wall.

As the two ventricles operate in series, left ventricular output decreases when right ventricular output decreases. Mechanical ventilation with positive end-exspiratory pressure (PEEP) impacts on both right and left ventricular function. The increased intrathoracic pressure impedes venous return and at the same time decreases AL by facilitation of aortic flow from the thoracic into the abdominal compartment [38]. The simultaneous reduction in PL and AL during PEEP will be of particular benefit for patients with ischemic heart disease. Cardiac output during PEEP will be the net effect of the simultaneous reduction in PL and AL.

Nonuniformity and asynchrony

In the normal heart, a physiological nonuniformity of activation, distribution of load, and inactivation exists [39,40]. Electrical activation starts in the right atrium, is delayed in the AV-node, and then spreading in the ventricles from apex to base. This physiological nonuniformity of electrical activation guarantees an optimal efficiency of filling and contraction, finally directing blood towards the outflow tract during ejection. In the presence of regional myocardial dysfunction, nonuniformity is enhanced. Such increase in nonuniformity is observed during myocardial ischemia and reperfusion when the ischemic and nonischemic myocardial regions contract asynchronously and the dysfunctional region reaches the maximum of wall deformation after the end of systole [41,42]. Systolic hyperkinesis develops in the normal region surrounding an ischemic area. This hyperkinesis can probably not be classified as compensatory as it occurs mainly during isovolumic contraction when the nonischemic zone stretches the ischemic zone [43]. Thus, blood is redistributed within the ventricle rather than being ejected through the aortic valve [44]. It is unclear, whether the increased deformation of normal myocardial regions during systole really represents increased myocardial work or merely results from altered regional loading conditions.

Techniques for the assessment of cardiac, ventricular, and regional myocardial function

While neglecting work spent for internal deformation and for the acceleration of blood during ejection, the assessment of pressure-volume loops would nevertheless be desirable in the clinical setting. However, the generation of pressure-volume loops implies invasive measurements of left ventricular pressure and sophisticated techniques for the assessment of volume (e.g., cine computertomography). Therefore, measures of cardiac, ventricular, and regional myocardial function are often derived from measurements of pressure and ventricular or regional myocardial dimensions.

Indicator-dilution techniques, in particular the thermo-dilution technique, are widely used in clinical practice to measure cardiac output. The thermodilution technique does not require an arterial puncture and uses saline as an inert, inexpensive indicator [45,46] (Table 19.1).

Intravascular pressure can be measured by a fluid-filled catheter-transducer system [47], which is, however, subject to artifacts (Table 19.1). Catheter-tip manometers provide much higher fidelity pressure wave forms and thus allow more precise measurements [48] (Table 19.1). Cine magnetic resonance imaging (MRI) [49–51] and cine computertomography (CT) [52–54] permit scans at various anatomical levels with a temporal resolution of 20 to 50 msec. The cine MRI/CT scanner allows cardiac imaging in real time without the need for ECG gating. By spatial reconstruction of the ventricular chamber from the single scans [53] ventricular volume is fairly accurately measured (Table 19.1). With the gating mode, MRI/CT scan data and ECG are recorded simultaneously [49,55]. Subsequently, the image is reconstructed at selected time points. Both cine and gated MRI/CT scanning provide information on dynamic wall motion and on changes in wall thickness. The conductance catheter continuously determines changes in ventricular volume over time [56] (Table 19.1).

Different from techniques that directly measure absolute (cine MRI/CT) or relative changes (conductance catheter) in ventricular volume, volume is estimated from measurements of cavity deformation with the assumption that the ventricular cavity is shaped like an ellipsoid with one major and two minor diameters [57]. However, following changes of the geometrical configuration (e.g., with regional wall motion disorders, or mitral valve

Table 19.1. Techniques for the assessment of cardiac, ventricular, and regional myocardial function.

Measure	Device	Limitations
cardiac output	indicator-dilution catheter	**invasive**, artifacts due to indicator injection
pressure	fluid-filled catheter-transducer system	**invasive**, artifacts due to micro-bubbles and oscillations
	miniature pressure transducer	**invasive**, artifacts due to motion of the catheter
volume directly assessed	magnetic resonance imaging (cine mode)	**non-invasive**, limited availability, artifacts due to motion and rotation of the ventricle, expensive
	computertomography (cine mode)	**non-invasive**, radiation, limited availability, artifacts due to motion and rotation of the ventricle, expensive
	conductance catheter	**invasive**, artifacts due to conductivity outside the ventricular blood pool
volume calculated from cavity deformation using geometrical assumptions	magnetic resonance imaging (gated mode)	
	computertomography (gated mode)	see cine mode
	contrast ventriculography (cine mode)	**invasive**, radiation, reactions to contrast agent, no information on wall thickness
	radiopaque markers	**invasive**, radiation, traumatic implantation, limited use in patients
	sonomicrometry	**invasive**, traumatic implantation, limited use in patients
	transesophageal echocardiography	**semi-invasive**, artifacts due to motion and rotation of the ventricle
	echocardiography	**non-invasive**, artifacts due to motion and rotation of the ventricle, not applicable in a significant number of patients
	radionuclide ventriculography	**non-invasive**, radiation, artifacts due to motion and rotation of the ventricle, no information on wall thickness

replacement), these methods result in inaccurate estimates of ventricular volume [57]. Also the estimation of right ventricular volume is not possible, since the right ventricle is not shaped like an ellipsoid [58].

Selective cine contrast ventriculography is the standard tool for evaluating changes in wall motion [59]. Selective cine contrast ventriculography with small cut films provides a larger number of sequential observations (30–60 frames per sec). Larger cut films are exposed less frequently (6–12 frames per sec) with improved edge detection of the opacified chamber [59] (Table

19.1). Gated digital subtraction ventriculography [60] has not gained wide acceptance because of its methodological complexity and greater expense.

Radiopaque markers sutured to the epicardium in mammals and postoperatively in man render a more accurate assessment of both dynamic wall motion and wall thickness than selective cine ventriculography [61–63] (Table 19.1). Sonomicrometry is an invasive and rather traumatic technique to measure dynamic wall motion [57,64], wall thickness [65,66], and segment length [65,66] (Table 19.1). Wall thickening provides an integrated measure of regional transmural deformation, whereas segment shortening is a measure of changes within a specific layer of the ventricular wall. Improper alignment of the ultrasonic crystals with respect to the local fiber orientation results in an underestimation of regional myocardial function [67]. Recently, the use of sonomicrometry has been introduced for the postoperative assessment of wall thickening in patients [14]. Although the application of a Doppler probe is less traumatic than the implantation of subendocardial crystals for the measurement of wall thickness and segment length, this technique cannot provide data on absolute wall thickness because the Doppler probe measures tissue displacement. Therefore, regional myocardial function may be underestimated, since wall thickening of subendocardial layers which contribute most to transmural thickening is inadequately assessed [14].

Transesophageal echocardiography (TEE) is a semi-invasive technique for the intra- and perioperative assessment of both dynamic wall motion and changes in wall thickness [68,69]. The future development of biplane TEE probes with multiple ultrasound sources will permit a three-dimensional reconstruction of the heart, similar to the real time imaging of cine MRI/CT techniques [68,69].

Apart from MRI and CT techniques mentioned above, non-invasive methods for assessing cardiac deformation include M-mode-echocardiography [70], 2D-echocardiography [71], and radionuclide ventriculography [72]. In contrast to these echocardiographic techniques, radionuclide ventriculography yields only information on dynamic wall motion (Table 19.1).

Parameters for the assessment of systolic function

Clear consciousness, sufficient urine excretion and adequate oxygenation of peripheral tissues may be taken as indirect though unspecific evidence of adequate cardiac function. Of course, cardiac output, i.e. the volume ejected within systole (stroke volume) times heart rate, is a more accurate measure of cardiac function (Table 19.2). Cardiac index normalizes cardiac output to body surface and thus accounts for interindividual variations. Cardiac output is dependent on PL, AL, C, and HR, and is inversely related to the hematocrit [73].

The maximum developed pressure is used only in isolated heart preparations; it is markedly affected by changes in PL, AL, C, and HR [18]. Stroke

Table 19.2. Parameters of cardiac, ventricular, and regional myocardial function.

Parameter	Calculation	Limitation
cardiac output (global)	$(V_{ED}\text{-}V_{ES})*HR$	dependent on: PL, AL, C, HR
stroke work (global)	$\int_{ED1}^{ED2} (P - P_{min}) * V\, dV$	dependent on: PL, AL, C, HR
ejection fraction (global)	$(V_{ED}\text{-}V_{ES})/V_{ED}$	dependent on: PL, AL, C, HR
fractional shortening (global)	$(D_{ED}\text{-}D_{ES})/D_{ED}$	dependent on: PL, AL, C, HR
mean velocity of circumferential fiber shortening (global)	$(D_{ED}\text{-}D_{ES})/SI$	dependent on: (PL), AL, C, (HR)
wall thickening (regional)	$(WT_{ES}\text{-}WT_{ED})/WT_{ED}$	dependent on: PL, AL, C, HR
segment shortening (regional)	$(SL_{ED}\text{-}SL_{ES})/SL_{ED}$	dependent on: PL, AL, C, HR
mean velocity of wall thickening (regional)	$(WT_{ES}\text{-}WT_{ED})/SI$	dependent on: (PL), AL, C, (HR)
mean velocity of segment shortening (regional)	$(SL_{ED}\text{-}SL_{ES})/SI$	dependent on: (PL), AL, C, (HR)

AL: afterload, C: contractility, D: diameter (minor axis), ED: end-diastole, ES: end-systole, HR: heart rate, P: pressure, PL: preload, SI: duration of systolic interval, SL: segment length, V: volume, WT: wall thickness.

work is the product of pressure and volume integrated over the cardiac cycle and is represented by the area of the pressure-volume loop (Table 19.2). Stroke work depends on PL, AL, C, and HR, and does not account for the time component of contraction and the position of the loop with respect to the end-diastolic pressure-volume curve (Table 19.2).

To account for interindividual variations in end-diastolic volume or dimension, respectively, the extent of ejected volume or deformation occurring within systole is normalized to the end-diastolic volume or dimension, i.e. ejection fraction or fractional shortening [74,75] (Table 19.2). On the regional level, the extent of systolic deformation is normalized to the end-diastolic dimension and expressed as systolic wall thickening or systolic segment shortening. Ejection fraction, fractional shortening, systolic wall thickening, and systolic segment shortening are all affected by changes in PL, AL, C, and HR. The velocity of circumferential fiber shortening is the deformation within systole normalized to the duration of the systolic interval, and thus accounts for the time component of deformation. The correlate to the velocity of circumferential fiber shortening on the regional myocardial level is the velocity of systolic wall thickening or segment shortening (Table 19.2). Velocity parameters are affected to a minor extent by changes in PL and HR but remain sensitive to changes in AL and C. In contrast to mean velocities, peak velocities are more sensitive to artifacts since peak velocities are measured only at a certain time point during systole.

To specifically judge the success of an operative intervention on ventricular and regional myocardial function, parameters are preferable that are sensitive to changes in C only and not dependent on loading conditions.

The maximum first derivative of left ventricular pressure (dP/dt_{max}) is a standard reference for the assessment of ventricular C [76]. Although dP/dt_{max} is not a very specific measure for C, it is highly sensitive to changes in C [77–79] as long as dP/dt_{max} occurs during the isovolumic systole. In the case of an aortic insufficiency, dP/dt_{max} may occur after aortic valve opening and thus be no longer an isovolumic index. The maximum ratio of dP/dt to the corresponding pressure or the ratio of pressure change at a developed pressure of 40 mmHg to that pressure are isovolumic indices of C under all circumstances [76,79–81]. These indices of C are, almost by definition, insensitive to changes in AL, but remain sensitive to alterations in PL [77,79,82], HR [77], and muscle mass [77] (Table 19.3).

Based on simultaneous measurements of left ventricular pressure and ventricular dimensions and a number of geometrical and physiological assumptions, sophisticated calculations provide measures such as the maximal shortening velocity of contractile elements [81,83]. However, such measures are neither easily feasible nor free from substantial methodological problems (Table 19.3).

The slope of the end-systolic pressure-volume relationship [18] or the maximal slope of the pressure-volume relationship [84] have been used to assess C (Table 19.3). The pressure-volume relationship is obtained by varying PL and AL with infusion of vasodilating [85] or vasoconstricting agents [85–87]. Postoperatively, loading conditions can be manipulated using the heart-lung-machine [88]. The slope of the end-systolic pressure-volume relationship or the maximal slope of the pressure-volume relationship do not account for changes in muscle mass, and thus, make an interindividual comparison of these indices difficult. The slope of the end-systolic pressure-volume relationship is highly specific in measuring C, but of limited sensitivity [89].

The stroke work-end-diastolic volume relationship integrates systolic and diastolic properties and is largely independent of loading conditions [90,91]. The slope of the stroke work-end-diastolic volume relationship as a measure

Table 19.3. Parameters of ventricular and regional myocardial contractility.

Parameter	Calculation	Limitation
maximum first derivative of LVP (global)	dP/dt_{max}	dependent on: PL, (AL), HR, MM
ratio of pressure change at a developed pressure of 40 mmHg to that pressure (global)	$\frac{dP/dt(LVP_{ED}+40\,mmHg)}{(LVP_{ED}+40\,mmHg)}$	dependent on: PL, HR, MM
velocity of shortening of unloaded contractile elements (global)	extrapolation of the force-velocity relationship to zero force	dependent on: HR and numerous assumptions
slope of the end-systolic pressure-volume relationship (global)	dP_{ES}/dV_{Es}	limited to a single time point within the cardiac cycle
slope of the stroke work-end-diastolic volume relationship (global)	dSW/dV_{ED}	integrating systolic and diastolic properties
slope of the end-systolic presure-wall thickness relationship (regional)	dP_{ES}/dWT_{ES}	limited to a single time point within the cardiac cycle
slope of the end-systolic pressure-segment length relationship (regional)	dP_{ES}/dSL_{ES}	

AL: afterload, ED: end-diastole, ES: end-systole, HR: heart rate, LVP: left ventricular pressure, MM: muscle mass, P: pressure, PL: preload, SL: segment length, t: time, V: volume, WT: wall thickness.

of C is linear over a wide range of end-diastolic volumes. At low end-diastolic volumes, the slope of the stroke work-end-diastolic volume relationship represents mostly systolic properties, whereas at higher end-diastolic volumes diastolic properties predominate [92] (Table 19.3).

On the regional level, the slope of the end-systolic pressure-wall thickness or pressure-segment length relationship has been proposed as an index of regional myocardial C [93,94] (see also Appendix). The end-systolic pressure-wall thickness or pressure-segment length relationship is curvilinear but may be extrapolated linearly within a physiological pressure range (80–150 mmHg) [25,93,94] (Table 19.3).

Parameters for the assessment of diastolic function

The isovolumic pressure fall is characterized by the time constant τ derived from an exponential fit of pressure fall during isovolumic diastole. τ decreases with negative inotropic interventions, with a decrease in maximal ventricular pressure, and with asynchronous contraction [95,96].

Diastolic ventricular filling is commonly assessed by the maximum filling rate, the time from end-systole to maximum filling rate, and the mean velocity of rapid filling. On the regional myocardial level, the mean velocity of wall thinning or of segment lengthening are used to assess diastolic filling [97]. The extent and the velocity of filling are dependent on HR and the driving atrio-ventricular pressure gradient [98]. Furthermore, if isovolumic relaxation is not complete and extends into the filling phase, diastolic filling is impaired.

Assessment of cardiac, ventricular, and regional myocardial function following cardioplegic arrest – overview of the literature

The maintenance of an adequate cardiac function is the main goal in the postoperative phase following open heart surgery since an adequate cardiac function ultimately determines the survival of the patient. The success of the surgical procedure as such is reflected by the improvement of ventricular (e.g., cardiac valve replacement) and/or regional myocardial function (e.g., coronary bypass grafting). In order to determine the influence of the surgical procedure on the genuine muscle properties, C must be assessed.

The recovery of cardiac, ventricular, and regional myocardial function is largely dependent on the duration of the preceding cardioplegic arrest. In normal canine hearts *in situ*, cardiac and ventricular function were not different from control conditions following 1 h and 2 h of cardioplegic arrest with non-oxygenated crystalloid solution [99]. Following 2 h of cardioplegic arrest with non-oxygenated crystalloid solution, ventricular C was consistently depressed at 30 min of reperfusion [100–102], with a complete recovery of ventricular C within 60 min of reperfusion [100,102,103]. Following 2 h of cardioplegic arrest, the recovery of ventricular C was better with oxygenated crystalloid and blood cardioplegia than with non-oxygenated crystalloid cardioplegia [100,102]. With 3 h of cardioplegic arrest using non-oxygenated crystalloid solution in normal canine hearts, cardiac and ventricular function were significantly decreased at 30 min of reperfusion with no further recovery after 60 min of reperfusion [99].

In contrast to normal canine hearts, cardiac output, ejection fraction, and stroke work in patients undergoing coronary bypass grafting initially declined following 1 h of cardioplegic arrest using non-oxygenated crystalloid solution. Cardiac and ventricular function were most depressed between 2 h and 6 h postoperatively and subsequently normalized within 24 h to 7 days [104–110]. In another group of patients, postoperative ventricular function after 1 h of cardioplegic arrest decreased in half of the patients whereas in the other half of patients ventricular function increased in the postoperative phase. In all patients, parameters of ventricular function were back to preoperative values within 7 days [111].

More recently, Bolli *et al.* analyzed regional myocardial wall thickening with an ultrasonic Doppler probe in patients undergoing coronary bypass grafting. On average, regional myocardial function remained unchanged but a marked interindividual variability was observed. In half of the patients regional myocardial function was decreased whereas in the other half it was increased 4 h after the operation [14].

Studies looking particularly at C (as measured by the slope of the end-systolic pressure-volume relationship or the stroke work-end-diastolic volume relationship) revealed no impairment of left ventricular C following 1 h of cardioplegic arrest [88,112,113]. Thus, the impairment of postoperative ventricular or regional myocardial function following 1 h of cardioplegic arrest may result from changes in PL and AL associated with hypothermia and the artificial non-pulsatile perfusion during the extracorporal circulation rather than a depression of C.

Whereas left ventricular C seems to be well preserved with current cardioplegic techniques [88,112,113], this is not necessarily the case for the preservation of right ventricular C. After 1 h of cardioplegic arrest using non-oxygenated cardioplegic solutions, right ventricular C was significantly depressed [114–116], while left ventricular C remained unchanged. This different recovery of C in the right and left ventricle results in a substantial contractile asynergy between both ventricles and may contribute to a depression of overall cardiac function [117]. In contrast to the recovery of C, recovery of diastolic function, as assessed by end-diastolic pressure-volume curves, was equally well preserved after 1 h of cardioplegic arrest in the right and left ventricle [114,115].

Limitations of experimental and clinical studies in the assessment of cardioplegic arrest

The perfusion of isolated hearts [118–127] with Krebs-Henseleit or oxygenated Ringer solution subjects the heart to ischemic conditions already under basal resting conditions [121,128] resulting in a non-stable preparation. Thus, variations in the recovery of ventricular function following 2 h of cardioplegic arrest ranging from 30 to 80% of control [118–127] may be related at least partially to the instability of the preparation *per se*.

The *in vivo* model[99–103,129,130] is a more stable preparation. However, cardioplegic arrest in healthy animal hearts can only to a limited extent be extrapolated to cardioplegic arrest in the diseased heart of man. Postoperative recovery of ventricular and regional myocardial function in the diseased heart is always the net effect of the cardioplegic arrest, the type of underlying heart disease, and the success of the surgical intervention. Whereas the cardioplegic arrest potentially impairs postoperative ventricular and/or regional myocardial function, the operation *per se* is performed to improve ventricular and/or regional myocardial function. It is difficult, if not impossible, to compare pre-, peri-, and postoperative function adequately, as the recovery of ventricular and/or regional myocardial function is affected by the temperature of the heart [131], the depth of anesthesia [132] the formation of pericardial clots [133], the level of pharmacological intervention (i.e., inotropic support and/or vasodilator therapy) [134,135], and the intrinsic level of catecholamines [136,137].

Recovery of function versus recovery of metabolism, electrophysiology, and morphology following cardioplegic arrest

Depending on the duration of the cardioplegic arrest, high energy phosphates (ATP, creatine phosphate) and glycogen contents are reduced at the end of ischemia. At this time point, lactate consumption is converted to lactate production [113,138,139]. Creatine phosphate [4,112,119,139] and glycogen content [139] rapidly return to preischemic values within 30 min of reperfusion. A discrepancy between the fast recovery of creatine phosphate and the gradual recovery of ventricular and regional myocardial function following reversible ischemia has been previously reported [9,140,141]. ATP content decreases less markedly and at a slower rate than creatine phosphate content during ischemia and also recovers more slowly during reperfusion [9,119,125,126]. However, since the reperfused myocardium responds to inotropic stimulation, a limitation of energy supply can be excluded as the underlying mechanism for depressed ventricular or regional myocardial function [142–147]. Lactate production is reversed to lactate consumption within 30 min of reperfusion [113,138,139], whereas the recovery of ventricular function lacks behind. Following the removal of aortic cross-clamping, either ventricular fibrillation or spontaneous sinus rhythm with no detectable ST-T segment elevation may occur. Neither the occurrence of ventricular fibrillation nor transient ST-T segment elevations predict the subsequent recovery of ventricular function [13–15,148]. Elevated CK-MB levels following cardioplegic arrest indicate irreversible myocardial damage. Unless a perioperative infarction occurs, there is no enzyme leakage due to cardioplegic arrest *per se* [4,15,139,148,149]. With the current techniques of cardioplegia, structural alterations such as loss of mitochondrial granulation and a clarified mitochondrial matrix [150–152], as well as an increase in myocardial water content occur only to a minor extent [150,151]. Subcellular alterations are difficult to quantify with current morphometric techniques, and the time course of these alterations in the clinical setting is difficult to follow. Neither the myocardial water content nor mitochondrial alterations predict the recovery of ventricular or regional myocardial function in the reperfusion period [15,149] (Table 19.4). In the presence of reversible impairment of postoperative ventricular and regional myocardial function, i.e., with myocardial stunning, ventricular and regional myocardial function gradually recover upon reperfusion. However, the time course and the extent of functional recovery do not correlate with the recovery of metabolic, electrophysiological, and morphological parameters (Table 19.4). Whereas metabolic, electrophysio-

Table 19.4. Postoperative changes of ventricular function, metabolic, electrophysiological, and morphological parameters as compared to preoperative values following 1 h of cardioplegic arrest in patients.

	Cross clamp release	30 min R	2–6 h R	48 h-7 days R
ventricular function	–	–	–, +	ϕ
	[104–111]	[104–111]	[104–110] [111]	[104–111]
CP content (B)	–	ϕ	ϕ	ϕ
	[13,112,139]	[13,112,139]	[13]	[13]
ATP content (B)	ϕ, –	ϕ, –	ϕ	ϕ
	[139] [13,112]	[139 [13,112]	[13,112,139]	[13,112,139]
glycogen content (B)	ϕ, +	ϕ	NDA	NDA
	[139] [15]	[15,139]		
lactate consumption (CS)	production	ϕ	ϕ	ϕ
	[112,113,139]	[112,113,139]	[112,113,139]	[112,113,139]
ST-T segment	ϕ	ϕ	ϕ	ϕ
	[13–15,149]	[13–15,149]	[13–15,149]	[13–15,149]
CK-MB (PB)	ϕ	ϕ	ϕ	ϕ
	[112,149]	[112,149]	[112,149]	[112,149]
mitochondrial integrity (B)	ϕ	ϕ	ϕ	ϕ
	[15]	[15]	[15]	[15]

+ increased, ϕ = unchanged, – = decreased, ATP = adenosine triphosphate, B = biopsy, CK-MB = myocardial creatine kinase, CP = creatine phosphate, CS = coronary sinus blood, NDA = no data available, PB = peripheral blood, R = reperfusion.

logical, and morphological parameters are quickly normalized during early reperfusion, the depression of ventricular and regional myocardial function is more longlasting. Thus, the recovery of the heart from ischemic cardioplegic arrest is most sensitively characterized by parameters of ventricular and regional myocardial function, in particular ventricular and regional myocardial C.

Conclusions

Cardiac function ultimately determines the survival of the patient. Ventricular and regional myocardial function depend on both loading conditions and contractility. Loading conditions and contractility, in turn, are affected by the underlying disease, the cardioplegic arrest, the surgical procedure, and pharmacological interventions. The adequate assessment of cardiac, ventricular, and regional myocardial function requires a clear definition of terms, a thorough knowledge of physiological and pathological determinants of contractile function, and the use of adequate techniques and parameters to obtain valid information on the detailed problem under question. Using current cardioplegic techniques in the clinical setting, cardiac, ventricular and regional myocardial function are decreased during reperfusion if the time of cardioplegic arrest is extended beyond 1 h. Following 1 h of cardioplegic arrest, left ventricular C is well preserved with current cardioplegic techniques whereas right ventricular C is already depressed. When the duration of cardioplegic arrest in patients is extended beyond 1 h, C is also depressed in the left ventricle.

At present, functional recovery following cardioplegic arrest cannot be predicted by metabolic, electrophysiological, and morphological parameters. Thus, contractile function has to be evaluated as a separate entity.

Appendix

To evaluate a new technique of mitral valve reconstruction, experiments were performed in anesthetized dogs (in cooperation with H. Korb and A. Borowski, Dept. of Thoracic and Cardiovascular Surgery, University of Cologne). In 3 sham-operated dogs the effect of 1 h normothermic cardioplegic arrest using a single dose (300 ml/10 kg) of Bretschneider's HTK-solution on ventricular and regional myocardial function as well as C was studied during 240 min of reperfusion. Measurements were performed under resting conditions, during PL reduction (blood withdrawal from left ventricular atrium), during an increase in AL (inflation of an intraaortic balloon) and during an increase in C (epinephrine 1 mg/min i.v.). Left ventricular end-diastolic pressure, maximal left ventricular pressure, dP/dt_{max} stroke volume (SV), end-diastolic (V_{ED}) and end-systolic left ventricular volume (V_{ES}) and stroke work (SW) were determined in order to assess left ventricular function. To assess regional myocardial function, systolic wall thickening as percent of enddiastolic wall thickness (%WT) and the mean systolic wall thickening velocity (MV) were determined using sonomicrometry. During PL reduction and AL increase, end-diastolic and end-systolic left ventricular pressure-wall thickness relationships were generated. V_{ED} and V_{ES} were estimated using a method described by Schipke *et al.* [25] based on wall thickness analyses with sonomicrometry.

The slopes and intercepts of the end-diastolic left ventricular pressure-wall thickness relationship did not change significantly following 1 h of cardioplegic arrest. Thus, structural damage of the left ventricle did presumably not occur. Under resting conditions, load-sensitive parameters of ventricular function such as SV and SW were significantly decreased at 2 h and 4 h of reperfusion, whereas dP/dt_{max} remained unchanged. During reperfusion, load-sensitive parameters of regional myocardial function (%WT, MV) were unchanged under resting conditions (Table 19.5).

The slope of the end-systolic pressure-wall thickness relationship, as a measure of regional C, was significantly decreased at 2 h and 4 h of reperfusion. A depressed C following 1 h cardioplegic arrest is in contrast to studies cited above. This discrepancy is probably related to an enhanced myocardial stunning that occurs with suboptimal cardioplegia using only a

Table 19.5. Hemodynamic data during control conditions (CON), and at 2 h and 4 h reperfusion (REP) following 1 h of normothermic cardioplegic arrest.

	HR	LVP_{ED}	LVP_{max}	dP/dt_{max}	% WT	MV	SV	CO	SW
CON	114 ± 7	4.0 ± 0.1	99 ± 10	1384 ± 337	13.3 ± 3.7	5.00 ± 1.03	29.7 ± 2.2	3.58 ± 0.26	1.34 ± 0.34
60 min NORMOTHERMIC ISCHEMIC ARREST, HTK-CARDIOPLEGIA									
2 h REP	125 ± 25	6.0 ± 6.0	80 ± 7*	1300 ± 337	15.0 ± 5.0	5.58 ± 2.00	23.3 ± 1.2	2.99 ± 0.37	0.66 ± 0.20*
4 h REP	117 ± 24	7.6 ± 6.7	80 ± 2*	1213 ± 66	13.2 ± 4.4	4.63 ± 1.36	21.2 ± 2.3	2.47 ± 0.18	0.58 ± 0.03*

CO (l/min): cardiac output; dP/dt_{max} (mmHg/s): maximum value of the first derivative of left ventricular pressure; HR (beats/min): heart rate; LVP_{ED} (mmHg): left ventricular end-diastolic pressure; LVP_{max} (mmHg): maximum left ventricular pressure; MV (mm/s): mean systolic wall thickening velocity; SV (ml): stroke volume; SW (Nm): stroke work; %WT: systolic wall thickening as percent of end-diastolic wall thickness; data are mean ± SD, n = 3; * $p < 0.05$ vs. control.

single dose application during normothermia. During inotropic stimulation with epinephrine, the increases in dP/dt_{max}, %WT, and MV were significantly attenuated at 2 h and 4 h of reperfusion. Thus, despite a failure of load-dependent parameters to detect ventricular dysfunction under resting conditions, these parameters consistently indicated contractile dysfunction during an inotropic challenge.

References

1. Melrose DG, Dreyer B, Bentall HH. Elective cardiac arrest: Preliminary communication. Lancet 1955; 2: 21–2.
2. Bretschneider HJ. Überlebenszeit und Wiederbelebungszeit des Herzens bei Normo- und Hypothermie. Verh Dtsch Ges Kreislaufforsch 1964; 30: 11–34.
3. Hearse DJ, Stewart DA, Braimbridge MV. Cellular protection during myocardial ischemia. The development and characterization of a procedure for the induction of reversible ischemic arrest. Circulation 1976; 54: 193–202.
4. Follette DM, Mulder DG, Maloney JV Jr. *et al.* Advantages of blood cardioplegia over continuous coronary perfusion or intermittent ischemia. J Thorac Cardiovasc Surg 1978; 76: 604–19.
5. Engelman RM, Rousou JM, Vertrees RA *et al.* Safety of prolonged ischemic arrest using hypothermic cardioplegia. J Thorac Cardiovasc Surg 1980; 79: 705–13.
6. Floyd RD, Sabiston DC, Lee KL *et al.* The effect of duration of hypothermic cardioplegia on ventricular function. J Thorac Cardiovasc Surg 1983; 85: 606 -11.
7. Silverman NA, Wright R, Levitsky S *et al.* Efficacy of crystalloid cardioplegic solutions in patients undergoing myocardial revascularization. J Thorac Cardiovasc Surg 1985; 89: 90–5.
8. Bolli R, Hartley CJ, Rabinovitz RS *et al.* Clinical relevance of myocardial "stunning". Cardiovasc Drugs Ther 1991; 5: 877–90.
9. Guth BD, Martin JF, Heusch G *et al.* Regional myocardial blood flow, function and metabolism using phosphorus-31 nuclear magnetic resonance spectroscopy during ischemia and reperfusion. J Am Coll Cardiol 1987; 10: 673–81.
10. Ambrosio G, Jacobus WE, Bergmann CA *et al.* Preserved high energy phosphate metabolic reserve in globally stunned hearts despite reduction of basal ATP content and contractility. J Mol Cell Cardiol 1987; 19: 953–64.
11. Guth BD, Wisneski JA, Neese R *et al.* Myocardial lactate release during ischemia in swine. Relation to regional blood flow. Circulation 1990; 81: 1948–958.
12. Goto R, Tearle H, Steward DJ *et al.* Myocardial edema and ventricular function after cardioplegia with added mannitol. Can J Anaesth 1991; 38: 7–14.
13. Hearse DJ. The protection of the ischemic myocardium: Surgical success vs. clinical failure? Prog Cardiovasc Dis 1988; 30: 381–402.
14. Bolli R, Hartley CJ, Chelly JE *et al.* An accurate, nontraumatic ultrasonic method to monitor myocardial wall thickening in patients undergoing cardiac surgery. J Am Coll Cardiol 1990; 15: 1055–65.
15. Codd JE, Barner HB, Pennington DG *et al.* Intraoperative myocardial protection: a comparison of blood and asanguineous cardioplegia. Ann Thorac Surg 1985; 39: 125–33.
16. Rogers WJ, Coggin CJ, Gersh BJ *et al.* CASS Investigators. Ten-year follow-up of quality of life in patients randomized to receive medical therapy or coronary artery bypass graft surgery. Circulation 1990; 82: 1647–58.
17. Chaitman BR, Ryan TJ, Kronmal RA *et al.* CASS Investigators. Coronary artery surgery study (CASS): comparability of 10 year survival in randomized and randomizable patients. J Am Coll Cardiol 1990; 16: 1071–8.

18. Sagawa, K, Sunagawa, K, Maughan WL. Ventricular end-systolic pressure-volume relations. In Levine HJ, Gaasch WH (eds): The Ventricle. Boston: Martinus Nijhoff 1985; 79–82.
19. Waldman LK, Fung YC, Covell JW: Transmural myocardial deformation in the canine left ventricle. Circ Res 1985; 57: 152–63.
20. Trautwein W, Gauer OH, Koepchen HP *et al.* In Gauer OH (ed): Physiologie des Menschen. München Berlin Wien: Urban & Schwarzenberg 1972.
21. Bretschneider HJ, Hellige G. Pathophysiologie der Ventrikelkontraktion-Kontraktilität, Inotropie, Suffiziensgrad und Arbeitsökonomie des Herzens. Verh Dtsch Ges Kreislaufforsch 1976; 42: 14–30.
22. Frank O. Zur Dynamik des Herzmuskels. Z Biol 1895; 32: 370–447.
23. Alexander J, Burkhoff D, Schipke J *et al.* Influence of mean pressure on aortic impedance and reflections in the systemic arterial system. Am J Physiol 1989; 257: H969–H978.
24. Sonnenblick EH. Force-velocity relations in mammalian heart muscle. Am J Physiol 1962; 202: 931–39.
25. Schipke JD, Alexander J Jr, Harasawa Y *et al.* Interrelation between end-systolic pressure-volume and pressure-wall thickness relations. Am J Physiol 1988; 255: H679–H684.
26. Raff WK, Kosche F, Lochner W. Herzfrequenz und extravasale Komponente des Coronarwiderstandes. Pfluegers Arch 1971; 323: 241–9.
27. Covell JW, Ross J Jr, Taylor R *et al.* Effects of increasing frequency of contraction on the force velocity relation of left ventricle. Cardiovasc Res 1967; 1: 2–8.
28. Mahler F, Yoran C, Ross J Jr. Inotropic effects of tachycardia and poststimulation potentiation in the conscious dog. Am J Physiol 1974; 227: 569–75.
29. Ross J Jr. Afterload mismatch and preload reserve: a conceptual framework for the analysis of ventricular function. Prog Cardiovasc Dis 1976; 18: 255–64.
30. Lee JD, Tajimi T, Patritti J *et al.* Preload reserve and mechanisms of afterload mismatch in normal conscious dogs. Am J Physiol 1986; 250: H464–H473.
31. Jacob R, Gulch RW. Functional significance of ventricular dilatation. Reconsideration of Linzbach's concept of chronic heart failure. Basic Res Cardiol 1988; 83: 461–75.
32. Sasayama S, Ross J Jr, Franklin D *et al.* Adaptations of left ventricle to chronic pressure overload. Circ Res 1976; 38: 172–8.
33. Linzbach AJ. Heart failure from the point of view of quantitative anatomy. Am J Cardiol 1960; 5: 370–82.
34. Grossman W, McLaurin LP, Moos SP *et al.* Wall thickness and diastolic properties of the left ventricle. Circulation 1974; 49: 129–35.
35. Nikolic SD, Yellin EL, Dahm M *et al.* Relationship between diastolic shape (eccentricity) and passive elastic properties in canine left ventricle. Am J Physiol 1990; 259: H457–H463.
36. Burkhoff D, Yue DT, Franz MR *et al.* Quantitative comparison of the force-interval relationships of the canine right and left ventricles. Circ Res 1984; 54: 468–73.
37. Feneley MP, Olsen CO, Glower DD *et al.* Effect of acutely increased right ventricular afterload on work output from the left ventricle in conscious dogs. Systolic ventricular interaction. Circ Res 1989; 65: 135–45.
38. Peters J, Fraser C, Stuart RS *et al.* Negative intrathoracic pressure decreases independently left ventricular filling and emptying. Am J Physiol 1989; 257: H120–H131.
39. Brutsaert DL: Nonuniformity: a physiologic modulator of contraction and relaxation of normal heart. J Am Coll Cardiol 1987; 9: 341–8.
40. Antzelevitch C, Sicouri S, Litovsky SH *et al.* Heterogeneity within the ventricular wall. Electrophysiology and pharmacology of epicardial, endocardial, and M cells. Circ Res 1991; 69: 1427–49.
41. Heusch G, Guth BD, Widmann T *et al.* Ischemic myocardial dysfunction assessed by temporal Fourier transform of regional myocardial wall thickening. Am Heart J 1987; 113: 116–24.
42. Ehring T, Heusch G. Left ventricular asynchrony: an indicator of regional myocardial dysfunction. Am Heart J 1990; 120: 1047–57.

43. Lew WYW, Chen Z, Guth BD *et al.* Mechanisms of augmented segment shortening in nonischemic areas during acute ischemia of the canine left ventricle. Circ Res 1985; 56: 351–8.
44. Guth BD, Schulz R, Heusch G. Evaluation of parameters for the assessment of regional myocardial contractile function during asynchronous left ventricular contraction. Basic Res Cardiol 1990; 85: 550–62.
45. Ganz W, Donoso R, Marcus HS *et al.* A new technique for measurements of cardiac output by thermodilution in man. Am J Cardiol 1971; 27: 392–9.
46. Van Grondelle A, Ditchey RV, Groves BM *et al.* Thermodilution method overestimates low cardiac output in humans. Am J Physiol 1983; 245: H690–H697.
47. Li JK, Van Brummelen GW, Nordergraaf A. Fluid-filled blood pressure measurement system. J Appl Physiol 1976; 40: 839–43.
48. Wood EH, Lensen IR, Warner HR *et al.* Measurements of pressure in man by cardiac catheterization. Circ Res 1954; 2: 294–8.
49. Markiewicz W, Sechtem U, Kirby R *et al.* Measurements of ventricular volumes in the dog by magnetic resonance imaging (MRI). J Am Coll Cardiol 1987; 10: 170–6.
50. Gaudio C, Tanzilli G, Mazzarotto P *et al.* Comparison of left ventricular ejection fraction by magnetic resonance imaging and radionuclide ventriculography in idiopathic dilated cardiomyopathy. Am J Cardiol 1991; 67: 411–5.
51. Benjelloun H, Cranney GB, Kirk KA *et al.* Interstudy reproducibility of biplane cine nuclear magnetic resonance measurements of left ventricular function. Am J Cardiol 1991; 67: 1413–20.
52. Lipton MJ, Higgins CB, Farmer D *et al.* Cardiac imaging with a high-speed cine-CT scanner: Preliminary results. Radiology 1983; 152: 579–85.
53. Sinak, LJ, Ritman EL. Dynamic spatial reconstructor. In Sinak LJ, Ritman Lj (eds): CT of the Heart and Great Vessels. Mt. Kisco, NY: Futura Publishing Co 1983; 61–73.
54. Lessick J, Sideman S, Azhari H *et al.* Regional three-dimensional geometry and function of left ventricles with fibrous aneurysms. A cine-computed tomography study. Circulation 1991; 84: 1072–86.
55. Osbakken M, Yuschok T. Evaluation of ventricular function with gated cardiac magnetic resonance imaging. Cathet Cardiovasc Diagn 1986; 12: 156–62.
56. Boltwood CM Jr, Appleyard RF, Glantz SA. Left ventricular volume measurement by conductance catheter in intact dogs. Parallel conductance volume depends on left ventricular size. Circulation 1989; 80: 1360–77.
57. Rankin JS, McHale PA, Arentzen CE *et al.* The three-dimensional dynamic geometry of the left ventricle in the conscious dog. Circ Res 1976; 39: 304–13.
58. Tobinick E, Schelbert HR, Henning H *et al.* Right ventricular ejection fraction in patients with acute anterior and inferior myocardial infarction assessed by radionuclide angiography. Circulation 1978; 57: 1078–84.
59. Dodge HT, Sheehan FH. Quantitative contrast angiography for assessment of ventricular performance in heart disease. J Am Coll Cardiol 1983; 1: 73–8.
60. Kronenberg MW, Price RR, Smith CW *et al.* Evaluation of left ventricular performance using digital subtraction angiography. Am J Cardiol 1983; 51: 837–45.
61. Mitchell JH, Wildenthal K, Mullins CB. Geometrical studies of the left ventricle utilizing biplane cinefluorography. Fed Proc 1969; 28: 1334–43.
62. Shoukas AA, Sagawa K, Maughan WL. Chronic implantation of radiopaque beads on endocardium, midwall, and epicardium. Am J Physiol 1981; 241: H104–H107.
63. Maughan WL, Jenkins RE, Ebert WL. Multiple marker cineventriculogrammetry: a new technique for simultaneous measurement of regional wall motion and overall geometry in animals. In Sigwart U, Heintzen PH (eds): Ventricular Wall Motion. New York: Thieme-Stratton, 1984.
64. Bishop VS, Horwitz LD, Stone HL *et al.* Left ventricular internal diameter and cardiac function in conscious dogs. J Appl Physiol 1969; 27: 619–23.
65. Weintraub WS, Hattori S, Agarwal JB *et al.* The relationship between myocardial blood

flow and contraction by myocardial layer in the canine left ventricle during ischemia. Circ Res 1981; 48: 430–8.

66. Gallagher KP, Kumada T, Koziol JA *et al.* Significance of regional wall thickening abnormalities relative to transmural myocardial perfusion in anesthetized dogs. Circulation 1980; 62: 1266–74.
67. Bugge-Asperheim B, Leraand S, Kiil F. Local dimensional changes of the myocardium measured by ultrasonic technique. Scand J Clin Lab Invest 1969; 24: 361–71.
68. Deutsch HJ, Curtius JM, Leischik R *et al.* Diagnostic value of transesophageal echocardiography in cardiac surgery. Thorac Cardiovasc Surg 1991; 39: 199–204.
69. Seward JB, Khandheria MK, Oh JK *et al.* Transesophageal echocardiography: technique, anatomic, correlations, implementation, and clinical application. Mayo Clin Proc 1988; 63: 649–80.
70. Luisada AA, Singhal A, Portaluppi F. Assessment of left ventricular function by noninvasive methods. Adv Cardiol 1985; 32: 111–7.
71. Tortoledo FA, Quinones MA, Fernandez GC *et al.* Quantification of left ventricular volumes by two-dimensional echocardiography: A simplified and accurate approach. Circulation 1983; 67: 579–86.
72. Kronenberg MW, Parrish MD, Jenkins DW Jr *et al.* Accuracy of radionuclide ventriculography for estimation of left ventricular volume changes and endsystolic pressure volume relations. J Am Coll Cardiol 1985; 6: 1064–72.
73. Faris IB, Iannos J, Jamieson G *et al.* The circulatory effects of acute hypervolemia and hemodilution in conscious rabbits. Circ Res 1981; 48: 825–34.
74. Stamm RB, Carabello BA, Mayers DL *et al.* Two-dimensional echocardiographic measurement of left ventricular ejection fraction: Prospective analysis of what constitutes an adequate determination. Am Heart J 1982; 104: 136–41.
75. Quinones MA, Waggoner AD, Reduto LA *et al.* A new simplified and accurate method for determining ejection fraction with two-dimensional echocardiography. Circulation 1981; 64: 744–8.
76. Mahler F, Ross J Jr, O'Rourke RA *et al.* Effects of changes in preload, afterload and inotropic state on ejection and isovolumic phase measures of contractility in the conscious dog. Am J Cardiol 1975; 35: 626–34.
77. Furnival CM, Linden RJ, Snow HM. Inotropic changes in the left ventricle: The effect of changes in heart rate, aortic pressure and end-diastolic pressure. J Physiol 1970; 211: 359–87.
78. Morgenstern C, Goebel H, Lochner W. Die Beurteilung der Kontraktilität des Herzens. Dtsch Med Wschr 1972; 41: 1563–8.
79. Davidson DM, Covell JW, Malloch CI *et al.* Factors influencing indices of left ventricular contractility in the conscious dog. Cardiovasc Res 1974; 8: 299–312.
80. Mason DT, Braunwald E, Covell JW *et al.* Assessment of cardiac contractility. The relation between the rate of pressure rise and ventricular pressure during isovolumic systole. Circulation 1971; 44: 47–58.
81. Mehmel H, Krayenbuehl HP, Rutishauser W. Peak measured velocity of shortening in the canine left ventricle. J Appl Physiol 1970; 29: 637–45.
82. Peterson KL, Sklovan D, Ludbrook P *et al.* Comparison of isovolumic and ejection phase indices of myocardial performance in man. Circulation 1974; 49: 1088–92.
83. Hugenholtz PG, Ellison RC, Urschel CW *et al.* Myocardial force-velocity relationships in clinical heart disease. Circulation 1970; 41: 191–202.
84. Suga H, Sagawa K. Instantaneous pressure-volume relationships and their ratio in the excised, supported canine left ventricle. Circ Res 1974; 35: 117–26.
85. McKay RG, Aroesty JM, Heller GV *et al.* Assessment of the end-systolic pressure-volume relationship in human beings with the use of a time-varying elastance model. Circulation 1986; 74: 97–104.
86. Mehmel HC, Stockins B, Ruffmann K *et al.* The linearity of the end-systolic pressure-

volume relationship in man and its sensitivity for assessment of left ventricular function. Circulation 1981; 63: 1216–22.

87. Heyndrickx GR, Boettcher DH, Vatner SF. Effects of angiotensin, vasopressin, and methoxamine on cardiac function and blood flow distribution in conscious dogs. Am J Physiol 1976; 231: 1579–87.
88. Harpole DH, Rankin JS, Wolfe WG *et al.* Assessment of left ventricular functional preservation during isolated cardiac valve operations. Circulation 1989; 80 (Suppl III): III-1–III-9.
89. Kass DA, Maughan WL, Guo ZM *et al.* Comparative influence of load versus inotropic states on indexes of ventricular contractility: experimental and theoretical analysis based on pressure-volume relationships. Circulation 1987; 76: 1422–36.
90. Freeman GL, O'Rourke RA. Afterload dependent shifts of end-systolic pressure-volume relation in closed chest dogs. Circulation 1988; 78 (Suppl II): II-69 (Abstr.).
91. Glower DD, Spratt JA, Snow ND *et al.* Linearity of the Frank-Starling relationship in the intact heart: the concept of preload recruitable stroke work. Circulation 1985; 71: 994–1009.
92. Kass DA, Maughan WL. From "E_{max}" to pressure-volume relations: a broader view. Circulation 1988; 77: 1203–12.
93. Aversano T, Maughan WL, Hunter WC *et al.* End-systolic measures of regional ventricular performance. Circulation 1986; 73: 938–50.
94. Krukenkamp IB, Silverman NA, Illes RW *et al.* Assessment of the intrinsic contractile state within an area of myocardium. J Thorac Cardiovasc Surg 1989; 98: 592–600.
95. Brutsaert DL, Rademakers FE, Sys SU *et al.* Analysis of relaxation in the evaluation of ventricular function of the heart. Prog Cardiovasc Dis 1985; 28: 143–63.
96. Lew WYW, Rasmussen CM. Influence of nonuniformity on rate of left ventricular pressure fall in the dog. Am J Physiol 1989; 256: H222–H232.
97. Ehring T, Schulz R, Schipke JD *et al.* Diastolic dysfunction of stunned myocardium. Am J Cardiovasc Pathol 1992; 4: 358–66.
98. Ishida Y, Meisner JS, Tsujioka K *et al.* Left ventricular filling dynamics: influence of left ventricular relaxation and left atrial pressure. Circulation 1986; 74: 187–96.
99. Grover FL, Fewel JG, Schrank KP *et al.* Effect of various periods of cold potassium cardioplegic arrest upon myocardial contractility and metabolism. J Surg Res 1980; 28: 328–37.
100. Goldstein JP, Salter DR, Murphy CE *et al.* The efficacy of blood versus crystalloid coronary sinus cardioplegia during global myocardial ischemia. Circulation 1986; 74 (Suppl III): III-99–III-104.
101. Tabayashi K, McKeown PP, Miyamoto M *et al.* Ischemic myocardial protection. Comparison of nonoxygenated crystalloid, oxygenated crystalloid, and oxygenated fluorocarbon cardioplegic solutions. J Thorac Cardiovasc Surg 1988; 95: 239–46.
102. Coetzee A, Roussouw G, Fourie P *et al.* Preservation of myocardial function and biochemistry after blood and oxygenated crystalloid cardioplegia during cardiac arrest. Ann Thorac Surg 1990; 50: 230–7.
103. Illes RW, Silverman NA, Krukenkamp IB *et al.* The efficacy of blood cardioplegia is not due to oxygen delivery. J Thorac Cardiovasc Surg 1989; 98: 1051–6.
104. Roberts AJ, Spies SM, Meyers SN *et al.* Early and long-term improvement in left ventricular performance following coronary bypass surgery. Surgery 1980; 88: 467–75.
105. Phillips HR, Carter JE, Okada RD *et al.* Serial changes in left ventricular ejection fraction in the early hours after aortocoronary bypass grafting. Chest 1983; 83: 28–34.
106. Breisblatt WM, Stein KL, Wolfe CJ *et al.* Acute myocardial dysfunction and recovery: a common occurrence after coronary bypass surgery. J Am Coll Cardiol 1990; 15: 1261–9.
107. Kent KM, Borer JS, Green MV *et al.* Effects of coronary artery bypass on global and regional left ventricular function during exercise. N Engl J Med 1978; 298: 1434–89.
108. Rubenson DS, Tucker CR, London E *et al.* Two-dimensional echocardiographic analysis

of segmental left ventricular wall motion before and after coronary artery bypass surgery. Circulation 1982; 66: 1025–33.

109. Brundage BH, Maissie BM, Botvinick EL. Improved regional ventricular function after successful surgical revascularization. J Am Coll Cardiol 1984; 3: 902–8.
110. Rankin JS, Newman GE, Muhlbaier LH *et al.* The effects of coronary revasculatization on left ventricular function in ischemic heart disease. J Thorac Cardiovasc Surg 1985; 90: 818–32.
111. Reduto LA, Lawrie GM, Reid JW *et al.* Sequential postoperative assessment of left ventricular performance with gated cardiac blood pool imaging following aortocoronary bypass surgery. Am Heart J 1981; 101: 59–66.
112. Fremes SE, Christakis GT, Weisel RD *et al.* A clinical trial of blood and crystalloid cardioplegia. J Thorac Cardiovasc Surg 1984; 88: 726–41.
113. Fremes SE, Weisel RD, Mickle DAG *et al.* Myocardial metabolism and ventricular function following cold potassium cardioplegia. J Thorac Cardiovasc Surg 1985; 89: 531–46.
114. Mullen JC, Fremes SE, Weisel RD *et al.* Right ventricular function: a comparison between blood and crystalloid cardioplegia. Ann Thorac Surg 1987; 43: 17–24.
115. Christakis GT, Fremes SE, Weisel RD *et al.* Right ventricular dysfunction following cold potassium cardioplegia. J Thorac Cardiovasc Surg 1985; 90: 243–50.
116. Christakis GT, Weisel RD, Mickle DAG *et al.* Right ventricular function and metabolism. Circulation 1990; 82 (Suppl IV): IV-332–IV-340.
117. Rabinovich MA, Elstein J, Chiu RC *et al.* Selective right ventricular dysfunction after coronary artery bypass grafting (brief communication). J Thorac Cardiovasc Surg 1983; 86: 444.
118. Schubert T, Vetter H, Owen P *et al.* Adenosine cardioplegia. J Thorac Cardiovasc Surg 1989; 98: 1057–65.
119. Munfakh NA, Steinberg JB, Titus JS *et al.* Protection of the hypertrophied myocardium by crystalloid cardioplegia. J Surg Res 1991; 51: 447–56.
120. Avkiran M, Hearse DJ. Protection of the myocardium during global ischemia. Is crystalloid cardioplegia effective in the immature myocardium? J Thorac Cardiovasc Surg 1989; 97: 220–8.
121. Menasché P, Grousset C, Gauduel Y *et al.* A comparative study of free radical scavengers in cardioplegic solutions. J Thorac Cardiovasc Surg 1986; 92: 264–71.
122. Bolling SF, Olszanski DA, Bove EL *et al.* Enhanced myocardial protection during global ischemia with 5′-nucleotidase inhibitors. J Thorac Cardiovasc Surg 1992; 103: 73–7.
123. Haan CK, Lazar HL, Rivers S *et al.* Improved myocardial preservation during cold storage using substrate enhancement. Ann Thorac Surg 1990; 50: 80–5.
124. Bolling SF, Bies LE, Gallagher KP *et al.* Enhanced myocardial protection with adenosine. Ann Thorac Surg 1989; 47: 809–15.
125. Bolling SF, Bies LE, Bove EL. Effect of ATP synthesis promoters on postischemic myocardial recovery. J Surg Res 1990; 49: 205–11.
126. Bolling SF, Bove EL, Gallagher KP. ATP precursor depletion and postischemic myocardial recovery. J Surg Res 1991; 50: 629–33.
127. Myers CL, Weiss SJ, Kirsh MM *et al.* Effects of supplementing hypothermic crystalloid cardioplegic solution with catalase, superoxide dismutase, allopurinol, or deferoxamine on functional recovery of globally ischemic and reperfused isolated hearts. J Thorac Cardiovasc Surg 1986; 91: 281–9.
128. Becker BF, Gerlach E. Nachweis multiplier hypoxischer Areale in "normoxisch" perfundierten isolierten Herzen. Z Kardiol 1987; 76 (Suppl I): 72 (Abstr.).
129. Krukenkamp IB, Silverman NA, Levitsky S. The effect of cardioplegic oxygenation on the correlation between the linearized Frank-Starling relationship and myocardial energetics in the ejecting postischemic heart. Circulation 1987; 76 (Suppl V): V-122–V-128.
130. Melendez FJ, Gharagozloo F, Sun S-C *et al.* Effects of diltiazem cardioplegia on global function, segmental contractility, and the area of necrosis after acute coronary artery occlusion and surgical reperfusion. J Thorac Cardiovasc Surg 1988; 95: 613–7.

131. Greene PS, Cameron DE, Mohlala L *et al.* Systolic and diastolic left ventricular dysfunction due to mild hyperthermia. Circulation 1989; 80 (Suppl III): III-44–III-48.
132. Lundborg RO, Rahimtoola SH, Swan HJC. Halothane administration and left ventricular function in man. Anesth Analg 1967; 46: 377–85.
133. Reddy PS, Curtiss EI, O'Toole JD *et al.* Cardiac tamponade: Hemodynamic observations in man. Circulation 1977; 48: 265–71.
134. Kaplan JA, Jones EL. Vasodilator therapy during coronary artery surgery. J Thorac Cardiovasc Surg 1972; 64: 563–7.
135. Harrison DC, Kerber RE, Alderman EL. Pharmacodynamics and clinical use of cardiovascular drugs after cardiac surgery. Am J Cardiol 1970; 26: 385–92.
136. Roberts AJ, Niarchos AP, Subramanian VA *et al.* Systemic hypertension associated with coronary artery bypass surgery. J Thorac Cardiovasc Surg 1977; 74: 846–52.
137. Wallach R, Karp RB, Reves JG *et al.* Pathogenesis of paroxysmal hypertension developing during and after coronary bypass surgery: A study of hemodynamic and humoral factors. Am J Cardiol 1980; 46: 559–65.
138. Rosenfeldt FL, Rabinov M, Little P *et al.* The relationship between coronary pressure during reperfusion and myocardial recovery after hypothermic cardioplegia. J Thorac Cardiovasc Surg 1986; 92: 414–24.
139. Teoh KH, Christakis GT, Weisel RD *et al.* Accelerated myocardial metabolic recovery with terminal warm blood cardioplegia. J Thorac Cardiovasc Surg 1986; 91: 888–95.
140. Swain JL, Sabina RL, McHale PA Prolonged myocardial nucleotide depletion after brief ischemia in the open-chest dog. Am J Physiol 1982; 242: H818–H826.
141. Rosenkranz ER, Okamoto F, Buckberg GD *et al.* Safety of prolonged aortic clamping with blood cardioplegia. J Thorac Cardiovasc Surg 1984; 88: 402–10.
142. Becker LC, Levine JH, DiPaula AF *et al.* Reversal of dysfunction in postischemic stunned myocardium by epinephrine and postextrasystolic potentiation. J Am Coll Cardiol 1986; 7: 580–9.
143. Ehring T, Heusch G. Postextrasystolic potentiation does not distinguish ischaemic from stunned myocardium. Pfluegers Arch 1991; 418: 453–61.
144. Bolli R, Zhu W-X, Myers ML *et al.* Beta-adrenergic stimulation reverses postischemic myocardial dysfunction without producing subsequent deterioration. Am J Cardiol 1985; 56: 964–8.
145. Heusch G, Schäfer S, Kröger K: Recruitment of inotropic reserve in "stunned" myocardium by the cardiotonic agent AR-L 57. Basic Res Cardiol 1988; 83: 602–10.
146. Ito BR, Tate H, Kobayashi M *et al.* Reversibly injured, postischemic canine myocardium retains normal contractile reserve. Circ Res 1987; 61: 834–46.
147. Schäfer S, Linder C, Heusch G. Xamoterol recruits an inotropic reserve in the acutely failing, reperfused canine myocardium without detrimental effects on its subsequent recovery. Naunyn Schmiedebergs Arch Pharmacol 1990; 342: 206–13.
148. McDonough KH, Dunn RB, Griggs DM. Transmural changes in porcine and canine hears after circumflex artery occlusion. Am J Physiol 1984; 246: H601–H607.
149. Chambers DJ, Sakai A, Braimbridge MV *et al.* Clinical validation of St. Thomas' Hospital cardioplegic solution No. 2 (Plegisol). Eur J Cardio-thorac Surg 1989; 3: 346–52.
150. Mills SA, Hansen K, Vinten-Johansen J *et al.* Enhanced functional recovery with venting during cardioplegic arrest in chronically damaged hearts. Ann Thorac Surg 1985; 40: 566–73.
151. Singh AK, Corwin RD, Teplitz C *et al.* Consecutive repair of complex congenital heart disease using hypothermic cardioplegic arrest – Its results and ultrastructural study of the myocardium. Thorac Cardiovasc Surg 1984; 32: 23–6.
152. Schaper, J. Myocardial uitrastructure in ischemia. In Heusch G (ed): Pathophysiology and Rational Pharmacotherapy of Myocardial Ischemia. Darmstadt, New York: Steinkopff and Springer Verlag 1990; 11–36.
153. Jacob R, Kissling G. Ventricular pressure-volume relations as the primary basis for evaluation of cardiac mechanics. Return to Frank's diagram. Basic Res Cardiol 1989; 84: 227–46.

Index

H. M. Piper and C. J. Preusse (eds): Ischemia-reperfusion in cardiac surgery, 449–451.

Developments in Cardiovascular Medicine

1. Ch.T. Lancée (ed.): *Echocardiology*. 1979 ISBN 90-247-2209-8
2. J. Baan, A.C. Arntzenius and E.L. Yellin (eds.): *Cardiac Dynamics*. 1980 ISBN 90-247-2212-8
3. H.J.Th. Thalen and C.C. Meere (eds.): *Fundamentals of Cardiac Pacing*. 1979 ISBN 90-247-2245-4
4. H.E. Kulbertus and H.J.J. Wellens (eds.): *Sudden Death*. 1980 ISBN 90-247-2290-X
5. L.S. Dreifus and A.N. Brest (eds.): *Clinical Applications of Cardiovascular Drugs*. 1980 ISBN 90-247-2295-0
6. M.P. Spencer and J.M. Reid: *Cerebrovascular Evaluation with Doppler Ultrasound*. With contributions by E.C. Brockenbrough, R.S. Reneman, G.I. Thomas and D.L. Davis. 1981 ISBN 90-247-2384-1
7. D.P. Zipes, J.C. Bailey and V. Elharrar (eds.): *The Slow Inward Current and Cardiac Arrhythmias*. 1980 ISBN 90-247-2380-9
8. H. Kesteloot and J.V. Joossens (eds.): *Epidemiology of Arterial Blood Pressure*. 1980 ISBN 90-247-2386-8
9. F.J.Th. Wackers (ed.): *Thallium-201 and Technetium-99m-Pyrophosphate. Myocardial Imaging in the Coronary Care Unit*. 1980 ISBN 90-247-2396-5
10. A. Maseri, C. Marchesi, S. Chierchia and M.G. Trivella (eds.): *Coronary Care Units*. Proceedings of a European Seminar (1978). 1981 ISBN 90-247-2456-2
11. J. Morganroth, E.N. Moore, L.S. Dreifus and E.L. Michelson (eds.): *The Evaluation of New Antiarrhythmic Drugs*. Proceedings of the First Symposium on New Drugs and Devices, held in Philadelphia, Pa., U.S.A. (1980). 1981 ISBN 90-247-2474-0
12. P. Alboni: *Intraventricular Conduction Disturbances*. 1981 ISBN 90-247-2483-X
13. H. Rijsterborgh (ed.): *Echocardiology*. 1981 ISBN 90-247-2491-0
14. G.S. Wagner (ed.): *Myocardial Infarction*. Measurement and Intervention. 1982 ISBN 90-247-2513-5
15. R.S. Meltzer and J. Roelandt (eds.): *Contrast Echocardiography*. 1982 ISBN 90-247-2531-3
16. A. Amery, R. Fagard, P. Lijnen and J. Staessen (eds.): *Hypertensive Cardiovascular Disease*. Pathophysiology and Treatment. 1982 IBSN 90-247-2534-8
17. L.N. Bouman and H.J. Jongsma (eds.): *Cardiac Rate and Rhythm*. Physiological, Morphological and Developmental Aspects. 1982 ISBN 90-247-2626-3
18. J. Morganroth and E.N. Moore (eds.): *The Evaluation of Beta Blocker and Calcium Antagonist Drugs*. Proceedings of the 2nd Symposium on New Drugs and Devices, held in Philadelphia, Pa., U.S.A. (1981). 1982 ISBN 90-247-2642-5
19. M.B. Rosenbaum and M.V. Elizari (eds.): *Frontiers of Cardiac Electrophysiology*. 1983 ISBN 90-247-2663-8
20. J. Roelandt and P.G. Hugenholtz (eds.): *Long-term Ambulatory Electrocardiography*. 1982 ISBN 90-247-2664-6
21. A.A.J. Adgey (ed.): *Acute Phase of Ischemic Heart Disease and Myocardial Infarction*. 1982 ISBN 90-247-2675-1
22. P. Hanrath, W. Bleifeld and J. Souquet (eds.): *Cardiovascular Diagnosis by Ultrasound*. Transesophageal, Computerized, Contrast, Doppler Echocardiography. 1982 ISBN 90-247-2692-1
23. J. Roelandt (ed.): *The Practice of M-Mode and Two-dimensional Echocardiography*. 1983 ISBN 90-247-2745-6
24. J. Meyer, P. Schweizer and R. Erbel (eds.): *Advances in Noninvasive Cardiology*. Ultrasound, Computed Tomography, Radioisotopes, Digital Angiography. 1983 ISBN 0-89838-576-8
25. J. Morganroth and E.N. Moore (eds.): *Sudden Cardiac Death and Congestive Heart Failure*. Diagnosis and Treatment. Proceedings of the 3rd Symposium on New Drugs and Devices, held in Philadelphia, Pa., U.S.A. (1982). 1983 ISBN 0-89838-580-6
26. H.M. Perry Jr. (ed.): *Lifelong Management of Hypertension*. 1983 ISBN 0-89838-582-2
27. E.A. Jaffe (ed.): *Biology of Endothelial Cells*. 1984 ISBN 0-89838-587-3

Developments in Cardiovascular Medicine

28. B. Surawicz, C.P. Reddy and E.N. Prystowsky (eds.): *Tachycardias*. 1984 ISBN 0-89838-588-1
29. M.P. Spencer (ed.): *Cardiac Doppler Diagnosis*. Proceedings of a Symposium, held in Clearwater, Fla., U.S.A. (1983). 1983 ISBN 0-89838-591-1
30. H. Villarreal and M.P. Sambhi (eds.): *Topics in Pathophysiology of Hypertension*. 1984 ISBN 0-89838-595-4
31. F.H. Messerli (ed.): *Cardiovascular Disease in the Elderly*. 1984
Revised edition, 1988: see below under Volume 76
32. M.L. Simoons and J.H.C. Reiber (eds.): *Nuclear Imaging in Clinical Cardiology*. 1984 ISBN 0-89838-599-7
33. H.E.D.J. ter Keurs and J.J. Schipperheyn (eds.): *Cardiac Left Ventricular Hypertrophy*. 1983 ISBN 0-89838-612-8
34. N. Sperelakis (ed.): *Physiology and Pathology of the Heart*. 1984
Revised edition, 1988: see below under Volume 90
35. F.H. Messerli (ed.): *Kidney in Essential Hypertension*. Proceedings of a Course, held in New Orleans, La., U.S.A. (1983). 1984 ISBN 0-89838-616-0
36. M.P. Sambhi (ed.): *Fundamental Fault in Hypertension*. 1984 ISBN 0-89838-638-1
37. C. Marchesi (ed.): *Ambulatory Monitoring*. Cardiovascular System and Allied Applications. Proceedings of a Workshop, held in Pisa, Italy (1983). 1984 ISBN 0-89838-642-X
38. W. Kupper, R.N. MacAlpin and W. Bleifeld (eds.): *Coronary Tone in Ischemic Heart Disease*. 1984 ISBN 0-89838-646-2
39. N. Sperelakis and J.B. Caulfield (eds.): *Calcium Antagonists*. Mechanism of Action on Cardiac Muscle and Vascular Smooth Muscle. Proceedings of the 5th Annual Meeting of the American Section of the I.S.H.R., held in Hilton Head, S.C., U.S.A. (1983). 1984 ISBN 0-89838-655-1
40. Th. Godfraind, A.G. Herman and D. Wellens (eds.): *Calcium Entry Blockers in Cardiovascular and Cerebral Dysfunctions*. 1984 ISBN 0-89838-658-6
41. J. Morganroth and E.N. Moore (eds.): *Interventions in the Acute Phase of Myocardial Infarction*. Proceedings of the 4th Symposium on New Drugs and Devices, held in Philadelphia, Pa., U.S.A. (1983). 1984 ISBN 0-89838-659-4
42. F.L. Abel and W.H. Newman (eds.): *Functional Aspects of the Normal, Hypertrophied and Failing Heart*. Proceedings of the 5th Annual Meeting of the American Section of the I.S.H.R., held in Hilton Head, S.C., U.S.A. (1983). 1984 ISBN 0-89838-665-9
43. S. Sideman and R. Beyar (eds.): [3-D] *Simulation and Imaging of the Cardiac System*. State of the Heart. Proceedings of the International Henry Goldberg Workshop, held in Haifa, Israel (1984). 1985 ISBN 0-89838-687-X
44. E. van der Wall and K.I. Lie (eds.): *Recent Views on Hypertrophic Cardiomyopathy*. Proceedings of a Symposium, held in Groningen, The Netherlands (1984). 1985 ISBN 0-89838-694-2
45. R.E. Beamish, P.K. Singal and N.S. Dhalla (eds.), *Stress and Heart Disease*. Proceedings of a International Symposium, held in Winnipeg, Canada, 1984 (Vol. 1). 1985 ISBN 0-89838-709-4
46. R.E. Beamish, V. Panagia and N.S. Dhalla (eds.): *Pathogenesis of Stress-induced Heart Disease*. Proceedings of a International Symposium, held in Winnipeg, Canada, 1984 (Vol. 2). 1985 ISBN 0-89838-710-8
47. J. Morganroth and E.N. Moore (eds.): *Cardiac Arrhythmias*. New Therapeutic Drugs and Devices. Proceedings of the 5th Symposium on New Drugs and Devices, held in Philadelphia, Pa., U.S.A. (1984). 1985 ISBN 0-89838-716-7
48. P. Mathes (ed.): *Secondary Prevention in Coronary Artery Disease and Myocardial Infarction*. 1985 ISBN 0-89838-736-1
49. H.L. Stone and W.B. Weglicki (eds.): *Pathobiology of Cardiovascular Injury*. Proceedings of the 6th Annual Meeting of the American Section of the I.S.H.R., held in Oklahoma City, Okla., U.S.A. (1984). 1985 ISBN 0-89838-743-4

50. J. Meyer, R. Erbel and H.J. Rupprecht (eds.): *Improvement of Myocardial Perfusion.* Thrombolysis, Angioplasty, Bypass Surgery. Proceedings of a Symposium, held in Mainz, F.R.G. (1984). 1985 ISBN 0-89838-748-5
51. J.H.C. Reiber, P.W. Serruys and C.J. Slager (eds.): *Quantitative Coronary and Left Ventricular Cineangiography.* Methodology and Clinical Applications. 1986 ISBN 0-89838-760-4
52. R.H. Fagard and I.E. Bekaert (eds.): *Sports Cardiology.* Exercise in Health and Cardiovascular Disease. Proceedings from an International Conference, held in Knokke, Belgium (1985). 1986 ISBN 0-89838-782-5
53. J.H.C. Reiber and P.W. Serruys (eds.): *State of the Art in Quantitative Cornary Arteriography.* 1986 ISBN 0-89838-804-X
54. J. Roelandt (ed.): *Color Doppler Flow Imaging and Other Advances in Doppler Echocardiography.* 1986 ISBN 0-89838-806-6
55. E.E. van der Wall (ed.): *Noninvasive Imaging of Cardiac Metabolism.* Single Photon Scintigraphy, Positron Emission Tomography and Nuclear Magnetic Resonance. 1987 ISBN 0-89838-812-0
56. J. Liebman, R. Plonsey and Y. Rudy (eds.): *Pediatric and Fundamental Electrocardiography.* 1987 ISBN 0-89838-815-5
57. H.H. Hilger, V. Hombach and W.J. Rashkind (eds.), *Invasive Cardiovascular Therapy.* Proceedings of an International Symposium, held in Cologne, F.R.G. (1985). 1987 ISBN 0-89838-818-X
58. P.W. Serruys and G.T. Meester (eds.): *Coronary Angioplasty.* A Controlled Model for Ischemia. 1986 ISBN 0-89838-819-8
59. J.E. Tooke and L.H. Smaje (eds.): *Clinical Investigation of the Microcirculation.* Proceedings of an International Meeting, held in London, U.K. (1985). 1987 ISBN 0-89838-833-3
60. R.Th. van Dam and A. van Oosterom (eds.): *Electrocardiographic Body Surface Mapping.* Proceedings of the 3rd International Symposium on B.S.M., held in Nijmegen, The Netherlands (1985). 1986 ISBN 0-89838-834-1
61. M.P. Spencer (ed.): *Ultrasonic Diagnosis of Cerebrovascular Disease.* Doppler Techniques and Pulse Echo Imaging. 1987 ISBN 0-89838-836-8
62. M.J. Legato (ed.): *The Stressed Heart.* 1987 ISBN 0-89838-849-X
63. M.E. Safar (ed.): *Arterial and Venous Systems in Essential Hypertension.* With Assistance of G.M. London, A.Ch. Simon and Y.A. Weiss. 1987 ISBN 0-89838-857-0
64. J. Roelandt (ed.): *Digital Techniques in Echocardiography.* 1987 ISBN 0-89838-861-9
65. N.S. Dhalla, P.K. Singal and R.E. Beamish (eds.): *Pathology of Heart Disease.* Proceedings of the 8th Annual Meeting of the American Section of the I.S.H.R., held in Winnipeg, Canada, 1986 (Vol. 1). 1987 ISBN 0-89838-864-3
66. N.S. Dhalla, G.N. Pierce and R.E. Beamish (eds.): *Heart Function and Metabolism.* Proceedings of the 8th Annual Meeting of the American Section of the I.S.H.R., held in Winnipeg, Canada, 1986 (Vol. 2). 1987 ISBN 0-89838-865-1
67. N.S. Dhalla, I.R. Innes and R.E. Beamish (eds.): *Myocardial Ischemia.* Proceedings of a Satellite Symposium of the 30th International Physiological Congress, held in Winnipeg, Canada (1986). 1987 ISBN 0-89838-866-X
68. R.E. Beamish, V. Panagia and N.S. Dhalla (eds.): *Pharmacological Aspects of Heart Disease.* Proceedings of an International Symposium, held in Winnipeg, Canada (1986). 1987 ISBN 0-89838-867-8
69. H.E.D.J. ter Keurs and J.V. Tyberg (eds.): *Mechanics of the Circulation.* Proceedings of a Satellite Symposium of the 30th International Physiological Congress, held in Banff, Alberta, Canada (1986). 1987 ISBN 0-89838-870-8
70. S. Sideman and R. Beyar (eds.): *Activation, Metabolism and Perfusion of the Heart.* Simulation and Experimental Models. Proceedings of the 3rd Henry Goldberg Workshop, held in Piscataway, N.J., U.S.A. (1986). 1987 ISBN 0-89838-871-6

Developments in Cardiovascular Medicine

71. E. Aliot and R. Lazzara (eds.): *Ventricular Tachycardias*. From Mechanism to Therapy. 1987 ISBN 0-89838-881-3
72. A. Schneeweiss and G. Schettler: *Cardiovascular Drug Therapoy in the Elderly*. 1988 ISBN 0-89838-883-X
73. J.V. Chapman and A. Sgalambro (eds.): *Basic Concepts in Doppler Echocardiography*. Methods of Clinical Applications based on a Multi-modality Doppler Approach. 1987 ISBN 0-89838-888-0
74. S. Chien, J. Dormandy, E. Ernst and A. Matrai (eds.): *Clinical Hemorheology*. Applications in Cardiovascular and Hematological Disease, Diabetes, Surgery and Gynecology. 1987 ISBN 0-89838-807-4
75. J. Morganroth and E.N. Moore (eds.): *Congestive Heart Failure*. Proceedings of the 7th Annual Symposium on New Drugs and Devices, held in Philadelphia, Pa., U.S.A. (1986). 1987 ISBN 0-89838-955-0
76. F.H. Messerli (ed.): *Cardiovascular Disease in the Elderly*. 2nd ed. 1988 ISBN 0-89838-962-3
77. P.H. Heintzen and J.H. Bürsch (eds.): *Progress in Digital Angiocardiography*. 1988 ISBN 0-89838-965-8
78. M.M. Scheinman (ed.): *Catheter Ablation of Cardiac Arrhythmias*. Basic Bioelectrical Effects and Clinical Indications. 1988 ISBN 0-89838-967-4
79. J.A.E. Spaan, A.V.G. Bruschke and A.C. Gittenberger-De Groot (eds.): *Coronary Circulation*. From Basic Mechanisms to Clinical Implications. 1987 ISBN 0-89838-978-X
80. C. Visser, G. Kan and R.S. Meltzer (eds.): *Echocardiography in Coronary Artery Disease*. 1988 ISBN 0-89838-979-8
81. A. Bayés de Luna, A. Betriu and G. Permanyer (eds.): *Therapeutics in Cardiology*. 1988 ISBN 0-89838-981-X
82. D.M. Mirvis (ed.): *Body Surface Electrocardiographic Mapping*. 1988 ISBN 0-89838-983-6
83. M.A. Konstam and J.M. Isner (eds.): *The Right Ventricle*. 1988 ISBN 0-89838-987-9
84. C.T. Kappagoda and P.V. Greenwood (eds.): *Long-term Management of Patients after Myocardial Infarction*. 1988 ISBN 0-89838-352-8
85. W.H. Gaasch and H.J. Levine (eds.): *Chronic Aortic Regurgitation*. 1988 ISBN 0-89838-364-1
86. P.K. Singal (ed.): *Oxygen Radicals in the Pathophysiology of Heart Disease*. 1988 ISBN 0-89838-375-7
87. J.H.C. Reiber and P.W. Serruys (eds.): *New Developments in Quantitative Coronary Arteriography*. 1988 ISBN 0-89838-377-3
88. J. Morganroth and E.N. Moore (eds.): *Silent Myocardial Ischemia*. Proceedings of the 8th Annual Symposium on New Drugs and Devices (1987). 1988 ISBN 0-89838-380-3
89. H.E.D.J. ter Keurs and M.I.M. Noble (eds.): *Starling's Law of the Heart Revisted*. 1988 ISBN 0-89838-382-X
90. N. Sperelakis (ed.): *Physiology and Pathophysiology of the Heart*. (Rev. ed.) 1988 ISBN 0-89838-388-9
91. J.W. de Jong (ed.): *Myocardial Energy Metabolism*. 1988 ISBN 0-89838-394-3
92. V. Hombach, H.H. Hilger and H.L. Kennedy (eds.): *Electrocardiography and Cardiac Drug Therapy*. Proceedings of an International Symposium, held in Cologne, F.R.G. (1987). 1988 ISBN 0-89838-395-1
93. H. Iwata, J.B. Lombardini and T. Segawa (eds.): *Taurine and the Heart*. 1988 ISBN 0-89838-396-X
94. M.R. Rosen and Y. Palti (eds.): *Lethal Arrhythmias Resulting from Myocardial Ischemia and Infarction*. Proceedings of the 2nd Rappaport Symposium, held in Haifa, Israel (1988). 1988 ISBN 0-89838-401-X
95. M. Iwase and I. Sotobata: *Clinical Echocardiography*. With a Foreword by M.P. Spencer. 1989 ISBN 0-7923-0004-1

Developments in Cardiovascular Medicine

96. I. Cikes (ed.): *Echocardiography in Cardiac Interventions.* 1989 ISBN 0-7923-0088-2
97. E. Rapaport (ed.): *Early Interventions in Acute Myocardial Infarction.* 1989 ISBN 0-7923-0175-7
98. M.E. Safar and F. Fouad-Tarazi (eds.): *The Heart in Hypertension.* A Tribute to Robert C. Tarazi (1925-1986). 1989 ISBN 0-7923-0197-8
99. S. Meerbaum and R. Meltzer (eds.): *Myocardial Contrast Two-dimensional Echocardiography.* 1989 ISBN 0-7923-0205-2
100. J. Morganroth and E.N. Moore (eds.): *Risk/Benefit Analysis for the Use and Approval of Thrombolytic, Antiarrhythmic, and Hypolipidemic Agents.* Proceedings of the 9th Annual Symposium on New Drugs and Devices (1988). 1989 ISBN 0-7923-0294-X
101. P.W. Serruys, R. Simon and K.J. Beatt (eds.): *PTCA - An Investigational Tool and a Non-operative Treatment of Acute Ischemia.* 1990 ISBN 0-7923-0346-6
102. I.S. Anand, P.I. Wahi and N.S. Dhalla (eds.): *Pathophysiology and Pharmacology of Heart Disease.* 1989 ISBN 0-7923-0367-9
103. G.S. Abela (ed.): *Lasers in Cardiovascular Medicine and Surgery.* Fundamentals and Technique. 1990 ISBN 0-7923-0440-3
104. H.M. Piper (ed.): *Pathophysiology of Severe Ischemic Myocardial Injury.* 1990 ISBN 0-7923-0459-4
105. S.M. Teague (ed.): *Stress Doppler Echocardiography.* 1990 ISBN 0-7923-0499-3
106. P.R. Saxena, D.I. Wallis, W. Wouters and P. Bevan (eds.): *Cardiovascular Pharmacology of 5-Hydroxytryptamine.* Prospective Therapeutic Applications. 1990 ISBN 0-7923-0502-7
107. A.P. Shepherd and P.A. Öberg (eds.): *Laser-Doppler Blood Flowmetry.* 1990 ISBN 0-7923-0508-6
108. J. Soler-Soler, G. Permanyer-Miralda and J. Sagristà-Sauleda (eds.): *Pericardial Disease.* New Insights and Old Dilemmas. 1990 ISBN 0-7923-0510-8
109. J.P.M. Hamer: *Practical Echocardiography in the Adult.* With Doppler and Color-Doppler Flow Imaging. 1990 ISBN 0-7923-0670-8
110. A. Bayés de Luna, P. Brugada, J. Cosin Aguilar and F. Navarro Lopez (eds.): *Sudden Cardiac Death.* 1991 ISBN 0-7923-0716-X
111. E. Andries and R. Stroobandt (eds.): *Hemodynamics in Daily Practice.* 1991 ISBN 0-7923-0725-9
112. J. Morganroth and E.N. Moore (eds.): *Use and Approval of Antihypertensive Agents and Surrogate Endpoints for the Approval of Drugs affecting Antiarrhythmic Heart Failure and Hypolipidemia.* Proceedings of the 10th Annual Symposium on New Drugs and Devices (1989). 1990 ISBN 0-7923-0756-9
113. S. Iliceto, P. Rizzon and J.R.T.C. Roelandt (eds.): *Ultrasound in Coronary Artery Disease.* Present Role and Future Perspectives. 1990 ISBN 0-7923-0784-4
114. J.V. Chapman and G.R. Sutherland (eds.): *The Noninvasive Evaluation of Hemodynamics in Congenital Heart Disease.* Doppler Ultrasound Applications in the Adult and Pediatric Patient with Congenital Heart Disease. 1990 ISBN 0-7923-0836-0
115. G.T. Meester and F. Pinciroli (eds.): *Databases for Cardiology.* 1991 ISBN 0-7923-0886-7
116. B. Korecky and N.S. Dhalla (eds.): *Subcellular Basis of Contractile Failure.* 1990 ISBN 0-7923-0890-5
117. J.H.C. Reiber and P.W. Serruys (eds.): *Quantitative Coronary Arteriography.* 1991 ISBN 0-7923-0913-8
118. E. van der Wall and A. de Roos (eds.): *Magnetic Resonance Imaging in Coronary Artery Disease.* 1991 ISBN 0-7923-0940-5
119. V. Hombach, M. Kochs and A.J. Camm (eds.): *Interventional Techniques in Cardiovascular Medicine.* 1991 ISBN 0-7923-0956-1
120. R. Vos: *Drugs Looking for Diseases.* Innovative Drug Research and the Development of the Beta Blockers and the Calcium Antagonists. 1991 ISBN 0-7923-0968-5

Developments in Cardiovascular Medicine

121. S. Sideman, R. Beyar and A.G. Kleber (eds.): *Cardiac Electrophysiology, Circulation, and Transport.* Proceedings of the 7th Henry Goldberg Workshop (Berne, Switzerland, 1990). 1991 ISBN 0-7923-1145-0
122. D.M. Bers: *Excitation-Contraction Coupling and Cardiac Contractile Force.* 1991 ISBN 0-7923-1186-8
123. A.-M. Salmasi and A.N. Nicolaides (eds.): *Occult Atherosclerotic Disease.* Diagnosis, Assessment and Management. 1991 ISBN 0-7923-1188-4
124. J.A.E. Spaan: *Coronary Blood Flow.* Mechanics, Distribution, and Control. 1991 ISBN 0-7923-1210-4
125. R.W. Stout (ed.): *Diabetes and Atherosclerosis.* 1991 ISBN 0-7923-1310-0
126. A.G. Herman (ed.): *Antithrombotics.* Pathophysiological Rationale for Pharmacological Interventions. 1991 ISBN 0-7923-1413-1
127. N.H.J. Pijls: *Maximal Myocardial Perfusion as a Measure of the Functional Significance of Coronary Arteriogram.* From a Pathoanatomic to a Pathophysiologic Interpretation of the Coronary Arteriogram. 1991 ISBN 0-7923-1430-1
128. J.H.C. Reiber and E.E. v.d. Wall (eds.): *Cardiovascular Nuclear Medicine and MRI.* Quantitation and Clinical Applications. 1992 ISBN 0-7923-1467-0
129. E. Andries, P. Brugada and R. Stroobrandt (eds.): *How to Face 'the Faces' of Cardiac Pacing.* 1992 ISBN 0-7923-1528-6
130. M. Nagano, S. Mochizuki and N.S. Dhalla (eds.): *Cardiovascular Disease in Diabetes.* 1992 ISBN 0-7923-1554-5
131. P.W. Serruys, B.H. Strauss and S.B. King III (eds.): *Restenosis after Intervention with New Mechanical Devices.* 1992 ISBN 0-7923-1555-3
132. P.J. Walter (ed.): *Quality of Life after Open Heart Surgery.* 1992 ISBN 0-7923-1580-4
133. E.E. van der Wall, H. Sochor, A. Righetti and M.G. Niemeyer (eds.): *What's new in Cardiac Imaging*? SPECT, PET and MRI. 1992 ISBN 0-7923-1615-0
134. P. Hanrath, R. Uebis and W. Krebs (eds.): *Cardiovascular Imaging by Ultrasound.* 1992 ISBN 0-7923-1755-6
135. F.H. Messerli (ed.): *Cardiovascular Disease in the Elderly.* 3rd ed. 1992 ISBN 0-7923-1859-5
136. J. Hess and G.R. Sutherland (eds.): *Congenital Heart Disease in Adolescents and Adults.* 1992 ISBN 0-7923-1862-5
137. J.H.C. Reiber and P.W. Serruys (eds.): *Advances in Quantitative Coronary Arteriography.* 1993 ISBN 0-7923-1863-3
138. A.-M. Salmasi and A.S. Iskandrian (eds.): *Cardiac Output and Regional Flow in Health and Disease.* 1993 ISBN 0-7923-1911-7
139. J.H. Kingma, N.M. van Hemel and K.I. Lie (eds.): *Atrial Fibrillation, a Treatable Disease?* 1992 ISBN 0-7923-2008-5
140. B. Ostadel and N.S. Dhalla (eds.): *Heart Function in Health and Disease.* Proceedings of the Cardiovascular Program (Prague, Czechoslovakia, 1991). 1992 ISBN 0-7923-2052-2
141. D. Noble and Y.E. Earm (eds.): *Ionic Channels and Effect of Taurine on the Heart.* Proceedings of an International Symposium (Seoul, Korea , 1992). 1993 ISBN 0-7923-2199-5
142. H.M. Piper and C.J. Preusse (eds.): *Ischemia-reperfusion in Cardiac Surgery.* 1993 ISBN 0-7923-2241-X
143. J. Roelandt, E.J. Gussenhoven and N. Bom (eds.):*Intravascular Ultrasound.* 1993 ISBN 0-7923-2301-7

Previous volumes are still available

KLUWER ACADEMIC PUBLISHERS – DORDRECHT / BOSTON / LONDON